HANDBOOK OF PSYCHIATRY · 2
MENTAL DISORDERS AND SOMATIC ILLNESS

HANDBOOK OF PSYCHIATRY

General Editor: Professor M. Shepherd

Edited by: Professor N. Garmezy, Dr L. A. Hersov, Professor M. H. Lader, Professor P. R. McHugh, Professor G. F. M. Russell, Professor J. K. Wing, Professor O. L. Zangwill

Assisted by the Editorial Board and International Advisory Board of *Psychological Medicine*

Volume 1: General psychopathology
Edited by M. Shepherd and O. L. Zangwill

Volume 2: Mental disorders and somatic illness
Edited by M. H. Lader

Volume 3: Psychoses of uncertain aetiology
Edited by J. K. Wing and L. Wing

Volume 4: The neuroses and personality disorders
Edited by G. F. M. Russell and L. A. Hersov

Volume 5: The scientific foundations of psychiatry
Edited by M. Shepherd

Handbook of PSYCHIATRY Volume 2

MENTAL DISORDERS AND SOMATIC ILLNESS

Edited by M. H. Lader
Professor of Clinical Psychopharmacology
Institute of Psychiatry
London

CAMBRIDGE UNIVERSITY PRESS
Cambridge
London New York New Rochelle
Melbourne Sydney

Published by the Press Syndicate of the University of Cambridge
The Pitt Building, Trumpington Street, Cambridge CB2 1RP
32 East 57th Street, New York, NY 10022, USA
296 Beaconsfield Parade, Middle Park, Melbourne 3206, Australia

First published 1983

Printed in the United States of America by
Vail-Ballou Press, Inc., Binghamton, NY

Library of Congress catalogue card number: 82-14582

British Library cataloguing in publication data
Handbook of psychiatry.
Vol. 2: Mental and somatic illness

1. Psychiatry
I. Lader, M.H.
616.89   RC454

ISBN 0 521 24220 7 hard covers
ISBN 0 521 28535 6 paperback

v

CONTENTS

Contents

Contributors

D. Peter Birkett, MRCP(Ed.), FRCP(Can.), MRCPsych,
Medical Director, Riverside Nursing Home,
and
Research Associate, Center for Geriatrics and Gerontology,
Faculty of Medicine, Columbia University, and New York
State Office of Mental Health,
100 Haven Avenue,
Tower 3-29F,
New York, NY, 10032,
USA

Michael R. Bond, MD, PhD, FRCS(Edin.), FRCP(Glasg.),
FRCPsych, DPM,
Professor of Psychological Medicine, University of Glas-
gow,
University Department of Psychological Medicine,
6 Whittingehame Gardens, Great Western Road, Glasgow
G12 0AA

J. L. Crammer, MA, MRCS, FRCPsych, DPM,
Reader in Biological Psychiatry, University of London,
Institute of Psychiatry,
and
Honorary Consultant, the Bethlem Royal Hospital and the
Maudsley Hospital,
Institute of Psychiatry,
De Crespigny Park, Denmark Hill, London SE5 8AF

J. Cutting, MD, MPhil, MRCP, MRCPsych,
Senior Lecturer,
King's College Hospital Medical School and Institute of
Psychiatry,
Denmark Hill, London SE5 8AF

George W. Fenton, MB, FRCP(Edin.), FRCPsych,
MRCP(Lond.), DPM(Eng.),
Professor of Mental Health, The Queen's University of Belfast,
Department of Mental Health,
The Queen's University of Belfast,
Whitla Medical Building, 97 Lisburn Road, Belfast BT9 7BL

Marshal F. Folstein, MD,
Associate Professor of Psychiatry, The Johns Hopkins University School of Medicine,
Department of Psychiatry and Behavioral Sciences,
The Johns Hopkins University School of Medicine,
Baltimore, Maryland 21205, USA

A. Hamid Ghodse, MD, PhD, MRCPsych, DPM,
Consultant Psychiatrist,
St George's, St Thomas's, and Tooting Bec Hospitals,
St George's Hospital,
Blackshaw Road, London SW17 0QT

J. L. Gibbons, MD, FRCP, FRCPsych,
Professor of Psychiatry, University of Southampton,
Department of Psychiatry,
Royal South Hants Hospital,
Graham Road, Southampton, SO9 4PE

Kenneth Granville-Grossman, MD, FRCP, FRCPsych, DPM,
Consultant Psychiatrist, St Mary's Hospital,
Praed Street
London, W2 1NY

Barry J. Gurland, MRCP(Lond.), MRCPsych,
Director, Center for Geriatrics and Gerontology,
Faculty of Medicine, Columbia University
and
New York State Office of Mental Health,
and
Professor of Clinical Psychiatry,
Department of Psychiatry,
Columbia University,
100 Haven Avenue, Tower 3-29F, New York, NY, 10032,
USA

Anthony D. Isaacs, FRCP, FRCPsych,
Consultant Psychiatrist,
The Bethlem Royal Hospital and the Maudsley Hospital,
Denmark Hill, London SE5 8AF

R. Kumar, MD, PhD, MPhil, MRCPsych,
Senior Lecturer,
Department of Psychiatry,
Institute of Psychiatry,
De Crespigny Park, Denmark Hill, London SE5 8AF

M. H. Lader, DSc, PhD, MD, FRCPsych,
Professor of Clinical Psychopharmacology, University of London,
Institute of Psychiatry,
De Crespigny Park, Denmark Hill, London SE5 8AF

Paul R. McHugh, MD,
Henry Phipps Professor of Psychiatry,
The Johns Hopkins University School of Medicine,
Baltimore, Maryland 21205, USA

C. D. Marsden, MD, BS, MSc, FRCP,
Professor of Neurology, University of London,
King's College Hospital Medical School and the Institute of Psychiatry,
De Crespigny Park, Denmark Hill, London SE5 8AF

H. G. Morgan, MD(Cantab.), FRCP, FRCPsych,
DPM(Lond.),
Norah Cooke Hurle Professor of Mental Health,
University of Bristol,
39 St Michael's Hill, Bristol BS2 8DZ

Ian Oswald, MA, MD, DSc, FRCPsych,
Professor of Psychiatry, University of Edinburgh,
University Department of Psychiatry,
Royal Edinburgh Hospital,
Morningside Park, Edinburgh EH10 5HF

Derek Ricks, MD, MRCPsych, DPM,
Consultant Psychiatrist,
Children's Department,
Harperbury Hospital,
Shenley, Herts WD7 9HQ

Maurice Victor, MD,
Professor of Neurology, Case Western Reserve University School of Medicine,
and
Director, Department of Neurology,
Metropolitan General Hospital,
Cleveland, Ohio 44109, USA

Foreword

The idea of this handbook originated from a survey of the available British books on psychiatry in the late 1960s (1). It became apparent then that the post-war development of the subject as a major, independent branch of medicine had been accompanied by a spate of textbooks and specialized monographs from the rapidly increasing number of academic and clinical departments. The time seemed ripe 'to compile the comprehensive authoritative multi-authored handbook which has yet to appear in this country' (2).

In the event almost another decade was to pass before the enterprise was to be realized. During this time the climate of opinion has come to favour the appearance of a representative statement of what has been termed the 'Maudsley' approach to psychological medicine. Modern British psychiatry, as Lord Taylor has pointed out, is 'largely the product of the Maudsley Hospital' (3). It embodies not so much a national school of opinion as a continuation of the broad, central tradition of psychiatric theory and practice which originated on the European mainland, was transported through the psychobiology of Adolf Meyer to North America and returned to Europe via the United Kingdom, where its pre-eminent representative has been Sir Aubrey Lewis (4). At its core is an adherence to the principles of scientific enquiry in clinical and basic research, with due acknowledgement of the role played by social and psychological investigation as well as by the natural sciences.

The prospects for the production of a handbook were further improved by the creation in 1969 of *Psychological Medicine,* a journal devoted to research in the field of psychiatry and the allied sciences, which brought together an editorial board which has played an important part in this undertaking. The participation of the journal's international advisory board also helped to ensure a wide base for the work which, from its inception, has received sympathetic encouragement from Cambridge University Press.

Why call a handbook what is clearly so much more than a manual or guide which can be held in the hand? If the term is a misnomer it is one which has been blessed by tradition and usage. In the German-speaking countries, where so many of the roots of modern psychiatry are embedded, a *Handbuch* is much weightier than a *Lehrbuch* and the massive volumes associated with the names of Aschaffenburg and Bumke exemplify the fruits of German scholarship at its most diligent. The format has, of course, been applied to other medical disciplines in other languages, largely to meet a need which has been clearly expressed in the preface to the *Handbook of Clinical Neurology,* now comprising some forty volumes: 'only a Handbook designed on the principle of exhaustive, critical, balanced and comprehensive reviews written by acknowledged experts, is in the position of reflecting the state of neurology in the second half of the twentieth century' (5).

While the *Handbook of Psychiatry* has a similar objective, it is less expansive in content and more ambitious in form. An encyclopaedic compilation of all the theories and speculations which impinge on contemporary psychiatry would call for more than forty volumes, but would become outdated very soon. Here we have preferred to concentrate on the fabric of psychological medicine and the loom of observations and concepts on which it has been woven. Accordingly, volumes 2–4 contain the clinical substratum of the subject, flanked by one volume devoted to general psychopathology and another to the various scientific modes of enquiry on which the discipline is founded.

A full list of contents, with titles of chapters and names of authors, is provided in each volume. An outline of the material contained in all five volumes is as follows:

Vol.1 General psychopathology
Editors: M. Shepherd and O. L. Zangwill
Part I
The historical background

Part II
The clinical phenomena of mental disorders
Part III
Taxonomy, diagnosis, and treatment

Vol.2 Mental disorders and somatic illness
Editor: M. H. Lader
Part I
General medical disorders
Part II
Neurological disorders
Part III
Drug-induced disorders
Part IV
Severe subnormality

Vol.3 Psychoses of uncertain aetiology
Editors: J. K. Wing and L. Wing
Part I
Schizophrenia and paranoid psychoses
Part II
Affective psychoses
Part III
Psychoses of early childhood

Vol.4 The neuroses and personality disorders
Editors: G. F. M. Russell and L. Hersov
Part I
Concepts, assessments, and treatments
Part II
Disorders specific to childhood
Part III
Neurotic states, sexual disorders, and drug-dependence
Part IV
Personality disorders

Vol.5 The scientific foundations of psychiatry
Editor: M. Shepherd
Part I
Philosophy and psychiatry
Part II
Epidemiology and genetics in relation to psychiatry
Part III
Social science, psychology, and ethology in relation to psychiatry
Part IV
The neurosciences in relation to psychiatry

All the volumes are self-contained and edited separately, but they are intended to reinforce one another. Every effort has been made to avoid overlap and duplication of material and the inclusion of cross-references, some in the text and others at the back of each volume, should facilitate the process of integration. The whole is designed to be more than the sum of its parts.

Michael Shepherd
Institute of Psychiatry
October 1980

References

(1) Shepherd, M. (1969) British books on psychiatry, I & II. *British Book News*, Feb/Mar., pp. 85–8 and 167–70

(2) (1980) Psychiatry: personal book list. *Lancet*, i, 937

(3) Taylor, Lord (1962) The public, parliament and mental health. In *Aspects of Psychiatric Research*, ed. Richter, D., Tanner, J. M., Taylor, Lord & Zangwill, O.L., p. 13. London: Oxford University Press.

(4) Shepherd, M. (1977) *The Career and Contributions of Sir Aubrey Lewis*. Bethlem Royal & Maudsley Hospitals

(5) Vinken, P. J. & Bruyn, G. W. (1969) Preface to *Handbook of Clinical Neurology*, vol. I, p. v. Amsterdam: North Holland

Introduction

M. H. LADER

This volume of the *Handbook* covers that area of psychiatry contiguous with general medicine and in particular neurology. Most of the conditions dealt with fall under the rubric 'organic', that is, some bodily cause is apparent for the psychiatric abnormality. The cause may be genetic, vascular, neoplastic, degenerative, and so on, but it is recognizable in general medical terms. Of course, it is possible that some of the psychiatric conditions of unknown aetiology dealt with in volume 3 also have an organic basis as yet undiscovered by our relatively crude techniques for investigating the human central nervous system, but until such discoveries have been made, the distinction between the organic conditions and the euphemistically-termed 'functional' conditions is both valid and useful.

This area of psychiatry also raises general issues of a philosophical nature, especially with respect to fundamental problems of the mind–body relationship. These aspects are discussed in the first chapter on 'Mind and Body', together with the more practical topics of psychosomatic medicine, life events, and personality (see also vol. 5, the chapter dealing with philosophy and psychiatry).

The second chapter addresses itself to some of the general medical disorders of most relevance to psychiatry. These include vascular disorders, in particular, ischaemic heart disease and hypertension, peptic ulcers, bronchial asthma, and renal failure. The third chapter covers the endocrine disorders with their important implications for psychiatry. The thyroid, adrenals and pituitary are discussed, as well as hypoglycaemic conditions. The fourth chapter concludes these general topics in medicine as relevant to mental illness with a survey of the nutritional disorders. Vitamin deficiencies are given especial prominence.

There follows a discussion of an epoch of life of particular psychiatric interest: the reproductive period in women and the typical psychiatric conditions encountered. Pregnancy and the puerperium are examined in detail, and also the use of psychotropic drugs at these times.

Two symptom-complexes commonly found in psychiatric patients, but which may have an organic basis, namely disorders of sleep and pain, are then dealt with briefly.

A second epoch of life of special psychiatric interest is next considered: normal ageing, the presentation and assessment of mental disorder in the aged, and the management of the elderly mentally infirm.

Several subsequent chapters cover various aspects of what is generally termed 'neuropsychiatry', namely the interface between neurology and psychiatry. First, in chapter 9, head injury, electroconvulsive therapy, and psychosurgery are outlined, special attention being paid to changes in brain function secondary to these conditions and therapies. Other neurological conditions are examined in chapter 10 and include Huntington's disease, Alzheimer's disease, Parkinson's disease, hydrocephalus, and brain tumours. Chapter 11 deals with the common clinical problem of acute organic reactions with a detailed description of the clinical picture, aetiologies, and management. The next chapter moves on to some other common but chronic neuropsychiatric conditions, the senile and pre-senile dementias. These increasingly common illnesses are presented in detail, with particular emphasis on management.

Epilepsy is a major topic in neuropsychiatry and it merits a long and full discussion. The various types of epilepsy, their presentation and management form a substantial portion of this volume. Another major topic of increasing importance is the psychiatric complications of alcoholism. Chapter 14 is devoted to this topic with a detailed analysis of its various aspects. Chapter 15 also deals with mental disorders associated with chemical substances, drug dependence, and intoxication. The topics of tolerance, dependence, and addiction are discussed in relation to various groups of psycho-active drugs. The management of drug-dependent individuals is presented.

The final chapter covers selected aspects of severe subnormality. It does not purport to be a comprehensive account of all the various and rare causes of severe subnormality but concentrates on the practical management of the severely handicapped child and adult.

Throughout this volume, contributors have been at pains to provide a clinically relevant account of their topics. Some overlaps have inevitably occurred but it is hoped that the topics covered provide a comprehensive survey of the mental disorders associated with somatic illnesses.

PART I
General medical disorders

1
Mind and body

KENNETH GRANVILLE-GROSSMAN

That a complete volume of this *Handbook* has been devoted to the theme of mental disorders and somatic illness demonstrates the importance of the mind–body nexus in discussions of contemporary psychiatry. On looking at the link between mind and body, however, one very quickly comes across serious problems concerning its nature and one must conclude that it has no generally accepted theoretical basis. Indeed, there is considerable doubt that any approach – scientific or otherwise – will resolve the problem of the way in which physical and mental events appear to co-exist and interrelate. Nevertheless many attempts have been made to investigate the mind–body complex and in this introductory chapter three viewpoints are given: first, an examination of the empirically derived evidence that there may be an association between physical disease and psychiatric disorder; secondly, the psychosomatic point of view, particularly as it has developed over the past 50 years; and thirdly, an account of the various approaches made by Western philosophers, with especial reference to developments following the publication of the influential doctrines of René Descartes.

Psychiatric disorder and physical illness

For many years now evidence has accumulated that physical illness and psychiatric disturbance tend to occur in the same individual more often than would be expected by chance. Examination and investigation of consecutive in-patients admitted to psychiatric units consistently shows a high prevalence (30–60 per cent) of physical disease which is sometimes severe, often previously undiagnosed (particularly among patients who have not been referred by doctors) and frequently of aetiological importance. Physical disorder is most common among patients diagnosed as having an organic mental reaction, but even among those with functional disorders the prevalence seems to be greater than in the general population and with increasing age the association becomes more common (Maguire & Granville-Grossman, 1968). Investigation of other populations of psychiatrically disturbed individuals, in in-patient units, in day hospitals and in emergency clinics has also shown a large number of patients with physical illness often relevant to their psychiatric condition.

The investigation of physically ill people has also shown a relationship between physical and psychiatric disorder. Typical of the many such studies is that carried out by Maguire and his colleagues (1974) who investigated a series of patients admitted to medical wards, excluding those who had taken overdoses. Each patient completed a questionnaire about his health and if the replies suggested that he might be psychiatrically disturbed he was interviewed in a standardized way. Almost one-quarter of the patients studied were considered to be psychiatrically ill – mainly suffering from affective disorders – and this proportion would certainly have been higher had patients who had poisoned themselves been included.

Patterns of mortality in psychiatric populations

Consistent with the apparent association between physical and mental disorder is the markedly increased mortality rate among psychiatric patients. Numerous studies in various parts of the world have shown that long-term in-patients in psychiatric hospitals have a much higher death rate than people of the same age and background in the general population. Some of the reasons for this are fairly specific. Patients with dementia due to cortical atrophy have a considerably shortened life and a very considerable excess mortality (6–10 times that of the general population), perhaps because the cerebral changes may be associated with generalized degeneration throughout the body. Suicide and accidental death are also very much more frequent among psychiatrically ill people than in the general population; at least 10 per cent of patients who have previously had a schizophrenic or manic-depressive illness

commit suicide, and the suicide rate amongst alcoholics is almost as high. This is presumably directly related to the abnormal thoughts and feelings which these patients have. Since excessive deaths due to suicide (and to accident) are also seen among patients who are no longer in hospital it appears that the high mortality rate is more closely related to factors associated with the illness than to circumstances inside the hospital. That accidental death is also very common among patients with functional psychosis (almost as common as suicide) is not obviously explicable but may be due to faulty classification of the causes of death. Coroners may sometimes record an open verdict or a verdict of accidental death, even when the patient deliberately intended to kill himself. In one series of apparently accidental death in which some 60 per cent of deaths were due to poisoning, drowning, or falling from a height, there was evidence of mental illness before death (Holding & Barraclough, 1977). Traffic accidents, particularly fatal ones, in the psychiatrically disturbed may also be suicidally intended but wrongly classified, thus increasing the apparent correlation between accident and mental illness. However, it may be that mentally ill people tend to take less care of themselves and hence to have more fatal accidents than the general population.

Even when deaths associated with dementia and those due to suicide and accidental death are excluded, the mortality rate in psychiatric populations still seems to be much higher than in the general population. At least some of this excess mortality may be due to unhygienic conditions within psychiatric hospitals leading to the acquisition of infections. This is supported by the observation that, since the beginning of this century, as patient care has improved, the death rate in psychiatric institutions has fallen considerably and moreover that death from pneumonia, tuberculosis, and malnutrition has declined. Certainly there are good reasons for supposing that infectious diseases might be more common among psychiatric in-patients. These patients may eat badly and suffer from the effects of malnutrition and of lack of exercise, partly because their ability to look after themselves is impaired and partly because supervision by staff may be inadequate, but it has also been suggested that medication may predispose to infection by interfering with the regulation of body temperature and with the normal immunological defences of the body.

Studies of patients outside psychiatric hospitals, where there is no question that institutional conditions are responsible for excess mortality, have also demonstrated a reduced life expectancy. Sims and Prior (1978) shewed that among neurotic patients discharged from hospital there were about six times more deaths due to suicide and about five times more accidental deaths than expected, but also that the death rate from natural causes was high, particularly from diseases of the respiratory, cardiovascular and nervous systems. Among patients who have had a psychotic illness, the death rate from natural causes is also higher, but the reasons for this are not known with certainty.

The nature of the association

The finding that physical and psychiatric disorder appear to occur more often in the same individual than would be expected by chance probably indicates a true association although part of the explanation may be that there are biases in the populations studied. Emotionally disturbed people may seek advice concerning their physical illnesses more readily than those who are emotionally stable, while the need to investigate physical disorder among psychiatrically disturbed individuals may load mental hospital populations with patients who have bodily ailments. If bias is discounted there are a number of possible explanations for the association (Granville-Grossman, 1976):

(1) Some physical illness may be psychogenic, i.e. the mental disturbance is a cause of the physical illness.
(2) Physical illness may arise as an indirect consequence of the mental disorder, the bodily illness resulting from behavioural disturbances secondary to the psychiatric abnormality.
(3) Physical methods of treatment of psychiatric illness may sometimes cause somatic disease.
(4) The mental disorder may be an organically determined manifestation of the physical illness or an adverse effect of its treatment.
(5) The psychiatric disturbance may represent a psychological reaction to the significance of the physical illness and of its consequences for the patient and his environment.

Many of these associations are discussed in detail in subsequent chapters in this volume, but some elaboration seems warranted here.

Psychogenic physical illness. The idea that psychological stress may cause physical disease is widely held – and is the basis of much psychosomatic research – but evidence that mental *disorder* is associated with somatic illness is not strong and is sometimes equivocal. For example, Heine (1970) studied a group of 40 patients who had recovered from a severe primary depressive illness and noted that the average blood pressure was higher than in a control group; there was, moreover, some evidence suggesting that the degree of hypertension was related to the earlier severity of the depression. However, Mann (1977) demonstrated no difference in psychiatric morbidity between hypertensive and normotensive subjects.

Indirect consequences of psychiatric disorder. Disturbances of behaviour due to psychiatric disorder sometimes endanger physical health and this explains some of the correlation between physical and mental disturbances. The increased risk of suicide and of fatal accidents has already been discussed and attempted suicide and non-fatal injury are also commoner among the mentally disturbed than in the general population. Long-continued ingestion of alcohol – as seen almost only in chronic alcoholism – may cause physical illness such as cirrhosis of the liver while dependence on heroin and on other addictive drugs is also associated with an increased morbidity and mortality risk (see chapters 14 and 15).

Adverse somatic effects of psychiatric treatments. All physical methods used in psychiatric treatment are associated with some risk of untoward reactions, often reversible but sometimes not. For example, major tranquillizers such as phenothiazine and butyrophenone derivatives can cause both temporary and permanent extrapyramidal disturbances (e.g. Parkinsonism and tardive dyskinesia respectively) while the anticholinergic effects of tricyclic antidepressants often lead to impairment of visual accommodation, hesitancy of micturition, and constipation and may sometimes precipitate acute glaucoma, acute retention of urine, and paralytic ileus.

Symptomatic mental disorders. This group of conditions, comprising organically determined psychiatric disorders, is caused either by a physical illness or by the drugs used in its treatment. There is therefore an association between physical and mental disturbance and examples discussed in later chapters include mental disorders arising in endocrine disease, vitamin deficiencies, alcoholism, and drug intoxication.

New examples of this type of association may be recognized in the future; thus there is some current debate that affective disorders (particularly depression) may be an early direct manifestation of malignant disease. Kerr, Schapira and Roth (1969) and Whitlock (1978) have published evidence suggesting this, but the findings of Evans, Baldwin and Gath (1974) indicate no relationship between cancer and depression.

Psychological reactions to physical illness. Mental disturbance arising during the course of physical disease, particularly serious and chronic physical illness, is most commonly an emotional reaction to the illness. The meticulous study by Hinton (1963) demonstrates very clearly the extent to which dying patients are emotionally distressed and some of the causes of this distress. Depression and anxiety are common and often severe and the intensity of the emotional disturbance is related to the duration and severity of the physical discomfort.

Other relationships. That some correlations between physical and mental disorder may have bases unrelated to those discussed already is suggested by studies on grief which indicate that bereavement may be a cause of both mental disorder and physical disease. On the one hand, loss of a wife or husband during the six months prior to admission to a psychiatric hospital is some six times more common than would be expected from the Registrar-General's statistics (Parkes, 1964) while on the other hand the risk of dying, particularly from cardiovascular disease, is much greater among men who have recently lost their wives than among married men of the same age (Parkes, Benjamin & Fitzgerald, 1969). These findings suggest that the stress associated with bereavement not only can cause mental disorder but is aetiologically important in some physical disease.

Psychosomatic medicine

Physicians have always been concerned with the relevance of the body–mind relationship to clinical practice and have been aware of the far reaching effects of disturbances of one on the other. The term 'psychosomatic' was coined by Heinroth in 1818 to emphasize that both mind and body are important in psychiatry and medicine, but was popularized much later, after the first World War, by a group of German and Austrian psycho-analytically oriented psychiatrists, notably F. Deutsch, G. Groddeck, E.

Wittkower and F. Alexander (World Health Organization, 1964; Wittkower, 1977). These workers emphasized the need to consider patients as psychosomatic units and saw danger in perpetuating the concept of a mind–body dichotomy. Many pioneers of the psychosomatic movement left Europe in the 1930s to work in the USA where they developed their ideas with American psychiatrists such as Flanders Dunbar. After the second World War, Britain became an important centre for psychosomatic research and practice and later psychiatrists in all parts of the world were influenced by the new knowledge.

The field of study has gradually expanded over the past fifty years. In the 1930s there was much discussion on the nature and classification of psychologically determined physical disturbances and particularly on the differentiation between the symptoms of conversion hysteria and the somatic manifestations of emotional distress. At that time, the term psychosomatic disorder was introduced in relation to a small number of physical diseases where emotional conflict appeared to be aetiologically important. With the introduction of expressions such as 'psychosomatic medicine' and 'psychosomatics' the original fairly limited field which early workers studied increased enormously, and attempts to restrict the use of the word 'psychosomatic' have largely failed. Indeed nowadays the practitioners of the psychosomatic approach regard it as legitimate (and perhaps obligatory) to study not only the whole person but his social and cultural environment as well; this is the currently favoured holistic approach. The definition of 'psychosomatic medicine' is therefore difficult but Lipowski (1976) points out that it is incorrect to assert that it is merely the study of psychosomatic disorders, or of the part played by psychological factors in the causation of physical disease, or is even, as many people have asserted, just a humane approach to patients. Psychosomatic medicine according to Lipowski encompasses three separate activities: (1) it is concerned with the study of the relationships between psychological, biological, and social factors in illness and health; (2) it emphasizes the holistic approach in clinical practice; (3) it deals with clinical situations where psychiatrists can with benefit work alongside physicians and surgeons. Even this very wide definition may be too limited, and it seems possible that the word 'psychosomatic' has outlived its usefulness. Nevertheless, much useful information has been obtained (and will continue to be obtained) by applying both psychological and physical methods to medical problems, and some of this research is discussed below and in subsequent chapters.

Personality, conflict, and illness

Prominent among the methods used in psychosomatic research are those which are concerned with demonstrating that characteristic types of personality or of emotional conflict are associated with particular illnesses (Lewis, 1967). Psycho-analytically oriented research workers have found it helpful to assume that if emotions were persistently expressed in an inappropriate or inadequate way, the resulting chronic psychological tension would lead to increased activity of the autonomic nervous system and in time to structural changes in the tissues. This hypothesis stimulated the search for characteristic psychological profiles relating to specific physical diseases. Alexander and his colleagues at the Chicago Psychoanalytic Institute studied patients with bronchial asthma, rheumatoid arthritis, ulcerative colitis, essential hypertension, neurodermatitis, thyrotoxicosis, and duodenal ulcer and described characteristic emotional patterns for each. Thus the central conflict of the asthmatic subject appears to be an inhibition of crying for his mother because of a fear of rejection, while in rheumatoid arthritis there seems to be a characteristic difficulty in handling aggressive–hostile impulses (Alexander, French & Pollock, 1968). Alexander and his colleagues proposed a specificity hypothesis that only individuals with specific intrapsychic conflict patterns would develop these diseases in response to stress, but since these patterns were also sometimes observed in normal individuals it was necessary to postulate that patients had a constitutionally determined organ vulnerability as well (Alexander's 'X-factor').

The Western Collaborative Group prospective study on ischaemic heart disease (Rosenman & Friedman, 1971) tends to support the idea that specific psychological patterns are associated with specific diseases. In 1960, the Group examined 3500 men aged 39–59 years and noted that 3182 were physically fit at the time. They allocated each man to one of two groups on the basis of certain personality traits: type A men were aggressive, ambitious, and competitive and tended to be under pressure at work, while type B men lacked these characteristics. Follow-up over a mean period of 6½ years showed that 195 men had developed clinical evidence of coronary heart disease and that the morbidity of individuals showing type

A behaviour was more than twice that of those of type B. Of the men who had died and who had been examined *post mortem*, coronary heart disease as the cause of death was found to be about six times more common among type A than among type B individuals (Friedman *et al.*, 1968).

The specificity hypothesis is supported by other findings such as that of Greer (1979) who investigated the personality of 160 women coming to biopsy for a lump in the breast. A diagnosis of malignant neoplasm was found to be associated significantly with suppression of anger as a behaviour pattern; a possible reason for this association was indicated by the finding that serum IgA levels were consistently higher in women who habitually suppressed their anger, suggesting that emotions may modify host resistance to cancer by an effect on immunological mechanisms. However, an alternative to the idea that specific conflicts are related to specific diseases has been proposed by Sifneos and his colleagues at the Massachusetts General Hospital. These workers coined the word 'alexithymia' to describe the emotional characteristics of patients suffering from various psychosomatic illnesses. The central feature is a well-marked difficulty in finding appropriate words to express feelings and alexithymic patients present with long descriptions of their physical symptoms in contrast with neurotic patients in general who do not emphasize their physical complaints. Alexithymic individuals also fantasize little and rarely dream and they tend to express their emotions inappropriately. It has been postulated that the reason for the association between alexithymia and psychosomatic disorder is that the patient's inability to express his emotions appropriately leads to a misdirection of libidinal activity which causes physical damage (Nemiah & Sifneos, 1970; Sifneos, Apfel-Savitz & Frankel, 1977).

Life-event stress and illness

An important development of the holistic approach in psychosomatic medicine is the emphasis placed on ecology (the study of the relationships between living organisms and their environment), such as that given by Hinkle and Wolff (1958). These workers studied the health of some 3500 people over a period of 20 years, obtaining data from medical, work attendance, and personnel records, as well as from detailed medical histories, physical examinations, psychiatric evaluations, psychological testing, and laboratory investigation, and they found that episodes of illness were not randomly distributed but that certain individuals had much more illness than the average. Moreover, each of these individuals appeared to be susceptible to the whole range of illnesses, both physical and psychiatric, and these tended to occur in clusters, particularly at times when the individual perceived his life situation as threatening, unsatisfactory and productive of conflict. Thus, to Hinkle and Wolff, at least some illnesses (both psychiatric and physical) are inappropriate adaptive responses, mediated through the nervous system, and these authors emphasize that awareness of the environment and the perception of it as threatening is the essential primary aetiological feature of disease due to faulty adaptation.

Holmes and Rahe (1967), much influenced by the work of Wolff and his colleagues, used the 'life chart' device introduced by Adolf Meyer to develop a measure of life change. They noted that events which would normally be considered stressful (events such as death or illness in the family) were not the only ones of aetiological importance, but that apparently desirable environmental changes such as marriage or birth of children were also relevant, and even seemingly neutral changes such as a change of job or house were of importance. They found that, in each individual, life changes tended to cluster at certain points of time and that these clusters tended to be succeeded by illness or by a series of illnesses. Thus life change seems to cause disease and the sort of change which appears to be particularly relevant is one that demands some adaptive response from the individual.

Research on the contribution of life events to the causation of illness has been very active during the past 15 years. When the previous life events of patients who have developed a specific illness – physical or psychiatric – are compared with those of control subjects, there is usually a clear cut difference between the two groups with the patients reporting many more life events than the controls. Thus it seems that a large number of physical disturbances including myocardial infarction, injuries, tuberculosis, leukaemia, multiple sclerosis, and diabetes mellitus may be precipitated by stress due to life events. However, Andrews and Tennant (1978a) have pointed out that a number of large scale prospective studies have failed to shew any relationship between life event stress and physical illness, so that the matter is at present in doubt. Moreover although there is some evidence that schizophrenia, depression and neurotic illnesses seem to be preceded by an increase in life events, the methods used to demonstrate this have also been criticized (Dohrenwend & Dohrenwend, 1978; Andrews & Tennant, 1978b) and hence there is also some doubt concerning the relevance of life stresses to psychiatric disorder. The idea, however, that environmental stress causes disease is so attractive that research on this will undoubtedly continue.

The mind–body problem
Cartesian dualism

It is generally believed nowadays by ordinary men and women that some statements about people, such as that they experience emotions and perceptions, that they have fantasies, dreams, intentions, motives, hopes, fears, and memories, and perhaps above all that not only are they aware of their environment but that they are aware of being aware, can be applied convincingly only to human beings, perhaps to some animals, and not at all to non-living objects. We like to think that there is a major difference between people and ordinary objects: human beings have *minds* (or *souls* or *selves*) whereas things do not, or that in people there are mental as well as physical events. Moreover, it is commonly held that the mind and the body (particularly the brain) of an individual closely interact, that they intimately influence each other: mental events, such as an intention to carry out a bodily action, are causally related to the willed movement; and physical events such as peripheral sensory stimulation can cause a mental experience. This common-sense point of view finds its clearest philosophical expression in Cartesian dualism (formulated by René Descartes, 1596–1650), that mind and body are distinct (dualism) and that they influence each other (interactionism).

Attempts to describe the differences between mind and body have led to a consensus view that physical matter (including that of human bodies) is subject to physical laws whereas minds are not, that minds are not made of ordinary substance, that they are unextended (i.e. exist in time but not in space) and perhaps most important of all that each individual has direct access to his own mind but not to the minds of others. In addition, minds are continuous and persist throughout a person's lifetime whereas the body changes, albeit very slowly, so that at the age of 70 years there is hardly a single atom still present in the body which was there at birth.

There are a number of variations on the theme

of Cartesian dualism, for example that the mind (or soul) can exist independently after death, that it can then appear as an apparition and can influence matter, or that it can be reincarnated. It has also been suggested that mind can act directly on other minds (telepathy), or on itself (psychic determinism) and on other objects and bodies (telekinesis), while some writers, notably Franz Kafka in his short story *Metamorphosis*, have speculated on the possibility of one person's mind, entire and intact, becoming intimately related to a new body.

Although there have been attempts to investigate these problems scientifically, they have not clarified the issues which remain therefore essentially philosophical, and we cannot yet decide, using the scientific method, whether or not mind is made of 'mental substance' which interacts with physical matter in the pineal gland, as Descartes asserted. How do we choose between this view and that of David Hume (1711–76) who taught that mind was 'nothing but a bundle of different perceptions which succeed each other with an inconceivable rapidity and which are in a perpetual flux and movement', or that of William James (1842–1910) that it only makes sense to think of mind as 'a stream of consciousness'?

The modern philosopher Gilbert Ryle, in his book *The Concept of Mind* published in 1949, describes Cartesian dualism as 'the official doctrine', an appropriate term considering that most legal systems only make sense if there is a distinction between mind and body and if they interact. Thus, for many offences in English law, the jury must be satisfied, before giving a verdict of 'guilty' that not only did the accused actually carry out the illegal act (*actus reus*) but that he intended to do so (*mens rea*). Ryle also speaks of this view, in a deliberately disparaging way, as 'the dogma of the ghost in the machine'. He puts forward the view that dualism is absurd and that it is a philosopher's myth based on an elementary mistake in classification, and that it is no more helpful to postulate the existence of human souls than it is to assume that all self-propelling devices, such as motor cars, must have souls as well.

Nevertheless Cartesian dualism receives much support, not only from the man in the street who knows little of philosophy, but also from influential philosophers such as Karl Popper (well known to psychiatrists for his book *The Logic of Scientific Discovery*) and scientists, such as John Eccles. In 1977, Popper and Eccles published a remarkable book, *The Self and its Brain*, which presents powerful arguments

– not necessarily amounting to proof – in favour of a version of interactionism. Popper and Eccles extend dualism by proposing a triality in which there are three interacting forms of ultimate reality: mind, body, and self. Moreover, they argue that if the conscious activity of the self has any useful purpose, it must have evolved as a result of natural selection: if two similar lowly animal forms exist, one with primitive conscious experiences (such as of pain and pleasure) and one without, the former type will tend to survive and the latter to become extinct, but only if mental activity can actually influence the body and if this capacity can be transmitted to the next generation. But this seems to lead to a paradox because, since genetic information is transmitted physically, it is difficult to understand how mind can be separate unless it interacts with matter and, moreover, has a physical basis.

Alternatives to Cartesian dualism

Various alternatives to the interactionism of Cartesian dualism have been proposed. Some philosophers have suggested dualistic schemes in which mind and body do not interact in the way Descartes postulated. Thomas Huxley (1825–95), among others suggested that man is a conscious automaton, that mental events are completely causally dependent on bodily activity but are themselves never causes of physical events. Thus Huxley's view, often labelled *epiphenomenalism*, is that mind is an ineffective concomitant, a collateral product of physical events, a mere observer of the physical scene and an epiphenomenon. The converse idea, that mental events can influence the body but not vice versa has not been considered, since it appears self-evident that physical events do affect the mind.

Psychophysical parallelism is another reaction to Cartesianism but one which denies any interaction whatsoever between mind and body. One variety of this (*occasionalism*) explains the apparent correlation between physical changes and mental experiences on the basis of divine intervention, that God is the cause of every mental and physical event and that He arranges matters so that mind and body appear to work together. Gottfried Leibniz (1646–1716) also espoused *parallelism* but was dissatisfied with the need for the continuous miraculous intervention which occasionalism demanded. His solution was the doctrine of *pre-established harmony* which postulated that God, at the time of creation ensured that minds and bodies, though independent, would continue to run together without the need for constant readjustment.

Monism attempts to solve the mind–body problem by denying that there are two things to be related: *materialism* (as exemplified by *behaviourism*) asserts that whatever exists is physical, while *subjective idealism* denies the existence of matter, proposing that ultimate reality consists only of perceptions of so-called physical objects (including one's own body) or that what is claimed to be the physical world is really just an exceptionally vivid and coherent dream or hallucination.

Other monistic theories include the *identity theory* which asserts that mental processes and physical processes are identical and the *double-aspect* theory, proposed by Baruch Spinoza (1634–77), that mind and body are different aspects of something more fundamental which is itself neither mental nor physical. Spinoza suggested that Nature or God might be the underlying basis but Bertrand Russell (1872–1970) proposed something else which he called 'neutral stuff'. The double-aspect theory can be viewed as related to *panpsychism* which asserts that all physical entities (even elementary particles) have a mind-like aspect which becomes conscious only when organized in a particularly complex way, as in the brain of man and of some animals, and, perhaps, in non-living matter when arranged to form advanced electronic computers.

Of the non-interactionist views described in this section, two merit further consideration, namely *behaviourism* and the *identity theory* because each forms the basis for current approaches to psychiatric problems; they are discussed in the following paragraphs.

Behaviourism. This doctrine or policy of reducing mental events (which are private and not directly observable by others) to publicly discernible behaviour has been so influential during this century that the word *psychology* is now usually taken to mean the science of *behaviour* rather than the science of *mind* or of conscious experience. In its mildest form (*methodological behaviourism*) it merely eschews introspection as a valid method of study and insists on investigating physical phenomena only. Thus John B. Watson (1878–1958), the founder of American behaviourism, showed that useful information could still be obtained even when physiological investigation was substituted for the study of subjective experience and consciousness. *Logical behaviourism* is more

stringent and defines mental phenomena only in terms of behaviour and physiology, while *radical behaviourism*, the most rigorous form of the doctrine, rejects the very concepts of mind and of other hypothetical constructs or intervening variables. Professor B. Frederic Skinner of Harvard University is perhaps the most uncompromising contemporary behaviourist. He believes that an individual's actions are totally determined by his environment, that mental activity is irrelevant to outcome, and that human beings are mindless, lacking free-will, and indeed can be considered as nonpersons. He asserts that humans have no more control over their own lives than animals, that what goes on inside men's heads is no more important than what goes on in those of any other creatures, and that there is no such thing as knowledge. Skinner (1953) agrees with dualists that an individual can describe states of affairs which are accessible only to himself, but he denies that this indicates the presence of mind or of conscious experience. Thus, when someone says 'I was on the point of going home' this should be interpreted according to Skinner as being equivalent to his saying 'I observed events in myself which characteristically precede or accompany my going home'. Behaviourism, though dissatisfying to many psychiatrists and psychologists, does appeal to some and is probably the only version of materialism that is at all accepted nowadays.

Identity theory. This proposes that mental processes and physical processes are identical (in the same sense that light waves and photons are identical) and that concepts of separate minds and bodies have arisen only because human beings are consistently looked at from two differing points of view. For a mental and physical event to be identical it must be shewn that a particular mental phenomenon occurs if, and only if, some specific physical change, say in the brain, occurs, that is, that mental and neural processes are one and the same.

Identity theory has become very influential in recent years, particularly in psychiatry where it forms an indispensable part of the holistic approach. Thus the World Health Organization's Expert Committee on Mental Health in its 13th report (World Health Organization, 1964) states that 'When we speak of psychological processes and physiological processes, we are speaking of different ways of approaching one phenomenon. The phenomenon is not so divided'. Thus the holistic view seems to conflict with ideas of ordinary interactionism and of Cartesian dualism, but nevertheless has been welcomed by psychiatrists in general, and practitioners of psychosomatic medicine in particular. Holism may be placed alongside interactionism and behaviourism as the resolutions of the mind–body problem which are most favoured by contemporary psychiatrists; none of the other doctrines described in this section can command the support which these three have.

Conclusion

It seems reasonable to wonder whether the concepts of souls and minds have been invented to enable us to better understand human beings – much as the *luminiferous aether* was postulated in the nineteenth century to account for the propagation of light and of other electromagnetic radiation *in vacuo*. The problem here is that while we might be persuaded (albeit with great difficulty) that other people may be merely extremely complex automata, we ourselves, who know the vividness of our experiences and emotions and who are consciously aware of our own existences, find it impossible – unless we are committed behaviourists – to deny that there is a mental aspect to our own beings. Like Descartes, each of us may say, after doubting the existence of the external world, *'Cogito, ergo sum'*, 'I think therefore I am', or even like George Berkeley (1685–1753) *'Esse est percipi'*, 'to be is to be perceived', and we cannot doubt the existence of our own minds. But if we do accept a psychophysical dualism and believe that there are two-way interactions between mind and matter, we have to face a problem concerning the manner in which they interact. How is it possible that physical events such as electrical or chemical reactions in the brain can lead to a vivid perception of the world around us? How can a thought or an idea decide which nerve cells will come into action and if they

do, is the law of conservation of energy broken? How can anything physical interact with something that is not? Eccles (Popper & Eccles, 1977) suggests that the columnar organization of neurones in the cerebral cortex into modules allows the transmission and reception of messages to and from the self-conscious mind, but this proposal poses as many problems as Descartes' much more naive idea that the pineal is the 'seat of the soul'.

The mind–body problem may never be finally solved, since it seems likely that the study of brain and its mechanisms will just amplify a picture of something that remains wholly physical and may never explain conscious experience. However, what might reasonably be expected is that further investigation into psychophysical relationships will allow a more precise description of the ways in which bodily states influence the mind (and vice versa) even if the exact nature of the interaction may never be known. A similar situation, an inability to provide ultimate explanations, already exists in physical science. Physical laws (such as Newton's law of gravitation) merely describe what does happen, not why or how. Newton himself was puzzled by the 'action at a distance' of gravitation, which contrasts strikingly with the more familiar action by contact, as when two bodies collide. Thus perhaps all that can ever be understood about the relationship between mental and physical events is the mathematical way in which the two sorts of happenings correlate while the actual mechanism involved will always remain unknown. (For further discussion see in particular volume 1, chapters 1 and 3, volume 4, chapter 8, and volume 5, chapter 6.)

Acknowledgement

I wish to thank Christopher Mace for reading part of the manuscript and for his helpful comments.

2
General medical disorders
H. G. MORGAN

Introduction

Psychological processes can have a complex inter-relationship with systemic organic disease. They may have a causal role, either in the form of long-standing psychological predisposition which renders the individual vulnerable to a particular kind of organic illness, or they may act as precipitants of acute physical disease.

Such psychological causal factors may be sufficient in themselves, but more commonly they become pathogenic because they act synergistically with some kind of predisposing somatic vulnerability: the psychosomatic approach to organic disease is usually concerned with causation which is complex and multifactorial.

Organic disease may also itself lead to secondary psychological complications, either concomitant with the illness itself or as sequelae which develop during the process of rehabilitation. These commonly accentuate or perpetuate the organic disease process, thereby delaying recovery or provoking relapse: they may thus play an important role in leading to chronic organic illness, even though the primary causal factors may have resolved.

This chapter reviews those organic diseases in which psychological factors appear to be relevant in any of these ways. The approach will be primarily a clinical one, and emphasis will be placed on the psychological aspects of evaluation and treatment of such organic diseases, either in their acute phase or during rehabilitation. Early antecedents will also be examined, important as they themselves are in treatment, particularly in primary prevention. Close attention will be paid throughout to the methodological problems inherent in the psychosomatic approach, particularly with regard to the differentiation of those factors which antecede as opposed to secondarily complicate the illness, and the critical evaluation of their relevance to the organic disease process.

Vascular disorders
Ischaemic heart disease
Aetiology. The search for causative precursors of ischaemic heart disease (IHD) has concentrated upon somatic variables, socio-economic conditions, behavioural and psychological characteristics, and precipitating stressful events (Jenkins, 1971). True prospective studies are few, and it is probable that the inconsistencies in findings of various studies reflect to a considerable extent the use of retrospective techniques as well as major difficulties in defining the relevant variables, which themselves are usually interconnected in a complex way. The low specificity and predictive value of the supposed risk factors mean that prospective studies need to include large numbers of persons at risk in order to produce reliable findings. Bias in case selection may occur through failure to include fatal or asymptomatic 'silent' cases of infarction, or not distinguishing between angina pectoris and actual infarction.

Aetiology: Somatic. The increased incidence of IHD in conditions such as myxoedema and diabetes mellitus which are associated with raised blood lipids has long suggested that abnormality of lipid metabolism or high fat dietary intake may be important predisposing factors. There is now a considerable body of evidence for this, as well as for other somatic factors which include raised blood pressure, smoking, obesity, short stature, physical underactivity (Epstein, 1971; Keys, 1957; Dawber & Kannel, 1962; Paffenbarger, Notkin & Krueger, 1966; Paffenbarger, Wolf, Notkin & Thorne, 1966). The precise pathogenic role of these correlates of IHD remains uncertain: we cannot discuss them further here, but they are of obvious relevance to behavioural and psychological precursors which we will analyse in more detail.

Aetiology: Behavioural. An association between a particular kind of personality and IHD has long been

the subject of debate. Dunbar (1943) emphasized a personality characterized by compulsive striving, self-discipline, sense of propriety, and mastery of others. More recently Friedman and Rosenman and their colleagues in the Western Collaborative Group Study have presented a considerable body of research evidence aimed at defining and measuring behaviour (type A) which may signify increased risk of IHD, and conversely, type B, which in the absence of such behavioural characteristics implies some degree of immunity (Friedman & Rosenman, 1959; Brandt, Rosenman, Sholtz & Friedman, 1976). Type A behaviour is characterized by extreme competitiveness, striving for achievement, aggressiveness (sometimes repressed), haste, restlessness, tenseness, hyperalertness, feelings of being under pressure of time and responsibilities. Assessment of type A behaviour is by evaluation of verbal and behavioural responses. Prospective follow-up studies over a 4½ year period have shown that the incidence of IHD in type A is increased by factors of 6.5 and 1.9 in the age groups 39–49 and 50–59 years compared with men categorized as type B. Significant differences in risk were still found after 8½ years' follow-up (Brandt *et al.*, 1976) and type A behaviour accounted for 31 per cent of the increased risk of IHD.

Autopsy findings suggest that type A behaviour is associated with increased incidence of atherosclerotic deposits in coronary arteries. It appears to have a close association with other risk factors such as smoking, shortened clotting time, high serum lipid level, and increased diurnal secretion of adrenalin which increases the oxygen requirement of the myocardium and releases fatty acids from body fat. A true psychosomatic pathogenesis is therefore hypothesized, whereby type A behaviour, together with frequent affective and autonomic arousal due to environmental demands, leads to atheromatous deposits in coronary arteries and in turn to IHD.

It is claimed that type A behaviour can be assessed in a highly reliable way, for example by the Jenkins Activity Survey which is an extensively validated questionnaire (Jenkins, Zyzanski, Rosenman & Friedman, 1969; Jenkins, Rosenman & Zyzanski, 1974). Recently attempts have been made to define more closely the element of behaviour inherent in the type A life-style and to simplify the assessment procedure, for example by evaluating speech characteristics using tape recordings (Schucker & Jacobs, 1977) in order to widen its applicability in prediction of risk. However, it has been the subject of much controversy regarding problems of measurement and replication because its evaluation requires the acquisition of special interview skills: its validity has also been questioned because of the failure of various studies to control for social class variables.

Although type A behaviour when combined with other high-risk factors such as hypertension or the presence of abnormal serum lipoproteins can be useful in predicting IHD, the over-all efficiency of its predictive value is not high. Thus, in the Western Collaboration Study, 80 per cent of men who subsequently developed IHD had initially been categorized as type A, but so had 52 per cent of those who did not develop the disease. In terms of absolute numbers the 1774 false positives greatly outnumbered the 80 true positives (the latter comprising only 0.04 per cent of all positive responders). However, type A behaviour does permit delineation of certain very high risk groups: when it appears in combination with hypertension, the risk of IHD was shown to be 6 per cent over a 2½-year period. It may also prove useful in predicting relative immunity to IHD, for example in individuals with type B behaviour (as defined by the absence of type A characteristics) with low serum cholesterol, triglycerides and lipoproteins. Only 0.02 per cent of type B individuals later developed IHD. Though there has been some reluctance in many medical circles to accept the relevance of behavioural variables to risk of IHD (*Amer. J. pub. Health*, 1969, *Brit. med. J.*, 1969) these findings in this research field cannot be ignored and should form the basis of further enquiry.

Aetiology: Psychological. Most studies have been retrospective, and in view of the major secondary psychological impact which IHD is bound to have, there are severe limitations to such an approach: it is not surprising that the literature is inconsistent and difficult to interpret. Some studies report negative findings (Shekelle, Ostfeld & Paul, 1969; Verghese, 1967), others emphasize a variety of features such as extroversion, cyclothymic personality, excessive use of self-control, and inhibition of behaviour (Minc, 1965), compulsivity and repressed hostility or a prevailing attitude of apprehension, indecision, and fear of failure (Dreyfuss, Shanan & Sharon, 1966).

Prospective investigations are relatively few. The early follow up study of Paffenbarger and colleagues (1966a, 1966b) retrieved the college health records of 45 000 American university students. Those who later suffered fatal episodes of myocardial

infarction differed from others in previously having reported greater subjective feelings of exhaustion by having more evidence of anxiety and other mood disorders. Further interesting findings came from the study of Thomas (1951, 1968) who administered a check list concerning habits of nervous tension to medical students in a longitudinal prospective survey. A high level of anxiety was found to be associated with smoking and a family history of IHD. It was suggested that high anxiety might have been merely an indirect indication of high risk because of its association with other relevant factors, rather than necessarily having any direct causal significance itself. These important studies have continued (Thomas & Greenstreet, 1973). Other prospective studies have used more sophisticated methods of psychological assessment such as the MMPI and 16 PF schedule of Cattell (Brozek, 1966). Persons who later develop IHD, especially angina pectoris, were shown to have high scores on the Hs (hypochondriasis), D (depression) and Hy (hysteria) scales of the MMPI and on the C (emotional stability) scale of the 16PF.

Aetiology: Socio-economic. The social and economic correlates of IHD have recently been reviewed in detail (Jenkins, 1971). Findings regarding social class appear to vary from one country to another, some emphasizing high risk in upper socio-economic groups, others claiming the opposite, or that social class variation in incidence disappears when the degree of physical activity is taken into account. Both social mobility (change of environment such as house move, a change of job) and social incongruity (inconsistency in status relevant to various aspects of a person's life situation) have also been implicated as high risk factors.

Several authors have suggested that the increased prevalence of IHD in Western society may be related mainly to psychosocial factors. Groen (1976) points out that males with an exaggerated striving for dominance and who use work as a major outlet for aggression are more exposed to particular stresses and conflict and are more conditioned than females to control their emotions when dealing with such conflict. The relative immunity of females to IHD may be a reflection of psychosocial rather than biological differences between the sexes. The relatively low prevalence of IHD in underdeveloped countries may also, according to Groen, be related to the fact that work pressures of the type described have hitherto been less intense, and the still dependent position of women and children has not exposed the male to the frustrations associated with his position in the modern Western family (Groen, 1976). Minc (1960) hypothesized that Western civilization predisposes to IHD by imposing the need for self-discipline governed by intellectual control and distant goals rather than basic drives and their more immediate gratification. Friedman and Rosenman (1971) suggest that the modern environment encourages the high-risk type A behaviour pattern: it rewards haste, aggressive competition, and a constant excessive preoccupation with the demands of work schedules, all of these being challenges not experienced by earlier generations.

Precipitants. It is well recognized that stressful affective arousal is closely related to physiological cardiovascular changes such as increase in heart rates, blood pressure, cardiac output, and peripheral resistance. The psychophysiological correlates undoubtedly involve the hypophysioadrenal axis, leading to an increased secretion of adrenal catecholamines and corticosteroids (Levi, 1961).

Several studies have reported an increase in incidence and intensity of stressful situations experienced by individuals immediately before they develop myocardial infarction (Fisher, 1963; Culpan & Davies, 1959; Pearson & Joseph, 1963; Cay, Vetter, Philip & Dugard, 1972a; Engel, 1971). An increase in the numbers of life-change units immediately prior to myocardial infarction has been reported in two series of Swedish males who survived, and in a further group who suffered sudden cardiac death (Rahe & Lind, 1971; Rahe & Paasikivi, 1971; Rahe & Theorell, 1971). The sense of threat which a situation may present is related not only to the individual's personality characteristics, but its impact is also dependent upon the degree of available interpersonal and social support. An event or situation may pose a threat because of uncertainty of outcome, risk of physical or psychological harm, or the need for continued vigilance. Events reported as precipitants of acute IHD include excessive work under pressure (Fisher, 1963), conflict with others, chronic dissatisfaction and frustration, bereavement, over-control of emotional reactions, a sense of emotional drain due to chronic frustration, or a feeling of depression and fatigue. Chronic preceding stress has also been reported by persons with IHD more often than controls and they have been described as obsessional and stress-prone (Leigh, 1968).

Stress situations of the kinds described are of course closely related to the behavioural patterns described earlier: a driving competitive individual is likely to find himself in situations which are perceived as stressful, and the process is accentuated if he uses faulty secondary coping strategies. Stress situations are of course also likely to be relevant to episodic relapse of established IHD.

Concomitants. Between half and two-thirds of patients who have been hospitalized because of an acute episode of IHD exhibit clear evidence of anxiety and depression which is of sufficient degree to require treatment in its own right (Wishnie, Hackett & Cassem, 1971; Cay, *et al.*, 1972a; Leigh, Hofer, Cooper & Reiser, 1972). Some authors have suggested that admission to a coronary care unit may accentuate such emotional upset (Klein, Kliner, Zipes, Troyer & Wallace, 1968; Kornfeld, Zimbers & Malm, 1965), though it is difficult to draw general conclusions on this issue. Probably only a minority of patients, such as those who remain in such units longest because of severe cardiac disease, are made more anxious by the intensive care situations. What does seem important, however, is the degree of awareness of medical staff concerning the high incidence of emotional difficulties which IHD patients experience and the way in which these are dealt with, particularly at certain times, such as transfer to general wards or discharge home, when anxiety is likely to be accentuated (Cay, Vetter, Philip & Dugard, 1972b; Dominian & Dobson, 1969). Anxiety may also be reduced in the intensive care situation by ensuring that patients retain a certain degree of privacy and are not unduly aware of the crisis situations which necessarily occur from time to time in the management of other patients: on the other hand, regular close personal contact, especially with full reassurances and explanation from staff, is just as important.

The study of Cay and colleagues (1972a) is of particular interest because it demonstrates that patient distress and disability may be more related to psychological and social problems than to the severity of organic symptoms. In this study, 203 consecutive male coronary care unit admissions were assessed by means of semistructured interviews and formal psychological testing. It was found that psychological, social, and work difficulties were more common in patients with a presumptive diagnosis of cardiac ischaemia in which physical symptoms and signs were less severe, than in those who had unequivocal myocardial infarction. Significantly more of those patients who were perceived as psychologically disturbed following their heart attack had been under some kind of emotional stress in the preceding month than had those who were not upset during convalescence.

Emotional disturbance is also common in patients with IHD apart from acute episodes of myocardial infarction or angina pectoris. Mayou (1973a, 1973b) interviewed 40 male out-patients with a diagnosis of angina pectoris, about half of whom had a previous history of myocardial infarction. Using a semistructured interview and the General Health Questionnaire Mayou found that half had high levels of depression and/or anxiety. Common symptoms included insomnia, apathy, poor concentration and irritability sufficient to cause family upset, and feelings of fatigue which correlate closely with psychiatric disability. Emotional precipitants of angina, which included anger, excitement, or anxiety, were reported in 75 per cent of those regarded as having mild cardiac disease, compared with 90 per cent who had severe cardiac disability, and here again the individual personality and degree of psychological disturbance seemed important.

Some of the secondary psychological reactions to acute episodes of IHD may lead to attitudes and behaviour which impair treatment and rehabilitation. Excess anxiety may lead to over-caution and inactivity or agitation which make rest difficult; certain endocrine changes with which it is closely associated may increase the risk of cardiac arrhythmia. Marked changes in catecholamine excretion occur during the first few days after myocardial infarction (Miller & Rosenfeld, 1975). The level of noradrenaline appears to reflect the extent of cardiac damage and circulatory failure, but that of adrenaline may be more related to altered autonomic function secondary to anxiety itself (Valori, Thomas & Shillingforth, 1967; Wallace, 1968). When such a mechanism leads to marked and sustained increases in catecholamine levels the risk of serious arrhythmia during recovery from acute IHD is greatly increased.

During the acute stages of any serious physical illness, a patient may be able to achieve some useful reduction of anxiety by distraction of attention or suppression of unpleasant thoughts. When this process is taken further, however, gross minimization and denial of illness and disability may occasionally occur: this may lead to rejection of essential treatment measures. Denial seems to be a particularly

common feature of patients with acute IHD (Olin & Hackett, 1964; Wishnie *et al.*, 1971; Nagle, Gangola & Picton-Robinson, 1971; Croog, Shapiro & Levine, 1971; Miller & Rosenfeld, 1975). Even in those who have not suffered recent acute episodes (Mayou, 1973a, 1973b) as many as 60 per cent minimize their condition by doubting the diagnosis, underemphasizing or even failing to acknowledge symptoms and psychosocial problems during interview. There may be little correlation between the degree of denial and psychophysiological measures such as excretion of catecholamines (Miller & Rosenfeld, 1975); such extreme forms of 'awareness control' implicit in denial tend to do more harm than good through secondary management problems, especially in conflict with ward staff. Occasionally denial mechanisms may lead to considerable delay before the patient reports significant cardiac symptoms (Olin & Hackett, 1964; Hackett & Cassem, 1969). Denial also seems to be a common finding in patients who survive a cardiac arrest, making it difficult to discuss the illness; other symptoms such as violent dreams, insomnia, and irritability may be experienced for several weeks after the event (Druss & Kornfeld, 1967).

Secondary disabilities. During convalescence after an acute episode of IHD at least half of all patients experience psychological problems which interfere with their return to full activity: well over half experience major problems in getting back to work (Wynn, 1967; Wishnie *et al.*, 1971; Mayou, 1973a, 1973b; Cay, Vetter, Philip & Dugard, 1973; Cay, Philip & Aitken, 1976; Nagle *et al.*, 1971). Wishnie interviewed 24 (18 males, 6 females) out of 50 survivors three to six months after hospital treatment; of the others, eleven had died, ten refused to cooperate, and five were not available for interview. A uniform tendency to minimize symptoms was found; eleven did not return to work and in nine of these the reasons appeared to be psychological in nature. Relatives reported a tendency to irritability and to take offence easily in 21 of those who returned to a family situation, and in respect of 12 there developed excessive anxiety in close relatives, with marked attitudes of overprotection and secondary family discord. Arguments about the nature of IHD and misinterpretations of the physician's advice were also common. Only a third gave up smoking and five out of six who resolved to discontinue alcohol intake failed to do so.

Secondary disability must of course reflect the setting in which rehabilitation occurs and the amount of available personal and social support. The fact that very similar findings have also been reported by two studies carried out in the UK suggests that they represent difficulties relevant and somewhat specific to rehabilitation from acute IHD whatever the setting. Mayou's series (Mayou, 1973a, b) consisted of forty men aged 38–74 years attending a hospital clinic because of angina pectoris (the duration 6 months to 7 years); almost half had previous episodes of myocardial infarction. Twelve remained unemployed, 11 had taken lighter jobs, and 3 were on sick leave. Those who had returned to their jobs tended to work less efficiently because of anxiety, and to reduce their level of physical activity compared with previously. Work problems were most common in manual labourers who had to change their jobs more often than others and had more difficulty in finding alternatives. Restriction of leisure activities was common, with increased dependence on family support. Secondary family problems were moderate or severe in 70 per cent, relatives showing an ambivalent mixture of concern and resentment of the extra restrictions and demands placed upon them. Sexual difficulties were common: of those who had been sexually active previously, 50 per cent had stopped intercourse completely and a further 30 per cent decreased its frequency. These problems stemmed most commonly from a fear that sexual intercourse would accentuate IHD, though in some it was related to loss of libido. In 70 per cent there was dissatisfaction regarding medical advice, which was seen as inadequate and conflicting, though this was less common in relatives. Disability at work and leisure was not closely related to physical handicap, and it was concluded that the most important factors in satisfactory rehabilitation were the degree of psychological well being and the quality of family and medical support.

In their Edinburgh study, Cay and her colleagues (1973) report similar findings in 203 patients followed up after treatment in a coronary care unit. In the absence of a special treatment programme, return to work appeared to be closely related to previous personality, a history of work difficulties prior to the onset of cardiac symptoms, and the degree of initial emotional upset in hospital at the time of acute IHD (see table 2.1).

This study also emphasizes the importance of preceding psychological problems in rehabilitation: of those with psychological disturbance in convalescence, 71 per cent had experienced psychosocial

Table 2.1. *Return to work after heart attack (Cay et al., 1973)*

Initial emotional upset	Return to work (full activity)	
	Within 4 months	Within 1 year
Absent	52%	78%
Present	36%	31%
Previous personality		
Normal	58% working normally after 68 days' convalescence	
Difficulties present	20% working normally after 92 days' convalescence	

stress before admission, compared with 31 per cent of those who remained free from emotional problems. Again a general picture emerged in which the degree of secondary disability was in many patients far more related to psychosocial difficulties than to the severity of organic cardiac symptoms: those with mild angina took much longer to return to work than did patients with severe ischaemic heart disease.

A proportion of patients show extreme disability in convalescence: they complain bitterly of physical symptoms and have severe social and work difficulties in the presence of little or no objective evidence of organic heart disease. There may be a variety of reasons why this occurs. When chest pain has been atypical or mild in severity, the physician's response may have been equivocal and inconsistent, thereby leading to anxiety and lack of confidence on the part of the patient (Klein, Dean, Wilson & Bogdonoff, 1965; Mayou, 1973a, 1973b). Alternatively the reason may be found in previous personality difficulties: there may have been a longstanding pattern of over-concern about somatic symptoms, this continuing as excessive timidity in coping with physical disease. Occasionally a fragile personality may retreat into invalidism in the face of minimal cardiac disease as a way of avoiding and so resolving quite independent conflicts. It is then no longer necessary to attend a place of work where interpersonal problems may for long have been difficult to bear, or to engage in social activities which have been a major source of anxiety: when such preceding difficulties have been severe, their avoidance through cardiac invalidism may seem to the patient to be an acceptable price to pay.

Treatment and rehabilitation. Psychological difficulties are clearly important precursors as well as concomitants of IHD and in recent years there has accumulated a considerable body of evidence which demonstrates that adequate management of psychological and social problems can contribute considerably to a reduction in the incidence of secondary disabilities.

Wynn was amongst the first to point out the unwarranted emotional distress which so often hinders rehabilitation from IHD: it was present in half of the 400 patients described by him, and psychosocial factors were the main reason for prolonged unemployment (Wynn, 1967). In view of the complexities introduced by the need to treat physical, psychological, and social factors concurrently, the concept of planned systematic rehabilitation programmes has gained wide support. This ensures that close integration is constantly maintained between all those who play a part in treatment: such co-ordination increases the effectiveness of rehabilitation and in particular it reduces the likelihood that the patient will receive conflicting information, which we have already noted to be a major problem facing patients during convalescence. Wynn (1969) has described how a rehabilitation programme enabled 70 per cent of IHD patients who already had various degrees of disability to return to work; high family morale was achieved and sustained. Zohman and Tobis (1970) also showed that with a comprehensive team approach 80 per cent of patients returned to work within four months of a heart attack. Even in the absence of a special rehabilitation service, careful observance of the principles described can ensure that 66 per cent of patients will be back at work within four months (Hay & Turbott, 1970a).

The principles of team work in cardiac rehabilitation have recently been summarized by Cay and colleagues (1976). The ultimate aim in the younger patient is to return him to his job, without loss of status or undue fear of physical disability: in older individuals, return to work might not be so important as ensuring that social isolation and excessive restriction of day-to-day activity are avoided. Psychiatric intervention should be aimed not only at any significant psychological distress exhibited by the patient but should also take into account interpersonal, social, and economic factors which so frequently are closely related. During the acute illness, prompt attendance by the doctor can do much to reassure and lay the foundation for effective rehabilitation: Cay and colleagues (1976) conclude that the patient's emotional well being is closely related to the availability of adequate reassurance and encouragement, and no general rules can be laid down as to whether this is best achieved in hospital or at home. Recognition by the physician of the frequency of psychological difficulties during the acute illness should increase the likelihood that they will be treated appropriately. The use of benzodiazepine drugs can be a useful short-term expedient in severe anxiety, but phenothiazines are less satisfactory because of their potential hypotensive side effects.

Psychiatric assessment also aims to recognize the various psychological defence mechanisms which may become established even in the very early stages of acute illness. Regular contact with therapists whom the patient knows and can trust is of course important at all stages.

Early mobilization is now widely practised in cardiac rehabilitation and the patient needs to be prepared for symptoms such as weakness, dizziness, and faintness on first getting out of bed, which in themselves are usually of no serious importance, but which may accentuate anxiety. Constant reassurance which stresses the healing process is necessary, especially at such times as departure from an intensive care situation or on return home, when there may be resurgence of anxiety and loss of confidence. At an early stage the prospect of return home and to work should be discussed in an optimistic way, pointing out that there is every reason to expect a return to work three months later: effective liaison with employers should not be delayed. A clear-cut programme of gradual resumption of normal activities leads to considerable psychological benefit and confidence. This may be a good time to attempt breaking old habits such as smoking or alcohol misuse, and to reduce weight by attention to diet, although only about half seem able to maintain initial resolve for long (Hay & Turbott, 1970b).

The patient's response to rehabilitation is closely related to the quality of support which he receives from others. The role of relatives is of course of the greatest importance: they need to be involved at an early stage of treatment and this is particularly important in order to prevent family tension which tends to occur when the patient returns home. Conjoint discussion helps the key relative to understand as much about the rehabilitation programme as does the patient, and relatives are less likely later to feel misinformed or poorly advised. The family is also less likely to become over-anxious and too protective, a common source of disharmony when the patient returns home. A spouse who develops major psychological problems may need individual treatment. In their study of 65 wives of men who had survived myocardial infarction, Skelton and Dominian (1973) found that initial feelings of loss, depression, and guilt were common, and a quarter were still considerably upset one year later. Uncertainties often focus on the resumption of sexual intercourse. Usually this should be possible when the patient has returned to full general physical activity without symptoms or ECG changes (Hellerstein & Friedman, 1970). Sexual problems will be found in some to have preceded the acute illness, and their management will then necessitate a more radical reappraisal of the relationship difficulties.

Regular group physical training can also be useful in promoting resolve to adopt a more healthy lifestyle (Cay *et al.*, 1976). Group psychotherapy has also been advocated (Adsett & Bruhn, 1968; Bilodean & Hackett, 1971).

The primary prevention of IHD remains an immense challenge. The avoidance of excess in any aspects of one's physical and mental life may seem banal advice, but it is probably the best that can be offered in the present state of knowledge, and is likely to contain more than a grain of truth.

Cardiac surgery

Psychiatric complications are common after cardiac surgery, especially when this involves open heart bypass techniques. In some cases the post-operative clinical picture is dominated by affective disturbance. Depressive symptoms with or without anxiety have been reported in up to half of those patients who survive the operation (Morgan, 1971; Kimball, 1972). These may be transient, appearing on the fourth or fifth post-operative day and lasting no more than one or two days, or they may be more prolonged and accompanied by irritability and insomnia: some patients may be mildly euphoric and a small minority may have hysterical conversion symptoms. Post-operative delirium is the most striking complication and this has been reported to occur in 28–57 per cent of adult patients who survive open

heart surgery (Blachy & Starr, 1964; Egerton & Kay, 1964; Kimball, 1972; Morgan, 1971). The incidence of this complication appears to be much lower in children.

Delirium may present immediately after the operation, when it is usually accompanied by evidence of major organic complications of the central nervous system. In some the delirium may develop after a few days in which the immediate post-operative period has been satisfactory, with clear sensorium and good physical progress. Typical organic impairment of cardiac function then occurs, with disorientation, memory impairment with or without hallucinations, delusional ideas, agitation, and insomnia. The delirium tends to be self-limiting and clears after a few days, provided there are no major physical complications. Pre-operative factors which may predispose to the development of post-operative delirium include previous evidence of organic brain damage or severe social and marital problems. Prolonged bypass procedures with hypothermia (Tufo, Ostfeld & Shekelle, 1970) or metabolic complications such as hyponatraemia and dehydration also increase the risk of delirium. Some authors have emphasized the importance of post-operative environmental factors in the causation of delirium, particularly sensory overstimulation, sleep deprivation, or the use of drugs which impair cognitive function.

As in the case of ischaemic heart disease, there is evidence that the preceding psychological state may also be an important determinant of mental adjustment during the post-operative period. It is not surprising that faced with such a major life-threatening event the majority of patients may show some kind of emotional disturbance involving anxiety, depression, or denial, with inability to discuss the situation directly and objectively.

Subsequent depression is more common in those who show morbid pre-operative anxiety, with or without denial mechanisms. There is also evidence to suggest that patients with severe pre-operative depression, feelings of hopelessness or morbid anxiety may have a high mortality, raising the possibility that such affective disturbance may adversely affect cardiovascular function (Morgan, 1971; Kimball, 1972).

These findings suggest that psychiatric evaluation may usefully be included in the pre-operative assessment of candidates for open heart surgery: some reports suggest that subsequent complications may thereby be reduced (Kimball, 1969; Layne & Yodofsky, 1971). Regular evaluation of the mental state as soon as the patient regains consciousness may be useful in the early detection of cognitive impairment (Quinlan, Kimball & Osborne, 1974). Adequate symptomatic control of delirium may require the use of tranquilliser medication, though the importance of regular close personal support and reassurance should not be forgotten. It has already been noted that environmental factors inherent in the intensive care situation itself may play a part in leading to postoperative psychological complications.

Essential arterial hypertension

Essential arterial hypertension (EHT) may be defined as a condition in which the arterial blood pressure is persistently raised above the range 140–160/90–95 (WHO, 1959) in the absence of any demonstrable causal organic disease. The role of psychological causal factors can only be assessed adequately through the prospective study of representative samples of the general population: the majority of investigations have hitherto been concerned with the study of patients with well-established hypertensive disease, and this approach can of course be very misleading when psychological antecedents are sought. Our understanding of EHT has also been hindered by the fact that it is usually discovered only by chance during its early asymptomatic stages. Its incidence increases with age, it is more common in men than women, in urban areas rather than rural areas, and in the lower social classes (Boyle, 1970). Controversy has centered on whether it is merely a quantitative variant of the normal (Pickering, 1955) or a qualitatively different pathological state. A familial predisposition is found in 40–75 per cent of patients with EHT (Jörgensen, 1969), and there is some evidence that a genetically determined hyper-reactivity of blood vessels might be a causal factor (Doyle & Fraser, 1961). Whether or not this leads to hypertensive disease probably depends upon a variety of somatic, psychological, and environmental factors which are in any case closely interrelated. The well recognized association between obesity, high calorie intake, and EHT may similarly be due to a complex web of psychosomatic factors.

Psychological disturbance in patients with essential hypertension. An increased incidence of psychological disturbance in patients with EHT has been reported by several investigators. Dunbar (1954) described a lifelong pattern of anxiety, perfectionism, compulsivity, and difficulties in relating to authority figures. Lewinsohn (1956) showed that hypertensive patients scored higher than controls on the MMPI. Sainsbury (1964) and Robinson (1964, 1969), using the Maudsley Personality Inventory, found increased neuroticism scores in hypertensive hospital out-patients. Bulpitt, Hoffbrand, and Dollery (1976) found high scores for anxiety and depression using the Middlesex Hospital Questionnaire in a large series of hypertensive out-patients.

For several reasons these findings are difficult to interpret. It is not usually clear whether the patients under investigation have true persistent hypertension or merely labile blood pressure. The latter group have been shown to have high levels of psychological difficulties (Ostfeld & Lebovitz, 1960) even though they cannot be regarded as having hypertensive disease. When care was taken to measure true basal levels of blood pressure by ensuring that all subjects were at rest, Davies (1970) found that hypertensives did not exhibit any more psychological difficulties than did controls. There is also evidence that hypertensive patients who attend hospital have a greater degree of psychological difficulties than those who have not sought help, suggesting that hospital-based studies are inevitably concerned with a highly selective sample of all hypertensives (Robinson, 1964, 1969). Those who have high neuroticism scores have a much higher chance of being discovered than individuals with equally high blood pressure but lower levels of neuroticism. This is due in part to the similarity of symptoms associated with neuroticism and those used as an indication that the blood pressure should be measured. Thus in a dietary trial involving apparently healthy volunteers, Cochrane (1973) showed that hypertensives discovered incidentally on physical examination did not differ from normals in their neuroticism scores on the Eysenck Personality Inventory.

The increased incidence of psychological disturbance in hypertensive patients may of course be related to the side effects of hypotensive and other drugs, although Bulpitt and colleagues (1976) point out that it seems unlikely that a raised blood pressure *per se* leads to psychological disturbance, because of the poor correlation between the two. Knowledge of the diagnosis may itself provoke anxiety, however, and this raises important practical questions regarding the process of medical examination and the degree to which details concerning the level of blood pressure should be conveyed to the patient.

Bearing these points in mind, it is clearly hazardous to draw conclusions about possible psychological causes of EHT from the study of hypertensive patients. Nevertheless there is much to suggest that psychosomatic mechanisms may play an important part in the development of hypertensive disease, and we must now turn our attention to these.

Causal psychosomatic mechanisms in essential hypertension. The way in which emotional stress may lead to autonomic arousal and a rise in blood pressure as a result of overactivity of the sympathetic nervous system is an obvious focus of attention in the search for causes of essential hypertension. It is hypothesized that recurrent emotional stress may, in certain predisposed individuals, lead to abnormally large and sustained rises in blood pressure and eventually hypertensive disease.

Animal experiments show that adverse psychological stimuli and a stressful environment can lead to sustained hypertension (Herd, Morse, Kelleher & Jones, 1969; Harris & Forsyth, 1973; Henry & Cassel, 1969). There is some evidence that in man a stressful social environment may also lead to an increased risk of hypertension. Harburg, Schull, and Erfurt (1970) found that residents in areas of increased social stress in Detroit tended to have higher blood pressures than did residents elsewhere, whilst Kasl and Cobb (1970) observed that blood-pressure levels in workers anticipating loss of job were higher than subsequently in a more settled social situation. The close association in normals between situational stress, or even on the recall of unpleasant memories, and raised blood pressure has been demonstrated by von Uexküll and Wick (1962). The hypertension induced by psychological stress appears to be due to raised peripheral vascular resistance with only slight change in cardiac output, whilst in physical stress raised blood pressure is secondary to raised cardiac output with lowered peripheral resistance (Herrmann *et al.*, 1976).

An association between acute anxiety, depression or anger, and raised blood pressure in man has long been recognized (Alexander, 1902; Ax, 1953; Altschule, 1953). This may of course be no more than a transient secondary effect of emotional disturbance. However, the finding that falls in blood pressure with effective treatment of agitated depressive states are far less in patients who had recurrent pre-

vious episodes of depression, suggests that chronic emotional stress may play some part in the development of irreversible changes in blood-pressure regulation (Heine, Sainsbury & Chynoweth, 1969).

Hypertensive subjects appear to differ from normotensives by showing greater and longer lasting rises in blood pressure in association with affective disturbance (Jost, Ruilmann & Hill, 1952; Schachter, 1957; Innes, Miller & Valentine, 1959). This has also been found to apply to normotensive relatives of hypertensives (Shapiro, Rosenbaum & Ferris, 1951) and this suggests that the exaggerated reactivity is not merely a function of the hypertensive state itself. Emotionally charged situations may also play a causal role in precipitating malignant hypertension (Reiser, Rosenbaum & Ferris, 1951).

Many studies concerning psycho-dynamic causes of EHT (Wolf & Wolff, 1951; Wolf, Pfeiffer & Fipley, 1948; Wolff, 1953) emphasize the role of inhibited anger and hostile impulses. Alexander (1902) postulates that inhibited hostile impulses precipitated by conflict situations may lead to extreme fluctuations of blood pressure and, if these are recurrent, to a fixed pattern of hypertensive disease. He regarded the controlled competitiveness of western society as particularly liable to lead to emotional conflict of this kind and to hypertension in susceptible individuals. According to Groen, Van der Vack and Weiner (1971), inhibition of aggressive impulses leads to activation of the limbic system, hypothalamus, and sympathetic nervous systems with vasoconstriction in renal and splanchnic arterioles, increased peripheral vascular resistance, and hypertension. Individuals predisposed to act in this way are seen as rigid, sensitive, and with inhibited needs to dominate others.

Although there is a considerable amount of literature on this theme, it remains hypothetical: the problems of measuring the relevant psychological variables are immense, as are methodological difficulties such as the avoidance of bias in selection of subjects and difficulties in carrying out prospective studies as opposed to unreliable reconstruction of causes from the findings in hypertensive patients. When careful attention was paid to these important methodological issues, Cochrane (1973) found no evidence that repression of hostility is found more often in hypertensives than in controls.

Reiser, Weiner & Thaler (1957) have discussed the ways in which hyper-reactive pressor mechanisms may influence the development of psychological traits, and how pathogenic defensive patterns may be learnt from chance experience or familial styles of behaviour. A psychopathogenic role of close family and household relationships is suggested by the fact that non-related members of households of hypertensive patients appear to have an increased risk of EHT compared with the general population (Chazan & Winkelstein, 1964).

The complex relationships between the large feedback control system embracing the individual and the environment, and the smaller one involving physiological mechanisms within the organism in the development of EHT have recently been discussed by Herrmann and colleagues (1976).

Management of hypertension. The increased incidence of psychological disturbance in hypertensive patients indicates that some may need psychotherapeutic help. In view of the evidence that the process of medical diagnosis may itself be an important cause of subsequent anxiety and other affective disturbance, caution is required in conveying knowledge of increased blood pressure to the patient: in some individuals it may be best not to impart any details at all, particularly when it is difficult to distinguish labile blood pressure from hypertensive disease.

Psychotherapy which helps the patient to recognize and deal with situations which prove stressful may lead to symptomatic improvement, and it has been claimed by Shapiro and colleagues (1951) that such an approach may lead to amelioration of the hypertension itself. When hypertensive drugs are used, it is necessary to remember that they may themselves lead to affective disturbance, either through their direct pharmacological action (for example rauwolfia alkaloids and methyl dopa may lead to depression) or by causing secondary anxiety precipitated by unpleasant episodes of hypotension. The use of tranquillizers or antidepressant drugs is justifiable when affective disturbance is severe and may have a beneficial effect both on symptoms and the severity of hypertension (Groen *et al.*, 1971). Behavioural techniques involving control of blood pressure by operant conditioning have met with a certain amount of success (Benson, Shapiro, Tursky & Schwartz, 1971). The prevention of EHT remains an area of treatment which is practically uncharted, but there are sound reasons to suggest that the psychosomatic approach, for example involving family therapy with close relatives of hypertensive patients, is worthy of further exploration.

Gastro-intestinal disorders

The various ways in which psychopathological processes may be related to gastro-intestinal disorders have been summarized by Engel (1974). Those which are *psychogenic* may lead to abdominal symptoms of a hysterical or delusional nature in the absence of any organic gastro-intestinal disease. Alternatively, psychogenic mechanisms may be paramount in disorders of feeding or elimination consequent upon bizarre or even psychotic ideation. *Psychophysiological mechanisms* lead to changes in gastro-intestinal function in response to affective disturbance such as anger, anxiety or depression. Some postulate that pre-existing organic vulnerability determines the way in which such psychophysiological processes may later precipitate certain organic gastro-intestinal diseases. *Psychosomatic* relationships are involved in those disorders, such as peptic ulcer or ulcerative colitis, in which, although the primary aetiological factor is a somatic process or constitutional predisposition, some kind of specific circumstance which may include psychological stress is required to precipitate the organic disease itself. Inherent in this approach is the concept that predisposing organic vulnerability is acquired in infancy, and this itself has a specific influence, not only upon subsequent personality development, but also plays a part in determining the kind of psychological stress which is subsequently likely to precipitate organic disease. Finally, secondary psychological disturbance may develop as a *somatopsychic* complication of organic gastro-intestinal disease and may then become a major factor both in its perpetuation and in leading to any subsequent relapse.

More detailed consideration of organic gastro-intestinal disorders will be confined to peptic ulceration and ulcerative colitis in which psychological processes are most clearly understood.

Peptic ulcer

A great deal of research into the psychological aspects of duodenal and gastric ulceration has been inconclusive, and in reviewing the subject Kessel & Munro (1964) were forced to conclude that 'the epidemiological evidence for any form of direct relationship between personality factors or emotional status and the development of peptic ulcer is obscure'. Whilst the lack of any demonstrable relationship may merely reflect the fact that aetiology is highly complex and multifactorial, it is also clear that negative results may stem from defects of research methodology. Studies are usually confined to those persons who have made contact with medical services, and failure to include those who have not declared themselves in this way may lead to selective and biased findings (Sandberg & Bliding, 1976).

Aetiology: Physical variables. It has been suggested by Ackerman and Weiner (1976) that 'peptic ulcer disease' is a misnomer because it encompasses a group of diseases, and failure to recognize this may lead to confusion. Variables such as chronicity, site, histopathology, whether the ulceration is single or multiple, superficial or deep, may all reflect differences in causation and response to treatment. Gastroduodenal physiological mechanisms may also be more complex than has hitherto been suspected. The long-held view that gastric and duodenal ulceration are respectively associated with low and high levels of gastric acid secretion has itself recently been questioned. Johnson (1965) found that half of gastric ulcers are associated with gastric acid hypersecretion: these have an increased probability that they belong to blood group O and fail to secrete A, B, H blood group antigen in the saliva. Hyposecretors, in contrast, tended to belong to blood group A. Duodenal ulceration was also found to be characterized by marked variation in acid secretion both above and below normal levels.

Even when ulceration appears to be related to gastric acid hypersecretion, the causes of this may themselves vary, either through neurogenic influences or defective peripheral autoregulation. Variation in gastrin production may be important: chronic duodenal ulceration may result either from increased production of gastrin or from parietal cell sensitivity to it. Patterns of gastric motility and degrees of duodenal reflux, both of which are related to the way in which acid stasis occurs in the stomach, also need to be taken into account in seeking causes of peptic ulceration: and once again non-uniformity is the rule.

Aetiology: Psychosomatic mechanisms. Psychic factors may influence gastroduodenal function either directly through neural (vagal) innervation or by endocrine and biochemical factors. Animal studies have demonstrated that hypothalamic lesions or electro-stimulation may increase gastric acid secretion, and may lead to gastric and duodenal erosions, particularly when there is lack of information feedback regarding the correctness of avoidance and escape response.

In man the effects of mood state on gastric function and acid secretion (Wolf, 1953; Wolf & Wolff, 1947; Engel, Reichsman & Segal, 1956) have been amply demonstrated both in individuals with gastric fistulae and in normals. Duodenal ulcer patients tend to respond to the sight and smell of food with greater acid secretion than do normals, though whether this is secondary or primary to the actual ulceration is not clear. Gundry and colleagues (1967) found that whereas depression in duodenal ulcer patients was associated with low basal and maximal acid output, anxiety appeared to cause high basal and maximal levels. Whether ulcer patients in general respond to stress with increased gastric secretion is not certain (Wolff & Levine, 1955).

Psycho-analytic theory has implicated early developmental patterns especially those involved in feeding. Alexander (1902) claims that male ulcer patients are commonly in emotional conflict between persistent infantile desires to be cared for and the constraints of adult life. He proposed a psychological predisposition in the nature of chronic oral conflict which promotes chronic gastric hypersecretion mediated by the vagus nerve. It is suggested that faulty feeding and gratification patterns in infancy may lead to chronic unconscious oral dependent and oral aggressive impulses which, if not successfully gratified, are then accompanied by physiological changes in the stomach. When certain precipitating stresses supervene, especially those which threaten dependency needs, peptic ulceration is likely to occur. Weiner, Thaler, Reiser, and Mirsky (1957) claim to have found evidence in support of such a theoretical approach in a prospective study of army draftees in which peptic ulceration was predicted with some success on the basis of levels of gastric acid formation and Rorschach test procedures. Clearly these findings need to be replicated using more reliable psychological techniques. Others (Bonfils *et al.*, 1971) claim evidence in support of the concept that the degree of conflict regarding dependency may have a major influence on the level of gastric acid secretion.

Treatment. Whilst it cannot be claimed that psychological factors are necessarily paramount in the cause of peptic ulceration, there is nevertheless sufficient evidence to indicate that due care and attention to them is likely to hasten its remission and reduce the likelihood of relapse. The psycho-analytic approach emphasizes the need to gratify the patient's dependency needs without undermining self-respect. The long-recognized value of bed rest in hastening remission is probably related not only to the fact that it leads to reduction of gastric acid secretion, but also to the way in which it permits disengagement from a stressful environment which leads to secondary affective disturbance. Successful management not only must be directed towards the treatment of significant affective symptoms such as depression or anxiety but must also deal with relevant precipitating factors. Conjoint therapy is necessary when such stress is interpersonal, and when other life-situational factors are significant then these will also need to be resolved in successful treatment. It may be that surgical operative intervention for peptic ulceration will become less common with the advent of drugs such as cimetidine which effectively reduce peptic acid secretion. Surgery will undoubtedly continue to be required, however, in the small minority of patients who continue to develop chronic ulceration which is associated with disabling symptoms. Pre-operative psychological assessment is advisable in order to determine those individuals who might react adversely to surgery with prolonged invalidism even though the ulcer has healed: those who show longstanding passive dependency of extreme degree or chronic anxiety and affective disturbance out of proportion to the degree of organic disease are most likely to do so.

Ulcerative colitis

Onset of ulcerative colitis is most commonly between 20 and 40 years of age. It may follow an acute fulminating course, though a remitting pattern is more typical. Typical symptoms consist of colic and severe bloody diarrhoea: complications include haemorrhage, infection, and sinus formation, as well as those of a more generalized nature such as polyarthritis or erythema nodosum.

Aetiology. Organic causal factors are still not fully understood although the disease is variously attributed to infective, allergic, genetic, or vascular mechanisms.

Aetiology: Psychological mechanisms. In attempting to elucidate psychological causal factors in such a severe and life-threatening disease it is necessary to distinguish between onset and exacerbation of the primary pathological process as opposed to its secondary complications: psychological symptoms which accompany the illness may of course be secondary to it rather than causal. Detection of psychological factors must also depend on techniques which are reliable yet sensitive to the specific issues involved.

Engel (1974) claims that there is not only a consistent association between a specific type of psychological stress and the exacerbation of ulcerative colitis, but that these patients also share certain premorbid psychological characteristics which may become accentuated when the bowel disorder becomes manifest. Much of this work is based on projective techniques, which it is claimed are more specific and sophisticated than standardized tests such as the MMPI which have produced less consistent findings. It is claimed that a high proportion of ulcerative colitis patients have obsessional compulsive personality traits, are easily hurt, find it difficult to express anger, and whilst outwardly energetic, ambitious, and efficient, inwardly feel insecure and inferior. They also are said to show excessive dependency on a key other person, with whom the relationship is often ambivalent. Not infrequently the other person is the mother and tends to control and dominate: families as a whole tend to be restricted in their interactions and to show false solidarity. Engel (1974) points out that in order to elucidate the relationship between psychological distress and onset of disease, careful attention must be paid to the exact time-sequence of events: when this is done it is claimed that onset usually occurs within a specific kind of stress situation. This generally takes the form of real, threatened or fantasized interruption of a key relationship, expectation of performance which the patient feels unable to fulfil, or disapproval from a parental figure. A response characterized by hostility and rage together with feelings of helplessness, seems particularly relevant. The early study of Lindemann (1945) which emphasized the high incidence of recent bereavement in a series of patients with ulcerative colitis and the improvement which can occur with adequate resolution of the grief reaction, also illustrates the relevance of loss as a precipitating factor in this illness.

Management. The work of O'Connor, Daniels, Flood, Karnsch, Moses, and Stern (1964), and O'Connor (1970) has demonstrated the way in which attention to psychological problems can improve the long-term outcome in ulcerative colitis. In a retrospective evaluation of 57 patients who had received variable amounts of psychotherapy at the Columbia-Presbyterian Medical Center, substantial improvement was demonstrated after four to eight years compared with controls who had not received psychiatric help. Assessment was based on proctoscopic findings and current symptoms at the time of assessment rather than retrospective description of progress which was deemed to be unreliable. Psychotherapy is indicated when affective disturbance is overt and the patient feels unable to cope with his environmental difficulties. Insight therapy is more effective in those who demonstrate some potential towards independence, but in others it may be necessary to support, allow cathartic expression and indulge dependency needs in a controlled way over a limited period. Whilst psychotherapy cannot claim to offer a complete cure it can validly aim to render the patient less vulnerable to certain stresses and help him to develop relationship skills and to deal with early parental figures in a more satisfactory way. The themes of dependence, feelings of helplessness, and the use of symptoms as a substitute for more efficient ways of dealing with relationship problems generally need to be dealt with in the course of therapy. Conjoint and family approaches may be particularly appropriate. Close collaboration rather than competition between medical and psychiatric teams is essential and therapy in parallel should be maintained rather than an 'either/or' approach which merely produces in the patient further feelings of loss and rejection.

In severe disease, surgical intervention leading to colostomy may be necessary. The response to this is usually one of relief and significant improvement from both the psychological and physical point of view (Druss, O'Connor, Prudden & Stern, 1968; Druss, O'Connor & Stern, 1969), although adjustment to a colostomy depends as much on attitudes of the key relatives and employers as on the reaction of the patient himself. Group support from ileostomy clubs may be very beneficial, especially in the early stages of adjustment to ileostomy when there may be considerable anxiety over spillage accidents and their social repercussions.

Diseases of the small intestine

Although the role of psychological factors in the aetiology of disorders such as idiopathic steatorrhoea and Crohn's disease is by no means certain, it is at least clear that these conditions are regularly complicated by emotional disturbance. Goldberg (1970), using a standardized psychiatric assessment of 80 patients with small gut disorders attending outpatient clinics, estimated that 34 per cent could be deemed to be psychiatrically ill because of minor affective disorders. A previous history of psychiatric illness and depressive personality traits was more common in patients with idiopathic steatorrhoea than in those with Crohn's disease. Whybrow and Ferrell (1973) in reviewing psychic aspects of Crohn's disease, concluded that whilst psychological factors may contribute to the onset and clinical course of the illness these cannot be considered either necessary or sufficient in its aetiology. On the other hand it may be expected that the majority of individuals developing Crohn's disease will, at some point, also manifest psychiatric disturbance, indicating the need for continuing psychiatric appraisal and support in their management.

Bronchial asthma

Neurogenic, psychological, and biological mechanisms are closely interrelated in bronchial asthma both in its aetiology and as secondary manifestations of the illness itself. Typically episodic and chronic, the natural history of bronchial asthma is nevertheless subject to much individual variation. Onset may be in childhood or later, some patients tend to improve, others to deteriorate as they get older. Explanatory theories must therefore take into account the probability that bronchial asthma is not a single entity but a collection of syndromes, in each of which causation is probably multifactorial. Experimental investigation must of course be based on objective parameters and particular care should be taken to use pulmonary function tests which are independent of the patient's voluntary effort.

Aetiology

The fundamental physiological deficit in bronchial asthma is a reversible obstruction of the small airways although the precise sequence in the pathological process whereby this occurs is not fully understood: smooth muscle spasm, hyperaemia and oedema of bronchiolar mucosa, accumulation of mucus and compression from without of the larger bronchi are all likely to play some part.

Aetiology: Somatic factors. Allergic mechanisms have long been regarded as being implicated in the cause of bronchial asthma and this is supported by findings such as an increased family history of allergy in asthmatics, its close association with infantile eczema, a concentration of eosinophils in bronchial mucosa of asthmatics and, in certain individuals, precipitation of asthmatic attacks by specific allergens. Neurogenic mechanisms are also likely to be relevant, possibly in the form of an imbalance between autonomic bronchoconstrictor and bronchodilator mechanisms, or the presence of some kind of beta adrenergic blockade which leads secondarily to excessive sensitivity to a wide range of allergens. Groen (1976) has suggested that an abnormal use of the voluntary musculature involved in respiration is an important factor in asthma: when an attack occurs, the chest, abdominal, and cervical muscles contract forcefully during expiration and this leads to intermittent compression of the trachea and larger bronchi with resulting obstruction of the airway. Such a mechanism goes some way to explain why positive pressure breathing or breathing against pursed lips may reduce the degree of obstruction, and it could itself lead to mucosal oedema and mucus formation by obstructing venous return.

Aetiology: Psychological factors. Bastiaans and Groen (1955) have reviewed the concept of a common personality type in bronchial asthma and the psychological factors which may precipitate it. Psycho-analytic studies suggest that the asthmatic is commonly in conflict with some other key person, commonly a parent, yet is unable to express aggressive or hostile feelings in words or action. Excessive self-control of this nature means that emotional tension is not adequately discharged and the asthmatic attack represents release of tension along an abnormal pathway. French and Alexander (1941) coined the term 'suppressed crying' to describe this mechanism. The predisposing personality structure includes hidden powerful aggressive impulses and passive dependency traits with difficulty in vocalizing effective responses and conflict over crying. Related to these mechanisms is the well-recognized improvement which may occur in about half of asthmatic children on separation from parents and there is now an impressive body of evidence to suggest this is not merely due to removal from house allergens (Lamont, 1958). Such separation from parents presumably interrupts psychopathogenic interactions which reflect problems in both parent and child. Family studies suggest that the mother may vary from the engulfing to the rejecting, the father being aloof and ineffective in correcting the imbalance between mother and child.

Psychic suggestion can influence airway resistance both in atopic (allergic) and non-atopic (intrin-

sic) asthma (Tal & Miklich, 1976) as may experimental stress involving anxiety, especially when this involves personal criticism (Mathé & Knapp, 1971). Although animal experiments have produced evidence that true asthmatic response can be learnt (Schiavi, Stein & Sethi, 1961) such a response can usually be readily extinguished. The process of generalization can lead to asthmatic attacks in response to a wide variety of situations other than the original precipitating one, just as it may account for improvement with the use of placebo agents. Anxiety associated with an attack of asthma may of course itself subsequently lead to a conditioned response of airway obstruction in a wide variety of anxiety-provoking situations. Groen (1976) suggests that emotional factors may induce abnormal ventilatory behaviour which itself could be a conditioned response. The increased attention induced by the dramatic sick role inherent in recurrent asthma may at all ages act as a reinforcing factor. Parents who avoid upsetting the child for fear of provoking an attack may unwittingly provide the setting for operant conditioning of further asthmatic responses.

Treatment

Whatever theoretical approach is followed, close ongoing collaboration between physician and psychiatrist is essential. Groen (1976) recommended a multidisciplinary approach based on asthma treatment centres and emphasized the importance of making help available to the patient at all times. Interpretive psychotherapy is most helpful when clear emotional problems are present, and conjoint, group (Groen & Pelser, 1960), or family (Liebman, Minuchin & Baker, 1974) techniques also have a place in treatment. Adjuvants such as breathing and relaxation exercises seem to be most effective in the early stages of the disease, especially in children. Behaviour therapy involving desensitization in fantasy to the anxiety induced by an attack may also be beneficial (Moore, 1965). Biofeedback techniques in controlling airway resistance have also produced promising results (Feldman, 1976).

Hepatic encephalopathy

The term hepatic encephalopathy refers to a range of more or less distinctive neuropsychiatric disorders which are found in patients with hepatic insufficiency (Read, Sherlock, Laidlaw & Walker, 1967; Sherlock, 1977; Steigman & Clowdus, 1971).

Clinical features

Metabolic failure secondary to progressive massive liver disease leads to a chronic organic brain syndrome, punctuated by episodes of acute disorders of consciousness with or without delirium and ultimate coma. In the more chronic form the early stages may be characterized by wide fluctuation in the severity of the clinical features. At first there may be no more than exaggeration of previous personality traits with mood changes of depression or anxiety: sometimes there is a lack of concern and denial of illness. Hypersomnia with a reversal of sleep rhythm may also be an early feature with overpowering episodes of sleepiness during the day. Slowing of the EEG may at this stage be a useful indicator of early encephalopathy (Laidlaw & Read, 1961). Fluctuating changes of degree of awareness may at first amount to no more than difficulty in concentrating on intellectual tasks or a tendency to be inactive and appear somewhat dazed. At this stage constructional apraxia as measured by the quality of handwriting or the ability to draw simple geometrical figures may be a distinctive feature. As the disease progresses frank episodes of confusion and disorientation occur, perhaps with inappropriate behaviour and a tendency to wander and get lost. Occasionally frank delusional ideas may occur with hallucinatory experiences which involve visual, tactile, or other senses, and visual illusions such as macropsia.

Hepatic coma may be heralded by increased drowsiness, confusion, and stupor and in one-third of patients by epileptic fits. At this stage some patients develop a characteristic flapping tremor with irregular coarse flexion movements of wrists and metacarpophalangeal joints. There may also be hyperreflexia, clasp-knife rigidity of limbs, extensor plantar responses, or cog-wheel rigidity. Frank coma may develop after days or weeks of confusion. It may be short-lasting and reversible, especially when exogenous precipitants are removed, though retrograde amnesia may persist subsequently (Summerskill, Davidson, Sherlock & Steiner, 1956). Terminal and fatal coma is characterized by profound loss of consciousness and areflexia, occasionally with decerebrate posture with opisthotonus and a characteristic foetor hepaticus.

Causes

Hepatic encephalopathy is due to metabolic changes secondary to liver cell failure. The metabolites involved and the mechanism of their toxic episodes are not fully understood: raised blood ammonia is usually found, though its presence does not correlate closely with the degree of neuropsychiatric changes, and other more complex factors almost certainly are also involved (Phear, Sherlock & Summerskill, 1955). In some cases the shunting of portal blood into the systemic blood system through collateral blood vessels, either extra- or intra-hepatic, and which have developed secondarily to structural changes in the liver, may also be an important factor: again the precise mechanisms involved are not fully understood, though toxic products of protein breakdown (for example ammonia, methionine or other aminoacids, tryptophan metabolites) are clearly important in view of the fact that high protein intake is a well known precipitant of hepatic encephalopathy. Short chain fatty acids may also be relevant. Some of the manifestations of encephalopathy may be due to the accumulation of various neuro-transmitters (Fischer & Baldessarini, 1971) originating from biogenic amines produced by bacterial protein breakdown in the intestine which bypass the liver to reach the central nervous system. When portal systemic shunting is a major factor, hepatic coma tends to be most easily precipitated by exogenous factors. These include the use of diuretics (leading to electrolyte imbalance, particularly hypokalaemic alkalosis), the ingestion of ammonium salts or large amounts of protein, the presence of blood in the gastro-intestinal tract (commonly from bleeding oesophageal varices), or intercurrent infection. Portal systemic shunting (especially that which is surgically induced in order to treat portal hypertension complicated by bleeding oesophageal varices) has been directly implicated in a variety of neuropsychiatric complications, including delusional hallucinatory psychosis and various forms of central nervous system damage such as paraplegia, cerebellar and basal ganglion disease, epileptic fits, and cerebralcortical lesions. Chronic unremitting encephalopathy has been reported in 20 per cent of patients following portal caval anastamosis (Mutchnick, Lerner & Conn, 1974). Sedatives should be used only with great caution in patients with liver failure because they may induce stupor or coma (Laidlaw, Read & Sherlock, 1961). Phenothiazines may produce marked drowsiness (Read, Laidlaw & McCarthy, 1969). Monoamineoxidase inhibitors and antidepressants are also liable to cause cognitive impairment and EEG changes in the presence of liver failure: amitriptyline is less likely to do so but should only be used with caution (Morgan & Read, 1972).

Differential diagnosis

The precise cause of an organic brain syndrome in any patients with liver disease needs to be assessed carefully because it may be due to another coincidental and treatable condition. An alcohol addict may have liver failure but may also sustain a serious head injury through falling. Sedatives and tranquillizers, even in normal doses, can lead to loss of consciousness because of impaired metabolism by the liver. Haemorrhage is common in serious liver disease because of the development of a haemorrhagic diathesis as a result of hypoprothrombinaemia and the presence of oesophageal varices. If severe it leads to shock and anoxia, factors in themselves relevant to confusion and organic changes in the mental state. The differentiation of alcoholic delirium tremens from hepatic encephalopathy is also important if only because sedative replacement in the latter can be fatal. The patient with DTs has usually stopped alcohol a few days previously, is physically over-active, perhaps aggressive, has vivid visual hallucinations, and his tremor is coarse and rhythmic. This picture contrasts with that of liver failure which usually leads to a hypoactive apathetic state and with irregular 'flapping' type tremor. Progressive EEG abnormalities occur as hepatic encephalopathy advances: normal background rhythmic alpha activity is gradually replaced by slow frequencies in the beta and delta range, sometimes with high amplitude triphasic waves (Bickford & Butt, 1955; Laidlaw *et al.*, 1961; Laidlaw & Read, 1963). Precipitation of these changes by a protein dietary load may be a useful diagnostic test. Early hepatic encephalopathy may be difficult to distinguish from depression and both may be associated in the same patient. The need for caution in the use of antidepressant drugs has already been emphasized.

Treatment

Unfortunately there is as yet no way of ameliorating metabolic change inherent in liver failure, and dialysis techniques such as those used in renal failure are not of value. Management of hepatic encephalopathy involves the recognition and avoidance of precipitating factors, and the provision of prompt and vigorous treatment for episodes of coma with close attention to exogenous and removable causes. Most techniques are aimed either at reducing substrate for ammonia production or diminishing its absorption, by restricting dietary protein, avoidance of constipation, or the use of oral neomycin or lactulose (Fessel & Conn, 1973). Levo-dopa may benefit some patients (Parkes, Sharpstone & Williams, 1970; Lunzer, James, Weinman & Sherlock, 1974). In some centres hepatic transplants are being developed and psychiatric management may be necessary to provide pre-operative preparation and support for the patient. The principles of therapy involved are common to any situation in which the patient has to face a major life-threatening event.

(For further discussion, see chapter 14.)

Acute intermittent porphyria

This disorder of haem synthesis is inherited as a Mendelian dominant and it frequently leads to psychiatric complications.

Typically the clinical picture consists of a neuropathy which causes limb weakness and sensory loss or cranial nerve palsies. Multiple somatic pains may be a prominent feature: acute abdominal pain and vomiting is an important form of presentation because of the diagnostic problems involved. In acute intermittent porphyria freshly voided urine is colourless, though it contains excess urobilinogen and rapidly darkens in colour on exposure to light. Such urinary pigmentation with fever may suggest to the unwary that the abdominal pain is due to gall bladder pathology. The condition may also be confused with appendicitis or myocardial infarction, and intensive investigation may be carried out unnecessarily.

The psychiatric complications are legion, and when they combine with multiple somatic symptoms they may produce bizarre clinical pictures. There may be confusion, delirium, disinhibited behaviour, as well as depressive or paranoid features. Persistent requests for analgesics may wrongly suggest the diagnosis of drug addiction (Carney, 1972) and hysterical mechanisms may also be erroneously invoked in trying to explain puzzling combinations of symptoms and signs.

The course is usually a relapsing one, and crises may last for hours or days. They are liable to be precipitated by intercurrent infection, pregnancy, or drugs (barbiturates, sulphonamides, methyl dopa, or oral contraceptives). It is not clear whether the psychiatric complications are due to some toxic metabolic intermediary or are merely non-specific in nature: the porphyrins themselves do not appear to be toxic.

Phenothiazines may be useful in the treatment of psychiatric complications. Each relapse is self-limiting, although when muscle paralysis is severe, particularly if respiratory ventilation is affected, then appropriate intensive physical care techniques such as mechanically assisted respiration may be urgently required.

Renal failure
Clinical features

The symptoms and signs of renal failure reflect not only the uraemic state itself, but also changes due to the underlying disease process as well as its secondary physical and psychological complications.

Uraemic encephalopathy is essentially an organic brain syndrome: as renal failure increases in severity, so the mental state deteriorates, ending ultimately in coma. Psychological disturbance tends to be more marked in uraemia of sudden onset or exacerbation and it is present in some form in 75 per cent of patients with blood urea of more than 250mg/100ml (Stenbäck & Haapanen, 1967). In the early stages there may be apathy, fatigue, headache, and anorexia with ill-sustained concentration. Later the organic type of mental impairment becomes more marked: there may be episodic disorientation and confusion with subsequent amnesia for each episode. In one-third of cases frank delirium may occur.

Some physiological disturbance may be a functional reaction to the illness. This is often understandable in the light of previous personality and needs to be distinguished from clinical features which are a direct reflection of biochemical and physical disorder. The early stages of uraemia can be difficult to distinguish from depression, which in any case is a common complication. Anxiety symptoms, problems revolving around the sick role, and various forms of psychological defence mechanisms often occur.

Disorders of neurological function occur in parallel with disturbance of mental state (Tyler, 1976). Muscle cramps and myoclonic jerks are common; twitching of the face and tongue tends to be confined to more severe cases. Asterixis or metabolic flap may also be seen, usually when there is some degree of clouding of consciousness; it is best demonstrated when the upper extremity is extended with the wrist in dorsiflexion, sudden lapse of posture giving the appearance of flapping of the hands. Extrapyramidal rigidity and involuntary movements are also common. Various forms of uraemic neuropathy affecting both cranial and peripheral nerves have become more frequent as the longevity of patients who have renal failure has increased, and leads to painful leg paraesthesiae, 'burning foot' and 'restless legs' syndromes. There may also be proximal muscle weakness due to polymyositis, reversible episodes of amaurosis, and in a third of cases epileptic fits occur. Neurological complications of various kinds may of course be due to secondary arterial hypertension when this is severe. Most patients with blood urea nitrogen levels more than 60mg/100ml have some kind of EEG abnormality, with lowered voltage, progressive diffuse slowing, and episodic epileptic type disturbance.

Aetiology

Gross lesions of the central nervous system are rare in uncomplicated uraemia in which there is usually found no more than a certain degree of neuronal degeneration and loss. More commonly the neuropathological picture is overshadowed by complications due to secondary disorders, such as arterial hypertension. Urea is in itself non-toxic and there is no direct relationship between the level of blood urea and the degree of uraemic encephalopathy (Stenbäck & Haapanen, 1967; Tyler, 1976). The level of blood urea is however a useful way to monitor the progress of uraemia and in general the degree of neuropsychiatric disturbance is greater in the later stages of the disease. The precise aetiological factors are not fully understood, but probably include electrolyte and acid base changes, especially when these occur rapidly either towards the normal or deviating from it, water intoxication, brain permeability changes, impaired cerebral oxygen neutralization and blood flow (Heyman, Patterson & Jones, 1951). Some abnormality of neuro-transmitter metabolism has also been suggested in view of the ease with which involuntary movements are provoked in uraemia.

Severe complicating hypertension may, in its malignant stages, lead to cerebral haemorrhage and intravascular clotting. Secondary anaemia and infection may be severe, and intense headache may herald the onset of meningitis or encephalitis. Thiamine deficiency due to inadequate dietary intake may lead to Wernicke's encephalopathy and peripheral neuropathy (Lopez & Collins, 1968). Complications of drug therapy are a most important potential cause of neuropsychiatric complications (Richet, Lopez de Novales & Verroust, 1970). High doses of penicillin may cause fits (Tyler, 1976; Bloomer, Barton & Maddock, 1967) and diuretics may lead to marked hypokalaemia and water depletion with resulting severe apathy and weakness (Tyler, 1976).

Peritoneal or haemodialysis usually leads to a gradual clinical improvement with restoration of biochemical normality, especially when the procedure is carried out slowly. Occasionally dialysis precipitates a 'disequilibrium syndrome', usually when it is carried out rapidly or when severe metabolic abnormality was present at the start. The patient then develops headache and confusion as dialysis proceeds, and in severe cases there may be fits, coma, and brain stem compression (Mawdsley, 1972). The underlying cause of this syndrome may be cerebral oedema induced by an osmotic gradient which develops between the blood and central nervous system when urea is removed too rapidly from the extracerebral body tissues. Reactive hypoglycaemia has also been suggested as a causal factor, provoked when glucose in the dialysing solution enters the central nervous system.

Wernicke's encephalopathy has been reported as a complication of chronic haemodialysis (Lopez & Collins, 1968), though perhaps more important is dementia dialytica, a state of chronic intellectual impairment often accompanied by dyspraxia, orofacial grimacing, other involuntary movements, and fits (Alfrey, Le Gendre & Kaehny, 1976; Mahurkar *et al.*, 1973). In this condition there is usually progressive degeneration and death over a period of six months. Its cause has until recently been obscure because it does not appear to be related to the degree of biochemical disturbance or dietary deficiency, nor is it improved by further dialysis. Recent reports both from the United States and the United Kingdom suggest that such dialysis encephalopathy, which is often associated with osteomalacia and multiple bone fractures, may be due to the accumulation of aluminium in the brain, the metal originating from the water used in the dialysis process. Such reports emphasize the potential neurotoxicity of aluminium in man (Alfrey *et al.*, 1976; Platts & Hislop, 1976; MacDermott *et al.*, 1978).

Some complications appear to be specifically related to renal transplantation. The use of immunosuppressants or high dosage steroid therapy predisposes to infections. There is, as a result, an increased risk of bacterial, viral, or fungal meningoencephalitis as well as reticulo-endothelial tumours, especially involving the central nervous system (Pierce, Madge, Lee & Hume, 1972; Tyler, 1976).

Management

Although neuropsychiatric complications of uraemia are most commonly due to an underlying organic brain syndrome and the various complicating somatic or biochemical disorders, other psychogenic mechanisms may also be important and need to be distinguished from those of cognitive defect. Environmental factors such as sensory deprivation, particularly at night, or heightened anxiety due to coincidental loss of personal support may accentuate confusion and even precipitate delirium or a paranoid reaction. Antibiotics and other drugs must of course be used with the utmost caution in view of the increased risk of toxicity in patients with renal failure.

Renal transplantation: donors, recipients and their families

In recent years the introduction of renal transplantation in the treatment of uraemia has raised challenging clinical and ethical problems: these have been reviewed by Cramond (1970). The decision-making process about donorship also needs careful evaluation; it by no means always follows a pattern of fully informed consent, and there is always a danger that it may be based on an instantaneous, irrational response which may later be regretted. Powerful coercive forces may act in family networks, and these too need to be assessed. It is particularly important to screen out potential donor relatives who have had a markedly ambivalent relationship with the proposed recipient in order to reduce the possibility of adverse psychological sequelae such as a state of hostile, unhappy interdependency. Recipients also may develop psychological problems. The immediate post-operative period, during which the patient may have to be physically isolated in some degree, is particularly likely to engender anxiety, and requires perceptive, sympathetic attitudes on the part of staff concerned. In the longer term, many adjustment demands will be made upon other family members: not only may family dynamics become markedly altered, but the more vulnerable members, especially children, themselves develop psychological difficulties. Such family stresses are of course more common in cases of chronic haemodialysis, especially when this is carried out at home.

Autoimmune disease

Some kind of immune reactivity against a component of an individual's own body tissue is thought to have a causal role in a wide variety of somatic dis-orders which includes rheumatoid arthritis, systemic lupus erythematosus, myasthenia gravis, polyarteri-tis nodosa, thyroiditis and acquired haemolytic anaemia. In other conditions such as multiple scle-rosis, thyrotoxicosis and ulcerative colitis evidence of autoimmune mechanisms is less certain but may well also in due course prove to be important. Even in neoplastic disease immunological mechanisms may contribute to the onset and subsequent course of the disease (Solomon, 1970). There is some evidence that autoimmune disease is connected in some way with immunological deficiency, and this is suggested by the fact that it tends to occur more commonly than expected in association with conditions such as agranulocytosis and the lymphomas. Stress and hypothalamic function, both of which are important in affective disturbance, may themselves be immuno-suppressive, and it is therefore clear that psychoso-matic factors have a potential role in autoimmune disease.

Rheumatoid arthritis has long been the subject of controversy regarding possible psychosomatic fac-tors, rheumatologists tending to deny the impor-tance of psychological factors either in relation to its cause or clinical course. Some of the research prob-lems involved have been summarized by Moldofsky (1970). Apart from the usual difficulties in evaluating the significance of life events and observer bias, it is by no means easy to assess the physical disease itself, particularly in its early stages: so much depends on items such as stiffness, pain, fatigability or malaise, themselves subjective and likely to be related to psy-chological factors.

The early literature regarding psychological associations of rheumatoid arthritis has been reviewed by Solomon (1970) and it is clear that in many studies failure to use adequate controls renders detailed interpretation difficult. Retrospective assessment of personality suggests such themes as perfectionism, dependence, conscientiousness, and over-control of aggression. Evidence for precipita-tion by such stresses as recent real or threatened loss or marital disharmony has been found in up to half of cases. Conflict situations with difficulty in dis-charging aggression may be particularly common in rheumatoid patients whose illness is of sudden onset and when a family history of the disease is lacking (Rimon, 1969; Solomon, 1970). Moos and Solomon (1964) used carefully matched sibling controls in

assessing female patients with rheumatoid arthritis and found that the latter were judged to be more duty-orientated, conscientious, self-sacrificing, tending to deny hostility, and unable to express anger. They were regarded as always having been more anxious, tense, and moody. In order to circumvent the obvious problem of trying to decide whether such psycholog-ical factors antedated the physical illness and hence might then be considered as potentially causal in a primary way, these authors carried out a control assessment of persons who, though free from arthritic disease were nevertheless positive for rheumatoid factor, a gamma globulin which predisposes to the illness. They were found to score significantly higher than controls on scales reflecting inhibition of aggression, though otherwise they were psychologi-cally more healthy. Solomon explained this on the basis that given a genetic or constitutional predis-position to rheumatoid arthritis, only those individ-uals with significant emotional conflict and psycho-logical distress go on to develop the disease. Under the conditions of his study he presumed that such persons would have already done so. Only long-term prospective large scale studies of the general popu-lation commencing before the age of significant mor-bid risk can really clarify this issue.

Psycho-dynamic concomitants of rheumatoid disease are probably complex. Moldofsky (1970) in a prospective study was able to distinguish two groups of patients: those in whom mood and joint pain occurred synchronously contrasted with the remain-der who showed an asynchronous or paradoxical pattern of a relationship between mood and pain. The paradoxical group appeared to adapt less well to the disease. Successful rehabilitation of rheumatoid arthritis is probably dependent in some degree on psychological factors such as adequate motivation, absence of depression, apathy, or an excessive com-plaining attitude, and the ability to make construc-tive use of social contact and support.

Sensory deficit
Deafness
Our knowledge of the relationship between deafness and psychological disturbance is limited by the fact that studies have hitherto been concerned with small selected series of deaf persons as opposed to full scale community surveys. The psychopatho-logical effects of deafness will depend upon its sever-ity, chronicity, and the age of onset.

Prelingual deafness. Onset of deafness in infancy and early childhood constitutes a sensory deficit which hinders language development and may have a profound effect on psychological growth. Such prelingual deafness tends to be associated with an increased tendency to impulsive aggressive behaviour; the child may be mistakenly regarded as inattentive or even mentally handicapped (Denmark, 1966) or develop a secondary behaviour disorder (Altshuler, 1971).

Adventitious deafness. Even when deafness begins after speech has been acquired there is good evidence that it is associated with an increased incidence of psychiatric illness. Mahapatra (1974) studied a series of 49 patients who had been admitted to hospital for surgical treatment of bilateral severe deafness, the onset of which had been in adolescence or adult life. An increased incidence of depressive illness (73 per cent), paranoid schizophrenia (21 per cent) and anxiety state (4.6 per cent) was found, compared with a control series of patients who were unilaterally deaf. Common symptoms included social ineptness, fears of appearing stupid or of saying the wrong thing, and occasionally marked suspiciousness and hostility. Although there is no clear relationship between severe deafness and schizophrenia in young adults (Altshuler, 1971), the possible pathogenic effects of less severe forms of deafness still remain to be clarified.

In contrast there is abundant evidence (Cooper, 1976) to suggest that paranoid hallucinatory psychoses in the middle-aged and elderly may be a secondary complication of chronic deafness. In one series of patients with late paraphrenia, nearly 40 per cent were found to have severe bilateral deafness (most commonly due to chronic middle ear disease) and this has been suggested as a major aetiological factor acting together with ageing and social isolation (Kay, Cooper, Garside & Roth, 1976).

Closely associated with deafness itself is of course the problem of tinnitus which may lead to considerable distress and depression, especially when it is severe, persistent, and complicated by giddiness due to concomitant vestibular disturbance. Occasionally tinnitus becomes the source of illusional secondary elaboration or ideas of reference; less commonly it may be incorporated into more organized auditory hallucinatory experiences when late-onset paranoid psychosis develops as a complication.

Pathogenic mechanisms. These have been reviewed by Cooper (1976). Psychological disturbance secondary to deafness may arise from the adverse response which it elicits in others. Whereas blindness tends to be regarded as a tragic disability, the deaf tend more often to be the subject of ridicule and social stigma: their disability is more likely to be ignored or misperceived, for example a deaf child sometimes regarded as deliberately inattentive or even mentally handicapped. Deafness is met with impatience and irritability when others are required to make an extra effort in order to communicate effectively. Such hostility may also manifest itself as a tendency to regard deafness as selective, perhaps used deliberately by the deaf person in certain circumstances in order to avoid unwanted communication or to achieve some other secondary gain. Whilst this undoubtedly may occur it is probably invoked far too often and on the basis of inadequate evidence.

Acute deafness constitutes a sudden loss which, like other events in this category, may lead to severe depression, feelings of isolation, and insecurity. On the other hand, the relationship between chronic deafness and paranoid hallucinatory states in the elderly suggests that adaptation processes inherent in a longstanding disorder of communication are relevant. Interference with verbal communication might lead to projective mechanisms which are not capable of correction by further environmental stimuli, and so possibly to ideas of reference or delusions of persecution in certain vulnerable personalities: the adverse social response from others may of course reinforce such psychopathological mechanisms. The possible role of perceptual defect as a cause of schizophrenia has been reviewed by Kirk (1968). Minor deafness, for example that which may lead to misinterpretation of speech sounds, in particular seems to warrant further investigation (Bull & Venables, 1974).

Treatment. The aims must be to improve the degree and quality of interpersonal communications and social contact at an early stage in order to prevent adverse psychological sequelae. Otological assessment should not be delayed and resistance to the use of hearing aids should be recognized and discussed adequately. Psychiatric assessment of the deaf can be particularly difficult, requiring patience and persistence in order to elicit the necessary information: the ancillary use of standardized self-rating assessment schedules may be particularly useful. Counselling and psychotherapy are of course time-consuming and demanding. Adequate health education regarding the full extent of disability inherent in deafness may to some extent reduce the general tendency to see the problem in derisory or hostile terms.

Visual impairment

The psychological impact of partial or complete blindness depends of course on the suddenness and circumstances of onset, as well as the duration of the disability. Also relevant are the resilience of the patient in terms of personality and liability to psychiatric breakdown, as well as the quality of interpersonal and social support.

Late onset psychosis. In contrast to deafness, the relationship between visual impairment and psychotic illness in the elderly is not very clear cut. Kay and Roth (1961) did not find visual defect to be more common in late paraphrenia compared with controls, though Herbert and Jacobson (1967) estimated that 47 per cent of their series of paraphrenics had significant visual defects. More recently Cooper and Porter (1976) found that paranoid patients did not have visual impairment sufficient to lead to significant social handicap any more commonly than did patients with affective disorders; although they had a significantly greater degree of impairment of distant vision in the eye with poorer sight.

It is difficult to evaluate the causal role which visual impairment might have in late onset psychosis because its severity preceding the onset of psychosis is not easy to evaluate retrospectively in a reliable way. On *a priori* grounds however visual impairment must be regarded as a significant potential barrier to effective communication and one which is relevant to mental breakdown. The general tendency for blindness to elicit sympathy rather than hostility in others may protect the blind individual to some extent.

Visual distortion. Illusional visual misinterpretation is common even in normal individuals, more so when the general anxiety level is high. Visual distortions due to organic eye disease may themselves precipitate acute psychological disturbance. A patient who had never experienced any previous psychiatric illness was admitted to hospital with bilateral glaucoma and severe impairment of vision which led to distortion of the facial appearance of others. He became very agitated and within a short time believed the medical staff and his family were impostors who were there with the intention of tricking him into having an operation. Management was initially very

difficult and he refused to accept operative intervention which would save his sight, but fortunately this paranoid reaction responded rapidly to reassurance and medication.

Visual hallucinations are common in psychotic states, whether these are schizophrenic, affective, or organic in nature: they are much less frequent in paranoid states (Lowe, 1973). In a series of psychiatric outpatients, visual hallucinations, distortions and illusions were found to be the best symptomatic discriminators between physical and functional psychiatric disorder, indicating that in non-psychotic individuals, physical illness should be suspected in those who complain of visual hallucinations (Hall *et al.,* 1978). Common causes include infective states, especially in the elderly, cardiovascular impairment, toxic effects of drugs such as tricyclic antidepressants, bromocriptine, or anticholinergic agents, as well as drug withdrawal states.

Hysterical blindness. In certain cases of visual impairment due to organic disease, superadded hysterical mechanisms may accentuate the degree of visual impairment: a correct evaluation of such a problem calls for a high level of clinical skill. When hysterical blindness occurs in the absence of organic disease then the clinical picture is less difficult to evaluate. Physical assessment will demonstrate no physical signs consistent with relevant organic disease. A normal chequer-board visually-evoked potential recorded over the cerebral occipital cortex in the midline in a person who professes blindness is highly suggestive of a functional as opposed to organic disorder. An important exception might be a patient with visual agnosia due to an occipital lobe lesion, but even here some asymmetry of evoked responses can usually be detected with more lateral recordings. In hysterical blindness clinical assessment usually reveals some relation between onset and an upsetting life event, and an element of secondary gain such as a compensation litigation may also be evident: such clinical assessment requires considerable skill because a relationship to environmental upset may be fortuitous, and apparent motivation merely a reflection of the observer's value judgement. A previous history of hysterical blindness or vulnerability to stress similar to that which is concomitant with the present disability may provide useful leads.

Hysterical blindness may recover spontaneously, especially when acute in onset and when the acute stress situation has resolved. It tends to be intractable when the underlying cause is persistent, especially when prolonged compensation litigation is involved.

Adverse reaction to eye surgery. Bilateral bandaging of the eyes after eye surgery is liable to produce adverse psychological reaction in certain vulnerable individuals. Usually beginning on the second post-operative day (sometimes developing immediately after the operation or as late as the seventh day) there may be disorientation, restlessness, suspiciousness, manic overactivity, and auditory or visual hallucinations. The syndrome is probably closely related to the process of sensory deprivation and is usually worse at night. It is more common in the deaf, elderly, or brain-damaged individuals, and particularly in those who have been alcohol-dependent or who show sig-nificant pre-operative anxiety. Complications of drug therapy may also be directly relevant. Removal of the bandages may lead to dramatic improvement, although this effect is less marked in the elderly or in those with poor vision in the other eye.

Adequate pre-operative preparation should include a period of trial bandaging with full explanation and maintenance of close personal support by familiar persons. When an adverse reaction has developed the emphasis must be on reassurance, explanation, and encouragement by those whom the patient knows well: discussion of favourite topics or pleasant past memories may be effective in reducing anxiety and hastening resolution of such a reaction, but in severe cases medication with psychotropic drugs may be necessary to control disturbed behaviour.

3
Endocrine disorders

J. L. GIBBONS

Introduction

Associations between psychiatric symptoms and endocrine disorders have aroused interest since the first description of the latter and have stimulated many case reports. The prevalence of psychiatric disturbance in an endocrine disease obviously cannot be determined from series of cases chosen because of psychiatric abnormality. There are reports of unselected series of patients with various endocrine disorders, but psychological disturbance is rarely described in detail. A statement that '20 per cent of patients were depressed' could mean that they were rather sad rather than that they showed features of frank depressive illness. Reference to the frequency of psychosis may also be ambiguous: is the author referring to organic or functional psychosis or merely to disturbed behaviour? Even when unselected series have been examined by psychiatrists, standardized methods of assessment have rarely been used. Control groups are exceptional in spite of the frequency of psychiatric disorder, usually affective, in physically ill patients in hospital.

Many investigators have looked for associations between particular endocrine diseases and specific psychosyndromes. The most frequently observed psychiatric disorders are cognitive impairment (sometimes with florid features of delirium) and affective disturbance (sometimes resembling affective psychoses). Manfred Bleuler (1954) described the 'endocrine psychosyndrome', essentially a mixture of symptoms of neurotic anxiety and depression. The psychosyndrome seems non-specific, occurring in neurotic patients seen in general practice and in patients with physical disease.

General reviews of the psychiatry of endocrine disease include those by Michael and Gibbons (1963), Smith, Barish, Correa and Williams (1972) and Sachar (1974).

A clear association between a psychiatric syndrome and an endocrinopathy may be explained in several ways.

(1) The endocrine disorder may cause the psychiatric disorder by its effects on brain function. This explanation is more likely when successful treatment of the endocrine disorder is accompanied by rapid resolution of the psychiatric disturbance. Even then, placebo responses can presumably occur. A direct causal relationship seems even more likely when interruption of treatment of the endocrinopathy is followed by both physical and psychiatric relapse. The disturbance of brain function may be a direct hormonal effect (as in hypothyroidism, where EEG changes reflect the severity of the hormonal defect), or may be due to derangements of metabolism or electrolyte distribution that result from the hormonal excess or deficit (as in hypersulinism where psychiatric abnormalities are due to hypoglycaemia).

(2) The association may be a more subtle one, with the endocrine disease acting as a 'stress'. The patient's psychiatric state may be an understandable reaction to a disfiguring or life-threatening illness. In that case improvement in the physical disorder should alleviate emotional distress. On the other hand, the onset or the detection of the endocrinopathy may be a 'life event', in the way that an event may precipitate a schizophrenic episode or cause a depressive illness (Brown, Sklair, Harris & Birley, 1973). Treatment of the endocrine disease might then not lead to prompt resolution of the psychiatric syndrome.

(3) The endocrine disease may be precipitated by the psychiatric disturbance. This explanation, only plausible when psychiatric symptoms precede the endocrinopathy, has been proposed in some cases of hyperthyroidism and of Cushing's syndrome.

(4) The association may be due to chance. Hypothyroidism is relatively common in the elderly, in whom both depression and dementia are common. If either psychiatric syndrome occurs in an elderly hypothyroid patient, age may be more relevant than the thyroid defect.

In an individual case it may be impossible to decide which explanation is the most appropriate. In general it is wise to treat the endocrine disorder first, unless the psychiatric symptoms are so severe or distressing that symptomatic relief is an urgent need. If amelioration of the endocrine disorder is not accompanied by psychiatric improvement, the patient should receive treatment appropriate for the psychiatric syndrome. However, psychiatric treatment is often ineffective as long as the endocrine disease remains untreated.

Thyroid

Psychiatric symptoms are commonplace in both thyrotoxicosis and hypothyroidism. Severe psychiatric disturbance occurs in association with both disorders, more frequently in hypothyroidism. Clower, Young and Kepas (1969) have reported the case of a young woman who developed a severe agitated depression during an exacerbation of thyrotoxicosis. Both disorders responded to subtotal thyroidectomy. A year later she became depressed again and was found to be hypothyroid. Her depression resolved during the first week of maintenance treatment.

Thyrotoxicosis

The commonest form is primary hyperthyroidism, Graves' disease, in which there is diffuse thyroid enlargement as the result of abnormal circulating immunoglobulins. Less common is secondary hyperthyroidism, when hyperactive nodules in the gland produce excess hormone.

The clinical picture of thyrotoxicosis is well-known and includes anxiety, irritability, and emotional lability. Many patients with anxiety neurosis are suspected to be hyperthyroid, and occasionally a thyrotoxic patient is wrongly diagnosed as neurotic. Wayne (1960) produced a diagnostic index that is helpful in the differential diagnosis. Features indicative of thyrotoxicosis include a preference for cold, increased appetite, weight loss, a palpable thyroid with a bruit, lid lag, hot hands, hyperkinetic movements, and a casual pulse rate of more than 90 per minute.

In a psychiatric study of 10 unselected cases of hyperthyroidism Whybrow, Prange and Treadway (1969) found high levels of anxiety in 8 and depressive symptoms in only 2. There was evidence of mild to moderate cognitive impairment in 5. All of these abnormalities improved with treatment of the thyrotoxicosis.

Sometimes, in older patients, the characteristic hyperkinesis of thyrotoxicosis is replaced by inactivation. Such patients usually have small goitres, with apathetic facial expression, considerable muscle weakness and marked weight loss. Depression of mood is frequent and a misdiagnosis of primary depressive illness is not uncommon. This disorder, known as apathetic thyrotoxicosis, responds well to antithyroid treatment (Thomas, Massaferri & Skillman, 1970).

Psychoses in Thyrotoxicosis. Among 1206 psychiatric in-patients in Glasgow the prevalence of thyrotoxicosis was 0.7 per cent, no higher than in the general population (McLarty *et al.*, 1978). Biochemical evidence of hyperthyroidism was found in only 5 of 662 consecutive admissions to a psychogeriatric unit in Adelaide (Henschke & Pain, 1977). Prevalence rates of psychosis in unselected series of hyperthyroid patients have varied from 0 per cent to 20 per cent, but the latter figure comes from American workers with wide criteria for the diagnosis of psychosis (Michael & Gibbons, 1963).

Reports in the literature of psychoses in thyrotoxicosis have been reviewed by Greer and Parsons (1968). The commonest types of psychosis are delirium (often with schizophrenia-like symptoms) and affective disturbance, especially mania, but including agitated depression. There are occasional reports of schizophrenic syndromes without disturbance of consciousness.

In thyroid crisis (Ingbar, 1966), when a sudden aggravation of the clinical features of thyrotoxicosis occurs, marked emotional lability is characteristic, clouding of consciousness is frequent and frank delirium not uncommon.

Laboratory diagnosis. In hyperthyroidism the serum thyroxine (T_4) is raised (above 150 nmol/l). It is also raised in any condition (including the use of an oral contraceptive and treatment with phenothiazines) in which the concentration of thyroxine-binding globulin (TBG) is increased. If the tri-iodothyronine (T_3) uptake is measured as well, the free thyroxine index (FTI) can be calculated. The FTI, which is not affected by changes in TBG, is abnormally high in hyperthyroidism. In the rare disorder known as T_3-toxicosis, serum T_4 concentration is normal but serum T_3 is raised. If repeated test results are equivocal, a thyrotrophin-releasing hormone (TRH) test can be performed. A normal result excludes hyperthyroid-

ism. For an excellent succinct account of laboratory tests of thyroid function, see Hoffenberg (1978).

The mechanisms responsible for the production of psychoses in hyperthyroidism are unknown. A direct effect of thyrotoxine on certain neurons has been suggested. Additional hypotheses include an alteration in central tryptophan metabolism and the enhancement of the functional effects of adrenergic (and possibly dopaminergic) neurons in the brain.

Treatment. In the treatment of thyrotoxicosis the advice of an experienced physician should be sought. Whatever definitive form of treatment is decided on, initial treatment is with an antithyroid drug, usually (in the UK) carbimazole 30–60 mg/day. Subjective improvement begins in a week, definite objective improvement after about a month. When rapid symptomatic improvement is needed, propranolol (40 mg four times a day) may be given as well.

As thyroid function returns to normal, organic psychoses can be expected to remit. Resolution of a functional psychosis may also occur, but sometimes depressive or paranoid or schizophrenic symptoms persist and require appropriate psychiatric treatment.

If a psychosis is so severe that immediate symptomatic psychiatric treatment is needed to relieve distress or to lessen behaviour disturbance, a combination of propranolol and chlorpromazine or haloperidol may be effective.

There are three reports of the acute onset of psychosis after 1–2 months of treatment of thyrotoxicosis with antithyroid drugs. Two were cases of organic psychosis and occurred when the patients had become hypothyroid. In the third case the patient, by then euthyroid, developed a schizophrenic syndrome which slowly subsided with phenothiazine treatment over 4 months. (For references, see Bewsher, Gardiner, Headley & Maclean, 1971.)

Hypothyroidism

Hypothyroidism is usually primary, the result of autoimmune disease, but iatrogenic cases occur following radioiodine or surgical treatment for thyrotoxicosis and lithium treatment for affective disorder. Hypothyroidism may also be due to pituitary failure.

Clinical picture. Many symptoms of hypothyroidism occur also in neurosis. Wayne (1960) has shown that the most characteristic symptoms are cold intolerance, decreased sweating, gain in weight, and 'mental lethargy' (a disinclination to undertake familiar tasks together with an inability to concentrate). Important signs include hoarseness, slow cerebration, slowness of movement, dry, coarse, cold, and yellow skin together with puffiness about the orbits and in the supraclavicular fossae and at the wrists. A combination of general pallor and a malar flush is characteristic.

Most patients complain of memory loss and somnolence. Reaction time is increased. Several studies have found cognitive dysfunction in a high proportion of patients. In a study of 30 consecutive cases Jain (1972) found significant depression present in 13 patients, which was confirmed by the Hamilton Depression Rating Scale and the Beck Depression Inventory. In addition, 10 patients were anxious, 8 had marked cognitive dysfunction and only 8 were psychiatrically normal. In this study there was no correlation between severity of psychiatric symptoms and severity of hypothyroidism. Although there was significant improvement in these symptoms after 4–6 weeks of replacement treatment, several patients still had depressive symptoms.

The cognitive defect in hypothyroidism may be severe enough to resemble dementia. Hence assessment of thyroid function is part of the routine investigation of patients with suspected pre-senile dementia. In some cases thyroxine treatment restores intellectual function to normal (Olivarius & Röder, 1970), but in others, especially when untreated hypothyroidism is of long duration, considerable intellectual deterioration may persist, sometimes amounting to severe dementia (Jellinek, 1962).

However only 5 of 662 consecutive admissions to a psychogeriatric unit had evidence of hypothyroidism severe enough to warrant replacement treatment, and only one depressed patient improved (Henschke & Pain, 1977). The authors suggest that dementia in a hypothyroid patient over 65 is only rarely due to hypothyroidism, so that no psychiatric response to thyroxine is to be expected.

Psychoses in hypothyroidism. This topic has been reviewed by several authors, including Michael and Gibbons (1963), Whybrow and colleagues (1969), Olivarius & Röder (1970).

The prevalence of major mental disorder in hypothyroidism is unknown, but it is thought to be significantly greater than in hyperthyroidism. Writers in the English language have generally been more impressed by the frequency of the association of psychosis and hypothyroidism than writers in German. This association is much less common in mental hospital populations than Asher (1949) suggested. The prevalence of hypothyroidism was only 0.5 per cent among in-patients in two psychiatric hospitals in Glasgow (McLarty *et al.*, 1978).

If one can judge from case reports in the literature, the commonest form of psychosis is organic, with florid symptoms such as hallucinations and paranoid delusions occurring in a setting of clouded consciousness. On the other hand typical mania, depressive psychosis, and schizophrenia have all been described in patients with no evidence of disturbance of consciousness. (For references see the reviews already mentioned.)

Laboratory diagnosis. In established hypothyroidism the serum T_4 concentration and the T_3 uptake will confirm the diagnosis: the FTI is abnormally low. In early cases (except those due to pituitary deficiency) the most sensitive single test is the serum TSH concentration, which is always raised, usually above 20 mu/l. A normal serum TSH (0–10 mu/l) excludes primary or iatrogenic hypothyroidism. For a more detailed account see Hoffenberg (1978).

Treatment. Treatment should begin with 100 μg of thyroxine a day. Few patients need more than 200 μg daily. In elderly subjects and in patients with angina, the initial dose should be 50 μg or less daily. Treatment may be monitored by serial measurements of serum T_4 or, better still, serum TSH. In a few cases too large a dose of thyroxine has produced an acute organic psychosis.

The response of psychiatric disorders to thyroxine treatment is variable. Organic psychoses, with clouding of consciousness, respond well. Sometimes the first sign of response to treatment is improvement in mental state. There are numerous case reports of successful treatment of manic, depressive, paranoid, and schizophrenic psychoses with thyroxine alone (references in Michael & Gibbons, 1963 and Olivarius & Röder 1970). On the other hand, symptoms of functional psychosis may persist in spite of euthyroid status. In such cases, psychiatric treatment which was ineffective in the hypothyroid state may be affective in the euthyroid patient (Pitts & Guze, 1961).

Adrenal
Cushing's syndrome

This is the result of prolonged excessive secretion of cortisol (and perhaps other steroids) by the adrenal cortex. It is about five times commoner in women. The commonest form is pituitary-dependent, due to excess ACTH secretion, but it is not clear whether the primary defect is in the pituitary or the hypothalamus. Cushing's syndrome may also be due to an adenoma or a carcinoma of the adrenal. Ectopic ACTH secretion by a benign neoplasm, especially a bronchial adenoma, may also cause typical Cushing's syndrome.

Clinical picture. The textbook description is well known: plethoric face, hirsutism, obesity of the trunk, and so on. However Ross, Marshall-Jones and Friedman (1966) found that the fully developed picture was unusual and remarked that the majority of obese, red-faced, hirsute women are not suffering from Cushing's syndrome. The commonest features in their series were obesity (often generalized), rounding of the face, hirsutism, muscle weakness, backache, amenorrhoea or oligomenorrhoea, reduced libido, and hypertension. Except in florid cases, a definite diagnosis is not easily made on clinical grounds.

Psychiatric aspects. Granville-Grossman (1971) cited several published reports of large series of cases, 795 in all. The frequency of psychiatric symptoms ranged from 21 per cent to 66 per cent. There are four reports of unselected series where psychiatric assessment was carried out. In three, totalling 94 cases, the severity of any psychiatric symptoms was stated (Trethowan & Cobb, 1952, Cohen, 1979, Jeffcoate, Silverstone, Edwards & Besser, 1979). Severe symptoms were present in 17, moderate in 24, mild in 28. In 25 there was no significant psychiatric abnormality. By far the commonest disorder was depression: sometimes severe with depressive and paranoid delusions; sometimes moderate sustained depression with sleep disturbance, tearfulness, irritability, hypochondriasis, and so forth; sometimes less severe or variable depression. Of the 94 patients, 3 showed a manic syndrome, 1 a delirious state, 1 a schizophrenic syndrome. In another study of 13 unselected patients, Furger (1961) reported persistent depression in 4, fluctuating depression in 5, euphoria in 2. He particularly stressed the emotional over-reactivity of the patients.

Symptoms usually develop early in the course of Cushing's syndrome, often before the physical stigmata are fully developed.

There are many case reports in the literature of psychoses in Cushing's syndrome. Some, especially in older patients, are deliria (Regestein, Rose & Williams, 1972). Affective psychosis, especially depressive, appears to be the most common, but paranoid and schizophrenic syndromes also occur. Often there are marked fluctuations in severity with lucid intervals (Michael & Gibbons, 1963).

Laboratory diagnosis. Definitive diagnosis of Cushing's syndrome requires admission to a specialized unit. Besser (1978) advocates the use of any two of the following screening tests to exclude the diagnosis.

(1) Low dose dexamethasone suppression test: 0.5 mg dexamethasone by mouth 6-hourly for 48 hours from 9 a.m. Blood is drawn for estimation of fluorigenic corticosteroids at 9 a.m. on days 1 and 3. Cushing's syndrome is excluded if the plasma concentration falls below 170 nmol/l.

(2) Basal urinary cortisol excretion, measured by the competitive protein-binding technique: the diagnosis is excluded if excretion is less than 335 nmol/day in men, 280 in women.

(3) Insulin tolerance test: in normal subjects plasma corticosteroids should rise by at least 220 nmol/l after symptomatic hypoglycaemia occurs.

In severe depressive illness biochemical findings suggestive of Cushing's syndrome may occur. Besser (1978) recommends the insulin tolerance test to distinguish between the two, because he has always found a normal cortisol response to symptomatic hypoglycaemia in depression. However Carroll (1969) reports that this response is impaired or absent in some depressives. Once the patient has recovered from depression, his adrenocortical function returns to normal.

Treatment. In most cases definitive treatment of Cushing's syndrome relieves psychiatric symptoms that have developed during the illness. Relapse of Cushing's syndrome is likely to be accompanied by reappearance of psychiatric symptoms. Where a psychiatric disorder, such as schizophrenia, has been present long before the Cushing's syndrome, it is likely to persist.

Recently Jeffcoate and colleagues (1979) have

observed the effect of initial treatment with metyrapone, which inhibits the synthesis of cortisol and reduces its plasma concentration. There was complete remission of psychiatric symptoms in all the 5 patients with severe depression, in 3 of the 4 with moderate depression, and in 6 of the 12 with mild depression. There was rapid improvement in a delirious patient. Of 2 manic patients, one showed partial improvement and one no improvement.

Mechanism of symptom production. The frequency of depression in comparison with other psychiatric disorders and the good reponse to treatment suggests that the psychiatric disturbance is directly due to the increase in circulating corticosteroids. Euphoria seems to be less common in Cushing's syndrome than during treatment with corticosteroids, and Sachar (1974) postulated that euphoria might be commoner in non-ACTH dependent Cushing's syndrome, i.e. adrenal adenoma or carcinoma, with depression more likely in the ACTH-dependent syndrome. However, what little evidence is available from other reported series does not support this view.

Addison's disease

In this disorder there is a deficiency of both cortisol and aldosterone. The two principal causes are autoimmune adrenalitis and tuberculosis: the former is three times as common as the latter.

Clinical picture. The early symptoms of adrenocortical insufficiency may be mistaken for neurotic symptoms: tiredness, lassitude, weakness, loss of appetite, and dizziness. However, marked weight loss, postural hypotension, and the development of brownish pigmentation in the buccal mucosa and in those parts of the skin exposed to sunlight or subject to pressure should suggest the diagnosis.

In Addisonian crisis, which may follow infection, trauma, or surgery, the patient becomes acutely ill with vomiting, dehydration, hypotension, and often hypoglycaemia.

Psychiatric aspects. Papers on the psychopathology of Cushing's syndrome continue to appear, but there have been few reports on Addison's disease in the last 15 years. The older literature was surveyed by Michael and Gibbons (1963).

In untreated Addison's disease most observers have stressed the appearance of apathy or depression, poverty of thought, and lack of initiative. Most of these reports date from the pre-cortisone era. Stoll (1953) studied 29 cases of Addison's disease of 4–5 years duration, finding definite psychiatric abnormalities in 27. The predominant mood was apathy in 25 per cent, depression in 25 per cent, and shallow euphoria in 50 per cent. In most cases there was evidence of cognitive defect, particularly impairment of memory.

In Addisonian crisis an organic psychosis may occur, which may subside slowly, as in the case described by Cohen and Marks (1961). A woman of 36 presented with hypoglycaemic coma due to Addison's disease. After recovery of consciousness she showed a fluctuating organic psychosis, which finally resolved two months later. Otherwise more severe psychiatric disturbance is unusual, although there are case reports of paranoid–hallucinatory psychoses in clear consciousness. An exception is provided by the experience of Knowlton (1971), who reported a personal series of 63 cases of Addison's disease treated for at least 5 years. No less than 7 developed a psychosis at some stage. In 2 patients it appeared to be a steroid psychosis. In the remaining 5 cases a diagnosis of paranoid schizophrenia was made and admission to a psychiatric hospital was needed. In 2 patients the psychosis appeared after several years' treatment of the adrenal deficiency.

Laboratory diagnosis. An excellent account is provided by Besser (1978). A low plasma cortisol at 8–10 a.m. (less than 170 nmol/l of fluorigenic corticosteroids) supports the diagnosis. The patient should then have plasma cortisol estimations before, and at 30 and 60 minutes after, the intramuscular injection of 250 μg of tetracosactin. The plasma concentration in a normal subject should rise by at least 190 nmol/l and should exceed 580 nmol/l. A diminished response is suggestive of Addison's disease.

If both tests suggest the diagnosis, more specialized investigation is required.

Treatment. Replacement treatment is with cortisol (usually 20 mg in the morning, 10 mg in the evening) and with fluorocortisone if aldosterone deficiency is severe. Cortisol produces rapid improvement in mood and in cognitive impairment. Organic psychoses following crisis will also resolve with maintenance treatment, but may persist for several weeks. It is usually said that a functional psychosis in untreated Addison's disease will respond to cortisol, but Knowlton (1971) has shown that this is not always so with schizophrenic syndromes, which may need appropriate psychiatric treatment as well.

Patients with Addison's disease are liable to develop steroid psychoses with large doses of glucocorticoid, and they may be more sensitive in this respect than subjects with normal adrenocortical function.

Phaeochromocytoma

This tumour is usually found in the adrenal medulla, but in 10 per cent of cases it occurs in other parts of the sympathetic chain in the neck, thorax, or abdomen. The tumour cells secrete adrenaline and noradrenaline in varying proportions.

Clinical features. The vast majority of patients present with attacks (Ross, 1972). Attacks last from a few minutes to a few hours, always have the same features and may be precipitated by exercise, change of posture, or emotion (Reid, 1978). An indescribable, alarming sensation is followed by palpitations, epigastric fullness, profuse sweating, and headache. Anxiety may be severe and the attacks mistaken for anxiety attacks. Afterwards exhaustion and weakness occur. Hypertension is invariable during the attacks and persists between attacks in 50 per cent of cases. Phaeochromocytomas are thought to be responsible for 0.5 per cent–2 per cent of cases of hypertension.

Diagnosis. This depends on the demonstration of increased concentrations of noradrenaline or adrenaline in the plasma, or of increased excretion of their metabolites in urine. Excretion of vanillyl mandelic acid (VMA) or metanephrine in the normal range in two 24-hour urine collections makes the diagnosis very unlikely (Reid, 1978).

A patient who has recurrent circumscribed anxiety attacks with marked physical symptoms should be screened for phaeochromocytoma, especially if he is hypertensive. However, most patients in whom the diagnosis is suspected are suffering from some other disorder.

Pituitary
Acromegaly

In this disorder excessive production of growth hormone, by a slowly growing acidophile tumour of the pituitary, causes enlargement of many organs. The established clinical features, with enlargement of nose, tongue, jaw, and hands, can be recognized at a glance. Associated disorders include hypertension, diabetes, and muscle weakness.

Very little has been written in English on the psychopathology of acromegaly, although such a disfiguring disease might be expected to cause emotional disturbance. Reports on series of cases do not mention psychiatric abnormalities. Bleuler (1951) described the psychiatric status of 28 acromegalic patients, noting personality change with lack of initiative and spontaneity. He found no evidence of cognitive impairment in uncomplicated acromegaly.

Schulte (1976) has reviewed the considerable German language literature on the psychopathology of acromegaly. He concludes that memory impairment and 'psycho-organic personality change' are common, but that paranoid–hallucinatory psychoses are rare. The latter are sometimes organic in type, but sometimes occur in clear consciousness and resemble schizophrenia. Presumably all of these psychiatric abnormalities are related to the pituitary tumour rather than to the excess secretion of growth hormone.

An excellent summary of the diagnosis and treatment of acromegaly is given by Sönksen and Lowy (1978).

Hypopituitarism

It is now known that deficiencies of individual pituitary hormones can occur. Thus TSH deficiency causes hypothyroidism which resembles primary hypothyroidism, except that the disorder is less severe and actual myxoedema is exceptional. In panhypopituitarism, with which this section is concerned, there are deficiencies of several hormones, including ACTH.

The commonest cause of panhypopituitarism used to be post-partum necrosis of the pituitary (Sheehan's syndrome), but its incidence has declined with advances in obstetric care. A chromophobe adenoma is now the commonest cause in adults. There is a good discussion of other causes by Sönksen and Lowy (1978).

Clinical features. The history of Sheehan's syndrome is characteristic, although the diagnosis may not be made for years. After circulatory collapse during or after labour, there is failure of lactation, and menstruation does not recur. In other forms of hypopituitarism, gonadotrophin deficiency occurs early, leading to amenorrhoea in women and impotence in men, and gradual loss of secondary sexual characteristics. There is a gradual development of chronic ill health with general weakness, lack of energy, and increased sensitivity to cold. Pubic and axillary hair are lost, the skin becomes thin and dry, the facies expressionless. Marked weight loss is not a feature of hypopituitarism, except as an occasional terminal event.

Psychiatric aspects. The early literature on this topic is misleading, because hypopituitarism and anorexia nervosa were confused (Sheehan & Summers, 1949). Kind (1958) reviewed all cases of proven hypopituitarism in the literature and described a personal series of 22 adult cases. Loss of initiative, interest, and drive occurred early, together with definite disturbance of mood: apathy or mild depression with occasional bouts of irritability. In untreated patients memory deficit could often be demonstrated and Kind mentioned a nurse who had to resign because of her inability to remember instructions.

Symptoms of an acute organic psychosis may accompany physical crises and patients who recover from hypopituitary coma may show such symptoms for several weeks (Blau & Hinton, 1960).

There were no affective or paranoid psychoses in Kind's series, and these are rare in hypopituitarism, although instances have been described. Some cases respond to maintenance treatment, others do not. Kitis (1976) described a woman with Sheehan's syndrome and a paranoid depressive psychosis which responded rapidly to cortisone and thyroxine. On four subsequent occasions psychotic symptoms reappeared after she stopped her maintenance treatment; on each occasion the psychiatric disorder cleared with hormone treatment. Ball & Grounds (1974) described a man of 40 with a 3-year history of schizophrenic symptoms and a 20-year history of hypopituitarism following head injury. With prednisolone and thyroxine his physical condition improved, but his psychosis became more florid. Later he became symptom-free after treatment with electroconvulsive therapy and trifluoperazine.

Diagnosis. Laboratory diagnosis depends on the demonstration of low circulating levels of pituitary hormones and of thyroid, adrenocortical and gonadal hormones. For details see Sönksen and Lowy (1978).

Although Sheehan pointed out the dissimilarity of the two disorders as long ago as 1949, even modern textbooks of endocrinology devote paragraphs to the differential diagnosis of anorexia nervosa and hypopituitarism. The weight loss, the overactivity and the characteristic psychopathology of anorexia nervosa are in marked contrast to the minimal weight loss, the apathy, anergia, and loss of pubic and axillary hair of hypopituitarism. Hormonal findings are also quite different with, for example, the plasma cortisol concentration high in anorexia nervosa and low in hypopituitarism.

Treatment. The cause of the hypopituitarism, such as a tumour, may require surgery or radiotherapy. Otherwise treatment is by hormone substitution therapy, initially with cortisol (or a synthetic corticosteroid) and thyroxine. Some authorities recommend depot injections of testosterone esters for men and a cyclical oestrogen-progestogen preparation for women to restore sexual function and to protect against osteoporosis (Sönksen & Lowy, 1978). Cortisol alone, or a combination of cortisol and thyroxine, produces rapid symptomatic improvement, while the mood disorder and lack of initiative respond more slowly. Some patients, despite prolonged and adequate treatment, still show some apathy and lack of drive; this is most likely if the symptoms have been severe and of long duration (Kind, 1958).

As already mentioned, the rare affective or paranoid psychoses complicating hypopituitarism may or may not respond to maintenance treatment, a situation analogous to that seen in primary hypothyroidism.

Hypoglycaemia

In their important monograph Marks and Rose (1965) define neuroglycopenia as the symptoms and signs which develop when the supply of metabolizable carbohydrate to the nervous system is inadequate for normal function.

(1) Acute neuroglycopenia occurs most often after insulin overdose. It is characterized by malaise, anxiety, derealization, palpitations, and restlessness. Tachycardia, facial flushing, profuse sweating, and an unsteady gait occur. Consciousness is clouded and coma may ensue. The entire attack is aborted by administration of glucose.

(2) Subacute neuroglycopenia is especially characteristic of insulinoma. Anxiety, restlessness, flushing, and palpitations are absent or only very mild. The patient's spontaneous activity is reduced, his performance is impaired, and he may appear drunk. Insight is usually absent and the patient's

general attitude is negativistic. All of the symptoms are relieved by glucose.

(3) Chronic neuroglycopenia occurs rarely, almost always with insulinoma. Insidious personality change occurs, memory is impaired, intellectual function deteriorates. Symptoms are unrelieved by food. Gradual improvement follows removal of the tumour but recovery is rarely complete. Marks and Rose suggest that chronic neuroglycopenia should always be considered in cases of suspected presenile dementia.

Any of these syndromes may lead to brain damage.

Causes of hypoglycaemia

Conventionally hypoglycaemia is said to occur when the true blood glucose falls to less than 2.2 mmol/l. There are many disorders in which hypoglycaemia can cause symptoms due to subacute (and less often acute) neuroglycopenia (Marks, 1975).

The commonest cause is iatrogenic: the administration of too much insulin or oral hypoglycaemic agent. The term factitious hypoglycaemia refers to the deliberate self-induction of hypoglycaemia, whether by diabetics (usually young women) or by non-diabetics (usually doctors or nurses).

From the point of view of the psychiatrist, the three other important disorders are insulinoma, alcohol-induced fasting hypoglycaemia and essential reactive hypoglycaemia.

Insulinoma. Insulinomas are insulin-secreting tumours, usually benign. The vast majority occur in or near the pancreas. Rarely an insulinoma may be accompanied by other endocrine tumours, the pluriglandular syndrome.

The natural history of insulinoma has been well described by Marks and Samols (1974). Almost always the diagnosis is made as a result of investigation of symptoms referable to the central nervous system, and often the symptoms have been present for years.

The commonest symptoms are episodes of odd behaviour or of disturbance of consciousness, but almost any psychiatric or neurological syndrome may be simulated. Attacks of subacute neuroglycopenia occur for months or years, sometimes with long remissions, but generally increasing in frequency and severity. During the attacks actual complaints by the patient are mild, but cognitive and/or motor impairment may be severe. Between attacks patients look and feel well. Comas are a late development, but may be the first recognized sign of organic disease. Symptoms may occur before breakfast, but also later in the day and after unusual exercise.

In very occasional patients the picture is one of chronic neuroglycopenia, preceded by a history of subacute episodes which may be overlooked.

Symptoms occur at any age, most commonly in the forties. The disorder is rare, with an annual diagnosed incidence in Western Europe of 1–2 per million.

Diagnosis depends on the demonstration that hypoglycaemia exists and is the cause of the symptoms. In Mark's experience, 90 per cent of proven cases have hypoglycaemia at least once after an overnight 15-hour fast, provided that at least 3 tests are carried out and that an accurate and specific method is used to measure blood glucose. The finding of inappropriately high plasma insulin levels during the hypoglycaemia makes the diagnosis of insulinoma very likely. A detailed account of methods of diagnosis is given by Frerichs & Creutzfeld (1976). Treatment is by surgical removal of the tumour.

Alcohol-induced fasting hypoglycaemia. This develops 6–36 hours after the ingestion of a moderate to large amount of alcohol by a previously malnourished person, who lapses into stupor or coma. If the hypoglycaemia is not recognized, and the patient is assumed to be 'dead drunk', death is likely.

Essential reactive hypoglycaemia. Patients with this disorder are said to develop episodes of acute neuroglycopenia 3–4 hours after a carbohydrate meal. Neuroglycopenia is not provoked by fasting. In order to establish the diagnosis it is necessary to demonstrate hypoglycaemia during a spontaneous attack, and also to demonstrate that the symptoms are relieved by intravenous glucose, but not by intravenous saline. Usually, however, the diagnosis is based on a hypoglycaemic rebound to a large dose of oral carbohydrate. As Marks (1975) points out, this is a perfectly normal phenomenon. In his view, the majority of sufferers from this over-diagnosed syndrome are really suffering from neurosis.

4
Nutritional abnormalities

J. L. CRAMMER

Nutrition is a neglected dimension in present-day psychiatric thinking. Vitamin deficiencies, notably of the B vitamins thiamine, pyridoxine, nicotinamide, cobalamin, or folic acid, may give rise to mental symptoms, posing questions of the mechanistic relationship between cerebral dysfunction and psychiatric illness. The clinician concerned with the elderly, or the rural poor, particularly in a remote or under-developed country, or with the restrictions of orphanages, hospitals for the chronically sick, and prisons, is usually aware of the risks of deficient or unbalanced food intake. He knows too that adequate diet means something different for foetus, child, adolescent, pregnant or lactating woman, active adult, or postmenopausal elderly person. But these are group requirements and group risks, with nutrition as a social problem. Psychiatry is concerned with individuals, and here nutrition means very much more than simply an adequate availability of vitamins, minerals, proteins, fats, and starches.

What an individual eats depends not only on what is available, which he knows how to cook and can chew, but on what appeals to appetite and tastes well, and conforms both to his idiosyncrasies of life experience and to the taboos of his society. What he takes as food is a mixture of substances in a variety of physical forms; some may be harmful rather than purely nutritive (caffeine, alcohol), others (fibre, phytin) may alter gastro-intestinal function or the availability of calcium.

Eating is a social cultural act, sometimes an act of individual relationship (the baby at the breast, the woman who cooks for her man), a long series of learned acts modulated by emotion. When, how much, and what one eats are determined more by habit, ritual, the state of one's emotions, than by the fuel consumption of the physiological machine.

Of course, metabolic requirements do play some part, and these fluctuate with the nature of one's life and activities, the balance of different substances in the diet, and the previous chemical experience of one's body. For while the individual's metabolic machinery is to a large extent genetically determined (and hence arise some individual differences of nutritional demand) part of it is modifiable by recent (chemical) environmental exposure. A few days' high carbohydrate diet, for instance, results in a flatter blood glucose curve in a glucose tolerance test and increases the need for the vitamin thiamine. Semi-starvation, or a fatty diet have the opposite effects and are thiamine-sparing. Severely depressed patients newly admitted to hospital with anorexia and weight loss may show a diabetic type of glucose tolerance curve, which in some circumstances disappears after a short period of carbohydrate feeding (Herzberg *et al.*, 1968; but see discussion in Weil-Malherbe & Szara, 1971), and such patients may need more thiamine as their recovery begins. (For the effects of increased exercise on human metabolism, see Rennie *et al.*, 1981.)

It is well known that late-onset diabetes mellitus may occur in a setting of obesity, and its symptoms can sometimes be controlled by diet alone. Hypothyroidism can be due to a deficiency of iodine in the diet or to the ingestion of excessive amounts of vegetables of the cabbage family which contain goitrogenic substances. Here are just two examples of changes in metabolic function brought about by diet: both of them may have behavioural consequences, diabetes in relation to dementia, and hypothyroidism to depression.

Nutritional treatment has other influences on psychiatric symptoms. Sleep may come with greater difficulty, be more broken and shorter in total duration, when the calorie intake is inadequate (Crisp & Stonehill, 1976), whereas bedtime feeding may be better than a hypnotic (Brezinová & Oswald, 1972). In institutions the amount of hypnotics used at night, and the amount of aggressive behaviour seen by day, can be altered by attention to the adequacy and the timing of meals. Anxiety and depression, particu-

larly in patients under average weight, can be treated with injections of insulin which stimulate appetite and glucose intake: weight gain and improvement in mood go hand-in-hand (Sargant & Slater, 1963).

The possibility that with some psychiatric illnesses the onset may be triggered or the severity determined by nutritional deprivations rather than by psychological stresses is rarely considered. Eating and drinking are such universal daily matters that they are often taken for granted. Every patient is assumed to follow the same eating behaviour and custom at all times, and lack of appetite, or over-eating, or the development of special appetites or food fads are seen as voluntary desires which may or may not be satisfied indifferently without consequence. But such behaviour could sometimes be the patient's unconscious physiological responses to his perception of alterations in his bodily functioning, as it appears to be in animals (*Handbook of Physiology*, 1967). Choice and satisfaction in food are complex variables, hardly examined in relation to mental functioning.

There is a close but obscure relation between the effect of psychotropic drugs on psychological state and on appetite. Chlorpromazine and lithium carbonate may give rise to obesity, and long-term amitriptyline likewise increases weight. One of the earliest signs that desipramine is going to benefit the mood of a depressed patient is an immediate arrest in the downward drift of weight observed in the untreated: this is not seen in patients who fail to improve with the drug (Crammer & Elkes, 1969).

Amphetamines are well known as drugs which impair appetite but also produce euphoria in the normal and a relief of symptoms in some who are depressed. Disturbances of food or fluid intake or balance in the presence of an adequate supply are not only brought about by drugs but may occur spontaneously as a distinct part of the course of some psychoses or neurological conditions.

Life implies change over time. Psychiatry is concerned with changes in the individual over time, and changes in the individual's growth rate or weight, haematocrit or haemoglobin, or other biochemical variables which are used as indices of nutritional state may be the result of changes either in nutrient availability or in the individual's behaviour and metabolic capacities for making use of nutrients. Nutritional abnormalities in psychiatry involve consideration of lack or excess of particular food substances (and the possibility of toxicity) or of imbalances in the proportions of two or more foods at the same time, and also of the factors in the individual which alter these requirements quantitatively. Each patient must be regarded as a changeable physical body as well as a behavioural unit, family member, and participator in a cultural group. Assessment must be biochemical as well as psychological and sociological, and the formulation should be a synthesis of these diverse approaches.

While textbooks of nutrition such as Davidson and colleagues (1975) or Goodhart and Shils (1973) should be consulted where appropriate, or the help sought of dietician or biochemist, a summary account will be offered here of clinical assessment, the physiological background of appetite and of metabolism which modifies nutritional demand, and the principal nutritional deficiencies likely to be encountered in psychiatric practice.

Assessment

The basic question is whether the individual's food intake is responsible for some unusual feeling or behaviour. It is necessary to consider both past chronic peculiarities of diet and also recent changes in diet. A general deficiency of food is much less common than a lack of certain specific substances in it, and the pattern of deprivation over time can determine the symptoms produced. A recent acute deprivation superimposed on a long milder chronic lack is most likely to precipitate illness. Many nutritional deficiencies produce no clinical symptoms, or only somatic symptoms of the most general kind, and special laboratory tests may be needed to identify the specific deficiency at work in a given case. Where psychiatric symptoms do result (which will be in a minority of patients), they may be of the vaguest and most non-specific, a restlessness, some apathy or mild depression, perhaps some anxiety, and may be regarded as neurotic; but more severe depression, or an acute brain syndrome, or a psychosis can occur.

Assessment of the individual's nutritional state therefore proceeds from certain general indicators, such as bodily growth or shrinkage, pallor, mucosal change, or peripheral neuropathy, to clinical and then laboratory tests for specific physical disorder. Body weight is such a simple direct indicator of over-all metabolic function that it must have a special discussion among clinical indicators of nutritional state. Blood is a tissue which continually renews itself and can be readily sampled for proteins and vitamins, and therefore has pride of place among laboratory aids.

General physical examination may reveal some reason why the individual's nutritional demands have risen. Adequate nutrition is a state where all the individual's different specific requirements, with the life-style at that time, are balanced by an intake of the appropriate quantities of the different nutrients. Apart from certain areas of the world where for social reasons nutritional deficiencies are endemic, nutritional abnormalities occur sporadically, widely but rarely, as a consequence of a very great variety of different circumstances. This emphasizes the importance of the individual assessment.

History

Just as the individual's psychological development is examined through childhood history, adolescent experiences, work and marriage records, so the nutritional history must be looked at over time. In view of evidence that protein deficiency in early foetal life may permanently depress brain development (Wurtman & Wurtman, 1977; Falkner & Tanner, 1978), this could logically start with a statement of the mother's nutrition in early pregnancy before the patient's birth. More often the childhood experience of food will be relevant, its quantity or style (the learning of habits of regular eating, the emphasis on starchy foods or vegetables, parental attitudes to the importance of eating, the emergence of food fads), and adult practice in relation to religious belief, economic position, and residence.

Changes in nutrition in the previous month or more before interview may also be significant. They may, of course, be a consequence of the onset of psychiatric symptoms (e.g. the anorexia of depression) but also the result of social changes. A new job may require an early start from home and the consequent omission of breakfast, or a change to the night shift and a new meal schedule. It may be necessary to eat a midday meal in a works canteen, or to take sandwiches, or to go out to some local café or pub, and these different environments with their different costs and opportunities may result in a change in total intake, or a shift to a greater carbohydrate and calorie intake, or to more alcohol or tea. The lonely housewife may get into a habit of extensive coffee-drinking, which can cause anxiety symptoms (Greden, 1974). The man whose wife has left him may live on sandwiches, the recent widow not bother to cook for herself, the old person who is toothless, lacking taste discrimination, and on a small pension, grudge money on food. Immigrants, whether from European, African, or Eastern countries, may find it difficult to get the foods to which they are accustomed, and have problems in cooking or eating what is on local offer. Vegetarianism, or religious prohibitions, or carnival excitement may limit balance. Smoking tobacco, drinking alcohol, and taking drugs of dependence diminish food intake. The chronic use of laxatives, certain steroids, and psychotropic drugs may affect nutritional state. Drugs in general must be viewed with suspicion (Macgregor *et al.*, 1979).

If there are suggestions of unusual dietary intake, it may be worthwhile if a relative (for outpatients) or a nurse (for in-patients) keeps a daily food diary, listing what is eaten and drunk throughout the day, preferably with estimates of quantity (the weights of eggs, meat, bread, potatoes; the number of cups of tea). If all served is not eaten, it is of course necessary to weigh what of each foodstuff is left. If the weight of cooked and raw foods consumed per day is known, a book of analytical tables can be consulted to work out estimates of the daily calorie, mineral, and protein intakes (Paul & Southgate, 1978). It is surprising how often the patient's or relative's general impression of adequacy is disproved by a detailed diary.

Body weight

Body weight in the adult often has a remarkable constancy over long periods. This was the basis of the practice in long-stay psychiatric hospitals of weighing chronic patients every month. After years of the same weight, plus or minus at most 1 kg, a weight-drop month by month was an early signal that something might be organically wrong, and a physical examination might then bring to light tuberculosis or an early carcinoma.

It must be understood that the constancy is a mean value, with constant fluctuations around it, depending partly on time of day, meals, and the state of fluid balance. Thus a good meal may immediately add 0.5–0.75 kg to a person's weight, the voiding of 300 ml of night urine reduce weight by 0.3 kg, the passing of a firm stool subtract 0.1 kg; depending on climate, sweating may be responsible for losses of over 1 kg. Even when care is taken to allow for such influences, the weight still fluctuates because the body water (the glycogen–water pool, Garrow, 1974) fluctuates – to the extent of about 0.5 per cent of the body weight, or somewhat more in the obese.

To get the most information from body weight it must be measured carefully and frequently, pref-

erably daily rather than weekly or monthly, because the short-term pattern of change, whether a rise or a fall or a coarse oscillation, may be very informative as an objective indicator of poor appetite, impaired fluid balance, or metabolic disturbance. Experimental studies of starvation (Keys *et al.*, 1950) have shown that a weight loss of more than 0.4 kg per 24 hours must be due to body-water loss and not loss of body fat or muscle mass alone. Likewise forced feeding of chronic schizophrenics (Anderson *et al.*, 1957) has shown that a weight rise of more than 0.25 kg per day must be due to fluid retention. This information enables us to interpret the weight chart in terms of food or water intake (with the possibility of confirmation by measuring fluid intake and urine output), and to reveal short-term disturbances of diagnostic importance (see p. 51, Taste and appetite).

The following precautions in weighing are suggested.

(1) It should not be done by the patient, particularly if he or she has a bias towards a particular result (e.g. in anorexia nervosa). It should be done by someone who is motivated to do it properly, understands its purpose and possible errors, and preferably can do it every day (to minimize observer error).

(2) It should not be on bathroom platform scales, which work by squeezing or stretching a spring linked to a needle on a dial, because the tension of the spring can vary considerably and falsify the weighing. A machine with weights in a pan or on a slider should be used, and its zero reading checked each time before weighing the patient.

(3) It should be at the same time every day, to improve comparability, and preferably around 7–8 a.m., i.e. shortly after rising and voiding the night urine and before breakfast, and if possible naked or dressed only in the same thin dressing gown. Where the patient is weighed in clothes, an attempt may be made to standardize from time to time what is worn, but on no account should some arbitrary value for clothing be subtracted before recording a weight. To take off 2 or 3 kg every time as some nurses do, simply adds a new error of considerable size to what is already not entirely exact, and brings no benefit.

Where changes in body weight are revealed it may be desired to analyse them further, and while it is ideal it is not essential to have a metabolic ward for this purpose. What is essential is to have sufficient nursing assistance to observe the patient closely throughout the 24 hours and to record everything eaten and drunk and excreted each day. Again, a special diet kitchen is inessential, especially for short studies (e.g. up to one week.) If a diet of known or standard composition is necessary, a simplified one using milk fortified with a protein food such as 'Complan' or 'Casilan', with rice, sugar, cheese, eggs, and fruit may be very adequate, and prepared on the spot.

Clinical examination

The skin is an important indicator of past nutrition. It may be loose and thin over bones, with prominent veins, or taut and smooth over fat or oedema, or show striae from previous rapid stretching. Discolouration and rash, or a dry eczema, may be suggestive, if symmetrical: the butterfly-shaped dermatitis on the face around the nose is a well-known sign of pellagra (nicotinamide–tryptophan deficiency.) Fat pads and oedema are sometimes confused: but only the latter can be dispersed by continued pressure on the skin. Oedema is a sign of increased *extracellular* fluid (with sodium retention), and increase in total body water without sodium retention allows the fluid to be held intracellularly without the production of oedema. Oedema may result from inappropriate thirst and sodium retention, or from hypoalbuminaemia or capillary damage resulting in disturbed hydrostatic relations in the tissue circulation.

Amenorrhoea can be linked with general weight loss. Pallor may point to anaemia; a red tongue with papillary necrosis and angular stomatitis to a vitamin deficiency; a peripheral neuropathy to a metabolic disturbance of some kind. It is important to remember that failure to absorb adequate nutrients may arise after a partial gastrectomy or intestinal resection, or as a consequence of mucosal change in ulcerative colitis, or simply in any illness where there is chronic diarrhoea. Carcinoma of visceral organs, and endocrine disturbances such as diabetes mellitus, thyrotoxicosis, or adrenal cortical hyperplasia may likewise modify absorption or metabolism. Intestinal parasites, such as the protozoan *Giardia*, or tapeworm *Diphyllobothrium latum* which interferes with the metabolism of vitamin B_{12}, must not be overlooked. Starvation amidst plenty, nutritional deficiency on a normal diet, implies physical illness.

Laboratory aids

Obviously a wide range of tests may be helpful in the diagnosis of physical illnesses generally. However certain blood tests are particularly relevant in the assessment of aspects of nutrition, because the blood is an easily accessible tissue with a rapid cellular turnover. Sampling its enzymes and coenzymes in erythrocytes is well established, and tests on leucocytes (vitamin C) are also known. Lack of red cell haemoglobin may be a sign of poor diet (a lack of iron, copper, vitamins); a lowered red cell folate is a better indicator of chronic folic acid deficiency than a *plasma* folate which responds quickly down or up to acute changes in folic acid intake. The red cell enzyme transketolase depends for its activity on the presence of thiamine pyrophosphate. If vitamin B_1 dietary intake has been adequate, the measured enzyme activity will not increase by more than 16 per cent at the most, when additional thiamine pyrophosphate is added to the blood sample *in vitro*. This is a more sensitive test for thiamine deficiency than measuring thiamine itself in the blood, or the pyruvate in the serum. Aspartate transaminase activity depends on pyridoxal phosphate, derived from dietary pyridoxine (vitamin B_6), and the vitamin can be similarly assessed. Red-cell glutathione reductase is riboflavin-dependent, and its activity is sometimes used as a test of general nutritional level. Plasma hypoalbuminaemia can be another pointer to general nutritional (protein intake) poverty (Thomson, 1978; Fink & Rosalki, 1978; Carney *et al.*, 1979).

Bone radiology may show osteoporosis from calcium deficiency. Paper chromatography of urine may show an aminoaciduria or indoluria. The EEG may show a generalized abnormality consistent with metabolic disorder, perhaps with rapid change in response to injection of vitamin. Discussion with the laboratory about these and other tests may be helpful.

Physiological aspects

Nutritional status is obviously a product of behaviour, constitution, and the available food, and each of these components is itself complex. The behaviour may be willed and deliberate, or unthinking but voluntary, or even compulsive or automatic; while as part of an illness it may be cause or result or epiphenomenon. Constitution implies something dynamic at several levels, metabolic machinery (including adaptive enzymes), capacities of organ systems, such as the somatic–muscular, the renal, hepatic, or cardiovascular, and the loads that current life-situations put on them, but also the sensitivity of sensation and the learned responses to perception (see p. 51, Taste and appetite; p. 53, Digestion, absorption, metabolism). Thus a nutritional disturbance can be simply an incidental part of a psychiatric syndrome, can be a prime cause of psychiatric illness, or may contribute to only some of the clinical features. Since the symptoms of psychiatric illness are non-specific and may arise from many causes, the psychiatric picture of itself cannot incriminate any particular organic factor. One must be alert to relative likelihoods and investigate the pathology of the individual case, remembering that the appearance of neurotic symptoms such as anxiety can (among many other possibilities) be the consequence of vitamin deficiency.

It is important to realize two things in this. One is the occult nature of many nutritional deficiencies. There will be biochemical signs of deficiency months before clinical signs begin to appear: more people show metabolic disturbances on test than ever appear ill. The second is that only a small minority of the different nutritional disturbances can lead to psychiatric illness. Most clinically evident nutritional failure is somatic only. Thus of the nine amino acids essential to human growth and maintenance (leucine, isoleucine, valine, lysine, threonine, methionine, histidine, phenylalanine and tryptophan) only the last-named can give rise to mental disturbance through lack or excess. Of the essential dietary minerals manganese, copper, zinc, cobalt, chromium, and molybdenum (Davies, 1972), only excess of manganese, and possibly of copper in Wilson's disease, have neuropsychiatric interest, although cobalt in the specific form of cobalamin (vitamin B_{12}) is important. Many vitamins – vitamins A, C, D, E, K, biotin, pantothenic acid, and so on – have no neuropsychiatric interest either. Many of these substances play important parts in brain chemistry (zinc in carbonic anhydrase, pantothenic acid as part of coenzyme A involved in the synthesis of acetyl choline, for instance), but the critical effects of deficiency are felt in skin or blood and not in the central nervous system. It is of course always possible that rare individuals will be found by future research to be psychiatrically sensitive to deficiency of one or other of what are commonly seen as somatic nutrients. There is a further point here. Straightforward lack of food in general, or starvation, does not cause mental illness (though it may lead to preoccupation with food and the disappearance of moral feelings), it is *imbalance* between *component nutrients* which precipitates symptoms, and more will be said about imbalance later.

The vitamin deficiencies which can matter in psychiatric practice are thiamine, nicotinamide, pyridoxine, cobalamin, and folate. In general an acute deficiency produces more cerebral symptoms than a chronic one, and in practice illness is most usually the result of a sudden acute deficiency superimposed on a pre-existing chronic lack, either because of a sudden food change or a sudden increase in bodily demand through exercise or infectious disease, for example. A chronic lack may be the consequence of a limited diet. Thiamine intake may be low in people who do not eat meat, because the vitamin goes along with animal protein in many foods. Heavy beer drinkers who get their calorie requirements largely by drinking and eat little else either because of gastritis or cost are therefore liable to chronic deficiency. So are some vegetarians, or those who from economy eat mainly polished rice. Reliance on maize as a staple food may result in nicotinamide lack. Sometimes the deficiency arises through a failure of food preparation – the nutrient is destroyed by cooking, or not released in digestible form. An unusual individual habit is the eating of raw fish, containing a thiaminase which destroys vitamin B_1. When considering nutrient substances that foods may lack, one should remember that food may also contain toxins. Caffeine poisoning from excessive coffee-drinking has presented before now as neurotic symptoms puzzling in cause until the dietary had been explored (Greden, 1974; Winstead, 1976). Modern food technology involves adding a whole series of dyes, antioxidants, sequestrants, emulsifiers, stabilizers, maturers, bleachers, and texturizers. The nitrogen trichloride ('agene') process of maturing flour was abandoned thirty years ago when such flour was found to cause fits in dogs because of the methionine sulphoxide formed by the process, although no positive evidence of harm in man was forthcoming. It is not impossible that other food chemicals may prove toxic to some individuals though not to the mass of their fellow-citizens.

Taste and appetite

It is instructive to look at the reasons why people sometimes drink large volumes of water. There are those who do it because they feel almost continuously thirsty, or because their mouth is dry, the physiological group; there are those who do it 'to wash away poisons', the paranoid psychotic group; and those who seek attention by frequently calling for water, or who aim at water intoxication or the sick role, so-called compulsive water-drinkers, the deviant personality group. The physiological group can be subdivided into those with some form of diabetes insipidus, in which the kidney continually leaks a dilute urine and the uncontrollable water loss creates the thirst, and those where the thirst mechanism is itself astray, sometimes because of a drug such as lithium carbonate. Patients with severe untreated depression quite commonly become dehydrated, although fluids are freely available, and the same thing is sometimes seen in schizophrenia and in acute brain syndrome. In such cases it seems likely there is a thirst failure, that the central nervous perception of hypertonic body fluids is blunted. In some manic patients one sees the reverse, a brief experience of unslakable thirst.

The taking of food is determined by greater complexities, in which taste and appetite (hunger and satiety) play parts. Depressed patients often complain that their sense of taste is dulled or strangely altered, and this can be set beside the observation that in some metabolic disorders the threshold for tasting salt (adrenal cortical failure) or glucose (diabetes mellitus) is raised, and indeed the threshold for salty and bitter things is also raised in pregnancy. It is possible that the normal woman's special cravings for sweet or pickled foods in the first three months of pregnancy are related to taste impairment, and her sudden aversions to tea and coffee connected with temporary changes in olfaction (Dickens & Trethowan, 1971).

Pica, the name given to the tendency to eat inappropriate things, such as earth, or even faeces, seen among children, some chronic schizophrenics, and some mentally handicapped, may have a different explanation. Studies on the appetite for thiamine in rats, for salt in sheep, for phosphate in cattle suggest two phases (*Handbook of Physiology*, 1967) in this behaviour, one of exploration, the other of increased well-being. Animals deprived of some essential nutrient start to widen their eating habits, casting around as if experimenting. If they hit on a new food which supplies the missing nutrient they continue to eat it, presumably aware of some feeling of bodily well-being it provides. There is evidence that children who eat clay and earth may have an iron deficiency, and that the earth is a source of iron: the pica is said to stop if they are given adequate iron treatment (*Lancet*, 1959; Carlander, 1959). Some animals, e.g. rabbits, eat their faeces as a source of vitamins. On this basis the chronic psychotic or ament with pica should be investigated for mineral and vitamin deficiencies. It is worth noting that learning about tastes is very rapid, selective, and persistent in man (Garb & Stunkard, 1974).

Appetites are regulators of intake, and appear to have both a hunger component and a satiety component, a turning on and turning off, which must be very finely tuned as far as calories are concerned because in the normal adult body weight is often remarkably constant over many months or years (Garrow, 1974, p. 183) in spite of many variations in the carbohydrate, fat, and protein contents of different meals. In psychiatric patients, however, weight fluctuations are often seen in the course of their illness, and the pattern of weight change may be characteristic for the illness and repeat with the mental symptoms in those who have recurrent attacks. There is clearly here either an appetite disturbance or a change in the control of sodium and water excretion: both types of disturbance can be demonstrated. The weight change is not in any way causative of psychiatric symptoms, it is simply an indicator of physiological disorganization. However, in the special case of an individual who has been on a chronically deficient diet for a long time, sudden cessation of all eating, especially with increased activity as in an agitated depression, could precipitate additional nutrient deficiency symptoms.

Figs. 4.1 and 4.2 show weight charts of some schizophrenic men, which illustrate both the overall constancy of weight level, and the possibility of a patterned fluctuation. In fig. 4.3A, an attack of depression in a drug-free elderly woman was associated with a rapid weight loss, with adjustment of weight at a lower level which lasted for the rest of the depression – about 11 weeks. When the depression spontaneously lifted and mood became normal, the weight rose rapidly to its old level. In fig. 4.3B, at the next attack in the same patient full meals ('diet') were provided and pushed for four days. This arrested the weight loss, and the weight then steadied until spontaneous recovery – and again a rapid weight gain. Clearly the weight loss seen at the start of each depressive episode was due to a sudden loss of appetite, which however recovered after about three weeks; and the weight gain at the end was probably from *a limited period* of excessive appetite or partial loss of satiety. Fig. 4.4 shows a different phenomenon, a fluctuating weight due not to any change in appetite, but to alternating natriuresis and oliguria in step with the mood changes (Crammer, 1957, 1959; Crammer & Elkes, 1969).

Anorexia (and weight loss) is so common in depressive illnesses as to be taken for granted and not investigated. In contrast, hypomania and mania are usually not associated with any body-weight change. A few depressives show a reverse of the usual, putting on weight whenever they are depressed. Weight gain, leading to obesity is discussed elsewhere, but it should not be forgotten that hypothalamic lesions and syndromes such as the Pickwickian and Kleine-Levin (see Lishman, 1978) may have voracious eating (not necessarily with hunger) and obesity with somnolence as their clinical presentation. Such patients seem to lack the normal feelings of fullness and consequent aversion for the time being from further food. What determines normal satiety is obscure. Robinson and colleagues (1979) in an interesting survey and study of the effects of gastro-intestinal surgery propose gastric motility and speed of emptying as an important control. This requires further study in psychiatric patients: depressives are often constipated, a sign of intestinal inactivity, and their anorexia may therefore perhaps be linked with this, but other conditions also require exploration.

Digestion, absorption, metabolism

Of the major components of the human dietary, protein is the most likely to be in short supply, and of the component amino acids tryptophan is one of the scarcest. Tryptophan is the essential raw mate-

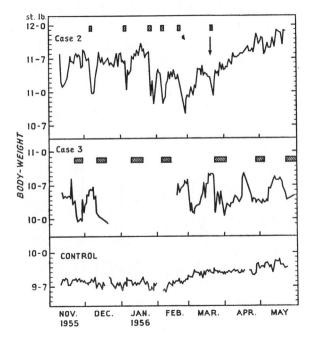

Fig. 4.1. Body weights of three schizophrenic men in the same ward: control suffered from chronic paranoid schizophrenia, cases 2 and 3 from catatonic schizophrenia with recurrent excited phases marked by rectangles. Arrow indicates start of treatment with chlorpromazine.

Fig. 4.2. (*below*) Daily body weight of an old man with recurrent catatonic stupors (marked by rectangles), and no treatment except general nursing care.

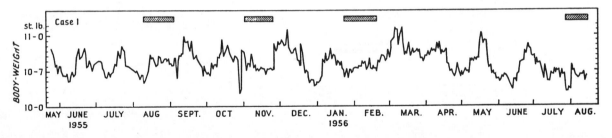

rial for brain serotonin, and is also an important source in man for the synthesis of nicotinamide (vitamin B₂), which in diphospho- and triphospho-pyridine nucleotides forms important and widely distributed coenzymes of respiratory and carbohydrate metabolism. It is not surprising therefore that deficiencies or excesses of tryptophan can produce psychiatric symptoms.

Vegetable proteins mostly contain less tryptophan than animal proteins, and zein, the chief protein of maize corn, contains none at all. Pellagra ('rough skin') with its skin lesions, chronic diarrhoea, and acute or chronic brain syndrome, has been a scourge of those condemned to live on a diet almost confined to maize, which in addition supplies little pre-formed nicotinamide. The human being is not capable of synthesizing more than about 40 per cent of the daily nicotinamide requirement, and the rest must be supplied in the diet.

Tryptophan is freed from dietary protein by intestinal digestion with the help of enzymes (trypsin) from the pancreatic juice. It is absorbed through the gut wall largely by an active metabolic transport process. In the rare genetically-determined condition of Hartnup syndrome this is lacking, insufficient

tryptophan enters the body in spite of a good diet and unless extra large amounts of nicotinamide are given pellagrous symptoms can develop. This rare individual requirement of a large vitamin intake has been termed 'vitamin dependency'. Seakins (1974) in

Fig. 4.4. Recurrent mood and weight swings marching together: weight loss is associated with sodium, excretion or polyuria, weight gain with oliguria and sodium retention, as shown by controlled dietary and water balance.

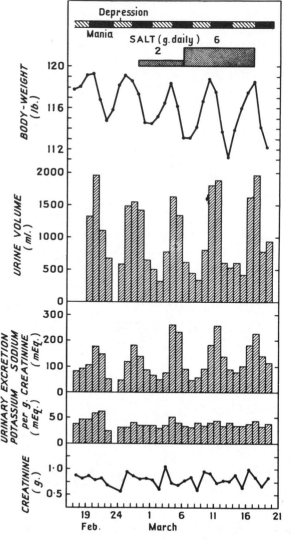

Fig. 4.3. Two depressive illnesses in an elderly woman not on any physical treatments: A shows the spontaneous weight chart, B the weight chart when 4 days of full diet were given near the start of the illness.

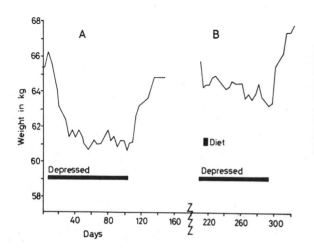

his survey of 54 cases notes that 3 were first seen for mental symptoms, and that one-quarter of them had anxiety, depression, hallucinations, and an acute brain syndrome.

Active transport of tryptophan occurs not only in the gut wall and the renal tubule, but at other tissue sites, including the brain, in particular the synaptosomes of nerve endings, and the system is not unique to one amino acid but carries also phenylalanine, tyrosine, methionine, and leucine, which can compete with tryptophan for passage (Green, 1978). This means that great excess of one of these other amino acids could prevent the entry of tryptophan, and reduce the production, for example, of serotonin. In untreated phenylketonuria, an inherited inability to metabolize phenylalanine by conversion to tyrosine, phenylalanine rises in the plasma and may have such a cerebral effect (and, of course, successful treatment of phenylketonuria depends on very careful dietary control, almost completely eliminating phenylalanine from the food during the early years of life).

When excesses of one of the essential amino acids have been administered to chronic schizophrenics in daily doses of 15–20 grams methionine and tryptophan are the only two found (with or without concomitant monoamine oxidase inhibitor) to produce fresh psychiatric symptoms (Park *et al.*, 1965). In the case of methionine these symptoms have been regarded by some as schizophrenia, by others as an acute brain syndrome, but the primary interest is that only these two amino acids disturb brain function, and the possibility exists that methionine is acting by competing in tryptophan transport. Other explanations are that it increases transmethylation, and also strongly acidifies the urine so that many biogenic amines are washed out of the body. Tryptophan in excess (3–7 g daily) is euphoriant and hypnotic, and may have some anti-depressant effect in depressed patients when given with pyridoxine and a monoamine oxidase inhibitor. These observations serve to emphasize how at the tissue level nutrients interact, and it is specific imbalances between them which may result in symptoms, rather than an overall lack of food. (For a discussion of transport competition between amino acids see Sprince, 1967; Daniel *et al.*, 1977; Davison, 1973; Gopelan & Rao, 1975.)

Homocystinuria is another rare inherited metabolic deficiency (usually lack of the enzyme cystathionine synthetase) in which, most commonly, methionine metabolism is blocked after the demethylation stage. Reducing methionine in the diet enables affected infants to develop successfully. Mudd and Freeman (1974) described an alternative variant of homocystinuria in two families, where one adult sufferer showed catatonic withdrawal and hallucinations which disappeared whenever she was given large doses of folic acid, and recurred twice within 6–9 months of stopping the folate. This particular form of vitamin dependency was due to inherited deficiency of the enzyme N-methylene tetrahydrofolate reductase which can methylate homocysteine as well as other metabolites, and might result in a cerebral lack of methionine.

A further example of vitamin dependency is the unusually big requirement of some individuals for pyridoxine, without which they rapidly develop epileptic fits. Pyridoxine (vitamin B_6), metabolized to pyridoxal phosphate, is the coenzyme for glutamic acid decarboxylase, amongst others, and this is responsible for brain synthesis of inhibitory transmitter GABA (gamma-amino butyric acid). The value of specific vitamin supplements in rare cases has given rise to the idea that large doses of vitamins might be generally therapeutic in psychiatry. Megavitamin therapy has particularly claimed gram daily doses of nicotinamide to be useful in schizophrenia, a claim which has not stood up to careful clinical trial (see Pauling, and others, 1974), and is indeed somewhat improbable when many studies suggest that schizophrenic illnesses are not a single pathological entity, and that vitamin dependencies manifest themselves as rare and specific. Any beneficial effect of a 3 g dose of ascorbic acid on manic-depressives (Naylor & Smith, 1981) could be through a change in the metabolism of psychotropic drugs taken about the same time, for instance, and not in cell metabolism.

The importance of gastro-intestinal function in maintaining normal nutritional status is shown particularly in the physiology of vitamin B_{12}. Deficiency states could arise in very strict vegetarians, since the vitamin is only available in animal foods or in foods contaminated by bacterial action, where bacteria synthesize the vitamin. In practice, the deficiency only manifests itself when there is failure to absorb B_{12}, which is by an unusual active process. A glycoprotein (intrinsic factor) is secreted by the parietal cells of the stomach, combines with dietary cobalamin, and the complex is absorbed through the wall of the ileum. This process can fail at two distinct anatomical sites, stomach and intestine, in a number of ways. Surgery may have removed too much of the stomach or intestine (or by-passed the absorptive zone). Antibodies to the parietal cells, and less commonly to the intrinsic factor itself, may have developed, as in pernicious anaemia, with atrophic gastritis and achlorhydria, so that the absorption complex cannot be formed. And on the other hand, the small gut may have a variety of diseases in which the absorptive surface is partially lost; there may be an abnormal bacterial flora taking up the vitamin, and there is intestinal hurry and diarrhoea. Crohn's disease, giardiasis, tropical sprue, and gluten-sensitive enteropathy are examples of such conditions.

Such intestinal disease can also affect the absorption of folate, and other nutrients, while chronic diarrhoea can be a continuing unsuspected loss of proteins and minerals making for an overall deficiency. Malabsorption syndromes, in particular steatorrhoea or coeliac disease, which appears to be an enteropathy caused by gluten, a dietary protein from wheat flour, in those predisposed to its action, have been assigned a place in the aetiology of schizophrenia. Dohan (1966, 1969, 1978) has produced evidence that diets avoiding wheat cereal and milk may be beneficial to psychiatric patients, but amid the difficulties of precise psychiatric diagnosis, spontaneous variations in mental state, and response to observer interest, the matter remains very controversial. The evidence that undigested protein (and of course polypeptides, including endorphins) can be absorbed from the gut into the circulation is, however, good (Hemmings, 1978; Klee *et al.*, 1979) and this has led to the idea that allergy to some of these proteins expresses itself in psychiatric symptoms, or that peptides derived from proteins excite neural effects. The ideas are interesting but so far there is no satisfactory evidence of their truth (see also Marsh, 1981).

Constitutionally, therefore, the brain availability of nutrients and their biologically active derivatives depends on a very heterogeneous collection of metabolic processes, and the symptoms of functional failure can result from a whole range of rare unrelated specific defects. The lesser degrees of metabolic deficiency have no clinical symptoms and are detected only by special tests. Such deficiency may be purely coincidental with a psychiatric illness, or may complicate its clinical course; but sometimes it will play a direct causative role. Only clinical study of the individual in the light of physiological fact can clarify aetiology.

Clinical features

There are no psychiatric syndromes or symptoms which point to any particular biochemical disturbance. Increased irritability, anxiety, fatigue, forgetfulness, depression ('neurotic' symptoms) may occur early, and frank delusions and hallucinations or a severe mood disturbance ('psychotic' symptoms) later in the development of a nutritional deficiency; but these symptoms in themselves are no different from those of other neurotic or depressive illnesses, or other acute brain syndromes or deliria. Organically-caused psychiatric syndromes often fluctuate in severity from day to day or even hour to hour, but this will not be a reliable guide here; nor will the clinical picture necessarily be that of an acute brain syndrome ('toxic confusional state', dysmnesic state, 'subacute delirium'). Diagnosis therefore depends on awareness of the possibility, on direct questioning to bring out disorientation or memory impairment, on the presence of skin, peripheral neural, or blood signs as well in some patients, and on laboratory tests. Neurotic illness appearing only late in life, depressive illness which does not respond to customary treatment, dementia appearing before the age of sixty, may rouse suspicion of nutritional factors. A history of finicky eating, of chronic diarrhoea or gastro-intestinal surgery, of carcinoma or malabsorption syndrome, or of chronic alcoholism, may strengthen the need to apply biochemical tests (see Assessment, p. 48). Manic-depressive or schizophrenic episodes, with their changed activity and appetite, may secondarily precipitate nutritional deficiency symptoms, and so may chronic drug treatment (Carney *et al.*, 1979).

Plain starvation produces irritability and intolerance of noise, a hypochondriacal self-concern with a callousness to others, a mental restlessness and physical apathy, and a loss of all social and family feelings. This (reversible) personality change has to be born in mind by those treating the patient, who may be awkward and paranoid. Sodium depletion, as in the dehydration of heat exhaustion, gives rise to a well-marked mental apathy, with loss of appetite, weakness, and vascular signs such as low blood pressure, collapsed veins, and rapid pulse. However, this section will concentrate on the vitamin deficiencies. It is noteworthy that vitamins A, C, D, E, K, pantothenic acid, biotin, and riboflavin are not associated with any psychiatric disorder.

Thiamine (vitamin B₁)

Deficiency is responsible for beri-beri, Wernicke's encephalopathy and some cases of Korsakow's psychosis. It arises insidiously where highly milled rice or wheat flour (e.g. white bread) without other fresh food is the staple diet. It also arises where the diet has been very restricted because of alcoholism, or (rarely) because of carcinoma of the stomach, or (even more rarely) after severe prolonged vomiting of pregnancy or severe prolonged dieting. Sometimes an unwonted exertion or a minor infection is the last straw in starting the symptoms – anorexia, ill-defined malaise, heavy weakness of the legs – or bringing on a sudden deterioration from this stage to the wet form of beri-beri with oedema, dyspnoea, and congestive cardiac failure. Alternatively, particularly where there is concurrently a lack of other nutrients, there may be a sudden onset of cerebral symptoms, particularly Wernicke's encephalopathy.

Clinical symptoms

Studies of thiamine depletion in volunteers, with blind periods of reintroduction of thiamine, have shown that neurasthenia is an early result of vitamin B₁ lack. Generalized weakness, anorexia, fluctuating irritability, and moodiness (depression) appear after a few weeks. Insomnia is common, and the sufferer may become forgetful and apathetic. Reintroduction of the vitamin quickly improves appetite and outlook. Such a neurasthenic picture also appears during epidemics of beri-beri which classically present with peripheral neuritic or cardiac signs.

Prolonged incomplete thiamine deficiency may be tolerated if resulting only in a general impairment of physical and mental work ability, without physical signs, although it has been claimed that institutionalized chronic psychotics may show worsening of the psychiatric clinical picture in consequence of thiamine lack. The major psychiatric risk is the imposition of a sudden acute thiamine deficiency on top of a chronic incomplete one, with the sudden onset of Wernicke's encephalopathy – clouding of consciousness, ataxic gait, and oculomotor disturbances, often with a marked disorder of memory. The clouding of consciousness, often a quiet disorientated apathy, may reach delirium and dominate the picture, and the neurological symptoms and signs may be less obvious or fleeting. Wavering field of vision, double vision and photobia may be linked with nystagmus, and external rectus palsy (sixth cranial nerve). The ataxia may be mild or result in inability to stand without support. Peripheral neuritis is of course common.

Setting

The vitamin is derived primarily from animal foods, including fish and poultry, and is in short supply for the pure vegetarian. The need for it is greater on a high carbohydrate diet – which is why a glucose infusion in a sick person with unrecognized B₁ deficiency can precipitate acute mental symptoms, as can the increased metabolism of an acute fever or infection.

Dietary peculiarities can produce the deficiency in individual cases. Raw fish contains a thiaminase, an enzyme destroying this vitamin, and a habit of eating raw fish, found particularly among cooks and waiters, may result in trouble. Heavy consumption of beer or other alcoholic liquor without taking solid food may provide sufficient daily calories, and thereby result in a deficient thiamine intake. Drugs of addiction, including nicotine, often lead to anorexia. Children, the elderly, the mentally handicapped, and the inmates of impoverished institutions are all at greater risk of nutritional deficiency.

The risk is also greater where there is prolonged gastro-intestinal upset, preventing the absorption of thiamine – as in gastric carcinoma, dysentery, typhoid – or frequent vomiting as in hyperemesis gravidarum.

Mechanism

Thiamine is not stored. Tissue deficiency results in carboxylase deficiency, and a partial failure of the tricarboxylic acid cycle: pyruvate accumulates instead of being decarboxylated to acetate (a step not needed in alcohol metabolism). This has led to the measurement of serum pyruvate levels and their response to a glucose load (pyruvate tolerance test), as well as serum thiamine assay, as laboratory aids to diagnosis. The modern test is the assay of the enzyme transketolase in erythrocytes.

Although carbohydrate metabolism occurs all over the body, the brain is unusual in that glucose is its sole source of energy, and yet it is an organ with a high metabolic rate. Therefore it is particularly vulnerable to a partial failure in glucose metabolism, generating unusual amounts of organic acid locally.

Treatment

The daily adult requirement of thiamine is of the order of 1 mg. It is chiefly absorbed from the small intestine by an active transport process of limited capacity (its upper limit is about 10 mg per day). Treatment of deficiency must always start therefore with intravenous or intramuscular doses of 100 mg daily, and can be converted to oral treatment (say 10 mg thrice daily) when thiamine is appearing in the urine. Actual thiamine requirement is greater with greater metabolic activity (0.5 mg thiamine per 1000 kcal) and giving glucose, particularly intravenously, may put the thiamine requirement up dangerously. Sudden refeeding, a burst of exercise, or hot baths are also risky. Infection and electrolyte imbalance may need attention.

Niacin (vitamin B₂)

Clinical features

The early symptoms are those of neurasthenia – fatigue, lassitude, irritability, poor sleep, depression – often without diarrhoea or any skin lesion. Later, often suddenly, an acute brain syndrome appears, even subacute or acute delirium, or an agitated depression, but occasionally retardation to stupor, or a schizophrenic picture. There may be some dysarthria, but neurological signs are minimal or absent. The tongue may be red and raw, less often diarrhoea and a symmetrical dermatitis may appear, the latter especially on exposure to sunlight, and spread over the face, neck, head, hands, and feet.

The condition tends to be variable or intermittent, and is worst in the spring. Both sexes are affected equally.

Setting

The poor, the elderly, the institutionalized, the alcoholic (although beer contains nicotinamide and riboflavin, but is lacking in thiamine) are at risk, particularly (though not exclusively) in maize-, millet-, or rice-eating countries, where animal protein is in short supply. Nicotinic acid is not available in digestible form in maize, and is very low in rice. Part of the daily bodily requirement is met by synthesis from dietary tryptophan in which maize is very lacking (rice is somewhat better). Synthesis is partly hepatic but also to some extent by the gut microflora, whence it is absorbed. This helps to explain why malabsorption syndromes, (including the inherited failure of tryptophan transport, Hartnup syndrome),

infections of the gut, and previous gastro-intestinal surgery predispose to the onset.

Mechanism

Although nicotinamide in the form of diphospho- and triphosphopyridine nucleotides (or coenzymes I and II) plays a very wide role in many processes of tissue respiration and metabolism, the brain appears particularly at risk, possibly because of its extremely active respiration and glycolysis. Deficiency, however, is very different from deficiency of thiamine, and tryptophan disturbance may play some additional role.

Treatment

Man needs about 6 mg nicotinic acid per 1000 kcal diet daily, and 60 mg tryptophane are roughly the equivalent of 1 mg niacin. For deficiency symptoms 50 mg doses of niacin repeated several times daily should produce dramatic improvement within 24 hours. Intravenous doses of 25 mg repeated once or twice may be used if the oral route is unsuitable. Where there are neurological signs, multiple deficiency is probably present, and thiamine will also be needed.

Cyanocobalamin (vitamin B₁₂)

Clinical features

The presentation is rarely psychiatric. Most commonly deficiency results first in a megaloblastic anaemia, and later the neurological picture of subacute combined degeneration develops. Sometimes, however, the neurological picture appears first, or alone – numbness and tingling in the hands and feet, with loss of vibration and position sense in the legs, a feeling as of walking on cottonwool. Where the presentation is psychiatric, neurological signs or anaemia may be discovered later. The psychiatric picture is similar whether it occurs early or late, and can take many forms (Eilenberg, 1960) but most commonly that of an acute brain syndrome or a depressive illness unresponsive to the usual treatments. Hypomania, schizophrenia, dementia are also described. There is no correlation between the severity of the blood disorder, the neurological symptoms or the psychiatric symptoms: they are three independent pictures with a common cause.

The EEG is abnormal in 60 per cent of all cases and may change quite quickly (within 7 days) of injection of a big dose of the vitamin.

Setting

Surveys of psychiatric populations, particularly the elderly, often show low vitamin B_{12} levels in the serum. This by itself is not evidence of serious vitamin deficiency, and treatment with the vitamin is disappointing. Only when there is positive evidence in history, physical examination, and other laboratory measures of deficiency should a course of cobalamin injections be embarked upon, i.e., dietary or surgical history, raw tongue, anaemia or neurological signs, achlorhydria, serum antibodies to gastric parietal cells or intrinsic factor, signs of dementia.

Dietary deficiency of the vitamin is unusual, and failure of the special absorption mechanism in the gut, as in pernicious anaemia, is the usual cause (see below).

Mechanism

The cobalamins are a whole group of substances, of which cyanocobalamin is the natural vitamin, which are extremely active in tiny amounts in the enzymatic processes of growth (nucleotide and amino acid metabolism) and in the maintenance of myelin in nervous tissue. The vitamin is not present at all in plant food (unless affected by bacterial action), whence a certain risk to extreme vegetarians. It is available to man only in animal products, but it arises in nature (is synthesized) only by bacteria, including those of the human colon.

However, the synthesized vitamin cannot be absorbed from the colon, and is simply excreted in the faeces.

The absorption of the vitamin from the food is curious. It must first, by cooking or digestion, be split from the protein to which it is bound, and must then combine with a glycoprotein secreted by the parietal cells of the gastric mucosa – the intrinsic factor. This complex is then absorbed through a special zone of the ileum, and cobalamin liberated into the blood, where it travels attached to various proteins. The serum level of vitamin B_{12} is therefore a reflection of binding conditions as well as the balance between vitamin availability and loss. Body stores may amount to 2–5 mg while the daily requirement is less than 1 μg, due to loss in the stool. Most cobalamin is excreted into the bile but if intrinsic factor is present 80 per cent is reabsorbed into the blood again.

This deficiency is normally very slow to develop, but is speeded when in the disease, pernicious anaemia, the intrinsic factor is missing, or when gastro-intestinal circumstances modify either stomach or ileum.

Treatment

This must be by intramuscular injection: hydroxocobalamin is now usually used, 2 mg every three days for six occasions, and then 1 mg every two months.

Folic acid
Clinical features

Deficiency causes a megaloblastic anaemia, glossitis, diarrhoea, and weight loss, very like the symptoms of cyanocobalamin lack, but there are *never* any neurological signs, and some doubt whether there really are psychiatric symptoms, except in rare inherited metabolic disorders such as the folate-dependent family described by Mudd and Freeman (1974). However, irritability and forgetfulness have been claimed as early symptoms, and the suggestion made that depressive illness and dementia may sometimes be caused or aggravated by folate lack (Reynolds *et al.*, 1970; Carney *et al.*, 1979).

Setting

There is little doubt that epileptics under treatment with phenytoin can develop a megaloblastic anaemia which responds to folate, the administration of which may diminish control of fits while generally brightening the patient up. This may, however, be a drug interaction effect, since phenytoin, phenobarbitone, and folic acid are all acidic substances, protein-bound in the plasma, but able to compete for binding. Old people admitted to hospital, and to a lesser extent psychiatric admissions at all ages, may have low serum folate levels, but this need not imply deficiency. Clinical improvement in mental state should be demonstrable under blind treatment with folic acid alone if the vitamin has a psychiatric value: this is still awaited. There is no clear EEG change with folate as there is with cyanocobalamin. The vitamin is extremely widely available in food.

Mechanism

Folic acid is a monoglutamate, but occurs in food, whether plant or animal, usually as polyglutamates, which are not well absorbed. Once a polyglutamate is split down to monoglutamate, however, it is rapidly and completely absorbed by direct diffusion. In the blood it travels partly (two-thirds) bound to plasma protein. Normally body stores (half in the liver) hold about 5–10 mg of the vitamin, but the daily requirement is only 50 μ.

Folic acid in the form of tetrahydrofolate acts as a co-enzyme, an acceptor and donor of methyl groups and other one-carbon fragments in enzymatic synthesis of purines and pyrimidines for nucleotides, methionine from homocysteine, and so on. Cyanocobalamin also plays a role in some of these syntheses, but has an additional function with myelin.

Treatment

If a trial of folate is to be made, it will be best given intramuscularly in case there is some gastrointestinal cause for deficiency. A dose of 1 mg i.m. daily for several days and then 0.1 mg orally daily should be tried, with monitoring of blood count and body weight.

Folate should not be used if there are any neurological signs, or any possibility that vitamin B_{12} may also be needed, because folate is useless in the treatment of subacute combined degeneration of the cord.

Pyridoxine (vitamin B₆)
Clinical features

There are uncertainties about the psychiatric significance of this vitamin. Experimentally, in adults lack of the vitamin has resulted in irritability, lethargy, and disorientation (Fabrykant, 1960).

Epileptic fits in infants (and adults) have been recognized as occasionally due to pyridoxine deficiency. The vitamin has been advocated in women who become depressed while on oral contraceptive (oestrogen), in patients who develop peripheral neuritis while on monoamine oxidase inhibitor drugs, and in association with oral tryptophan in the treatment of depression.

However, pyridoxine deficiency is more certainly a cause of seborrholic skin lesions on the face, with glossitis, and of anaemia, and probably of peripheral neuritis.

Setting

Pyridoxine is widespread in foods, and nutritional deficiency in man normally does not occur. The need is greater, however, the greater the animal protein intake, and is also increased by treatment with some drugs (hydrazides, oestrogens). It is likely that deficiency symptoms, giving rise to therapy-resistant anaemia or to epilepsy, result from various metabolic defects, often familial, and always rare.

Mechanism

The vitamin is readily absorbed and is converted into pyridoxal phosphate, the co-enzyme for many transaminases and amino-acid decarboxylases, including those involved in the synthesis and destruction of the inhibitory neuro-transmitter GABA. Free pyridoxal is converted by the liver to pyridoxic acid and excreted in the urine.

Treatment

Pyridoxine should not be given to patients being treated with levo-dopa for Parkinsonism because the co-enzyme enhances the activity of the peripheral decarboxylase converting levo-dopa to dopamine and less levo-dopa is then available to enter the brain.

Pyridoxine 2 mg per day is a normal adult requirement. For treatment, 100 or 200 mg a day may be tried.

5

Reproduction and psychiatric disorders in women*

R. KUMAR

Introduction

Many explanations have been advanced to account for differences between the sexes in the manifestation of common psychiatric disturbances such as depression and anxiety. For example, men and women, irrespective of whether they are patients or doctors, may have acquired different concepts of health and sickness. There may be very particular cultural and social factors which shape the housewife's and the working woman's behaviour and, very importantly, constitutional factors may markedly influence the predispositions of the two sexes to certain kinds of disorder. More women than men consult their doctors or use the available health services for both physical and psychological problems and the prevalence of neurotic disorder amongst women is generally found to be about twice that in men, although there are variations due to age, culture, social class, and the type of disorder. Such broad generalizations are derived from surveys of whole populations (Essen-Möller, 1956; Hagnell, 1970), of general and representative samples (Ingham, Rawnsley & Hughes, 1972; Taylor & Chave, 1964; Dunnell & Cartwright, 1972) and of attenders in general practice (Kessel & Shepherd, 1962; Shepherd et al., 1966). Studies of psychiatric outpatient populations (for example, Ingham et al., 1972; Johnson, 1973) show,

* The survey of literature for this review was completed in July, 1979

however, that disproportionately more men than women are referred on to hospital although, of course, there are differences between types of clinic.

Anorexia nervosa occurs almost exclusively in women; states of anxiety and depression are found roughly twice as often in women, but the pattern of sex differences is influenced by factors such as age and severity. Although men complain less of depression, they are more likely to commit suicide (Kreitman, 1978). Guze and Perley (1963) have characterized hysteria as a 'feminine' disorder but the incidence of conversion symptoms and dissociative states in the sexes is roughly equal (Reed, 1971). Obsessional states occur about as often in men as in women (Carr, 1974) and though social phobias are as prevalent in either sex, women suffer more often from agoraphobia and from animal phobias (Marks, 1969). There are no obvious sex differences in the incidence of schizophrenia, but in the case of manic-depressive disorders, it has been suggested (Winokur, Rimmer & Reich, 1971) that an increased prevalence of alcoholism in male relatives of alcoholic patients may be matched by an increased occurrence of depressive disturbances in female relatives. Cloninger, Christiansen, Reich and Gottesman (1978) have, however, pointed out that the development of such differences may more readily be explained by social and environmental factors than by genetic transmission.

Previous reviewers (Seiden, 1976; Tonks, 1976; Weissman & Klerman, 1977; Clare, 1978) are agreed that the detailed study of sex differences will be of considerable importance in psychiatry. One important aspect of this subject is those disorders to which *only* women are susceptible. These are the major psychiatric disturbances that are specifically associated with female reproductive functions. Disorders of adolescence and of the involutional period are dealt with elsewhere in this series (vols 1, 3, 4, 5; vol. 2, chaps. 3 and 8–13; and see cross-references) and this chapter focuses on the psychiatric disturbances which arise in pregnant and parturient women. These disturbances which are peculiar to women are of course intrinsically important, but they do not necessarily differ in their clinical manifestations from psychiatric disorders in other contexts. Studies of the psychological impact of reproduction in women may therefore have some general as well as specific implications.

Psychiatric aspects of pregnancy

(1) *Psychosis*

Pregnancy, particularly the first one, is a psy-

chological watershed for a woman. The transition to motherhood is a creative process in which fundamental changes in the concept of self and of role are negotiated against a background of resolved and still unsettled developmental 'crises'. The psychological and physical demands of the infant are an essential ingredient in this process of maturation which begins, however, long before the baby is born. For the pregnant woman, becoming a mother means becoming a different sort of child to her own parents, a different sort of sexual partner, and, indeed, a different sort of mother if there are already other children. Temporary or permanent changes of career and of social role can be a direct consequence of pregnancy and are sometimes a source of major difficulty. Given the psychological and physiological upheavals which begin after conception, it is surprising that severe psychiatric disturbances are relatively uncommon in pregnant women (Kendell, Wainwright, Hailey & Shannon, 1976; Paffenbarger, 1964; Pugh, Jerath, Schmidt & Reed, 1963). It has even been suggested that schizophrenia is ameliorated during pregnancy (Baker, 1967; Horsley, 1972; Priest, 1978) but the evidence is anecdotal. There are occasional reports of pre-partum psychosis and of associated harm to the foetus or of subsequent infanticide (e.g. Seymour-Shove, Gee & Cross, 1968; Bucove, 1968) but, fortunately, such catastrophes are rare.

(2) *Neurosis*

The psychological disturbances which occur in the context of unwanted pregnancy are discussed later (p. 64, (6)) and, apart from such specific problems, earlier surveys of women attending general practice (Shepherd, Cooper, Brown & Kalton, 1966) or antenatal clinics (Nilsson & Almgren, 1970) have not provided any evidence of an increased incidence of neurotic disorder amongst pregnant women. It is, however, necessary to carry out prospective, serial assessments beginning early in pregnancy but, even so, the subject's 'base-line' state before pregnancy has to be evaluated retrospectively. A recent study of primiparae has shown that there is an increased incidence of depression during the first trimester (Kumar & Robson, 1978a,b). The subjects had mostly planned their pregnancies and none had sought a termination. They were, however, more likely to be depressed in the first trimester if they had considered having an abortion or, independently, if they had previously had an induced abortion, suggesting that there were underlying psychological problems in maternal adaptation. Ante-natal depression was also associated with a previous history of medical consultation for psychological problems and with concurrent reports of increased marital tension and conflict, which is in keeping with the findings of surveys of the mental health of women in the community. It is notable that after one such survey (Brown & Harris 1978) the authors concluded 'As things turned out in our series there is no evidence that childbirth and pregnancy *as such* (their italics) are linked to depression'. The series to which they refer is a sample of 114 psychiatric in- and out-patients, seventeen of whom were pregnant or had given birth in the previous nine months. These women were contrasted with 382 women who comprised the 'normal' segment of the community sample. Hospital patients are a highly selected population and the stated conclusions might have been more sound had Brown and Harris compared 'cases' in the community with their normal subjects. Returning to their seventeen patients, five had very bad marriages, five lived in grossly inadequate housing, one was unmarried and one had had a miscarriage. In contrast only 6 of 37 pregnant 'normal' women had similar problems. Comparisons of larger groups of childbearing and non-childbearing psychiatric hospital patients may confirm or refute the suggested absence of a link between having a baby and being a depressed *patient* of a mental hospital. Brown and Harris juxtapose marked social adversity and childbearing in twelve of their seventeen patients and then make the generalization that their results 'clearly suggest that it is the meaning of events that is usually crucial: pregnancy and birth, like other crises, can bring home to a woman the hopelessness of her position'. The supporting evidence for such a statement is rather thin and an alternative view is that the process of reproduction may be linked with depression at levels of meaning that extend beyond social adversity (see p. 66, Psychiatric aspects of the puerperium).

(3) *Pseudocyesis*

The syndrome of false pregnancy is rare, and among the symptoms which it comprises are amenorrhoea or hypomenorrhoea, abdominal enlargement, breast changes, reported foetal movements, softening of the cervix and sometimes enlargement of the uterus, nausea and vomiting, and weight gain (Bivin & Klinger, 1937; Moulton, 1942; Fried, Rakoff, Schopbach & Kaplan, 1951). Obstetricians are often taken in by such patients and although there are no characteristic endocrine changes, early studies have shown elevated titres of gonadotrophins and oestro-

gens and reduced FSH (Fried *et al.*, 1951; Steinberg *et al.*, 1946). The diagnosis of pseudocyesis is based upon the presence of a firmly held belief by the patient that she is pregnant and the co-existence of one or more 'physical' symptoms. The diagnosis is confirmed by the presence of an inverted umbilicus (in pregnancy there is effacement of the umbilicus), the absence of a foetus on ultra-sound tests, and the subsidence of the abdominal enlargement during anaesthesia. The differential diagnosis, of course, includes organic causes of abdominal enlargement. In a comprehensive review, Barglow and Brown (1972) note that there are differing views about the true nature of pseudocyesis – it has been looked upon as an illusion, a conversion symptom, a delusion, an hysterical identification, and as a manifestation of a fear of, or a wish for pregnancy, a form of mourning, or as a defence against psychotic breakdown. The symptoms (and signs) typically subside following psychotherapy and unless there is firm evidence of other overt psychological disturbance, medication with psychotropic drugs is not indicated.

(4) *Psychosomatic changes in normal pregnancy*

The traditional (male) concept of the pregnant woman who blooms is occasionally upheld but much the most common picture is presented by women who report a range of unpleasant subjective and somatic disturbances. The early months are a time of almost universal tiredness and reduced energy. Changes in appetite and in food preferences are very common but marked cravings and pica are unusual (Trethowan & Dickens, 1972). Over 50 per cent of pregnant women experience some degree of nausea and a proportion may vomit, but hyperemesis is infrequent (Fairweather, 1968; Tylden, 1968). Libido is typically reduced in early pregnancy and many women report a fear that sexual intercourse will harm the foetus or induce miscarriage. Anxieties about the foetus are universal and can be unnecessarily exacerbated, for example, when medical investigations are carried out without adequate explanation. The ultimate reassurance can only be obtained after the birth of a healthy baby, but sympathetic acceptance and sharing of worries can be of great help to mothers-to-be, particularly if the anxieties are of pathological severity, as can happen in a proportion of women with histories of previous induced abortions (Kumar & Robson, 1978a).

Relationships have been sought between the presence or absence of somatic symptoms of pregnancy, such as vomiting, and a woman's underlying 'acceptance' of her foetus. Two related propositions have been advanced: hyperemesis is a sign of 'rejection' of the foetus and, alternatively, complete lack of nausea is an indication of denial of the pregnancy (Deutsch, 1945). Studies of the extent and severity of normal vomiting and nausea in pregnancy (Uddenberg, Nilsson & Almgren, 1971; Wolkind & Zajicek, 1978) suggest an association between the absence of nausea and the occurrence of emotional disturbance during pregnancy and after childbirth, but possible mechanisms remain obscure. Understanding of underlying psychological factors in hyperemesis is mainly derived from individual case reports.

One clinical reason for psychological investigations of pregnant women is that such enquiries may uncover reliable predictors of post-partum breakdown. Links between excess anxiety during pregnancy and post-natal depression have been described (Tod, 1964; Meares, Grimwade & Wood, 1976) but, in general, there has been little systematic, prospective research into the ante-natal predictors or precursors of post-natal psychiatric disorders. Allowance must be made in such research for various sources of possible bias, for example, the processes of selection which operate when a sizeable minority of pregnant women obtain abortions each year and thus drop out of the population 'at risk.'

(5) Still-birth

The difficulty of coping with stillbirth, particularly by staff is now well recognized (Lewis, 1976; Lewis & Page, 1978) and 'denial' by staff exacerbates parental reactions to the still-birth where there is a lack of a real baby to mourn. It is suggested that the loss be made as tangible as possible and the parents be encouraged to grieve for the death of their baby. Further psychological support may be needed both afterwards and in the special circumstances of a subsequent pregnancy. Similar principles apply when babies are born with congenital malformations.

(6) Termination of pregnancy

Changes in social attitudes, in the law, and in medical practice. In the short place of ten years several nations have executed a remarkable U-turn in their policies concerning the problems of unwanted pregnancy. A discussion of the reasons behind such changes is outside the scope of this review but some of the relevant factors are: improvements in contraception, developments in methods of early abortion,

a more permissive approach to sexual *mores*, a trend towards recognition of women's rights, an increasing awareness of over-population, and a gradual acknowledgement that unwanted pregnancy is a psychological and a social problem. Since the Abortion Act (1967) became effective, about 100 000 legal abortions have been obtained every year by residents of England and Wales and, presumably, there has been a compensatory fall in the illegal abortion rate. A falling birth rate and a steady demand for abortion (DHSS, 1977) illustrates how difficult it is to analyse the efficacy and use of contraceptive measures and it is very likely that many unwanted pregnancies are the outcome of more than just simple errors in contraception. For example, Beard and colleagues (1974) found that only about a third of their sample of 360 women who obtained legal abortions had a poor knowledge of contraception.

The psychiatrist's role. Whereas, ten years ago, a psychiatrist was typically asked to assess whether continuation of a pregnancy to term was likely to have disastrous consequences for the mother's mental health, questions nowadays are much more frequently asked about the extent of a subject's ambivalence and the possibility that, for her, abortion may be a maladaptive way of coping with intrapsychic and interpersonal problems. Such changes are a direct consequence of the decriminalizing of abortion and of removing the necessity to justify the termination on medical grounds. Previously, a doctor was required to be confident that not to terminate the pregnancy could result in the woman becoming a 'physical or mental wreck' (*British Medical Journal*, 1938).

As a profession, psychiatrists have, in general, recognized that it is impossible to evaluate a person's physical and psychological health in isolation from social factors (RMPA, 1966) and have been in favour of liberalizing the laws on abortion. Repeated and regular contact with women in the sort of crisis caused by an unwanted pregnancy leads many doctors to acknowledge that there are very wide grounds for induced abortion. Thus, they hope to prevent the humiliation and risk of illegal procedures and to move away from the need to subject healthy women to unnecessary and detailed psychiatric interviews. Dissenting voices (Sim, 1963; Stafford-Clark, 1967) have argued for much more restraint and, indeed, have maintained that there are very few, or even no, psychiatric indications for terminating a pregnancy and have explicitly discounted severe depression or threat of suicide as grounds. Like-minded gynaecologists (McLaren, 1967) have observed that in their opinion there are *no* valid social grounds for terminating a pregnancy, and other gynaecologists have been quick to point out that it is they and not the psychiatrists who must actually do the operation.

Any pregnant woman seeking abortion needs support and if she is manifestly ambivalent she may need time and help to reach a decision which, in such cases, is often in favour of going to term. Sometimes abortions and requests for repeat abortions overlie major sexual problems and personal as well as marital conflicts, and counselling and psychotherapy may be indicated whatever the decision. The question of competence and responsibility is a particularly difficult one – for example, in cases of subnormality or severe mental illness where there is doubt about a pregnant woman's ability to decide. Fortunately, such cases are rare and, as far as possible, the woman's own wishes must be given prime consideration, but other factors such as possible foetal complications, the presence or absence of a partner, the support and wishes of her family, the woman's ability to cope with a baby and the environment into which the baby will be born, must all bear upon the decision.

In a study of women with mental illness who were refused abortion (Arkle, 1957) it was subsequently noted that while their mental states were little changed, many of the subjects (mental defectives, psychotics, psychopaths) were quite unable to look after their children or their homes. Where there is a history of relevant previous psychiatric disorder and a high risk of relapse, as in women who have previously had puerperal psychotic breakdowns, it is important that the risks are fully explained so that the pregnant woman, and her partner if she wishes it, can reach a very difficult personal decision with the maximum amount of information available. It is estimated that the risks of a recurrence of psychosis are a hundredfold greater in a subsequent pregnancy, i.e. between 10 per cent and 20 per cent as compared with the general rate of 1–2 per 1000 deliveries (Granville-Grossman, 1971).

In a summary of the changes which have been made internationally in laws on abortion, Cook and Dickens (1978) note that the criteria upon which the abortion decision is based vary greatly from country to country and they range from the strictly medical down to simple request during the first trimester, as in Austria, Denmark, East Germany, France, Singa-

pore, Sweden, Tunisia, and the United States. Some countries, Bulgaria, Czechoslovakia, and Hungary, which previously allowed abortion 'on demand' have tightened up their regulations and there are also repeated attempts in England and Wales to amend (restrict) the Abortion Act of 1967. The comparative ease with which abortion can be obtained places an obligation on doctors to provide informed support at a time of crisis for a woman and her family and to acknowledge that they are not alone in their respect for human life.

Terms of the Abortion Act (*1967*). The decision to terminate a pregnancy can be part of an emergency procedure to save the mother's life but in all other circumstances the law requires two doctors to certify that they are 'of the opinion in good faith' that in the case of the patient the pregnancy meets one or more of the following conditions:

(1) continuance would involve risk to the life of the pregnant woman greater than if the pregnancy were terminated;

(2) continuance would involve risk of injury to the physical or mental health of the pregnant woman greater than if the pregnancy were terminated;

(3) continuance would involve risk of injury to the physical or mental health of the existing child(ren) of the family of the pregnant woman greater than if the pregnancy were terminated;

(4) there is a substantial risk that if the child were born it would suffer from such physical or mental abnormalities as to be seriously handicapped.

The act stipulates that the abortion must normally be carried out in an NHS hospital or other approved place. The gynaecologist who performs the abortion need not be one of the two doctors who have certified that abortion is indicated, and a gynaecologist can object on conscientious grounds to performing the operation in which case the patient may be referred elsewhere.

Between 1971 and 1977, 60 per cent of women have regularly gone outside the NHS for their terminations. In some instances this has been because of marked regional variations in the provision of services in the NHS (Coles, 1975; Fowkes, Catford & Logan, 1979) but there are some other important general differences. Women treated in the private sector have always had a quicker service and, consequently, a greater number of abortions in the NHS have been done at a later gestational stage. Thus only some of the delays can be explained on strictly clinical grounds. More single women and multiparous women obtain private sector abortions and a multiparous woman with two children who has her pregnancy terminated is much more likely to be simultaneously sterilized if she is treated in the NHS than in the private sector (36 per cent v. 3 per cent of such women respectively were sterilized in 1975). As Fowkes and colleagues (1979) observe, the time of abortion may not be the optimum occasion for a woman to make major decisions about her future fertility.

There is no easy solution to the moral dilemma posed by abortion and the problem is made even more complicated by recent medical advances. The criteria for independent life of the embryo/foetus need to be clarified. Younger and younger foetuses are surviving and demonstrations that the fertilized ovum can be temporarily maintained outside the uterus have underlined the difficulties facing lawyers who would like clear definitions about the status of the embryo. The law is similarly murky about the distinction between contraception and abortion (Tunkel, 1979).

Psychological sequelae of induced abortion. Moderate to severe guilt feelings are commonly recorded after legal and illegal abortion (Ekblad, 1955; Simon & Senturia, 1966; Osofsky & Osofsky, 1972; Greer *et al.*, 1976) but, typically, such feelings are shortlived. Feelings of grief and guilt can, however, persist and in some cases they remain dormant until they are 'reawakened' by a subsequent pregnancy (Kumar & Robson, 1978a). Severe mental illness, for example, psychotic breakdowns analogous to puerperal psychosis, are virtually unknown (Brewer, 1977), and most investigators have found that states of depression and anxiety lift once the pregnancy has been terminated. Much of the early research into the impact of abortion in women with prior psychiatric disturbance is suspect because women often had to manifest a degree of disorder that was sufficient to convince doctors that abortion was indicated. As a general rule, women are more likely to experience psychiatric disturbances after an abortion if they already have a previous history of psychiatric disorder, but several studies have shown that the incidence of depression after legal abortion is low (Ekblad, 1955; Pare & Raven, 1970; Lask, 1975; Greer *et al.*, 1976). Many more women are depressed after childbirth (Pitt, 1968; Nilsson & Almgren, 1970; Kumar & Robson, 1978b) than after abortion but such direct comparisons are compli-

cated by the way in which the populations have selected themselves.

Psychological sequelae of refused abortion. Illsley and Hall (1976) draw attention to three reasons why studies of refused abortion must be interpreted with caution: subjects who are refused abortion may be more 'stable' than those whose requests were granted; those refused may obtain abortions elsewhere, legally or illegally; follow-up is likely to be incomplete, particularly when subjects associate the research staff with the people who originally refused the abortion.

Among the adverse psychiatric sequelae which have been noted in studies of refused abortion are an increased risk of suicide (Whitlock & Edwards, 1968; Tylden, 1966; Visram, 1972) increased likelihood of depression (Höök, 1963; Pare & Raven, 1970), persistent regrets about the refused abortion in a proportion of subjects, and problems in accepting the originally unwanted baby, as well as subsequent repercussions in the child – e.g. antisocial behaviour and incidence of psychiatric disturbance (Forssman & Thuwe, 1966). There can be few more cogent arguments for not making it more difficult to obtain an abortion than the concluding comments in the review by Illsley and Hall (1976), 'it seems that, although many women who are refused abortion adjust to their situation and grow to love the child, about half would still have preferred abortion, a large minority suffer considerable distress and a small minority develop severe disturbance'.

Psychiatric aspects of the puerperium
(1) *Post-partum or maternity 'blues'*

Many recently delivered women experience transient episodes of tearfulness, emotional vulnerability and mild depression four or five days after the birth of their babies (Yalom, Lunde, Moos & Hamburg, 1968). Pitt (1973) noted that there was no obvious basis for their worries in a large proportion of subjects with the 'blues' and he had an impression of mild impairments of concentration, memory, and learning which led him to suggest that there might be a hormonal basis for these brief psychological disturbances. Subsequent investigations (Stein *et al.*, 1976; Handley *et al.*, 1977) of possible underlying neuroendocrine and neuro-transmitter mechanisms have been inconclusive and Gelder (1978) has drawn attention to the risks of making connections between parallel events, in this case mood changes and variations in biological functions. The importance of the 'blues' as warning signals of more serious disturbance in the offing, for example post-natal depression or psychotic breakdown is compromised by their ubiquity – they occur in up to two thirds of mothers. Apart from post-delivery hormonal and other metabolic changes, factors which may contribute to the blues include psychic trauma following 'separation' from the baby, the changes associated with lactation, pain and soreness, lack of sleep, and the effects of hospitalization.

(2) *Post-natal depression*

The incidence of depression is believed to be raised during the first few months after childbirth (Tod, 1964; Pitt, 1968; Nilsson & Almgren, 1970; Dalton, 1971; Meares *et al.*, 1976; Kumar & Robson, 1978b) but differences in methods of sampling and data gathering and in criteria for depression are probably responsible for considerable divergences in the rates reported by different investigators. Pitt (1968) found that about 11 per cent of women participating in his survey became depressed in the six weeks or so after delivery, a rate of occurrence which has been broadly confirmed in a subsequent study by Kumar & Robson (1978b).

Investigations of possible metabolic causes of post-natal depression have so far been inconclusive (Coppen, Stein & Wood, 1978; Nott, Franklin, Armitage & Gelder, 1976) and in a proportion of cases, at least, it is possible to point to psychological and social contributory factors – for example lower social class, marital disharmony, poor housing, and so on (Brown & Harris, 1978). In a survey of primiparae (Kumar & Robson, 1978b) it was found that post-natal depression occurred more frequently in women who had originally entertained doubts about continuing with their pregnancies or in those who had described difficulties in their relationships with their parents. The women were also more likely to become depressed if they were aged 30 or more years or if they had experienced problems in conceiving.

The clinical picture of post-natal depression is similar to depression in other circumstances and it is striking how few women either seek, or are seen as being in need of, support and perhaps medication. The course of such depression is also similar to depression unrelated to childbirth in that the majority of cases improve relatively quickly, but a small proportion may persist for up to a year (Pitt, 1968).

Post-natal depression may have repercussions on the child. Any difficulties in adjusting to being a mother are likely to be exacerbated by the symptoms of depression, for example increased irritability, lowered self-esteem, guilt, inability to cope. There have not been any systematic prospective studies of the ways in which the children of depressed mothers may be affected.

Management of post-natal depression. Depressions of moderate severity typically remit within a few months and in puerperal women the process of remission may be considerably facilitated by simple supportive measures – for example reduction of isolation, identification of sources of stress and hence their avoidance or mitigation. Adjustment of sleeping patterns and sharing of feeding responsibilities can often be of great help, but there are mothers who express their inner conflicts by an inability to allow their infant a separate existence; they scrutinize the baby's every movement and, although they complain of exhaustion and misery, they are resistant to counselling and support. Maternal depression is very often present when a mother consults repeatedly on behalf of her (usually healthy) baby. In cases of severe or persistent depression, marked improvements can be obtained upon treatment with antidepressants (see p. 71).

(3) *'Puerperal psychosis'*

The heading for this section is qualified by quotation marks because the official view, which is embodied in the International Classification of Diseases, 8th revision and associated Glossaries of mental disorders (WHO, 1974 and HMSO, 1968) is that, as a clinical entity, puerperal psychosis does not exist. This view is presumably not shared by the one or two in every thousand recently delivered women who are often unexpectedly, and usually catastrophically, afflicted with a severe mental illness.

The original descriptions of puerperal insanity are ascribed to Hippocrates although it is likely that he was documenting instances of toxic confusional states and delirium in cases of puerperal sepsis. Some comments by earlier observers may convey a flavour of the history of the controversy surrounding puerperal psychosis.

> In women, blood collected in the breasts indicates madness.
> Hippocrates (400 BC; transl. Adams, 1939)

> It is needless, here, to give a minute and detailed description of mania and melancholia

in child-bed or suckling women; it is generally like mania and melancholia under other circumstances . . . there is no end to the diversity which the symptoms are capable of assuming.
Robert Gooch (1820)

There is a 'lacteal diathesis' which modifies all the secretions of the female and impresses upon them its own character.
E. Esquirol (1838)

Affections of the uterus and its appendages afford notable examples of a powerful sympathetic action upon the brain, and not infrequently play an important part in the production of insanity, especially of melancholia.
H. Maudsley (1899)

People often speak of 'puerperal mania' in the sense of a particular form of insanity produced exclusively by the puerperium . . . The puerperium cannot be regarded as the cause, but as the last impulse to the outbreak of the disease (manic-depressive insanity). As a rule the pictures of disease which develop in the puerperal state are not maniacal at all . . . katatonic states of excitement are particularly common.
E. Kraepelin (1906)

Brockington, Schofield, Donnelly & Hyde (1978) reviewed a series of studies carried out between 1911 and 1978 in which patients with post-partum psychoses were assigned to particular diagnostic categories. They found, as might be expected, that toxic psychoses had become much less common in the past thirty years and, while American investigators had continued reporting a preponderance of schizophrenic disorders, British psychiatrists were more likely to make a diagnosis of affective psychosis. Such differences are in keeping with national differences in diagnostic habits (Cooper *et al.*, 1972), and Brockington and colleagues (1978) concluded, 'the truth is that hospital diagnostic concepts are far too variable and unstable (geographically and historically) to be capable of resolving a difficult nosological problem such as that of post-partum psychosis'. A hundred years before, Savage (1875) had been lamenting 'We have not yet got beyond what Dr. Hughlings Jackson calls the market gardeners classification; we have not been able to form natural orders like the botanists, or at least we have not many natural orders yet'.

Another reason advanced for eschewing the concept of puerperal psychosis as a clinical entity was that psychiatrists disagreed over the correct defini-

tion of the puerperium, i.e. the time interval after the birth during which a psychosis could properly be called 'puerperal'. Investigators varied between 6 weeks, 6 months, and a year in their definition of the puerperium (Granville-Grossman, 1971) and, not surprisingly, they disagreed in their assessments of the incidence of psychotic illnesses. As a result, it was recommended that the existence of puerperal psychosis was best denied and its occurrence should only be diagnosed *in extremis* when the condition could not be fitted in, for example under the label of schizophrenia or manic-depressive psychosis.

Paffenbarger (1964), Pugh and colleagues (1963) and, more recently, Kendell and colleagues (1976) have, incidentally, all pointed to a clear relation with childbirth and a peak incidence within the first three months, or even the first two or three weeks (Brockington *et al.*, 1978; Hamilton, 1962). Because the appropriate clinical diagnosis, for example schizophrenia or manic-depressive psychosis, is not qualified in most coding systems with the further information that the illness followed childbirth, as childbirth is not a disease, it immediately becomes very difficult to identify cases. Retrospective epidemiological surveys of this relatively rare condition are therefore now largely restricted to places which keep case-registers (see Kendell *et al.*, 1976). Nevertheless, the application of standardized interviewing techniques and of improved methods for making psychiatric diagnoses may eventually help to locate puerperal psychosis in its correct slot in the 'market gardener's' classification – perhaps as a rare species on its own.

Clinical features. In a comprehensive survey of puerperal psychosis, Hamilton (1962) observed that the illness typically never began before the third day post-partum. After a lucid interval, many patients began to show their first symptoms towards the end of the first week, and over half were manifesting some symptoms by a fortnight after delivery. The asymptomatic latent period and the early prodromal symptoms are rarely, if ever, directly observed by psychiatrists since there is no cause for alarm at this stage. Nevertheless, it is generally accepted that the early manifestations include symptoms such as insomnia, restlessness, exhaustion, depression, irritability, headache, and changeability of mood. The similarity between such a clinical picture and the 'blues' suggests that the transient mood disturbances which occur in the majority of recently delivered women may have been mistakenly and retrospectively assigned special significance as prodromal symptoms. Only prospective studies can resolve such questions but they are unlikely to be undertaken when the incidence of 'cases' is estimated as one or two per thousand deliveries.

The later onset of symptoms such as suspiciousness, confusion, incoherence, and irrationality, and of unusual reactions to the baby, are more sinister warnings of impending psychosis. The clinical picture may take the form of an affective psychosis, manic or depressive in type, or of a schizophrenic illness, or it may take a mixed 'schizo-manic' form. Brockington and colleagues (1978) have attempted a detailed analysis of symptoms based upon carefully edited transcripts of the mental states and behaviours of post-partum patients from which 'all non-psychopathological clues to the post-partum state had been removed'. In comparison with controls, such patients manifested significantly more agitation, lability of mood, loss of social reserve, and 'clouding' or confusion of thinking. It is acknowledged that methodological problems inevitably complicate such studies and the nosological status of puerperal psychosis is still a major clinical challenge, as is the almost total lack of understanding of underlying biological mechanisms. Some clues may be found in observations that women who have suffered previous puerperal psychotic illness have a hundredfold greater risk of breakdown following a subsequent pregnancy (Paffenbarger, 1964) and that women with a previous history of manic-depressive illness have a similar high risk (about one in five) of developing puerperal psychosis (Bratfos & Haug, 1966; Reich & Winokur, 1970).

Treatment. The choice of physical treatment for puerperal illness depends upon the predominant clinical picture. Women with manic or schizo-manic symptoms respond to medication with neuroleptic drugs and/or lithium. Antidepressants may be given initially but many severely depressed women eventually require ECT (Freeman, 1979). Patients with a primarily schizophrenic disorder may require maintenance therapy with neuroleptics (see p. 71). The immediate response to treatment is usually good and most such women are discharged within 2–3 months but still require very careful out-patient supervision. A subsequent relapse that is unrelated to any future pregnancies is estimated to occur in about 30 per cent to 50 per cent of subjects.

Ideally, all mothers should be admitted to specialized mother-and-baby units where particular nursing skills are available and attempts can be made to preserve mothering capabilities and to foster the 'bond'. Special attention is also needed when mothers express infanticidal impulses or when they are in acute and disorganized psychotic states. Nursing apart from the baby, with supervised and graded mother-and-baby contact is the general rule in such cases until remission allows more freedom (Protheroe, 1977). Administrative flexibility may be needed if there are other young siblings to be cared for and whenever possible, fathers should be involved in the treatment programme both in hospital and after discharge. The number of places provided by specialized mother-and-baby units falls far short of demand, but while the provision of 'centres' allows for the concentration of skills and resources, there are inevitable disadvantages associated with increased distance from the patient's home. In hospital, mothers are often nursed in side rooms of wards where extra facilities can be provided to meet their needs but the amount of contact with the baby may depend less upon the mother's condition and more upon the availability of staff and the state of the other patients on the ward.

Forensic aspects of puerperal psychosis. The Infanticide Act 1938 states 'where a woman by any wilful act or omission causes the death of her child under the age of 12 months, but at the time of the act or omission the balance of her mind was disturbed by reason of her not having fully recovered from the effect of giving birth to the child or by reason of the effect of lactation consequent upon the birth of the child, then notwithstanding that the circumstances were such that but for this Act the offence would have amounted to murder she shall be guilty of an offence, to wit of infanticide, and may for such offence be dealt with and punished as if she had been guilty of the offence of manslaughter of the child'.

Although the law seems to be concerned with puerperal insanity, and indeed even cites the lactational hypothesis, it appears that diagnoses such as personality disorder or reactive depression are much more commonly made in cases where mothers kill their babies than is the diagnosis of puerperal psychosis which applies to about 5 per cent to 15 per cent of cases (Bluglass, 1978; d'Orban, 1979). As Bluglass (1978) observes, the offence of infanticide has some unique features – the defence is not required to demonstrate that the killing was the result of the mother's disturbed state of mind, simply that there was disturbance. As with other kinds of manslaughter, the judge is able to exercise complete flexibility, in his sentencing of the woman, from absolute discharge to life imprisonment.

Psychotropic drugs, pregnancy and the puerperium

(1) *Early pregnancy*

There are two main periods during pregnancy when the foetus is particularly vulnerable to the placental transfer of drugs: in early pregnancy when the drugs may exert a teratogenic action and just before and during labour and delivery. The breast-fed neonate is also vulnerable to chemicals which appear in its mother's milk.

Teratogenicity. The literature is patchy and, while there are often reports of undesirable effects in animals, extrapolations to man are heavily qualified by differences between species in their ways of absorption, distribution, metabolism, and excretion of drugs as well as in their susceptibilities to particular actions. Many animal reports have been derived from toxicity studies in which very large doses of drugs have been used.

There appears to have been an increasing clinical and client awareness of the dangers of drug-taking in pregnancy, and so it may appear somewhat alarming that pregnant women consume more prescribed drugs than over-the-counter preparations (Forfar & Nelson, 1973; Hill *et al.*, 1977) and that psychotropic drugs comprise the fourth largest category of drugs taken by pregnant women (see review by Lewis, 1978). However, the great majority of these drugs are prescribed for other than psychiatric purposes, for example phenothiazines for nausea and barbiturates for high blood pressure. Thus the actual psychiatric prescribing in the first trimester is very small and it is encouraging to see that both patients and doctors can in some circumstances resist the pressures which have led to the present levels of over-consumption of psychotropic drugs.

There have been isolated case reports linking congenital abnormalities with almost all psychotropic drugs. Slight associations between benzodiazepine use and cleft palate have been described and between phenothiazines and butyrophenones and a range of abnormalities, but firm evidence is lacking in the case of neuroleptics. Isolated reports of malformations in babies of mothers who took antidepressant drugs in early pregnancy have not been substantiated by controlled studies, but lithium use in the first trimester has been linked with an increased incidence of cardiovascular abnormalities. Monoamine oxidase inhibitors are even less safe in pregnancy than at other times because of the possible interactions which may occur, should, for example, the mother require anaesthesia or sympathomimetic drugs – for example if an operation is necessary or she is in premature labour or threatens abortion. Anticonvulsants are linked with a small increase in congenital malformation and research with these substances illustrates the difficulties of teasing out the contribution of the drugs and possible effects due to the underlying illness itself (see reviews by Forrest, 1976; Tylden, 1977; Cooper, 1978; Lewis, 1978).

Apart from the patients who misuse drugs or those who take overdoses in early pregnancy, there is one very small group of patients who can pose extremely difficult problems for the clinician. Very occasionally a pregnant woman may require urgent treatment with drugs; this may be necessary if a psychotic illness develops during pregnancy or if the woman conceives while she is acutely ill, for example during a hypomanic episode. Each patient has to be assessed on her own merits but appropriate medication should not be withheld because the woman is pregnant. Electroconvulsive therapy is best avoided because of problems associated with anaesthesia, muscle relaxation, and possible anoxia. There may, however, be overriding clinical reasons for prescribing ECT and in such cases the expert contribution of an anaesthetist is essential.

The problem of what to do about maintenance therapy depends as much upon the relevant clinical history of a patient who becomes pregnant as it does upon the drugs she is taking. Against the risk of relapse in the common neurotic disturbances, where antidepressants and benzodiazepines are usually prescribed, must be balanced the rapidly changing biological and psychological state of the subject, as well as her peace of mind. It is usually better to withhold such drugs as well as hypnotics, after full discussion with the patient. Phenothiazines and related drugs are cleared very slowly, and stopping maintenance therapy, for example, in a schizophrenic woman who becomes pregnant, is like leaving the stable door open and finding that the horse will not bolt. Lithium, on the other hand, is rapidly excreted and, where possible, treatment should not be restarted or continued during the first trimester of pregnancy. Starting long-term lithium prophylactic treatment in women of childbearing age should not therefore be lightly decided upon.

Occupational and environmental hazards to the foetus. The large-scale use of defoliant, herbicidal, and pesticidal chemicals is alleged to be responsible for both increased rates of abortion as well as of malformation. Particular professions that are 'at risk' include anaesthetists and operating theatre staff who are regularly exposed to volatile anaesthetics, radiographers and other individuals exposed to irradiation, and certain workers in industry where careless exposure to chemicals, for example pharmaceuticals, might lead to an increased chance of abortion or foetal malformation.

(2) *Late pregnancy, labour and delivery*

The foetus is susceptible to most psychotropic drugs which cross the placenta with ease because they are lipophilic and hence also penetrate the foetal brain tissue. Analgesics, sedative/hypnotics, and anxiolytics all depress foetal cerebral functioning and a 'drugged' neonate is more likely to manifest respiratory problems, feeding difficulties, and poor temperature regulation. Benzodiazepines, for example, are poorly metabolized by the neonate and they result in the 'floppy infant' syndrome (Patrick, Tilstone & Reavy, 1972). Overdose with opioid analgesics can cause respiratory depression in the neonate which is reversible by naloxone. Naloxone is, however, contraindicated in the opioid-dependent neonate.

Prolonged use of phenothiazines during pregnancy has been reported in isolated instances to cause foetal hepatitis (Beecham, Braun, Clapp & Lucey, 1973) and extrapyramidal signs in the neonate (Hill, Desmond & Kay, 1966; Levy & Wisniewski, 1974) and long-term imipramine medication is said to be associated with neonatal 'irritability' (Eggermont, Raveschot, Deneve & Casteels-Van Daele, 1972).

Subtle behavioural and psychological sequelae in children of women who take certain drugs in pregnancy may be suspected on the basis of animal studies (reviewed by Lewis, 1978) and one instance of 'behavioural teratogenicity' may emerge out of the controversy surrounding the consequences for the infant of maternal smoking during pregnancy.

(3) *Puerperium: psychotropic drugs for lactating women*

Tricyclic antidepressants appear in very small amounts in breast milk and no adverse effects seem to have been described. Benzodiazepines are found in breast milk in appreciable quantities and regular daily medication can produce sedative/depressant effects in the breast-fed infant. Propranolol is also found in breast milk and associated neonatal respiratory and cardiovascular difficulties have been reported (Forrest, 1976; Savage, 1976). Lithium appears in the maternal milk at about one-third to one-half of the concentration found in the mother's serum (Schou & Amdisen, 1973) and the babies of such mothers should be bottle-fed. Certain phenothiazines and butyrophenones have been detected in human and bovine milk in relatively large concentrations (one-third and two-thirds of those in the maternal serum (Vorherr, 1974; Ziv *et al.*, 1974) but adverse effects in babies have not so far been described. It seems more appropriate, anyway, to bottle-feed infants when the clinical condition of the mother is such that large doses of neuroleptic drugs are indicated.

(4) *The pregnant addict*

Pregnancy multiplies the clinical problems which arise in patients who abuse drugs. Addicts are often unreliable historians and are erratic in their attendance at clinics and the obstetrician may therefore find that he has to contend with uncertainty over dates, dietary deficiencies, intercurrent infections, such as hepatitis caused by needle-sharing, and increased risks of spontaneous abortion and later of toxaemia.

Teratogenicity. Multiple, or poly-drug abuse is very common and it is therefore difficult to make generalizations about the risks of teratogenicity, but prematurity, low birth weight and obstetric complications are common in addicts. Drugs of abuse with known, or suspected teratogenic properties include barbiturates, opioids, hallucinogens, cannabis and amphetamines. The status of the foetal alcohol syndrome is controversial (Kessel, 1977) (see also chap. 14, p. 207), and it is probably wise anyway for pregnant alcohol users to refrain or to reduce their consumption. Tobacco smoking is strongly discouraged on account of the adverse effects on the foetus. One problem which affects drug users and abusers alike is that they may have continued taking psychotropic drugs for a time before realizing that they were pregnant. Advice and reassurance is often sought in such circumstances but relatively little is known about the timing, nature, and extent of risk to the pregnancy and to the foetus from a wide range of psychotropic and other drugs.

Toxic and withdrawal effects. Opiate addicts have an increased risk of spontaneous abortion and they also present special problems because their babies may develop an opiate withdrawal syndrome soon after delivery. Planned induction can ensure that the delivery takes place in a hospital where the mother's drug-intake is known and a special care unit is available for the baby (Fraser, 1976). The infant's opioid abstinence syndrome is characterized by tremors, sneezing, watery stools, yawning, shrill crying, hypersensitivity to stimulation, and, sometimes, convulsions. Benzodiazepines or phenothiazines have been recommended to 'cover' the abstinence syndrome but the rationale for this is unclear and these drugs have adverse effects of their own. Opioid drugs appear in breast-milk and if, for example, the mother is maintained on methadone she should be advised to bottle-feed her baby. There are, incidentally, insufficient quantities of opioids in breast-milk to prevent, or substantially mitigate, the abstinence syndrome in the infant. Administering opioids in decreasing doses to the neonate is one way of managing the withdrawal syndrome but respiratory depression can easily develop as a result of inaccurate dosage, and prophylatic treatment with methadone should be avoided (Ghodse, Reed & Mack, 1977).

Salicylate abuse in late pregnancy can result in haemorrhagic disorders in the newborn. Barbiturates if taken in large doses around the time of delivery can cause respiratory depression and there are occasional reports of barbiturate-dependent neonates who develop withdrawal convulsions. As already mentioned, excessive use of benzodiazepines results in the 'floppy-infant' syndrome, but no abstinence phenomena seem to have been described, probably because of the slow rates of clearance of these drugs.

The pregnant addict exemplifies above all the importance of preventive measures. The need to develop methods of prevention as well as effective treatments is, of course, a general problem in all health programmes. Improvements in maternal and infant mortality and morbidity in recent years have not been matched by similar improvements in maternal mental health, but there are some signs of gathering momentum to investigate and hopefully to try and alleviate the psychological problems of mothers and the problems which may lie in store for their offspring.

PART II
Neurological disorders

6
Disorders of sleep

IAN OSWALD

The doctor's commonest act in psychological treatment is the prescription of a drug that promotes sleep. This is true even if it is nominally intended to ease anxiety by day, for the drugs are the same, and diazepam taken this morning is so long-acting that it will still be there tonight, and tomorrow night too.

Some patients complain of too little sleep, a few of too much. Those who are deviant in either of these ways have a higher death rate in the next few years than those who describe a conventional eight hours (Kripke, Simons, Garfinkel & Hammond, 1979). Psychiatrists associate the complaint of too little sleep with anxiety and depression, but it is as often found with organic brain disorders, alcoholism and personality disorders (McGhie, 1966).

Not enough sleep

Complaints of insufficient sleep become commoner with increasing age, and are commoner among females and those of nervous temperament (McGhie & Russell, 1962; Karacan et al., 1976). Young adults complain especially of difficulty in falling asleep and older folk of repeated awakenings.

The psychiatric history may reveal the source of anxiety. Enquiries should be made about the habits of life, such as the times of going to bed and getting up. Many young people drink coffee in the evening and yet sleep well. As they grow older they go on drinking it, not realizing that it keeps the older brain awake (Březinová, 1974). A 50-year-old businessman from West Africa recently explained how he could not sleep. In his hot country he was drinking eight bottles of Coca-Cola each evening, a drink full of caffeine. A young woman hesitated to explain how she could not get to sleep because of an itchy anus. She had threadworms.

Some will say they are so tired because they 'just can't fall asleep' that they don't get up till nine or ten in the morning. Of course they cannot get to sleep. The hour when we get sleepy is determined by our biological clock. Those who regularly get up at six to milk the cows are sleepy by ten at night, those who get up at ten are not. It is the time when we get up that is important, not when we go to bed, and if the person flew to live in India she would soon find she was getting up five hours earlier and falling asleep five hours earlier than the time she does now by her British clock. We learn the hour for falling asleep and the hour for waking up. The transition to a new clock schedule is easy for some, difficult for others. The disorganization of bodily rhythms associated with shift work is often associated with increased emotional lability, to a point where shift work may have to be abandoned.

Depressive illness is associated in clinical practice with reports of early morning waking. Electrophysiological recordings show sleep to be fragmented and light at all times of night (Mendels & Hawkins, 1971) and it is probably the black cloud of depression, descending at about two in the morning, that makes the later awakenings memorable. Many people wake early, but the psychiatrist wants to know the mental content while awake: 'Happy thoughts or unhappy thoughts?', 'Morbid thoughts?', 'Wondering how to face the day?' The hypomanic patient does not complain, but may agree she was up at four, singing and whistling about the house.

Alcohol is a common cause of broken sleep. It first makes us sleepy and then its withdrawal causes rebound insomnia. The insomnia is extreme in delirium tremens, but in a less dramatic way this rapidly-metabolized hypnotic and anti-anxiety drug is followed by agitation six or seven hours after ordinary intake, by irritability during the day, or sleeplessness at five in the morning, with or without gastritis. The harassed businessman taking short drinks at lunch and in the evening should stop drinking rather than resort to benzodiazepines for his symptoms. The 60-year-old labourer, in the general ward for physical investigation, who is noisy and restless at night, who says the nurses are trying to poison him and that a relative was laughing at him from the ward door this morning, will cause the doctor to think of unaccustomed abstinence from alcohol.

Hypnotic drugs likewise perpetuate, if they do not cause, poor sleep. The short-acting ones, such as sodium amylobarbitone will, like alcohol, make sleep less restless in the early night and more broken during a late-night rebound. Regular intake of the long-acting, cumulative drugs, such as flurazepam, or phenobarbitone, give patients about as high a tissue level by day as by night. The biological clock that would strive to make the patient sleepy by eleven at night, and not at eleven in the morning, is swamped into insignificance by compounds the actions of which are constantly present.

Respiratory deficiency, heart failure, pain, and the anxiety of illness all cause insomnia, especially in an unfamiliar, general hospital environment. Chronic bronchitis and emphysema are common, 'sleep apnoea' is not, but it disturbs sleep, and is discussed below. Loss of weight causes broken sleep. Fat people are less anxious and sleep longer (Crisp & McGuiness, 1976; Adam, 1977). Worst is the short, broken sleep of the patient with anorexia nervosa, whose sleep returns to normal after return to normal weight (Lacey *et al.*, 1975). Crisp and Stonehill (1973) studied 375 psychiatric out-patients. One observer rated any recent sleep change, another independently rated weight change, another mood change. Loss of weight was associated with broken sleep, independently of mood. Weight loss may play a role in the broken sleep of depressed patients and of the wasted patient with early dementia.

Old age and dementia are associated with broken sleep and wanderings in the night. Laboratory studies have shown that the degree of cognitive deterioration, the diminution of REM sleep, the degree to which sleep is broken by periods of wakefulness and the degree by which cerebral oxygen consumption is reduced, are closely correlated (Feinberg, Koresko & Heller, 1967). It all begins as we enter our thirties.

Chronic primary insomnia is a term used when the symptom cannot be understood as secondary to other disorders. I believe that for many it is a matter of attitudes: because unbroken sleep was enjoyed in younger years it must imply that tonight's broken sleep represents a disorder deserving of treatment. But we did not have wrinkles or grey hair in our twenties either! Hypnotic drugs should be used rarely and briefly, although some patients seem to believe that the drugs are like telephones – features of modern life that are asked for and need not be denied.

Certainly, those patients who say they do not sleep a wink all night usually sleep for six or seven hours when investigated. In the laboratory, chronic insomniacs on average do sleep worse than controls, though no worse than many others of the same age who have no complaints. Those workers who have found a difference from controls wrote that their insomniac out-patients agreed to give up hypnotic drugs two weeks (Gaillard, 1978) and four weeks (Frankel, Coursey, Buchbinder & Snyder, 1976) in advance. My patients too will agree to stop their drugs, but sometimes nevertheless continue them in secret. I therefore wonder if what has been reported might have been partly the poor sleep of more immediate drug withdrawal. At present it is easier to measure the minutes of sleep than its restorative qualities.

The doctor should seek to treat the primary disorder if, as with depression, he has an effective treatment. He should encourage the patient to adopt a sensible rhythm of sleep–wakefulness habits, to take more and regular physical exercise, for exercise by day promotes sleepiness in the evening (and more growth hormone during sleep), and to regulate the intake of caffeine and of alcohol. He will recognize that there are a few individuals, among the blind, (Miles, Raynal & Wilson, 1977) or among those who reject social conventions, whose biological clocks are not entrained to a 24-hour cycle and who will claim that they cannot conform to that clock by sleeping regularly, no matter the conflict with those around them (Kokkoris et al., 1978).

The doctor will think of prescribing sleeping pills. He likes to see himself as a kindly helper to his patient, who is usually a female. His own emotions become involved through her appeals for his help, and he may be reluctant to face the truth, that he cannot change her dissatisfaction with her family, her life by day, or her sleep by night. If he cannot resist the impulse to prescribe, he should remember that his pills may be taken in overdose and so should be safe, that they should be active in small dosage and be as non-cumulative as possible, that they could impair her skill and discretion by day (Oswald, Adam, Borrow & Idzikowski, 1979) and perhaps render her more prone to ill-judged aggression (British

Medical Journal, 1975) or even to shoplifting. He should especially remember that the older patient's brain is more sensitive to benzodiazepines (Castleden, George, Mercer & Hallett, 1977), and that what the patient says about her sleep after use of the drug may depend more on her personality than on its pharmacology (Oswald, Březinová & Carruthers-Jones, 1975). He should try to prescribe, not because of the patient's cajolings, but because of stress from which he can foresee recovery, and should from the outset share with the patient his expectation of an early end to the prescriptions (Clift, 1972).

Too much sleep

The psychiatrist less often meets the patient who complains of being too sleepy, but a proportion of those who complain of lack of energy, of tiredness, or of difficulty in concentration, or who have fallen foul of employers through unpunctuality or erratic work, are sufferers from unrecognized disorder of sleep. Poor sleep at night can mean a genuine lack of restoration, and fatigue by day.

Idiopathic narcolepsy is the easiest syndrome to recognize. The patient falls asleep for 10–15 minutes, two or three times a day, especially when conditions favour drowsiness, as during boredom or rhythmic activity. He fails to get off the bus at the appropriate stop, or he falls asleep at the meal table, at the cinema, or across his desk at work, to the annoyance of his wife, girl-friend, or employer. The secretary's typing tails off into nonsense, the driver runs into the back of the vehicle in front (Broughton & Ghanem, 1976). Walking down the street he may see double, and as he becomes drowsier people take him for drunk. One of my patients thus walked under a bus.

With the onset of the sleep attacks, he probably gained weight, and a year or two later, or occasionally as a first symptom, came to have cataplectic attacks, with brief loss of muscle tone, in response to a social situation that provokes laughter, anger, fear, or triumph. One patient will have to sit down before a friend tells a joke, another will crumple up when feeling he has outsmarted someone, or when he has a good hand at cards. There may be a falling in the street, a sudden sagging of the jaw, or just 'a funny, weak, trembly feeling in my arms'.

The two other classical features of idiopathic narcolepsy are sleep paralysis (a feeling of having woken but being then unable to move, as we all have with occasional nightmares) and hypnagogic hallucinations, or dreamlets associated with the times of sleep and drowsiness. An afternoon or evening EEG recording with concomitant electro-oculogram will catch the patient falling asleep, and on a proportion of occasions he will pass directly into REM (paradoxical) sleep. Normal people only do this if they take a nap in the first part of the morning.

The cataplectic attacks can be abolished by clomipramine 50–100 mg daily, a drug that prevents the loss of muscle tone that accompanies REM sleep. Patients get fat on it, however. The sleep attacks are more of a problem. They are traditionally treated with dexamphetamine or methyl phenidate, but narcoleptics are as prone as any to become dependent on the drugs for elevation of mood, to become tolerant and, with their organic brain disorder, perhaps more prone than most to become irritable or paranoid. I avoid prescribing such drugs. It is important to discuss the disability with the family, and, if possible, the employer, to explain that it does not imply slothfulness or lack of interest, that driving should cease, and that it is a good idea to plan deliberate naps during the morning coffee break, at lunch time and in the afternoon tea break. Planned naps mean fewer unplanned naps.

Hypersomnia: other patients fall asleep by day and have no REM sleep peculiarities. Most are obese, a few have a history of what could have been encephalitis. They will describe falling asleep for 30 minutes or more, once or twice a day, or falling asleep very early in the evening and then sleeping all night. Caffeine and rigorous dieting will relieve some. I have never met an underweight patient who was too sleepy by day in this way.

It is important to enquire of a spouse or relative about snoring or snorting by night, because a proportion of these patients, usually obese (and then called Pickwickian) have periods of apnoea during sleep. Their nights are so disturbed by repeated respiratory obstruction that they have difficulty staying awake by day (Guilleminault & Dement, 1978). The story, and the witnessed picture, is characteristic. Nocturnal sleep consists of sequences of 20–30 seconds, each made up of abortive respiratory movements, grunting noises, and a final crescendo of violent snorts or braying noises that accompany three or four deep breaths. With his snorts he almost wakes himself, he may kick and slap around, and the bed may come to look like a battlefield. His wife has to sleep in a separate bed, and by day he can be sleepy,

irritable, aggressive, and paranoid. In a child the cause can be large tonsils and adenoids, in adults the tongue may be falling back or the pharynx going into spasm. Rigorous loss of weight, or tracheostomy open only at night, allow normal sleep again and prevent progress to pulmonary hypertension.

Sleep drunkenness or post-dormitial confusion: some of us are 'larks', bright and alert early in the day; others are 'owls', lively at night but sluggish in the morning. A few are very sluggish. They get irritable when their wives try repeatedly to rouse them, remain unable to think clearly all morning, and lose their jobs on account of lateness (Roth, Nevsimalova & Rechtschaffen, 1972). Plenty of strong coffee for breakfast, an afternoon or evening job, an understanding doctor, and a tolerant spouse are needed.

Strange events in the night
'The borderland of sleep is haunted by hallucinations . . . voices . . . distressingly real visions . . . sensory shocks', wrote Weir Mitchell (1890). When drowsing we hear the voices of others and of ourselves, forming strange phrases and constructing neologisms, all of which we forget unless we promptly rouse and record them, as did Emil Kraepelin (1906), whose interest lay in the parallels with dementia praecox. Sensory shocks include the feeling of a sudden jerk after a fall, an explosion in the head, a pistol shot, an electric feeling from abdomen to head, a flash of light, or several of these concurrently. They are normal events. Patients receiving MAOIs have more twitches and jerks at night.

Snoring is a subject for hilarity, but a cause of distress to the partner. It is more common among the obese and after alcohol. There have been many treatments because there is no cure. It can form the focus, or excuse given by a wife, for deriding and leaving her husband.

Enuresis, night terrors, and sleep walking: these three disorders that occur in the early night, and arise out of EEG slow wave sleep, more often face the psychiatrist who works with children, but occur among occasional adults. Enuresis is a handicap to a girl of marriageable age and she will be grateful if the buzzer technique helps her.

Night terrors usually involve fear of attack by persons or animals, fears of entrapment, of falling, dying, or choking, and leave little lasting memory (Fisher et al., 1974). A few strangled words or cries precede blood-curdling shrieks. The youth sits up and stares wide-eyed. He may stumble out of bed, move around with a distressed expression and then slowly return to bed and sleep. In some the sleep-walking arises silently and on its own. A 23-year-old patient of mine has learned in the morning that he has urinated into his own wardrobe, or his sister's bedroom, or tried to get back into his parents' bed. Some will fall down the stairs or otherwise injure themselves and simple precautions come first in management.

Sleep walking, excessive sleep talking, and night terrors run in families (Bakwin, 1970; Hällström, 1972) and arise in adult life following recent waking anxiety, as among battle-front evacuees (Pai, 1946) or sporadically for no obvious reason. The EEG usually shows a large measure of arousal, but not to full wakefulness, during the walking (Kales *et al.*, 1966) and the state of automatism provides a successful, if not always convincing, defence to a charge of homicide, or other crime (Legal Correspondent, 1970). In one instance where I gave evidence in court there was only an 18-month history. The middle-aged man's family had erected a portcullis to stop him falling down the tenement stair, he had once been found staring out of the window at night, pointing to a street lamp and saying, 'That light's evil', and had now improperly driven a car in the small hours. For that same 18-month period he had taken not only his usual evening wine but also the narcotic DF118 (dihydrocodeine tartrate) pills prescribed for his sister-in-law, but taken for his own backache. Reassurance and support through the period of worst night terrors and sleep walking are my usual choice, but diazepam is effective.

Rhythmic movements that take place in sleep include scratching, tooth grinding (here again let us remember that drugs, such as fenfluramine, may be a cause), and head-banging or body-rocking (Oswald, 1964). It is a piquant experience for the bed partner to find her 110 kg man frenziedly hurling himself from side to side or hammering his brow up and down on the mattress for half a minute without awakening and doing so recurrently through the night. Usually it started in early childhood and has become less frequent since and always it is a challenge to therapeutic ingenuity. Fig. 6.1 illustrates the head-bangings and tooth grinding during sleep of a 26-year-old married professional man.

Nightmares, or anxiety-dreams, are part of normal life. Unlike night terrors they are extended dream adventures, and not brief ideas of elemental terror. They arise late in the night, during REM (paradoxical) sleep, and are accompanied by the motor paralysis characteristic of that state. They become common when daytime anxiety levels are higher (Gentil & Lader, 1978) or when alcohol or hypnotic drug withdrawal is in progress. Nightmares diminish with successful general management. Indeed, it is a fairly general rule that happy days mean happy nights.

Fig. 6.1. Excerpts at 0253 h and 0300 h of a recent night's recording of sleep from a 26-year-old man, showing examples both of his rhythmic tooth grinding and rhythmic head-banging, without awakening. (The help of Dr Pauline Skarrott is acknowledged.)

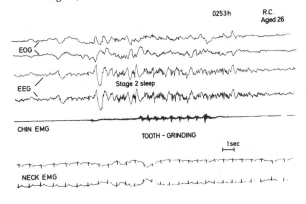

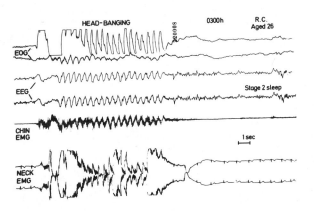

7

Pain, as illustrated by the problems of headache and facial pain

C. D. MARSDEN

Introduction

Pain is an emotion, not a nervous impulse. This comment may be obvious, but needs emphasis. Any noxious stimulus causing tissue damage evokes a train of neuronal discharges in nerve fibres known to be concerned with appreciation of pain (and in many other neuronal systems), but whether such information is registered as a painful experience depends upon the circumstances of the injury, memory, emotional content of the event, and other factors. The classical example of painless tissue injury is the soldier wounded in battle who does not feel pain until he notices blood trickling into his boot.

Since pain is an emotion, it is not surprising it is often encountered as a complaint in patients with psychiatric disease. This may occur in one of four settings.

(1) Concurrent psychiatric illness may provoke organic conditions causing pain, for example, when depression provokes attacks of migraine.

(2) Concurrent psychiatric illness makes the pain of an existing organic illness worse, for example, when depression intensifies cancer pain.

(3) Organic pain causes psychiatric illness, for example, when chronic unrelieved sciatica provokes depression.

I do not propose to consider these three aspects of the inter-relation between psychiatric illness and pain further in this chapter, for concepts of psychosomatic disease are considered elsewhere, as is the psychiatric management of chronic pain syndromes (chap. 1; vol. 4, chap. 8; vol. 5, chap 6). I will concentrate on the fourth relationship between psychiatric and physical illness, namely

(4) Psychiatric illness presenting with the complaint of pain.

It is inevitable that patients whose illness is primarily psychiatric, but whose main complaint is one of pain, should initially be referred to the physician appropriate to diseases causing their pain. Thus, every organ specialist recognizes a pain syndrome which is due to psychiatric illness, but which mimics common physical conditions within their specialty. The cardiologist, for example, has to separate chest pain due to anxiety from true angina, the gastro-enterologist is constantly investigating abdominal pain of no known cause, and likewise, the gynaecologist has problems with undiagnosed pelvic pain. The neurologist, too, has his particular problems of which headache and pain in the face are the commonest.

Headache, and to a lesser extent pain in the face, are common physical complaints. Also, they are widely assumed by patients with a variety of behavioural and emotional disturbances as a means of gaining access to the 'medical ear'. A significant proportion of such patients turn out not to have physical illness, but are believed to suffer from the psychiatric conditions of tension headache, or atypical facial pain. A proportion of these latter individuals will be referred to psychiatrists for further evaluation and treatment, and the psychiatrist must be in a position to judge the validity of the referral diagnosis. This problem may be approached by the application of a number of simple general principles which are applicable whether the patient's complaint of pain is referred to his belly, his chest, or his head. The purpose of the present chapter is to develop the background to these principles and to illustrate it by the approach to the problems of a headache and pain in the face, which are used as appropriate examples of the general problem.

Headache

Acute, or subacute, headache is not a problem that often involves the psychiatrist, but chronic recurrent headache is a different matter. Some one in five of the population is said to suffer chronic or recurrent headache, and 99 per cent of such individuals will have no abnormal physical signs on careful examination. The diagnosis of the cause of their headache rests therefore on careful history-taking, which aims to match the details of their complaint with one of the patterns of a known illness. Such pattern recognition depends upon defining exactly the site of the pain and its radiation, its incidence and time course, its associated features, and those factors aggravating and relieving the pain. All these features establish the picture of a pain in the head which can then be compared with that of known diagnostic entities, each of which has a typical pattern. However, the typical picture of a common illness is not sufficient for accurate diagnosis: rather it is necessary to appreciate the range of variation of presentation of known entities for comparison with an individual patient's complaints, and experience is the tool of the diagnostician. This is not the place to detail all the various patterns of headaches encountered in clinical practice, but common types will be described.

(a) *Referred pain* may be due to disease of the eyes, ears, sinuses, teeth, or neck. Usually the cause is evident, but some conditions require further comment.

Refractive error does not directly cause headache, but some patients with failing vision may develop tension headache consequent upon the effort of trying to read. 'Eye-strain headache' is thus a form of tension headache following visual effort and can be relieved by glasses. Angle-closure glaucoma may cause pain in the eye, radiating into the forehead, and is not always accompanied by the typical history of failing vision and coloured haloes around lights. Unexplained pain centered in an eye and radiating into the forehead in a middle-aged or elderly patient always should raise the suspicion of glaucoma, and should prompt appropriate ophthalmological assessment.

Chronic headache is often blamed on sinusitis, but this is a misconception. Patients with chronic sinus disease (often diagnosed on X-ray appearances) may get recurrent attacks of acute sinusitis, with typical local pain and tenderness exacerbated by bending, lying, coughing, or sneezing, but do not generally complain of chronic unrelieved pain. Likewise, dental disease is not a cause of chronic headache, although abnormalities of bite due to temporo-mandibular joint abnormality (Costen's syndrome) may cause pain radiating into the temple on chewing. Degeneration of the upper cervical disc spaces, or malformation of the first two or three cervical vertebrae, can cause compression of emerging posterior roots leading to radiation of pain in the neck and back of the head in the distribution of C2 and 3. This is uncommon, because degenerative cervical spondylosis preferentially affects lower cervical levels. High cervical symptoms suggest another diagnosis such as rheumatoid arthritis, or congenital malformation.

(b) *Raised intracranial pressure* may be caused by a mass of tumour, blood or pus, may be due to hydrocephalus as a result of obstruction to CSF flow, or may occur in the syndrome of benign intracranial hypertension. Headache due to these causes usually has been present only for a matter of weeks or a few months, not for years. The classical features pointing to a diagnosis of raised intracranial pressure, such as the presence of headache that wakes the patient in the morning, increase on coughing and straining at stool, and vomiting, often are not present. Suspicion frequently is aroused by the development of headache for the first time in a previously healthy person not prone to such a complaint. Examination of the optic discs is of critical importance in such patients, but difficulty in interpreting their appearance is very common. Pseudo-papilloedema, which refers to the presence of a swollen disc due to local changes and not raised intracranial pressure, is frequent in the normal population usually as a result of either hypermetropia or drusen. Perhaps the most valuable sign to look for in assessing disc changes as possibly indicating papilloedema is venous pulsation. By focusing on to the edge of a vein as it dips into the optic disc, it is commonly possible to see pulsation of the wall in time with the arterial pulse. This is due to the pulsation of the carotid artery within the venous lake of the cavernous sinus into which such veins drain. If venous pulsation is seen, intracranial pressure is not raised.

Headache on coughing or exertion requires further comment. Both may occur with raised intracranial pressure, but frequently this is not the case. Cough headache may indicate cerebellar ectopia, or frontal sinus obstruction as by mucocoele, but commonly no cause is found. Benign headache on exertion also is common, and although subarachnoid haemorrhage may occur during sexual intercourse, no cause usually can be demonstrated for orgasmic or other forms of exertional headache.

(c) *Giant cell arteritis* deserves separate consideration because of its serious complications and need for urgent treatment. Anyone over the age of 55 presenting with headache should be suspected of having giant cell arteritis, especially if there is associated constitutional disturbance and ill-health. The patient may have noted a tender scalp when combing the hair, and may have experienced pain on chewing due to claudication of muscles. Superficial temporal arteries and other cranial vessels may be unduly prominent, tender, and non-pulsatile. Malaise, weight loss, and night sweats, sometimes with fever, often are conspicuous. The ESR is raised above 45 mm/hour in virtually every patient. Biopsy of an affected artery does not always pick up the characteristic histological abnormalities, which are patchy in distribution. The commonest severe complication is blindness due to involvement of the optic nerve, but other neurological problems occur that are due to ischaemia elsewhere including diplopia due to cranial nerve palsies, transient ischaemic attacks usually in vertebrobasilar territory, visual disturbance due to posterior cerebral artery insufficiency, and dementia. Suspicion of the presence of giant cell arteritis demands immediate investigation and treatment with steroids.

(d) *Post-traumatic headache* persists in about one-third of those who suffer head injury of any severity. The problem is to decide how much is due to organic and how much to psychological factors in each individual patient. The persistence of headache does not correlate with the duration of coma, post-traumatic amnesia, skull fracture, or EEG abnormality. The incidence is higher in those with scalp laceration, pre-existing psychiatric disability, or pending litigation. Undoubtedly, a variety of factors contribute to post-traumatic headache. Head injury may precipitate migraine, scalp neuromas, or whiplash injury of the cervical spine. Concussion commonly causes persistent pulsating headache, made worse by movement, coughing, and straining, and often accompanied by other signs of organic origin, such as positional vertigo and mild intellectual impairment with memory difficulty. The impact of this organic post-traumatic syndrome is to interfere with concentration and working capacity. Premature return to normal activities, be they occupational or household, may reveal to the sufferer that he is not in a position to cope with his usual range of demands. This may lead to secondary depression with superimposed tension headache. The organic origins of this sequence of events are obvious in previously stable, successful individuals, but it is very difficult to be sure in others of less robust personality, particularly in those seeking legal compensation. Compensation-neurosis certainly exists, and frank malingering is well known to those engaged in medico-legal practice. There is no easy way to distinguish those in whom psychological factors are playing a major role in perpetuating their headache after injury. Often information must be sought from a wide circle of relatives and friends to build a picture of the normal behaviour of the individual when not under medical supervision, as well as to observe the patient closely and assess the significance of his complaints.

(e) *Migraine* probably occurs in around 1 in 10 of the population at some time of their life, but only about one-third of patients are referred to a neurologist. Migraine is now defined as a familial disorder characterized by recurrent attacks of headache of varying intensity, frequency and duration. Attacks commonly are unilateral, and are usually associated with anorexia, nausea, and vomiting. About a third of patients have classical migraine, in which headache is preceded by transient focal neurological symptoms such as the typical visual phenomena and speech and sensory disturbances. Common migraine refers to migrainous headaches without prodromal focal neurological symptoms. Individual patients may get episodes of classical migraine, interspersed with bouts of common migraine, and may be liable to episodes of focal neurological disturbance without headache or vomiting (so-called migraine equivalents). Almost any area of the brain may be subject to ischaemia in the half-hour to one hour prior to the onset of a classical migraine attack so that the varieties of prodromal neurological symptoms are protean. Those due to ischaemia in the distribution of the vertebro-basilar system (so-called basilar artery migraine) are of interest because not only do such patients develop diplopia, dysarthria and ataxia, but they may also experience complex psychological and memory disturbances as a consequence of hippocampal ischaemia (the posterior cerebral arteries supply the medial temporal areas). The diagnosis of migraine is established by the repetitive paroxysmal nature of the disorder, with attacks occurring at intervals of weeks or years, the patient being normal between intervals. It is rare for migraine to begin after the age of fifty.

Problems arise when headache in a migraine sufferer occurs very frequently, every few days, or even daily.

Ordinary migraine does not occur this frequently, although its incidence may be increased by development of hypertension, the administration of certain drugs, other intercurrent physical illnesses and occasionally pregnancy. Another cause for such frequent headaches in a migraine sufferer is the overusage of ergotamine-containing preparations, which themselves can provoke headache. In this situation patients may enter a vicious cycle in which increased headache prompts extra ergotamine intake which causes more headache and so on, until the patient ends up apparently in status migrinosus. The commonest cause for excessive headache in a migraine sufferer, however, is the concurrent development of tension headache due to anxiety or frank depressive illness. Treatment of this underlying psychiatric condition commonly relieves much of the extra headache complained of by such patients.

(f) *Tension headache.* Most individuals have suffered headache under conditions of stress from time to time. The ceaseless telephone in a busy office, the screaming of children, the barking of the dog in a busy home, or battling through rush-hour traffic or the local shopping centre on a Saturday morning are common situations in urban life which provoke tension headache. The pain is usually dull, generalized, and constant. A description of pressure or tightness extending as a band round the head is typical. In mild cases where the provocative stress is limited, the pain may be relieved by analgesia or a good night's sleep, but where stress persists the headache becomes continuous. Thus, tension headache may vary from the occasional few hours discomfort at the end of a busy day to a constant unremitting pain present 'all day and every day'.

The patient with an occasional tension headache rarely consults a doctor. It is those whose headaches recur frequently, or whose pain becomes continuous, that seek medical help. Amongst the latter, a considerable proportion, perhaps a third or more, also complain of the typical symptoms of depressive illness including loss of appetite, loss of weight, sleep disturbance, and diurnal mood variation. Appropriate treatment of their depression relieves the headache. As mentioned earlier, an intercurrent depressive illness may provoke tension headache in those with head injury or migraine, and antidepressant therapy again may relieve this aspect of their headache. Another group of patients with tension headache, again about a third, have obvious if unavoidable life stress which, while not provoking a frank depressive illness, generates chronic anxiety. Psychotherapy and social help may assist such individuals to cope with their problems and thereby relieve headache. The remainder of patients with tension headache do not have overt depression and deny severe stress. Amongst this last group of patients there are certainly some who will not admit to themselves or their relatives the existence of depression or concern, yet this emerges after careful and often prolonged interview. Such apparently masked depressive illnesses or anxiety states are common in neurological practice, so much so that even when patients with tension headache will admit to no such symptoms it is worth considering a trial of appropriate antidepressant therapy. Finally, there is a group of patients with the symptoms of tension headache in whom no psychiatric illness is evident but who appear to gain benefit from complaining of headache either to their doctors, or their relatives, or both!

Pain in the face

Pain in the face may be due to infection of the teeth, sinuses, ear, or eye. Such causes usually are self-evident, but eye pain due to glaucoma, and pain on eating due to temporo-mandibular joint arthritis or parotid gland dysfunction may be more difficult to diagnose. Pain in the face on chewing in an elderly unwell patient should raise the suspicion of cranial arteritis.

When abnormalities of sensation are found on examination of a patient with pain in the face, lesions compressing the Vth nerve usually are discovered after investigation. The most subtle test of Vth nerve sensory function is the corneal reflex, which may be lost without other obvious signs of Vth nerve involvement. The Vth nerve may be affected by lesions of the posterior fossa affecting the sensory root, such as tumours in the cerebello-pontine angle, in the middle fossa where tumours or aneurysms may compress the nerve or its ganglion or its peripheral branches may be involved by nasopharyngeal carcinoma or other neoplasms involving the air sinuses and adjacent structures. Good quality X-rays of the skull, particularly basal views, are often required to detect such lesions. The presence of definite Vth nerve sensory signs is a clear indication for full neuroradiological investigation.

The majority of patients, however, with pain in the face have no abnormal physical signs on examination or abnormal findings on simple X-rays. The diagnosis depends on the history, as is the case with headache. The common diagnoses encountered are trigeminal neuralgia, post-herpetic neuralgia, facial migraine, and migrainous neuralgia. There are also a variety of rarer neuralgias, such as glossopharyngeal

neuralgia, and dental neuralgia. When the patient's history does not match one of these recognized physical entities, a diagnosis of atypical facial pain commonly is applied. The latter, which is of interest to psychiatrists, is thus primarily a diagnosis of exclusion and can only be entertained comfortably when all physical causes of facial pain have been ruled out.

(a) *Trigeminal neuralgia* is usually, but not exclusively, a disease of the middle-aged or elderly. The pain consists of excruciating, stabbing, cutting, knife-like paroxysms, each lasting only a matter of seconds. Spasms of pain may occur at short intervals, but between each attack there is no pain, or, at most, a slight residual ache. The pain is always unilateral, and most commonly affects the second and third divisions of the Vth nerve. The jabs of pain usually start around the mouth, gums, or nose, and shoot towards the ear or orbit. Pain in mouth–ear distribution occurs in two-thirds of patients, while that in nose–orbit distribution occurs in about one-third. It is very rare for trigeminal neuralgia to start in the first division of the Vth nerve. The paroxysms of pain are provoked by external stimuli to Vth nerve territory and usually such triggers cause pain in the same division of the nerve. Touching the face, nose, gums, or teeth are obvious triggers; the paroxysms may also be caused by eating, washing the face, or teeth, shaving, blowing the nose, yawning, or even a cold wind on the face. At the height of a bad attack, the patient may be too terrified to speak or eat, lest it trigger off the pain.

The diagnostic features of trigeminal neuralgia (tic douloureux) thus are three-fold – paroxysms of pain, in Vth nerve territory, and triggered.

The prognosis of trigeminal neuralgia is one of repeated exacerbations and remissions. Most patients can expect a remission after the first attack has lasted a matter of days or weeks. This remission itself may last months or even years, but usually the pain recurs. The intervals between attacks tend to become shorter, and the duration of each episode becomes longer with the passage of time. Treatment initially is with carbamazepine, which will rapidly relieve pain in 70 per cent to 80 per cent of cases, at least in their initial episodes. However, with repeated attacks the drug often becomes less efficient, and injection or division of the Vth nerve may be required for pain relief.

(b) *Glossopharyngeal neuralgia* is much rarer than trigeminal neuralgia. The character of the pain, and its provocation by triggers (coughing, swallowing, chewing) are similar, but its site differs. Stabs of pain are felt in the throat, back of tongue, and deep in the ear. It is important to exclude structural causes such as carcinoma of the tongue by full visual and digital examination before accepting the diagnosis. Glossopharyngeal neuralgia also responds to carbamazepine or nerve section.

(c) *Post-herpetic neuralgia* occurs in about one in every ten patients who have herpes zoster. It appears to occur more severely and to last longer in the aged, and when the herpes affects the face, particularly the first division of the Vth nerve. Patients usually complain of a severe, constant discomfort, burning, boring, crushing, or tearing feeling in the area of skin previously affected by the rash, superimposed upon which are shoots of pain. The affected dermatomes, which carry the white scars of the rash, may be exquisitely sensitive to touch or other stimuli despite impaired sensation in the area. Such stimuli may provoke burning dysaesthesiae or spasms of lancinating pain similar to those of trigeminal neuralgia. Treatment of post-herpetic neuralgia is very difficult, and when established chronically, the condition becomes compounded by increasing reactive depression. Simple analgesics do not usually help, and nerve section or more elaborate surgical procedures are of no avail. Luckily, the pain remits eventually in most patients.

(d) *Migrainous neuralgia* is known by many other names including Horton's and Sluder's neuralgia, sphenopalatine neuralgia, cluster headache, and clockwork headache. The condition usually occurs in young men affected by recurrent, short-lived attacks of pain affecting one side of the head and face, often associated with changes in the conjunctiva and nasal mucosa. Pain is an intense, constant, and boring ache of great severity in and around the eye, spreading to the temple and cheek. It is always unilateral and affects the same side in each attack in 90 per cent of patients. During the attack, which lasts between one-half to two hours, the eye waters and goes red, the ipsilateral nostril runs or becomes blocked, and the affected skin may become swollen and red. A striking feature of the disease is the tendency of the attacks to occur at the same time of each day or night in any one individual. Pain often wakens the sufferer at exactly two o'clock each morning, and there is usually only one attack every twenty-four hours. Attacks occur daily for a matter of weeks or months, but then disappear during the remission, which may last for months or years. Such patients rarely give a history of typical migraine, and mi-

grainous neuralgia is not prefaced by any of the typical migrainous auras. However, it responds dramatically to treatment with ergotamine.

(e) *Facial migraine* refers to pain in the face which follows the typical frequency and time course of migraine headache, that is, occurring usually not more frequently than at intervals of two or three weeks, and lasting a matter of hours to days. Such attacks may be prefaced by the typical neurological aura of classical migraine, often accompanied by nausea and vomiting, and the affected individual may have attacks of typical headache on other occasions.

(f) *Other neuralgias* affecting the face not uncommonly follow dental treatment. While the vast majority of patients survive conservative dentistry without mishap, a very small number report the development of severe and sometimes crippling pain following local anaesthesia, tooth extraction, root fillings, or other such manoeuvres. Often this pain is referred to the affected tooth and jaw, occurs in excruciating paroxysms, and may be precipitated by cleaning the teeth and chewing. Presumably such dental neuralgia is related to partial nerve damage to dental nerves, causing something akin to causalgia. Similar sorts of neuralgic pain also may follow maxillo-facial trauma, leading to damage to supra-orbital, infra-orbital, or other such nerves.

(g) *Atypical facial pain* became established as an entity because many patients were encountered whose description of their facial pain did not match any of the recognized patterns of known causes. Certainly the entity can only be diagnosed by exclusion, but atypical facial pain does have many recognizable characteristics. Thus, the patient is commonly a middle-aged female, the pain is chronic and continuous, occurring throughout the waking hours, 'day in – day out', often it is not confined to the territory of the Vth nerve but extends into the neck and even into the arm, and it is quite resistant to treatment with analgesics.

Within this group of patients diagnosed as having 'atypical facial pain' some are obviously depressed, with typical mood, diurnal variation, early morning waking, and somatic symptoms, one of which in such cases is pain in the face. Treatment of these patients with antidepressants relieves their pain. Other patients with atypical facial pain deny depression and have none of the typical symptoms of the condition, but their pain is relieved by antidepressants. For this reason it is sensible to institute a therapeutic trial of antidepressant medication for an adequate period of time in all patients with atypical facial pain.

Still other patients with atypical facial pain are neither depressed nor respond to antidepressants. While some of these individuals may have an unrecognized physical cause for their pain, I believe that in most of them the pain is psychogenic. A number of subgroups of psychogenic facial pain can be detected. There are some for whom the pain remains an acceptable excuse for visiting doctors, and repeatedly confounding them! The clue to such behaviour often comes from interviewing the spouse, who reports that the patient appears only to complain of pain when visiting the doctor, but at other times appears quite happy, and unconcerned by the symptoms. Other patients may use their pain to gain sympathy from relatives or friends.

Implications for the psychiatrist

A patient with headache or pain in the face is referred for psychiatric evaluation when either he has obvious psychiatric illness which has not responded to simple therapy by the general practitioner or physician, or no organic cause has been found for his complaint: the question is asked whether this is due to psychiatric illness. What general principles can the psychiatrist employ when evaluating patients in the latter category?

The first question that arises is how to broach to a patient complaining of chronic pain the suggestion that he or she should consult a psychiatrist. Many such individuals immediately resent that advice, believing that it implies that either they are contriving their symptoms, or that they are 'mental', which even in this enlightened age still carries a stigma. Careful wording by the referring doctor and by the receiving psychiatrist can, however, often overcome even the most obstinate of refusals. One approach that I have found helpful for patients with headache, or pain in the face, is the following: I frankly admit that despite extensive clinical assessment and investigation, I can find no physical cause for their symptoms, but I then go on to reassure the patient that I know the pain is real, and that it is necessary to pursue every avenue of treatment to try to gain relief. At this point I draw attention to the fact that their chronic suffering has naturally led to secondary depression, and emphasize that this is exactly what happens to any patient suffering chronic pain due to physical illness such as cancer. The next stage is to draw attention to the effects of depression upon the suffering of

pain, pointing out that even a slight nagging ache may become a torment if one is down in spirits. This leads to the observation that successful psychiatric treatment of secondary depression caused by physical pain, may dramatically relieve the pain itself, perhaps by breaking a vicious cycle of pain causing depression, causing more pain. Since all other avenues of treatment have failed it must be worth pursuing a psychiatric approach.

The understandable secondary depression that occurs in virtually all patients with chronic unrelieved pain, does, of course, add to their suffering, but it also makes diagnosis difficult. The symptoms of the original physical illness become hidden in the superstructure of the added depression. In addition such patients usually have a long saga of repeated consultation, investigation, and opinion to relate to their physician. A sensible approach to discover whether a physical illness is behind the complaint, or whether a psychological disorder precipitated the situation is to go back to the *onset* of the illness. A careful history from the patient and the relatives about the initial complaints often is the best pointer to the origin of a chronic pain problem, for subsequent events distort and cloud the picture.

A prerequisite for the psychiatrist wishing to evaluate and treat a patient with chronic pain must be that he or she is convinced that all organic causes have been excluded as far as is possible. Almost by definition the patient under discussion will not have obvious physical signs and will not give a classical history of organic disease. These are, therefore, patients requiring careful assessment by an expert clinician experienced in the vagaries of physical illness. The psychiatrist cannot and should not attempt this task, for he has neither the experience nor the training necessary to elicit subtle signs, or evaluate bizarre histories. He must rely upon the wisdom of colleagues who say that they can find no evidence of physical illness. This is no different from, say, a neurologist accepting the conclusion of a wise psychiatrist who, from his extensive experience of mental illness, says in a difficult patient this cannot be a psychiatric disease.

A number of expert opinions may be required to exclude all possible physical causes of headache, or pain in the face. For instance, with regard to the latter it may be necessary for the patient to be seen by a dentist, an ophthalmologist, an ENT surgeon, and finally a neurologist before all physical avenues have been adequately explored.

Before embarking on extensive psychiatric assessment and protracted therapy, it is generally wise to have pursued every simple investigation relevant to the problem. Nothing can be more disconcerting for the patient, and disruptive to a programme of treatment, than to have second thoughts about the diagnosis, and then discover that some critical investigation was not undertaken initially. A typical example would be failure to obtain adequate views of the base of the skull in someone with facial pain. To arrange further physical investigation at this stage inevitably awakens doubts of the diagnosis in the patient, and may destroy his confidence in the planned psychiatric approach. It is best to ensure that all reasonable avenues of investigation have been thoroughly reviewed before embarking on extensive psychiatric involvement in a patient with problems such as chronic pain.

Having reviewed the diagnosis and accepted the patient with chronic pain for psychiatric evaluation and therapy it is prudent to set a time limit on how long to pursue this approach. Obviously this must be dictated by psychiatric indications, but if after a period of some months such a patient has gained no benefit there is little point in continuing.

Finally, once treatment of a patient with chronic pain has lifted depression and allayed anxiety, it is worth reconsidering the physical aspects of the condition in case some more can be done to help that. The management of such patients should involve a continued dialogue between psychiatrist and referring physician.

(The reader is referred to the references for full information on aspects of headache and facial pain.)

8
The senium

ANTHONY D. ISAACS

Introduction

The justification for giving special consideration to the psychiatric disorders of the aged must first be established. Virtually all the syndromes that arise in younger age groups can be found in the elderly, but nevertheless within the general field of adult psychiatry the sub-speciality of geriatric psychiatry has evolved. The term is worthy of careful definition because it can be interpreted in several ways. For the purpose of this section, the term is used to embrace all psychiatric disorders arising in an elderly person and this includes almost the entire psychiatric spectrum. It is thus analogous to child psychiatry, that is the delineation is based on the criterion of age alone rather than any specific clinical condition. The term geriatric psychiatry is preferable to 'psychogeriatrics' which, literally interpreted, means the coexistence of physical and psychiatric disability and thus includes a far wider range of clinical conditions than if the term is limited to predominantly psychiatric syndromes arising in the elderly. It is not unknown for the term 'psychogeriatric' to be used to describe an elderly patient with advanced dementia. The use of the term in that sense lacks any justification.

The emergence of geriatric psychiatry as a subject of special interest closely parallels the development of geriatrics within the broad context of general medicine. By the middle of the twentieth century, developed countries became more aware of the implications for health and welfare services of an

Table 8.1. *Population of England and Wales in thousands*

Year	Total	Aged 65+	Aged 75+
		%	%
1901	32 528	1518 (4.7)	442 (1.4)
1911	36 070	1878 (5.2)	518 (1.4)
1921	37 887	2291 (6.0)	648 (1.7)
1931	39 952	2963 (7.4)	821 (2.0)
1951	43 758	4824 (11.0)	1567 (3.6)
1961	46 104	5494 (11.9)	1976 (4.3)
1971	48 929	6496 (13.3)	2318 (4.7)
1974	49 195	6865 (13.9)	2437 (4.9)
1975	49 157	6967 (14.2)	2490 (5.1)
1976	49 142	7055 (14.4)	2545 (5.2)
1977	49 120	7145 (14.5)	2605 (5.3)
1978	49 104	7241 (14.7)	2673 (5.4)
1979	49 171	7330 (14.9)	2737 (5.7)
[a]1980	49 298	7427 (15.1)	2815 (5.7)

[a]These figures are provisional

ageing population. The combination of a general increase in the total population, together with a decline in birth rate which began towards the end of the nineteenth century, which has continued throughout the present century, has resulted in an increasing number of elderly people in the population who, in addition, represent an increasing proportion of that population. This is illustrated by the change in the population of England and Wales during the present century (table 8.1). It can be seen that the proportion of the population over the age of 65 has increased from 4.7 per cent in 1901 to 15.1 per cent by 1980 and, of greater significance, is the six-fold increase of people over the age of 75 during the same period.

It is predicted that by the end of the twentieth century the number of people in the population aged 85 and over will increase by some 60 per cent and those in the range 75 to 84 by 20 per cent. In both age groups women will outnumber men by some 3 to 1 (*Population Trends 11*, 1978). It is sometimes mistakenly believed that this dramatic expansion of the old age population is due to the fact that elderly people now live longer because of improvements in standards of health care generally, a concept of 'medicated survival'. In fact, the life expectancy of an elderly person is only slightly better than it was in 1841 (table 8.2). The improvement of standards of health care

during the twentieth century has substantially increased the survival prospects of younger people who are more likely to grow old and contribute to the ageing population as a whole.

During the 1930s an inevitable consequence of these population trends was the steady accumulation of substantial numbers of elderly people in a variety of institutional settings, many of whom were suffering from chronic physical disabilities and others from what later came to be recognized as the damaging effects of institutional care. One notable pioneer, Dr Marjorie Warren, tackled this legacy of neglect in a positive way with much innovation, and demonstrated the very real benefits that the elderly could derive from an active and enthusiastic regimen that was specially designed to meet their needs. The medical speciality of geriatrics steadily evolved from this early work and is now well-established in the United Kingdom.

Following the emergence of geriatrics as an important medical speciality, the significance of these population changes for psychiatry became evident, and the special features of mental disorders in old age were pointed out (Lewis, 1946; Roth & Morrissey, 1952). Like geriatrics, the speciality of geriatric psychiatry emerged slowly but by 1965 a British statistician commented: 'it is no longer an exaggeration to say that the problem of psychiatric care in this country is largely a geriatric one' (Brooke, 1965). The accuracy of this prediction is evident in psychiatric hospital statistics. Despite a steady fall in the number of patients resident in psychiatric hospitals and units in England, in 1977 49.6 per cent of patients were aged 65 and over while some 27 per cent were aged 75 or over. Similarly, some 23 per cent of all patients admitted were elderly.

It is clear that the elderly feature increasingly in clinical practice and as in the case of geriatrics, the needs of this group of patients are more adequately met by the provision of special services and, in particular, by the clinician becoming more alert to the interplay of psychiatric, physical, and social factors in such patients (Arie, 1973).

Normal ageing

The psychiatric disorders that arise in old age must be clearly distinguished from those psychological changes known to be associated with normal ageing: the age-related changes most relevant in clinical practice will now be summarized. It is noteworthy that certain changes develop in the ageing

Table 8.2. *Expectation of life in England and Wales*

	At birth		At 1 year		At 15 years		At 45 years		At 65 years	
	M	F	M	F	M	F	M	F	M	F
1841	40.2	42.2	46.7	47.6	43.4	44.1	23.3	24.4	10.9	11.5
1901–1910	48.5	52.4	55.7	58.3	47.3	50.1	23.3	25.5	10.8	12.0
1930–1932	58.7	62.9	62.3	65.5	51.2	54.3	25.5	28.3	11.3	13.1
1960–1962	68.1	74.0	68.0	74.4	55.3	60.9	27.1	32.1	12.0	15.3
1972	68.9	75.1	69.2	75.2	55.7	61.7	27.3	32.8	12.1	16.0

brain, the main features being senile plaques, neurofibrillary changes, and neuronal loss. Some measures of intellectual change correlate with the number of senile plaques in the brain (Roth, Tomlinson & Blessed 1966).

The main psychological changes related to intelligence, memory, personality, and social behaviour.

(1) *Intelligence*

It is usually assumed that with advancing age intellectual ability steadily declines, based on the finding that older people tend to perform less well than younger people on tests of intelligence such as the Wechsler Adult Intelligence Scale (Wechsler, 1958). It is clear, however, that performance is more impaired in respect of some of the subtests than others, and Wechsler has divided the subtests into a category that resists the effects of ageing and those that are more vulnerable. The former, known as 'hold' tests measure such skills as vocabulary, information, object assembly, and picture completion whereas the 'don't hold' tests include digit span, similarities, digit symbol substitution and block design. Cattell (1943) has drawn a similar distinction between abilities that depend on a person's ability to adapt to changing circumstances, apply new methods, or use innovation to solve problems, and those abilities that depend on previously acquired skills. The former are described as reflecting 'fluid' intelligence compared with the 'crystallized' intelligence of the second category. It can be demonstrated that the 'fluid' type of intelligence is more liable to decline with age.

The structure of intelligence in the aged has been reviewed by Savage (1971) who suggested that four major factors are involved: general intellectual level, verbal and performance intellectual level, general intellectual deterioration, and learning impairment. Normal ageing is characterized by changes in the first three of these factors.

The technical problems involved in psychometric studies cannot be under-estimated but it can be concluded that certain intellectual skills are slowly affected by the ageing process.

The subject has been approached in an entirely different way by the classical studies of Lehman (Lehman, 1953). He estimated the academic achievements of scientists of various ages and found that their output was maximal in the 30 to 34 age range with a progressive decline in subsequent years to almost zero after the age of 70. Despite methodological shortcomings of such work, these findings are compatible with other experimental studies of creative intelligence that show a similar decline with ageing.

(2) *Memory*

As in the case of intelligence, the effect of ageing on memory must be related to the components of the memory process, namely registration, retention, recall, and recognition. The apparent forgetfulness of some elderly people reflects their failure to adequately register concepts – perhaps because of inattention or perceptual difficulties caused by visual or hearing defects. It can, however, be demonstrated that elderly people do experience particular difficulty with short-term learning and memory. Long-standing memories are relatively well-preserved, a differential effect commonly known as Ribot's law.

(3) *Personality and social behaviour*

Personality change is not inevitable in old age but it is not unusual for the personality to become modified, resulting in a reduction of the intensity of traits that were prominent earlier in life, such as drive, aggressiveness, or meticulousness, producing a general mellowing of the personality. Alternatively, some traits might become more pronounced, producing a caricature of the earlier personality. The most consistent changes, however, of which some objective evidence exists, is in respect of cautiousness and rigidity (Botwinick, 1973). Chown (1962) has demonstrated that rigidity consists of various components, some of which are understandable as an adjustment to the decline of intellectual powers that supervene in an elderly person. Other studies have suggested that old people show a tendency to increased introversion (Eysenck, 1957). A gradual slowing down of both mental and physical activities is a further characteristic feature of old age and this in itself can account for some poor performance on tests that are timed.

Of particular clinical value is the approach to the study of personality changes in old age described by Bromley (1978). This leads to greater understanding of the difficulties that are commonly experienced when relating to an elderly person. With advancing age, non-verbal expressive behaviour and gestures become reduced, together with general slowing and less spontaneity, which gives the impression of poor responsiveness, almost indifference to the observer, and a feeling that rapport is lacking. Such features, when combined with an unattractive physical appearance can deter a younger person and this, in turn, can lead to the segregation of old people and the adoption of a patronizing, almost dehumanizing attitude towards them. Awareness of how such attitudes develop can lead to a more tolerant, compassionate attitude on the part of those younger people who are responsible for the care of the elderly.

A sociological view of successful ageing was first described by Cumming and Henry in 1961. This equated successful ageing with a progressive disengagement from involvement with other people and activities that might have been enjoyed in earlier life, leading to an increasing isolation and inactivity. An alternative view is that such changes are imposed on the elderly person rather than reflecting a successful adaptation and are thus to some extent avoidable. It can be argued that the needs of elderly people are essentially the same as those they experienced when young, and successful ageing should be measured by the extent to which old people are able to continue with their usual activities and interests, despite compulsory retirement from work and similar restrictions (Havighurst, 1968).

Prevalence and distribution of mental disorders in the elderly

Epidemiological surveys demonstrate not only the prevalence of various types of psychiatric disorders that arise in old age but also the distribution of patients between various types of residential institution and the community. They also provide a measure of the disability which these patients experience. Such information is needed to appreciate fully the significance of geriatric psychiatry as well as to provide a basis for the planning of psychiatric services of this group of patients. It is not proposed to provide a detailed and comprehensive account of the epidemiology of psychiatric disorders in the elderly, but to summarize some of the findings that are of particular relevance to the clinician.

The way the population at risk is distributed must first be established, and this can be illustrated by the position in England in 1976 (DHSS, 1974, 1975, 1977). Of 6 641 000 people over the age of 65, 257 177 (3.9 per cent) were in residential care, 0.6 per cent in psychiatric hospitals, 0.8 per cent in geriatric hospitals and the remaining 2.5 per cent accommodated in a variety of residential homes. Psychiatric disorders are prevalent amongst the residents of non-psychiatric institutions. A study of routine admissions to a geriatric hospital has shown that 65.9 per cent were suffering from a psychiatric disorder. Almost half had an organic condition while 15 per cent showed signs of an affective disorder (Copeland, 1978). A survey of the residents of homes for the elderly in Scotland revealed that 37.2 per cent were confused, and a similar study in England showed that 48 per cent of women and 35 per cent of men were similarly affected (Carstairs & Morrison, 1971; DHSS, 1976). Of those elderly people living in the community, 25 per cent suffer from some form of psychiatric disorder (Kay, Beamish & Roth, 1964).

Of particular significance is the fact that 5 per cent of all elderly people suffer from dementia and those living in the community outnumber those living in residential settings by some 6 to 1. A further 5 per cent suffer from milder forms of the organic syndrome. Inevitably, the prevalence of dementia rises with age. Thus, in the age range 65 to 70 it is about 3 per cent but rises to 20 per cent in those age 80 or over. Despite the high prevalence, it has been suggested that some 80 per cent of old people living at home suffering from moderate or severe dementia are not recognized as such by their general practitioners (Williamson *et al.*, 1964).

About 12 per cent of all old people suffer from neurosis or character disorder and the risk of suicide is far greater amongst elderly people suffering from depression than in the case of younger age-groups. The risk for men is some fourfold greater than for women, and physical illness and recent bereavement are important precipitating factors (Barraclough, 1971).

Of considerable practical importance is the way in which severely disabled elderly psychiatric patients are distributed between different types of residential settings, and the community. One study defined a group of patients requiring maximum nursing care (Pasker, Thomas & Ashley, 1976). These were either bedfast, chairfast or unable to move about without the help of another person; 41 per cent of such patients were apparently found in geriatric hospitals but 13 per cent were located in residential homes and no fewer than 21 per cent were living in private households cared for by community nurses and relatives, many of whom were themselves elderly. Such findings have obvious implications for the deployment of resources.

Finally, in view of the significance of social factors in the development of mental disorder generally, some of the social characteristics of elderly people living at home should be noted (Hunt, 1978): 30 per cent of elderly people live alone and 80 per cent of these are women, of whom a third are over the age of 75. Most have a low income. Housing tends to be old and amenities less adequate than in the case of younger people. Less than half of those aged 85 or over are able to go out alone and of all elderly people, less than half go to any social centre. Ill-health and loneliness are what they fear most.

In summary, it can be seen that mental disorder in the elderly is widespread both amongst the relatively few living in residential settings and the majority who live in their own homes. The prevalence rises with increasing age and socially the elderly tend to be a vulnerable and under-privileged section of the population.

The clinical assessment and presentation of psychiatric disorders in the elderly

The clinical assessment of an elderly psychiatric patient is based on the same principles that apply to younger patients (Leff & Isaacs, 1978). There are, however, some aspects that merit special emphasis.

The patient might be encountered in a variety of different settings but there are considerable advantages in assessing the patient in his own home. It has already been noted that with advancing age a person's ability to adapt to new circumstances and surroundings is diminished and the unfamiliar and possibly frightening effects of a psychiatric ward or clinic might distort the mental state. The other advantage of home assessment is the greater likelihood of an independent informant being available as well as the opportunity to make direct observations of the patient's social circumstances which can be of diagnostic significance.

The assessment follows the familiar sequence of a comprehensive history, careful psychiatric and physical examination, followed by relevant investigations. Of this sequence, the history is likely to provide the most helpful information and a patient's own account needs to be supplemented with that provided by a reliable informant. Old people fatigue easily and time and patience are needed, not only for establishing a trusting relationship with the patient, but also to enable him to provide the indispensable historical information.

Certain aspects of the routine psychiatric history merit special emphasis. It is best to concentrate initially on the presenting problems in case the interview should be prematurely ended by the patient, and it is not unusual for the history to extend over several short sessions. The time and mode of onset of the presenting problem should first be established. The observations of a friend or relative can prove invaluable here. The objective of the history should always be to establish diagnosis or, should that prove impossible, to define those areas that require further exploration by means of physical or psychiatric examination or some form of special investigation.

Major psychiatric disorders in the elderly commonly present with a sudden and often dramatic change in the patient's personality and behaviour. In these circumstances an account of his usual personality must be obtained, and any history of serious psychiatric or physical illness in the past. When a clear line exists between a previously well-adjusted elderly person and someone who has become acutely disturbed the diagnostic possibilities will usually rest between an acute organic disorder and a functional psychosis. An acute organic psychosis (*delirium or acute confusional state*) will lead to questions aimed at identifying the underlying physical cause. A recent head injury, no matter how trivial, can be followed by a subdural haematoma. Symptoms that might suggest an infectious condition, such as cough or shortness of breath, urinary symptoms, or the presence of another person in the household with an infectious disease might usefully be excluded. Cerebral neoplasm must be considered and it is particularly important to establish what drugs the patient might have been taking as many of those that are commonly prescribed can precipitate an acute confusional reaction. Such drugs as antihistamines, hypotensive agents, and anti-Parkinsonian drugs are relevant in this respect and, conversely, the abrupt withdrawal of some drugs may act in a similar way.

The possibility of *alcoholism* might be overlooked unless specifically excluded by direct enquiry as well as by discreet observations of the contents of the patient's home. Alcoholism is a recognized problem in the elderly (Rosin & Glatt, 1977) and two patterns have been described. The first is that of a person whose long-standing drinking habits extend into old age and, secondly, more moderate drinkers who, in old age, tend to start to drink excessively. This is commonly at the expense of an inadequate diet and failure to maintain a habitually high level of alcohol intake can precipitate delirium tremens (Glatt, Ross & Javhar, 1978).

Failure to continue adequate replacement therapy for disorders such as myxoedema and diabetes might also emerge from the history.

When the history suggests an acute confusional state, the mental state examination should concentrate on those features that are characteristic of this condition (see also p. 120). Firstly, the level of consciousness is 'clouded', that is the patient's awareness of his surroundings is diminished. The patient is usually restless, often terrified by vivid visual hallucinations. He is usually disorientated and bewildered and liable to misinterpret ordinary sensory experiences which tend to assume a terrifying or perplexing quality. The physical examination is of special importance if the patient is delirious as there may be signs of the physical condition that underlies the disturbance. Most obviously, the patient's body temperature must be measured for either a pyrexia or hypothermia are significant. Hypotension might suggest a 'silent' cardiac infarct but usually the presenting symptoms will provide a reliable guide to the likely physical basis of the condition. Appropriate special investigations will be required.

In the absence of the diagnostic features of a toxic confusional state, an acutely disturbed elderly patient might be suffering from an affective or schizophrenic psychosis. Both mania and depression are well recognized in the elderly but depression is especially common in the age range 65 to 74.

Most *depressive illnesses* in old age have a precipitating cause such as illhealth, bereavement, illness in a spouse, retirement and moving house. The history will frequently reveal these or similar precipitating factors. Relatives might have noted the patient becoming slower, more withdrawn and less communicative, as well as the typical biological features of severe depression, namely poor appetite, loss of weight, and disturbed sleep rhythm, characteristically early morning waking. Preoccupation with bodily symptoms, especially those relating to the bowels is a characteristic of depression in the elderly and when such hypochondriacal tendencies are prominent, the risk of suicide is increased (d'Alarcon, 1964). History of an earlier episode of affective illness will increase the diagnostic probability.

Examination of the patient's mental state will reveal evidence of a depressive mood change but this might be overshadowed by clinical features common in the elderly. These include somatic delusions – especially as noted above, those related to the bowel, and pathological guilt feelings. When nihilistic delusions predominate, the condition is known as Cotard's syndrome. The patient might be retarded and unresponsive, almost speechless. This condition can superficially resemble dementia and is known as depressive pseudo-dementia (Post, 1975). The apparent cognitive impairment is reversible once the underlying depressive illness has been treated.

Other conditions that can mimic some features of depression in the elderly are Parkinsonism, myxoedema, or any serious debilitating physical illness, all of which can produce retardation, apathy, and a general lack of responsiveness. Some patients suffering from cerebrovascular disease may show a lability of affect but the mood change is usually brief, intermittent, and tends to fluctuate rapidly from tearful depression to fatuous and often inappropriate laughter.

Manic illnesses are less common than in younger patients but both the history and mental state examination will reveal changes in behaviour that are a striking contrast to the patient's normal personality. The general lack of inhibition and over-activity might produce an uncharacteristic coarsening of behaviour but the various changes can be understood as arising from a basic elevation of mood. Grandiose delusions might be present but, more commonly, there is an admixture of depressive features together with the manic ones.

Less common in old age, an acutely disturbed patient might be suffering from a *schizophrenic illness* or the closely related schizophreniform psychosis or paranoid hallucinosis (Post, 1966). There will often be a history of early episodes and the behavioural change of recent onset can be attributed to the effects of the psychotic symptoms the patient experiences. In *paranoid* hallucinosis, the most prominent feature is the experience of auditory hallucinations in a setting of clear consciousness. This is elaborated by the patient as indicating some unwanted intrusion or interference, possibly dangerous, and he might take precautions to protect himself or complain to various agencies. Such beliefs become more diffuse and bizarre in *schizophreniform psychosis* whilst *schizophrenia* proper is diagnosed when the typical features of schizophrenia in younger life are present. The hallucinations assume the typical form of voices talking about the patient in the third person. There may be passivity phenomena, thought echo, or broadcasting, and delusions of influence from external sources. Less commonly, incoherent speech might arise.

The clinical examination of an acutely disturbed elderly patient must include an assessment of the patient's *cognitive function* as this is of considerable diagnostic importance in distinguishing an organic from a functional condition. A variety of clinical tests have been described and these assess memory, general information, orientation, and concentration. Such tests cannot replace the more extensive and sophisticated assessment carried out by a psychologist but some have been validated and are thus of diagnostic value. It is suggested the clinician should familiarize himself with the simple schedule, preferably brief, to avoid the distorting effects produced by fatigue which can affect both the patient as well as the examiner. It will also have the advantage of enabling the examiner to memorize the schedule and provides a more consistent basis for his clinical judgement than that which arises from a random series of questions. Perhaps the simplest of such tests is the '10 question' test (Quereshi & Hodkinson, 1974; Hodkinson, 1973). The questions are: (1) Age. (2) Time (nearest hour). (3) An address for recall at the end of test. (4) Year. (5) Name of institution (or home address). (6) Recognition of two persons (e.g. doctor, nurse, relative). (7) Date of birth (day, month). (8) Years of World War I. (9) Name of present monarch.

(10) Count backwards, 10 to 1. A score of 8 and above is normal, 6 and below is abnormal and 7 borderline. Similarly, the 'set' test (Isaacs & Kennie, 1973) has been shown to have diagnostic value for dementia. The patient is asked to name 10 objects in each of four categories or sets – colours, animals, fruits and towns. The maximum score is thus 40. A score of less than 15 corresponded closely with a diagnosis of dementia whereas no patient with a score of 25 or over was demented. Finally, there is a schedule that measures both memory impairment as well as disturbance of higher cerebral function, which has been shown not only to have diagnostic value in identifying organic conditions but also to provide a reliable basis for establishing the prognosis, especially when repeated after an interval of 4–6 weeks (Hare, 1978) (table 8.3).

The 'Mini-Mental Scale Examination' is a further useful clinical schedule that provides a quantitative measure of cognitive impairment (Folstein, Folstein & McHugh, 1975) and if necessary a more extensive and detailed scheme should be followed (for example Lishman, 1978). When the history suggests that the onset of the illness is *gradual* it is important to try and establish when the patient could last be described as being his usual self. Such information can easily be obtained from a reliable informant, who will also be required to describe the course of the illness over subsequent months or years.

Patients suffering from a *chronic organic brain syndrome* will have experienced personality and behavioural changes that are understandable in relation to the progressive impairment of cognitive ability that characterizes this condition. In the early stages, features reflecting memory impairment will be evident. The names of familiar people might not be recalled and there will be hesitancy in recalling personal information such as a telephone number or correct address. It would not be unusual for an address to be given where the patient lived many years previously. The hesitancy in simple calculations and a tendency to rely on written notes would similarly suggest cognitive impairment. There may then follow evidence of the development of disorientation, with the patient losing his way in familiar surroundings. An insidious change of personality can be a further manifestation of this condition. A general slowing down, apathy, and restriction of activities can be understood as enabling the patient to adjust to his declining powers. Usual traits tend to become exaggerated so that a usually shy, sensitive person may become frankly paranoid and, similarly,

Table 8.3. *Schedule for measurement of memory impairment and disturbancce of higher cerebral function*

Memory	Aphasia	Parietal signs
What year are we in?	What do you call this (a watch)?	Show me your left hand
What month is it?		Touch your left ear with your right hand
Can you tell me two countries we fought in the Second World War?	What do you call this (a wrist strap or band)?	Name the coin in hand (named as 10p or two shillings)
What year were you born?	What do you call this (a buckle or clasp)?	No tactile inattention present
What is the capital city of England?	What is a refrigerator for?	Normal two-point discrimination
	What is a thermometer for?	Draw a square
	What is a barometer for?	

a normally rather orderly meticulous type of person may develop definite obsessional symptoms and perhaps the most striking change is the type that reflects a loss of control due to the disinhibiting effect of the dementing process and antisocial patterns of behaviour in old age that were never apparent earlier in life. Explosive irritability, shoplifting, sexual offences, such as exhibitionism, or offences involving children are examples. As the process advances, disturbance of higher cerebral function can reduce the patient's ability to care adequately for himself. Clumsiness with dressing, putting on clothes back to front, feeding difficulties, and, ultimately, loss of bladder and bowel control can all develop.

Symptoms of organic origin will typically be more pronounced at night or when the patient is removed from his familiar surroundings.

Almost all the factors that can produce an acute confusional state can lead to dementia and the history must similarly explore the relevant areas that might result in the cause being identified. Again, the physical examination is concerned with the recognition of such conditions that are associated with a dementia.

When the history is suggestive of a slowly developing cognitive impairment, the mental state examination will be especially concerned with the assessment of the patient's cognitive ability. Tests of recent and remote memory, orientation, and concentration will be impaired as, on occasions, will those reflecting impairment of higher cerebral function such as dyspraxia, dysphasia, and dyscalculia. It has already been suggested that the assessment should be based on a simple but consistently applied schedule such as those referred to above.

A *functional psychosis* in an elderly person might develop gradually, with the history extending over a period of months or possibly years. The history of the patient suffering from chronic depression might superficially resemble that described for the patient suffering from dementia. Gradual slowing down, apathy, and social withdrawal can occur but in depression these changes can be seen as arising from a mood of despondency and hopelessness with associated expressions of unworthiness, feelings of inadequacy or pathological guilt. Hypochondriacal features are common as well as the biological features referred to previously. In these circumstances, a careful examination is of particular importance because of the known association between affective illness and physical ill-health in the elderly (Kay & Bergmann, 1966).

Symptoms arising from any of the three types of *paranoid psychosis* that occur in the elderly can be longstanding, and result in increasingly obvious abnormalities of personality and behaviour which informants will report as becoming more eccentric and bizarre on occasions. Other aspects of the history that are especially relevant to the development of a paranoid psychosis in the elderly include an association with deafness (Cooper *et al.*, 1974) and a schizoid type of morbid personality with shyness, a tendency to social withdrawal, and difficulties in sexual adjustment.

Mental state examination will usually show that cognitive function is well-preserved and the various psychotic features characterizing the three varieties of paranoid psychosis will be evident.

A characteristic feature of illness in the elderly is the finding of multiple pathology. Thus, depression can be the presentation of a physical illness, features of which might be overshadowed by the depressive symptomatology. Lifelong neurotic symptoms can be intensified by the development of a dementing process or affective illness. An apparently progressive dementing condition can be due to a reversible neurological disorder such as normal pressure hydrocephalus or a cerebral tumour (Marsden & Harrison, 1972). It has been demonstrated that elderly neurotic patients have increased mortality, raising the possibility of a significant relationship between neurosis and physical illhealth (Kay & Bergmann, 1966).

It thus becomes clear that an elderly person presenting with psychiatric symptoms requires very broadly-based assessment. This must include not only a conventional psychiatric assessment but careful evaluation of all possible physical and social factors leading to a comprehensive formulation of the patient's problem.

The management of elderly psychiatric patients

Successful management is always based on accurate diagnosis. When strict diagnostic criteria are not applied there is a tendency to over-diagnose irreversible organic states and the opportunity for effective treatment is lost. Treatment of the various psychiatric syndromes is considered in detail elsewhere in the *Handbook* (see in particular vols. 3 and 4) but this section will consider some of the principles that arise relevant to the treatment and management of elderly patients.

Physical treatment

The ageing process influences the way in which a person responds to drug treatment (Crooks & Stevenson, 1978). The factors that may change in advancing age include tissue sensitivity (pharmacodynamics) and the absorption, distribution, metabolism, and excretion of drugs (pharmacokinetics). There is also the question of the interaction of different drugs that the patient might be taking and perhaps, most important of all, is the question of the compliance with treatment unless the patient is closely supervised. In addition, the presence of physical disease necessitates caution in the use of certain psychotropic drugs. Thus, while care is required, the use of psychotropic medication in the elderly should not be restricted unduly to the point of depriving patients of the benefit that they undoubtedly can produce.

Insomnia and restlessness at night frequently arise with elderly patients. Barbiturates should never be prescribed. Drugs such as nitrazepam and flurazepam should be used with caution because of the increased sensitivity to benzodiazepine derivatives shown by some elderly patients (Castleden & George, 1978). Chloral hydrate and its derivatives are usually safe and effective as is chlormethiazole although both carry some risk of producing drug dependency. The same precaution should be applied to the use of drugs as anxiolytics or mild sedatives during the day.

Antidepressant drugs have an important part to play in the treatment of affective disorder in the elderly. Tricyclic drugs may cause hypotension in some sensitive individuals and the initial dosage should be low. The presence of heart disease necessitates caution but of the various tricyclic preparations available, doxepin has been shown to have the least toxic effects on the myocardium. Monoamine oxidase inhibitor antidepressants can be useful in some elderly patients but the patient's ability to adhere to the necessary dietary restrictions must be clearly established before treatment is commenced. The use of a dietary supplement of L-tryptophan should be considered when the use of more effective antidepressants is contra-indicated. As in younger patients, lithium has a prophylactic effect on recurrent affective disorders. Prior to commencing treatment it is particularly important to ensure that both thyroid and renal function are adequate. The latter declines with age and, if significantly impaired, lithium treatment is contra-indicated because of the risk of producing toxicity.

The major tranquillizer drugs (phenothiazines and butyrophenone derivatives) can be effectively used to treat psychotic disorders but elderly patients are especially sensitive to the extrapyramidal effects of these drugs. Brain damage increases the risk of producing tardive dyskinesia, a condition that does not necessarily remit once the drug is withdrawn. Other Parkinsonian side-effects can be controlled by adjustment or the dose of the use of anti-Parkinsonian drugs. The frequency of these and comparable side-effects is such that patients receiving long-term treatment need very regular supervision.

Although a number of drugs are available that are alleged to benefit patients suffering from senile or multi-infarct dementia, there is no convincing evidence that they are effective (*British Medical Journal*, 1979).

Contra-indications to the use of modified ECT in the elderly are relatively few and are factors that would increase anaesthetic risk generally, such as heart disease or a history of recent stroke. Unilateral treatment reduces the risk of memory impairment and confusion although the therapeutic effectiveness of this technique is probably less than when the electrodes are applied bilaterally.

Because of the availability of other effective measures, psychosurgery has a very limited place in the treatment of elderly patients. The main indication is for the relief of severe incapacitating intractable depressive symptoms, especially where tension and agitation are prominent associated symptoms (Post, Rees & Schurr, 1968).

Psychological treatment

In general, psychotherapy has only very limited scope in elderly patients although it is important to be aware of the specific problems with which elderly patients are faced (Bergmann, 1978). These include the need to cope with the prospect of approaching death, physical ill-health, as well as a general decline of physical ability, the problem of dependency on others, and an associated feeling of helplessness. There is also the need to cope with an altered role and status within the family. There are considerable and often unrecognized opportunities for psychotherapy with the families of elderly patients when the presentation of a problem concerned with an elderly relative might, in fact, be symptomatic of difficulties within the family and, in these circumstances, the focus of treatment should be on the family as a whole rather than the patient who has been referred.

There is a variety of other psychological techniques that have been developed including reality orientation, behaviour modification, and the provision of various environments in which the patient can continue to play a useful role and programmes that involve stimulation and activity (Woods, 1979; Woods & Britton, 1977; Brook, Degun & Mather, 1975).

Organization of services

The progressive ageing of the population, knowledge about the prevalence of mental disorders in the elderly, and the interplay between physical, psychological, and social factors has led to the recognition that psychiatric services for the elderly need to be organized in a way as to take full account of these and other relevant factors. Detailed accounts of the organization of such services have been given (e.g. Arie & Isaacs, 1978; Jolley & Arie, 1978; Roth, 1973) but the principles involved can be summarized as follows:

Care of elderly patients is best undertaken by specialized services in which their special needs are recognized. This includes the provision of a suitable environment in hospital and familiarity with the medical aspects of old age. The service must be flexible and mobile in the sense of being available to patients in a variety of settings which, in addition to the usual psychiatric ones, will include geriatric wards and residential homes for the elderly as well as the patients' own homes. A specialized service is more likely to achieve a better allocation of resources for the elderly than when they are competing with the needs of younger patients. Special commitment to the needs of elderly patients is likely to achieve a higher standard of care, which must include the maintenance of morale of all concerned. The needs and difficulties of relatives and staff involved in the management of elderly psychiatric patients must be recognized and understood and, wherever possible, met. Psychotherapeutic skills will be required for this supportive role. Disability in the elderly typically arises from multiple pathologies, and a problem-orientated approach is particularly appropriate. A multidisciplinary team is essential for the truly comprehensive management of elderly psychiatric patients.

9

Head injury, and changes in brain function secondary to electroconvulsive therapy and psychosurgery

MICHAEL R. BOND

Brain damage is often due to naturally occurring diseases of the central nervous system and may also be the result of direct trauma caused accidentally or deliberately in the course of everyday life. The brain-damaged person may be referred for psychiatric and psychological assessment, he or she may require medical or psychological treatments, and occasionally admission to hospital for short or long-term care. Furthermore, psychiatrists use, or collaborate in the use of, techniques designed to alter brain function by physical means; for example they frequently prescribe courses of electroconvulsive therapy and occasionally refer patients for psychosurgery. Therefore, it is important that psychiatrists are well informed about the consequences of brain injury for the patient and his or her family and, with this in mind three topics of central interest have been selected for description in this chapter:

(1) The natural history and psychosocial consequences of head injury.
(2) The effects of electroconvulsive therapy on mental functions.
(3) The psychological and social consequences of surgery for mental illness.

(1) The natural history and psychosocial consequences of head injury

Head injury is a common form of trauma and from those who are seriously injured approximately 1200 moderate to severely disabled survivors are added to the community each year. Most of the disabled are under thirty years of age and half will never work again (London, 1967). In Britain and other western countries men are injured more often than women in a ratio of 2–3:1 with the maximum preponderance of men during adolescence and early adult life. Children are at greatest risk between four and eight years and whereas road traffic accidents and home accidents together account for more than half their injuries, amongst adults road traffic accidents alone account for over half the injuries (Field, 1976; Jennett & MacMillan, 1981). Head injury is not a common cause of death and mortality has been reduced by substantial improvements in primary care, but with an increase in the number of severely disabled survivors.

Head injuries may be closed or penetrating depending upon the cause. Closed injuries, also known as acceleration/deceleration injuries, are commonest in peacetime and are associated with widespread effects in the brain which, apart from the most trivial injuries, result in unconsciousness and varying degrees of physical damage to brain tissues. Penetrating or open injuries are caused by projectiles, such as bullets and shell or bomb fragments. By their nature they cause focal brain damage although more generalized lesions are found in severe injuries.

Assessment of the severity of injury

The duration of unconsciousness is related to severity of brain damage and is still widely used as a means of assessing the severity of an injury (Carlsson, von Essen & Löfgren, 1968). However, it is very difficult to define the point at which consciousness returns and this has led to the development of a coma scale by Teasdale and Jennett (1974) which takes into account both the level of consciousness and certain neurological signs. It gives a highly accurate prediction of outcome in the early days and weeks after injury (Jennett & Teasdale, 1981). Unconsciousness is followed by a period of memory impairment or post-traumatic amnesia (PTA), the duration of which is also an index of the severity of a closed head injury. The period of PTA is defined as 'the period after injury during which the injured person does not have full and continuous memory for day to day events'. The use of this measure, which is of course a retrospective one, was first described by Russell (1932) and by Russell and Smith (1961) who concluded that if the duration of PTA is less than an hour the injury is mild, if 1–24 hours moderate, if 1–7 days severe, and

if more than 7 days very severe. Post-traumatic amnesia of 24 hours is approximately equivalent to coma duration of 6 hours as an index of the degree of brain injury. The end of post-traumatic amnesia may be detected, especially after mild to moderate injuries, using a test recently devised by Fortuny and colleagues (1980).

The severity of open or penetrating injuries is measured in terms of the quantity of brain tissue destroyed and the depth of penetration of the brain, assessed radiographically, at operation, and in terms of residual neurological deficits (Lishman, 1968).

Assessment of the consequences of injury

Three aspects of the consequences of all injuries are considered and they are, first, the nature and extent of any residual neurological deficits, next, mental deficits and, last, the social problems which they provoke. Until recently far more attention was paid to physical than to mental handicap, and indeed most rehabilitative services still attend chiefly to this aspect of injury giving scant attention to psychological and social difficulties (Bond, 1975), when in reality there is overwhelming evidence that it is the mental consequences of injury which give rise to the worst problems patients and their families have to face (Fahy, Irving & Millac, 1967; Thomsen, 1974). As a result of the latter observation assessments are now being made separately of each of the three areas mentioned (Bond, 1975; Eson, Yen & Bourke, 1978; Yen, Bourke, Nelson & Popp, 1978), or on a global basis combining assessments of physical, mental and social problems (Jennett & Bond, 1975). Recently workers have emphasized the need for intensive studies of patients and their families, including the assessment of the pre-morbid psychosocial status of both as a basis for planning rehabilitation. Regarding the former, there has been considerable debate about factors predisposing to injury. Jamieson and Kelly (1973) found that adult civilian head injury victims are characterized by their youth, most are young men with evidence of previous antisocial behaviour, a higher rate of domestic and industrial accidents, and a higher incidence of disturbances in family life than non-injured individuals from a similar social group.

The process of recovery from injury

There is a commonly held view that individuals continue to recover from moderate and severe closed head injuries for several years after the initial

Table 9.1. *Recovery from brain injury*

	Duration	Events in the brain	Management priorities
A. First stage	Days	Immediate physical reaction to injury	Intensive physical care for patient
			Counselling for relatives
B. Second stage (1)	Usually 6 months	Reorganization of mental processes subserving full consciousness	Physical rehabilitation for the patient
			Counselling for relatives
The end of post-traumatic amnesia (2)		Continued rapid recovery of processes basic to motor and higher mental functions	Increased need for psychological and social methods of rehabilitation for patient and relatives
C. Third stage	From 3–6 months onwards	Greater part of physical and mental handicaps established	Psychological and social methods of rehabilitation predominate
		Emergence of behaviour patterns constituting the coping response	

brain damage. However, work carried out on adult patients with closed or open injuries, and also after strokes, reveals that the greater part of recovery of physical and mental functions which are directly attributable to brain activity takes place within 12 months of injury. In other words neurological deficits (Roberts, 1976; Newcombe, Hiorns, Marshall & Adams, 1975) and disorders of intellect and personality are largely established within one year of injury (Bond & Brooks, 1976; Dikmen & Reitan, 1977). However, the rate of recovery of individual functions varies: for example, verbal ability is restored at a faster rate than non-verbal skills – perhaps because the latter is subserved by a number of other functions which are seriously disrupted whereas verbal activity is not and represents an 'overlearned' activity (Mandleberg & Brooks 1975). Therefore, how is it that recovery continues after a year has elapsed? It is now commonly believed that physical and mental deficits do lessen to a limited extent with time but that the greater part of any improvement centres upon the adaptation of the injured person to his or her deficits and the degree of success achieved depends on the personal and social resources available to the individual with which he or she can combat the problems of handicap. Three hypothetical states of recovery and

their relation to management priorities are given in table 9.1.

The mental effects of head injury

A wide variety of factors play a part in the aetiology of mental disorders after injury and they include physiological, psychological and environmental factors, but the part played by each is not always easy to determine as there is considerable interaction between them (Lishman, 1973). The main aetiological factors identified so far are given in table 9.2.

Mild injuries: the post-concussion syndrome and accident neurosis

Mental and physical symptoms are common after mild closed head injuries, even when consciousness has not been lost, and they are twice as common after an injury at work than in any other situation (Miller, 1961). Men are affected more often than women and the symptoms of which both complain most frequently include emotional tension with irritability, mild depression, fatigue, sensitivity to noise, headache, and dizziness. Hypochondriacal reactions, conversion disorders, and obsessional neurosis may also occur (Ota, 1969). From the many

Table 9.2. *Personal, family & environmental factors influencing the outcome of brain injury*

Personal factors	Family and environmental factors
Physical	Family attitudes to the injured
Amount and location of brain damage	Influence of 'role shifts' in family
Epilepsy	Attitudes of employers, friends
Mental	Availability of support services
Premorbid constitution	Compensation claims
Primary changes in personality and intellect	
Secondary responses to injury	

symptoms reported, three, namely headache, dizziness, and emotional instability, are held to constitute the 'post-concussion syndrome' though the exact composition of the symptom complex remains a subject for debate. Cartlidge (1978) investigated 372 mildly injured patients during a period of two years and taking headache, dizziness, and depression as essential features of the post-concussional syndrome discovered two quite separate groups in his population. The first consisted of patients who experienced headache and dizziness at the time of discharge from hospital and were symptom-free within two years although 45 per cent of the group had positional nystagmus initially. The second group were virtually symptom-free at discharge but when seen six months later many complained of dizziness, of whom only 5 per cent had nystagmus, and over one third said they were depressed. The number claiming industrial compensation was over twice as high in this group (51 per cent) as in the first (21 per cent).

It is clear that even after very trivial injuries physical symptoms and signs attributable to physical damage occur. A proportion of patients complaining of dizziness have nystagmus which, if not gross, will be revealed by electronystagmography and of these most are symptom-free and have lost their signs within twelve months of injury (Harrison, 1956; Toglia, 1969). High-frequency hearing loss may produce a condition resembling intellectual damage but without a defect in comprehension on psychological testing, and headache may be the result of a transient increase in cerebral blood flow (Taylor & Bell, 1966). Damage to cervical structures may also give rise to headaches and dizziness. If complaints of physical symptoms, in the absence of physical signs, continue for more than a year the condition of 'accident neurosis' has been established. It is most common in

those with an unstable pre-morbid personality, below average intelligence, low social and economic status, dull monotonous work giving little personal satisfaction, and an outstanding claim for compensation (Miller, 1961). It is generally believed that complete intellectual recovery occurs virtually in every case of mild injury (PTA < 1 hour) but recent studies by Jane and Rimel (1979) show that defects of memory occur in as many as 37 per cent of patients three months after injury when sensitive tests developed by Halstead and Reitan (Reitan & Davison, 1974) are used. However, whether this finding has any practical significance remains to be seen but it lends support to current opinion amongst neuropathologists that even trivial head injuries produce a degree of structural brain damage.

Moderate and severe injuries

The consequence of moderate and severe injuries may be considered in terms of the changes in intellect and personality in the injured person, his or her reaction to physical, emotional and social difficulties, and the impingement of all three upon family life, work, and leisure.

Traditional intelligence tests are of limited value, as quite often an individual's performance and behaviour in everyday life are not closely related to test results. Nevertheless they give an estimate of intellectual capacity and a baseline for assessment of the process of recovery. Furthermore, interpretation of test results may be difficult because a patient's performance may be hampered by impaired concentration, lack of motivation, distractibility, mental slowness, and mood changes, one or more of which occur often after moderate and even more often after severe injuries. Occasionally patients react 'catastrophically' with an outburst of weeping or anger when under the stress of test conditions (Goldstein, 1942, 1952). Although moderate and severe injuries are not always associated with a poor mental outcome, there is mounting evidence of a strong relationship between severity of injury and degree of intellectual impairment incurred (Levin, Grossman, Rose & Teasdale, 1979), and more specifically, that the level of memory deficit is related closely to the duration of PTA. Other cognitive deficits found in the moderate and severely injured include slowness of thinking, impaired judgement, and increased orderliness. In some, dementia is profound and a small number become non-sentient or vegetative (Jennett & Plum, 1972). Personality changes vary in form and severity and, unlike cognitive change, may be marked after only a very short period of PTA or coma. Nevertheless, almost all patients with very severe changes in personality have cognitive deficits. In the mildest cases patients, and their relatives, are aware of subtle changes usually involving increased irritability, feelings of insecurity, and reduced self-confidence, at times leading to withdrawal from social activities. Feelings of depression are commonly expressed especially in patients who have deficits of intellect or neurological function which prevent resumption of previous patterns of living; depression if persistent is therefore a secondary neurotic reaction developing out of an appreciation of personal losses and as such it is often severe in adolescents and young adults on the threshold of marriage and a career, and amongst those who exhibit premorbid neurotic traits (Lishman, 1973). After more severe injuries patients may become apathetic and mentally dull, at the same time lacking in initiative and spontaneity with little or no interest in previous social and leisure interests. Feelings of depression in this group tend to be transient. By contrast some patients become euphoric, disinhibited, facile, socially disruptive, verbally abusive, and violent, with or without sexual promiscuity. Patients unfortunate enough to have these deficits may require permanent mental hospital care. Virtually all patients who have had a moderate to severe injury have a substantial reduction in their tolerance to alcohol. Changes in libido are common at all grades of severity and are the cause of difficulty between spouses. Incontinence occurs occasionally and is usually evidence of frontal lobe damage. Interestingly, studies of focal brain-injured individuals show that dominant hemisphere lesions produce greater levels of psychiatric disturbance than those in the non-dominant hemisphere (Lishman 1966, 1973).

Families of the brain-injured find it harder to cope with mental than with physical problems in the injured person (Fahy, Irving & Millac, 1967; Thomsen, 1974; Bond, 1975; Oddy, Humphrey & Uttley, 1978). Considerable stress is experienced immediately after injury when the patient's denial of its severity is marked (Romano 1974), leading to unrealistic views about survival, levels of disability and later of capacity for work and leisure pursuits (Najenson, Mendelson, Schecter, David, Mintz & Groswasser, 1974). Husband and wife relationships are more stressed than parent/child bonds (Panting & Merry, 1970; Thomsen, 1974), with wives finding difficulty in coping with the loss of husband's supporting role, his loss of sexual potency, and alterations in his mood and personality. As a result they express feelings of loneliness, isolation and depression (Rosenbaum & Najenson, 1976). There is a close relationship between severity of injury and levels of stress experienced by relatives in the first three months of recovery but this rapidly diminishes and is absent in most cases after a year; even after very severe injuries. Therefore stresses experienced by families seem to be the consequence of certain types of problems – usually those produced by alterations in personality and behaviour (McKinlay *et al.*, 1981). Finally, Weddell, Oddy, and Jenkins (1979) have reported that family stresses are not closely linked to whether the injured person returns to work nor do they depend upon the duration of his or her time in hospital. Nevertheless, family stresses may first arise when the injured person returns to and has difficulty in coping with work as a result of physical or mental handicap.

(2) The effects of electroconvulsive therapy (ECT) on mental functions

There is undeniable proof that electroconvulsive therapy produces significantly greater improvement than simulated ECT, and that it is at least as effective as antidepressant drugs with the advantage of a faster response in the treatment of severe depressive illness, (Royal College of Psychiatrists Report, 1977; Kendell, 1978), typified by the features given in table 9.3 (Freeman, 1979). Nevertheless ECT has been subjected to criticism on the grounds that it has not been proved effective by currently accepted scientific means, that its mode of action is unknown, that it is frightening and sometimes dangerous and often produces permanent memory impairment.

It is not known precisely how ECT affects metabolism of the brain and relieves depression but recent work by Grahame-Smith, Green, and Costain

Table 9.3. *Clinical features of depression that predict response to ECT*

		Carney, Roth & Garside (1965)[a]	Mendels (1965)[a]	Hobson (1960)[a]
Favourable features	early waking	+	+	
	somatic delusions	+	+	
	paranoid delusions	+	+	
	retardation		+	+
	good insight		+	+
	weight loss	+		
	pyknic body build	+		
	family history of depression		+	
	previous ECT		+	
	sudden onset			+
	obsessional personality			+
	self-reproach			+
	illness of less than one year			+
Unfavourable features	hypochondriasis	+	+	+
	hysterical attitude to illness	+	+	+
	ill adjusted personality		+	+
	neurotic traits (child or adult)		+	+
	emotional lability		+	+
	fluctuating course		+	+
	depersonalization			+
	above-average IQ			+
	precipitating factors		+	
	worse in the evenings	+		
	anxiety	+		

[a]See Freeman, C. P. L. (March 1979). Electroconvulsive therapy: its current clinical use. *British Journal of Hospital Medicine*, 281–92. Reproduced with permission (see also References).

(1978) on rats revealed that it enhances post-synaptic responses induced by biological amines (5-hydroxytryptamine and dopamine). This observation is important because it accords with the amine theory of depression which is based upon the proposal that depletion of brain amines, or a reduction in sensitivity to them, at effector sites is associated with depression. Electroconvulsive therapy has complex effects upon other aspects of brain metabolism. For example, it causes an immediate rise in prolactin levels, (O'Dea, Gould, Halberg & Wieland, 1978), and has variable effects on follicle-stimulating hormone and luteinizing hormone depending upon the patient's age and sex. Thus conclusive proof regarding the role of ECT in relieving disorders of mood by altering brain metabolism remains uncertain; but this is also true of other physical treatments.

Patients do worry about the possible effects of ECT on memory (Gomez, 1975), and it is probably no accident that alterations in memory immediately after therapy and during the following weeks and months have been more closely studied than other aspects of intellectual function. Memory is least disturbed if electrodes are placed unilaterally over the non-dominant hemisphere and if the amount of current used to produce seizure activity is as small as possible: this point has not yet been fully appreciated in Britain because a recent survey of the indications for ECT and its use by senior psychiatrists revealed that only 40 per cent favoured the unilateral technique (Gill & Lambourn, 1979), perhaps because they felt it was less effective, a viewpoint absolutely contradicted by a recent report (Weeks *et al.*, 1980). Relief of depression depends on the effects of seizures and not the amount of electricity used to produce them (Ottossen, 1960; Valentine, Keddie & Dunne, 1968; Kiloh, Child & Latner, 1960). The immediate effect of ECT is brief post-ictal confusion in a small proportion of patients (16 per cent reported by Greenblatt, Grosser & Wechsler, 1964), and the incidence is reduced by unilateral treatment. Psychological tests reveal that in the vast majority of patients short-term verbal and non-verbal memory is disturbed in the post-ictal period and for up to four weeks (Cronholm & Molander, 1964), but many months later up to two-thirds of patients may feel that their memory is worse than before treatment, even though the most sensitive tests available do not reveal any measurable memory deficits (Squire & Chance, 1975; Freeman & Kendell, 1980). The reasons for the discrepancy between subjective and objective assessments of memory remain

a mystery, but part of the answer may lie in the fact that a greater number of patients who are not relieved of their depression complain about loss of memory, whereas those who have been fully restored to health ignore or cope with minor disturbances without complaint (Freeman, Weeks & Kendell, 1980). Disturbance of memory for isolated events months or years before treatment occurs only after bilateral electrodes have been used and then in only a small number of cases (Freeman, 1979). With regard to the EEG, after an initial brief post-ictal period of electrical silence, activity is disturbed for a period of eight to twelve weeks (Freeman, 1979). Finally, the mortality associated with ECT is very low and must be weighed against higher mortality rates for drug-treated depressions and untreated illnesses (Avery & Winokur, 1976). Barker and Baker (1959) from London give a figure of one death in 28 000 treatments, Perrin (1961) from the USA one death in 12 500 treatments, and very recently Heshe and Roeder (1976) quoted a figure of one death in 22 100 treatments in Denmark.

Thus, using modern techniques and with careful attention to present indications for its use, there can be no doubt that electroconvulsive therapy remains an essential treatment for mental disorder and that it very rarely produces permanent brain dysfunction or death (*British Medical Journal,* 1980).

(3) The psychological and social consequences of surgery for mental illness

Ten years after the introduction of standard leucotomy by Freeman and Watts (1942) and sixteen years after the description by Moniz (1936) of the first therapeutic use of frontal lobotomy in a group of twenty seriously disturbed schizophrenic patients there were decidedly mixed feelings about the value of surgery in the treatment of mental disorders. The feelings were succinctly expressed in a *Lancet* leader of 1952 which stated, 'The cured patient is likely to be emotionally blunted and may become friendless. The finer human relations depend on a delicate balance of feeling which cannot survive the tactless remark, the thoughtless act or the failure to show understanding. When are we therefore ethically justified in advising a procedure which, though it relieves the misery of neurosis or pain, will also dull the patient's sense of responsibility, conscience or feelings for others'. (Leader, 1952) It could also have mentioned a mortality of 6 per cent and a high risk of post-operative epilepsy. However, it was clear that the operation could be therapeutic (Tow, 1952), and the main surgical issue of the day was to find ways of achieving therapeutic success while at the same time avoiding the gross changes in intellect and personality that could follow leucotomy. These included a period of post-operative confusion and later the appearance of emotional emptiness, poor self-control, gross egocentricity, euphoria, aggressiveness, laziness, and lack of initiative.

The knowledge that the orbito-insulo-temporo-cingulate cortex, comprising part of the limbic circuit first described by Papez (1937), is concerned with emotional expression, and that the supero-lateral frontal cortex plays a major role in intellectual functions, produced increasing refinements in surgical techniques aimed at division of white fibre tracts in the inferior medial quadrant of the frontal lobes (Scoville, 1949; Knight, 1964), in the cingulate gyrus (Whitty, Duffield, Tow & Cairns, 1952; Le Beau, 1952), and more recently in both areas simultaneously as in the limbic leucotomy (Kelly, Richardson & Mitchell-Heggs, 1973). Greater accuracy in lesion placement has been a notable feature of improved surgery and at present about two thirds of all operations performed in Britain employ stereotactic methods (Barraclough & Mitchell-Heggs, 1978).

As a result of refinements in technique the risk of death has fallen to less than 1 per cent, and of epilepsy to less than 1 per cent. Adverse changes in personality are far less common though they still occur (Post, Linford Rees & Schurr, 1968; Knight, 1973; Bridges, 1972), and impairment of intellect is very uncommon, (Mitchell-Heggs, Kelly & Richardson, 1976).

Following standard leucotomy about 25 per cent of patients improved significantly, but with improved criteria for selection for operation and improved surgical techniques the success rate overall now ranges from 55 per cent to 85 per cent, depending upon the nature of the disorder being treated. In Britain at present the operations most favoured are the stereotactic/subcaudate tractotomy of Knight (1964) and stereotactic limbic leucotomy. Reporting on the former, Ström-Olsen & Carlisle (1971) and later Göktepe, Young & Bridges (1975) showed that about 58 per cent of patients treated were symptom-free or retained only mild symptoms and a further 25 per cent were improved after surgery. In no case did operation worsen a patient's condition. Depressed patients responded most favourably (67.9 per cent), next those with chronic anxiety or tension disorders

(62.5 per cent) and then those with obsessional neurosis (59 per cent). No disabling personality traits appeared post-operatively, though relatives complained of undesirable changes in 6.7 per cent of patients, including a tendency to excessive eating, volubility, extravagance, reduction in social standards, and lack of consideration for others. It has become clear that there is a need for pre- and post-operative counselling of relatives, not only because adverse changes in personality do occur occasionally, but also because changes regarded by clinicians as favourable may alter relationships and roles within a family to such an extent that marital breakdown may occur. In 1976 Mitchell-Heggs and her co-workers, following an earlier paper (Kelly & Mitchell-Heggs, 1973), evaluated the short- and longer-term effects of limbic leucotomy in the treatment of severe obsessional neurosis, anxiety states, depression, and states of increased tension in schizophrenia. Eighty-four per cent of patients with obsessional neurosis, 63 per cent of patients with chronic tension, depression, and schizophrenia became symptom-free or were substantially improved. In the first few days after operation, headache, lack of sphincter control, and extreme laziness were common but cleared rapidly although a small number of patients complained of continuing lethargy 16 months after operation. These changes are common to all forms of surgery. Disorders of memory were not produced, personality was not blunted, and aggressiveness, impulsivity, or irritability did not occur (Mitchell-Heggs, Kelly & Richardson, 1976). Of 66 patients reported by the latter group one became slightly more outspoken and one mildly euphoric and overactive. Measured levels of neuroticism, depression, and anxiety fell and there was a marked reduction in the resistance and interference phenomena present pre-operatively in obsessional patients. Despite the overall satisfactory reduction in symptoms and very low level of side effects it should be noted that the course of recovery fluctuates and that at times patients or their relatives may feel the operation has failed after an initial period of success. This is a dangerous moment in recovery because suicidal attempts may be precipitated by such feelings.

To conclude, improved surgical techniques allied with stringent methods of selection of patients, and a critical attitude towards results gained has, in the past decade, re-established surgery as a beneficial treatment for chronic mental illness (Bridges & Bartlett, 1977). Finally, although there is still widespread apprehension on the part of clinicians (Barraclough and Mitchell-Heggs, 1978; Donnelly, 1978), and considerable opposition to this form of treatment amongst certain elements of the general public, the benefits of psychosurgery have been shown, quite convincingly, to far outweigh risks. The reduction of suffering is rapid with successful treatment in two-thirds or more of those selected for treatment.

10

The neuropsychiatry of some specific brain disorders

MARSHAL F. FOLSTEIN*
PAUL R. MCHUGH*

Introduction

The brain is vulnerable to a multitude of pathologies: those common to all tissues such as infarction, neoplasia, trauma, vascular diseases, and some peculiar to it such as neuro-specific infectious processes, nutritional disorders that produce strategic lesions in brain, and some 'degenerative' changes with genetic or idiopathic aetiologies.

The discipline of neurology focuses on the identification of the clinical conditions emerging from such disorders with the time honoured concerns for diagnosis, prognosis and treatment. Psychiatry, and particularly that re-emerging subspeciality within psychiatry called neuropsychiatry attempts to amplify on these issues by focusing on the changes in mental life that such pathologies produce. Those general changes in mental life common to brain disease of all kinds are contrasted with those changes which seem more specific to particular brain diseases or strategically localized pathological change. The primary aim of neuropsychiatry, as for any clinical discipline, is practical in that information is sought to amplify the capacity for early accurate diagnosis, improved care and treatment, and informed prognosis. Its secondary aim of further comprehension of brain–mind relationships merge with the common interests of psychologists, neurophysiologists and neuroscientists in behaviour.

* Supported in part by NIH grant #1PO1–NS16375 and the Eleanor and T. Rowe Price Teaching Service.

Since all cerebral neurology could provide material for attention and thus exceeds the limits of any one chapter, we are considering here the neuropsychiatry of a rather heterogeneous group of pathological conditions that have as their common theme the production of cognitive disorders, although each of them shows emotional disturbances and other symptomatology.

We intend to present a comprehensive view of some of the disorders and also to clarify the ways in which the mental symptoms of one resemble and differ from those of others. We consider Huntington's disease, Alzheimer's disease, Parkinsonism, hydrocephalus and some features found with stroke, multiple sclerosis, and brain tumour.

Huntington's disease

Huntington's disease (HD) is a distinct clinical entity resting on a recognizable neuropathology, that is inherited in a Mendelian dominant fashion (Bruyn, 1968; Bruyn *et al.*, 1979). Its special interest to psychiatrists derives from the frequent occurrence of psychological disorders. These include a progressive dementia, a disruption of mood, a delusionary and hallucinatory condition, and a change in personality (Huntington, 1872; Bruyn *et al.*, 1968; Dewhurst *et al.*, 1969; McHugh & Folstein, 1975).

Although the interpretation of these psychological symptoms is debated, their recognition is critical for the management of the patient. Many of the psychological manifestations are seen in other disorders but some seem special to HD.

HD usually has its onset in the third or fourth decade, although juvenile forms occasionally occur. The course is of steady progression to death in 10–15 years in many families. Recent evidence from study of age of onset and mortality rates suggests several types of the disorder (Burch, 1979).

The psychopathology and the movement disorders do not run in complete parallel. In some families aspects of the psychopathology appear before the movement abnormalities. In a few families, no mental abnormality is seen even after the progression to severe motor disorder. The psychiatric symptoms, as with the motor symptoms, do change over time. Distinctions can be appreciated in the early, mid, and late stages of the illness (Streletzki, 1961).

The dementia syndrome

An intellectual decline (dementia) is a characteristic psychological problem in HD (Wilson & Gar-ron 1979). It varies in its severity from mild to severe in different families. It is occasionally the first symptom of the condition. In a study of 11 patients, the cognitive disorder appeared before the chorea in two (McHugh & Folstein, 1975).

Once cognitive difficulties do appear they tend to progress in a steady fashion. The cognitive disability expressed clinically in HD is the result of a variable mixture of impaired cognitive functions and a progressive intellectual and emotional apathy. These two features of the dementia syndrome in HD can be separately described.

Impaired cognitive functions. The earliest disturbance in cognitive capability can be mistakenly disregarded or explained away as the expression of fatigue, distraction, or discouragement. These early symptoms are reported as change in the patient's skill in thinking through problems with his accustomed efficiency either at home or at work. Problems that have been easy for him to solve now seem more difficult. He is less able to appreciate situations and to remember.

Although these difficulties may seem vague and unaccompanied by clear failures on casual mental status examination, formal tests such as the Wechsler Adult Intelligence Scale (WAIS) document the impairment with a decline in the performance scores. An early symptom is memory difficulty. Five out of eight patients seen in a psychiatric hospital for HD complained of their memory and these patients, studied with the Wechsler Memory Quotient, were found to have memory scores below their full scale intelligence test scores (McHugh & Folstein, 1975).

These observations have been confirmed by Butters, who has characterized the memory deficit in HD. Butters contrasts the memory disorder in HD with that of Korsakoff's psychosis and concludes that the memory impairment in HD is as severe but that in contrast to the Korsakoff patient, the HD patient's memory was not disturbed by the interference of previously learned material (Butters, Albert & Sax, 1979). HD patients have more difficulty in recording experience than they do in retrieving that which is recorded (Weingartner *et al.*, 1979).

As the dementia advances in HD, memory and cognitive problems become obvious, the patient will now have a difficulty in comprehension that can be demonstrated by his inability to speak to the point, to follow directions that are complicated, and to appreciate the gist of conversations.

His judgement will be poor. He is liable to misinterpret situations and other people's meanings and may react inappropriately and emotionally.

The bedside examination now clearly reveals the disorder in thinking. Although the patients are usually oriented in time and place, mental tasks that require attention and concentration, such as the serial additions or subtractions, are badly performed. The impression is not of a specific deficit in any particular cognitive function, but a general loss of efficiency in all aspects of thinking.

Psychological tests at this time show a worsening in the overall IQ with the lowering of both verbal and performance scores. Full scale WAIS IQs in the 70 to 80 range are common at this midstage.

The terminal stage of the dementia syndrome in HD occurs after 10–15 years of the illness. At this time the patient shows a very severe cognitive loss with disorientation, a collapse of verbal and performance test scores, and the severe memory impairment. However, because of the apathetic state that will be discussed below, it may be difficult to be sure of what the patient is aware of and what mental capacities could emerge with a vigorous stimulus. Many patients at the terminal stage still grasp the significance of certain events and respond to them surprisingly accurately.

There are several cognitive functions that are always spared in HD. These spared functions help to define the dementia syndrome as 'subcortical' and differentiate it from dementias seen with cortical brain diseases.

HD patients do not develop aphasia. They may have impaired word finding and difficulty with abstract words but these difficulties reflect their problems in attention, understanding, and interpretation. Most specifically, a patient with HD never develops a jargon paraphasia that is so characteristic of patients whose dementia syndromes involve cortical degeneration such as Alzheimer's disease (Bruyn, 1968, Sjögren, Sjögren & Lindgren, 1952).

Patients with HD also do not show cortical blindness or unilateral neglect. Such common cortical features as alexia and agnosia strictly defined are never seen in patients with HD.

Mental apathy. The other feature of the dementia syndrome which is apparent essentially from the onset of the difficulties in thinking and which both worsens the cognitive disturbances and makes them more difficult to measure accurately is the appearance and gradual progression of apathy. This affects such aspects as the patient's intellectual vitality, physical energy, emotional drive, and curiosity. It is usually first recognized by a lessening interest in work, appearance, current affairs, or even in the increasing disability. This apathy, inertia, or loss of initiative can result in a much poorer performance in daily affairs than would be thought likely from the modest difficulties found on formal intellectual assessment in the early stages of the syndrome. In the late stages of HD there is a marked progression of this apathy and inertia to the point of profound self-neglect, double incontinence, and mutism.

In this terminal stage the patient is barely accessible to examination and resembles a patient with the akinetic mute syndrome. As in that condition a sudden stimulus to the patient may lead him to give evidence that some capacities to remember and appreciate something of the situation are present but masked by apathy, inertia, and mutism.

Thus, there are three distinctive features of the dementia syndrome in HD. First, a slowly progressive dilapidation of all cognitive powers; secondly, a prominent psychic apathy and inertia that worsens to akinetic mutism, and thirdly, the absence of aphasia or alexia or agnosia.

Symptoms that resemble portions of this syndrome appear with localized cortical pathology, such as the apathetic state in patients with frontal lobe disease. However, the combination of the three features that form this syndrome is distinctive and is found most often in disorders with prominence of subcortical pathology. It is for this reason that we have referred to this syndrome as the subcortical dementia syndrome. This view has been also advanced and confirmed by Albert in his study of progressive supernuclear palsy ('Steel-Richardson syndrome') (Albert, Feldman & Willis, 1974).

We see certain advantages in this clinical distinction. The most obvious advantage is that it considers other parts of the brain than the cortex have a role in cognitive activity. Also the distinctions between dementia syndromes help us recognize at the bedside conditions that have different neuropathologies, treatments, and prognosis.

Affective and schizophreniform symptoms in Huntington's disease

At different stages of the disorder as it advances other psychiatric signs and symptoms emerge in patients with HD. We will attempt to describe both symptoms and their temporal appearance in relationship to one another and to the dementia syndrome.

Early in the course, a variety of disturbances of mood are seen in HD patients. Since this is the time of onset of the disease with all the implications this realization brings to the patient and his family, it is hardly surprising that it is difficult to differentiate symptoms which are a response to such realization from those symptoms which may rest upon and be intrinsic to the disease itself. However, it has become clear that a mood disorder with symptoms that resemble the manic depressive condition, occurs in many patients with HD and in fact can occur before the onset of the choreic movements or any other signs that the patient is carrying the abnormal gene. Its frequency amongst patients with HD was noticed by George Huntington himself when he said that these patients suffer from 'the insanity with a tendency to suicide' and in fact made that feature a distinguishing characteristic of the illness (Huntington, 1872). For these reasons we consider it to be a disorder intrinsic to the disease itself and will begin by describing it in detail.

Mood disorder. The disturbance of mood usually appears in the depressive form as episodes of depression that are associated with attitudes of hopelessness and guilt and often the appearance of delusions of sinfulness, blameworthiness, poverty or disease. It is from this state of mind that the ideas of suicide and suicidal efforts by HD patients appear to spring. The frequency of suicide was identified in Michigan as the cause of death in some 7 per cent of non-hospitalized HD patients (Reed & Chandler, 1958).

Along with the change in mood and these depressive delusions, the patients may show psychomotor retardation with slowing of verbal productivity and motor activity.

The episodes of depression last from weeks to months and then spontaneously resolve. They are responsive to antidepressant drugs and electroconvulsive treatment.

Although depression is the more common affective state, mania can appear either after an episode of depression or spontaneously and without prior affective change. The episodes of mania take the typical form of elation, expansiveness, overactivity, and garrulousness. The patient may show ideas of grandeur and self-importance, may be over-

active sexually, may overeat, or may overspend. The manic state can also affect the movement disorder by increasing the amount of the chorea.

Like the depressive state, the manic state can persist for weeks and either spontaneously resolve or switch to depression.

There is little, if anything, to distinguish this set of symptoms from the manic-depressive psychosis itself.

Other forms of depression such as those which are reactive to the situation or reflect the patient's demoralization are common amongst patients with HD and do not necessarily take this episodic and bipolar form. HD patients are often sad and discouraged and they report disorders in sleep, appetite, and activity. They usually point to their clinical symptoms as the cause for their discouragement. Since many of these symptoms can be relieved with antidepressant medication, even these symptoms may be related to a pathogenic process in HD. The most recent reports by Lieberman and Folstein consider that approximately 40 per cent of patients with HD have some form of affective disorder (Lieberman *et al.*, 1979, Folstein *et al.*, 1979).

Other mood disorders. Clinicians managing patients with HD report that a variety of other alterations besides elation and depression are seen. These include irritability, aggressiveness, and a general, unpredictable vulnerability to explosive emotional reactions.

It is difficult to interpret these symptoms. Some of them may be catastrophic reactions, others may be aspects of the original personality acting in a pathoplastic fashion, still others yet to be specifically described may be HD syndromes.

Delusionary and hallucinatory states

Early in the course of HD and more commonly amongst afflicted young women is a condition often considered schizophrenic-like. It also may appear before any of the neurological disabilities. Delusions and hallucinations are displayed but they seem more to be subsidiary symptoms to a more pervasive experience in which the patient senses a foreboding change in the world around him. With this come vague delusions of influence and control, usually associated with auditory hallucinations. Schneiderian first-rank symptoms occur. For example, patients feel that their mind is controlled by other agents and have auditory hallucinations in which these agents speak about the patient. The patients are convinced of the reality of these mental experiences and act on them occasionally.

The diagnosis of schizophrenia with paranoid and catatonic features will commonly be made in such patients particularly if these features occur before the onset of chorea (McHugh & Folstein, 1975).

The course

As is obvious many of these symptoms are hard to distinguish from the standard 'functional psychoses.' They can appear before any movement disorder signals the diagnosis of HD. They are, though, usually early symptoms of the disorder.

Our experience confirms that of Streletzki, that the first symptoms of Huntington's disease can present problems of differentiation from the endogenous psychoses, affective disorder, and schizophrenia (Streletzki, 1961). However, as HD progresses and the symptoms of dementia become more prominent, these psychotic features tend to be overshadowed by the dementia. A chronic, less syndromically characteristic set of emotional changes becomes stabilized in the form of irritability and depression, all in the context of an apathetic loss of comprehension. The terminal akinetic mute state supervenes over all the features of the condition.

Summation

The unique neuropsychiatric symptoms of HD include a particular dementia syndrome characterized by (1) a progressive decline in cognitive capacity, (2) a progressive apathetic, inertial state, (3) absence of aphasia, alexia or agnosia. We refer to this constellation of features as a 'subcortical dementia.' There are prominent symptoms that mimic both manic-depressive disorders and schizophrenia, particularly early in the course.

Alzheimer's disease

We discuss Alzheimer's disease at this point to contrast its dementia syndrome with the dementia seen with HD.

Alzheimer's disease is a degenerative disorder of the nervous system of unknown aetiology but one in which brain atrophy and characteristic microscopic neuropathological changes occur (Alzheimer, 1907; McMenemey, 1966). It is a rather common condition amongst the elderly, afflicting approximately 5 per cent at age 65 and 20 per cent above age 85 (Gruenberg, 1978). In institutionalized series, females seem twice as affected as males. The course has been described as beginning with cognitive impairment and ending in a severe dementia with seizures, gait disorder, and paralysis (Sjögren *et al.*, 1952; Constantinidis, 1978). Since, along with the dementia, the patient with Alzheimer's disease will often develop aphasic and apractic symptoms and yet retain features of prior personality and alertness long into the course, we have considered it a prototype of the 'cortical dementia' which also include Jakob-Creutzfeldt disease and kuru. For the purposes of this article pre-senile and senile dementia are considered to be the same disorder with varied age of onset (Newton, 1948; Lauter & Meyer, 1968).

Dementia of Alzheimer's disease

The prominent psychopathological feature of this condition is a slowly worsening dementia. The first symptoms are often hard to judge by anyone except those most familiar with the patient. They take the form of a difficulty in judgement and an easy fatiguing of intellectual activity. However, the impairment that is usually the first symptom mentioned to physicians is disturbance in memory for recent events. This amnesic difficulty is accompanied by some disorientation in time and place. The patient becomes forgetful, particularly of the events of the day, overlooks appointments, fails to remember conversations, and forgets the purposes of his errands. At this time other symptoms reflect the patient's bewilderment in the face of complexity. He becomes lost in attempting to find his way in the city, he fails to understand a conversation particularly if several people are involved, and he cannot follow directions that involve a series of steps.

Usually within one to two years of the onset of these symptoms other difficulties in cognition appear. These are disturbances in abstract reasoning, in comprehension, and in judgment.

At this time any standard mental status examination will reveal these impairments. The patient's difficulties in orientation, in attention, in abstraction, will be apparent. How these impairments show up in the daily life of the patient will vary with his occupation and way of life (McHugh & Folstein, 1979).

Other specific cognitive symptoms in Alzheimer's disease

As Alzheimer's disease progresses, symptoms that relate to cortical injury become more apparent. These include an aphasia, often with at first a simple naming problem but later the appearance of dysphasic jargon that severely disrupts communication. Apraxias and agnosias also become prominent and can progress to a complete incapacity to manage dress, feeding, and even such manipulations as switching on a light. An agnosia for faces is a late but common symptom amongst these patients, the family members often complaining that they are not recognized by the patient (Flekkoy, 1976).

Throughout the middle stages of this disorder a tendency of the patient to perseverate on words and on other tasks appears and progresses. This interferes with the examination and can, at first, be a distraction to the further appreciation of the mental impairment.

With further progress of the condition there is a profound dementia, with the patient totally disoriented and unable to sustain any kind of communication with the examiner or with others.

An intriguing feature of the Alzheimer patient that has often been commented on is the issue of his mental alertness. Alzheimer's patients do lose their intellectual drive but many of them sustain an alert appearance and responsiveness long into the course of their illness, losing this function only when dementia is profound and in its terminal phase.

Neurological signs

Although Alzheimer's disease usually begins with psychopathological symptoms, eventually some 3 to 5 years into the course a gait disorder in which the initiation of walking is impaired becomes apparent and will advance eventually to a paralysis. The frontal signs of the grasping and sucking reflexes appear along with a change in muscular tone in the direction of *Gegenhalten*. Myoclonic jerks and seizure disorders occur in 15 per cent of patients (Jacob, 1970). Increased deep tendon reflexes and extensor plantar responses appear late in the course and in the terminal stage. The patient displays a decorticate state with flexion contractures of all limbs and a profound dementia.

The fact that the neuropathology begins in the frontal and temporal regions and advances backward provides the most likely explanation of the course, in which there is early onset of psychological symptoms and only the late appearance of crippling motor changes.

Neuropathology

The neuropathology of this condition is its defining characteristic (McMenemey, 1966). There is a progressive change in the neurons, at first in the fronto-temporal region. Microscopically the cortex comes to contain many 'senile plaques' which are microscopic collections of granular and argyrophilic particles which tend to form a halo around an indefinite centre containing sudanophilic fat and an amyloid-like substance. These plaques are collections of neuron particles and other degenerative material. In addition, however, the neurons of the cortex show a very peculiar alteration of their neurofibrils, which are thickened and twisted into distinctive 'neurofibrilary tangles'.

The contention has always been that Alzheimer's disease is an atrophic process of the brain in which nerve cells disappear from the cortex. This concept has been challenged by nerve-cell counts and remains an issue for further investigation (Terry, 1979). However, the neuropathology is clearly a progressive process, afflicting in particular the neuron parenchyma of the cerebral cortex and its connections. It eventually affects all parts of the brain and even the peripheral nervous system (Levy, 1978).

The psychopathology seems to correlate with the extent and severity of the neuropathology. This correlation assumes significance where normal subjects are included. Among affected subjects the correlation between the pathology and the symptoms is less clear. The severity of the cognitive symptoms has been correlated with the quantity of plaques and tangles in a clinical pathological study by Blessed *et al.* (1968).

Parkinson's disease

Parkinson's disease, like Huntington's disease, is also a distinct clinical entity that rests upon a known neuropathology (Parkinson, 1817; Foix & Nicolesco, 1925). Unlike Huntington's disease its relationship to genes or to other pathogenic factors is still debated but, as with Huntington's disease, it is frequently associated with psychological disorders. These include a progressive dementia, disorders of mood, and a variety of hallucinatory states (Mindham, 1974; Loranger *et al.*, 1972; Sweet *et al.*, 1976; Mindham, Marsden & Parkes, 1976; Sacks, 1976).

The neurological symptoms are the easiest to describe. They appear in middle life but most commonly after the age of 50, as some variant of the classical triad of tremor, rigidity, and akinesia. The tremor or rigidity frequently begins unilaterally. The condition, though, progresses to a bilateral neurological disorder in which the tremor, rigidity, and akinesia produces in the patient a characteristic posture, facial expression and gait.

Psychopathology

Individual Parkinsonian patients endure a wide variety of psychopathological symptoms including disturbances in motivation and sleep rhythms, sexual disorders, and obsessions. We do not plan to discuss these but will focus on symptoms common to many patients and that appear in relationship to the onset of the illness and its progression. These are the dementia syndrome, the affective changes and the hallucinatory syndromes.

Dementia syndrome. Dementia occurs in Parkinsonism, in contrast to the opinion of Parkinson himself. However, as distinct from Huntington's disease, it is by no means a universal phenomenon. It occurs in approximately one-third of the patients. The dementia tends to occur late in the course of the illness after the motor symptoms have advanced significantly. It may be this appearance late in the very advanced condition where psychomotor retardation is so prominent that led to its being overlooked or mistaken for slowness to respond. However, if a careful cognitive status examination of the most affected patients is done, dementia will be evident in a significant number (Lieberman *et al.*, 1979; Marrtilla & Rinne, 1976).

The dementia syndrome does take the form of a subcortical dementia. That is, as in HD, the Parkinsonian patient is clearly lessened in his capacity to think, reason, and remember. However, at no time does he show a set of symptoms characteristic of cortical lesions like aphasia or a jargon aphasia or a cortical blindness.

The apathetic feature commented on earlier in this chapter in connection with HD is also very prominent in patients with Parkinsonism. It, too, produces a great slowness in response and an apparent lack of interest in problems or difficulties. It can advance, as with Huntington's disease, to an akinetic mute syndrome.

Thus, the dementia syndrome in Parkinson's disease is similar to that seen in HD but is different from the dementia in Alzheimer's disease. It differs from HD, however, in that it occurs late in the course of the neurological condition, afflicts only a fraction of the patients with Parkinson's disorder, and is easily overlooked because of its appearance in severely incapacitated, elderly infirm patients.

Affective disorder. Whereas dementia occurs late in the course of Parkinson's disease, irritability and depression are described as appearing early in the condition, and are hard to distinguish from emotional reactions to the disease. However, a depressive disorder that could be characterized as a clear syndrome, identical to that seen in affective illness and responsive to the usual treatments, including electroconvulsive treatment, is found in approximately one-third of patients with Parkinsonism (Asnis, 1977).

The severity of the affective syndrome is related to the severity of the motor defect (Mindham, Marsden & Parkes, 1976), but the motor deficit and depressive symptoms can be dissociated from one another (Asnis, 1977). It is often crucial to treat the depressive syndromes specifically, even though there has been a considerable improvement in the neurological syndrome with levo-dopa. A programme which combines levo-dopa and an antidepressant is often required for patients who have these symptoms (Lishman, 1978).

Although a bipolar course is unusual amongst patients with Parkinsonism, depression being by far the more common expression of their affective change, the patient can be provoked into a manic state occasionally in the course of treatment. This is more common with levo-dopa treatment but it has been seen with a neurosurgical chemo-pallidectomy (Goodwin, 1971).

Hallucinatory states. Perhaps the most common hallucinatory condition suffered by Parkinson patients occurs in the context of a delirium secondary to levo-dopa or anticholinergic medications. This delirious state has the customary features of disturbance in consciousness, disorientation, and the appearance of visual hallucinations and illusions. The diagnosis is made by the association of these several features together.

Distinguished from the delirium is another often observed phenomenon in Parkinson patients, namely visual hallucinations in clear consciousness. This usually occurs in association with a mild cognitive impairment and some disturbances of vision or hearing. However, the patients report vivid hallucinations involving people and small animals. Patients have reported a whole range of visual perceptions but many of the patients state that they usually see small and peculiarly dressed people that they call dwarfs, leprechauns, or fairies. The resemblance of these hallucinations to the so-called peduncular hallucinosis of Lhermitte is clear (Smith, Gelles & Vanderhaeghen, 1971; Lhermitte, 1922).

The hallucinations differ from those seen in patients with delirium in the sense that the patients often retain some insight into the fact that these vivid perceptions do not reflect reality. The patient however may complain about them as experiences, occasionally losing insight and fearing their actions. These symptoms appear refractory to treatment and have not responded well to neuroleptics in our experience.

Hydrocephalus

Although hydrocephalus had previously been thought of as a birth defect with prominent effects on growth and development, it is now known that adults with either an arrested hydrocephalus that had produced little prior impairment or the onset of some pathological process affecting the flow of spinal fluid, can present a neuropsychiatric syndrome that is quite characteristic. This combination of motoric and psychopathological features is sometimes referred to as occult hydrocephalus or normal pressure hydrocephalus (McHugh, 1964, 1966).

The motor features include a prominent disorder of gait and bodily stance in which the patient walks with difficulty, taking stiff steps in a fashion resembling a spastic paraparesis. On neurological examination, increased deep tendon reflexes in the legs and extensor plantar responses are often found.

The psychopathology takes the form of an apathetic dementia very similar to that seen in HD and in Parkinsonism. An occasional patient will have a Korsakoff syndrome without any other evidence of dementia.

Dementia

The dementia of these patients varies in severity from mild to extreme. As with all dementias, when early and mild, the family, and sometimes the patient, notices only that his judgement and his capacity to think on crucial issues is impaired, but as the dementia progresses there is a steady loss of all cognitive abilities and a decline in the Wechsler Adult Intelligence Scale.

As with all subcortical dementia, but very particularly in this condition, the apathetic features are prominent. This apathy at first is registered as concern by the family because of the lack of interest the patient shows in work, family life, and his clinical condition. As it increases, its resemblance to akinetic

mutism is progressively obvious, as it leads to a bedfastness, double incontinence, and unresponsiveness. The advanced state thus can find a patient with a neurological syndrome of a total paralysis of his lower extremities and in a mute state that can be confused with catatonic stupor. As with any akinetic mute condition the influence of the apathy upon the cognitive abilities is prominent; occasionally, with a sharp stimulus, the patient can be made to give a response that belies his unconscious appearance.

It is the severe apathy that is most responsive to the treatment for this condition which involves a shunting of the spinal fluid. With apathetic patients there can be a remarkable reawakening of mental life and even a resumption of full activities. Individuals that do recover in this way often persist in showing some injuries to their cognitive capacities, which may take the form of impaired performance scores on the Wechsler Adult Intelligence Scale. This psychological deficit is the result of the tissue destroyed by stretching as a result of the chronic hydrocephalus (McHugh & Folstein, 1979).

It is our clinical impression that to attempt to relieve a modest amount of cognitive disability in patients with hydrocephalus but without the apathetic akinetic feature is frequently unsuccessful. These are individuals who, despite their hydrocephalus and its injury to cognitive power, have reestablished themselves, and further shunting will not restore function.

An occasional patient without apathetic feature will report a memory disorder and particular inability to learn new things. This seldom is of such a degree that the patient is completely disoriented, but certainly can be shown to affect the Wechsler Memory Scale out of proportion to the Wechsler Adult Intelligence Scale. Occasionally, though, the memory disorder can reach proportions similar to that of Korsakow's syndrome. Again, without an apathetic feature there seems little to be gained by shunting spinal fluid in these recompensated hydrocephalics. The particular cause of the memory disorder in these patients is not known but may reflect the distension of the third ventricle.

The dementia syndrome of hydrocephalus, like all subcortical dementias, has associated apathy and no evidence of aphasia, apraxia, or cortical blindness. Again the apathetic feature has often been compared to the inertia that can be seen in patients with severe frontal lobe injury. Certainly individuals with a severe frontal lobe lesion due either to haemorrhage or to surgical procedure can resemble patients with subcortical dementia. The likely explanation would be the rich connections between the subcortical region and the frontal region.

Disseminated pathologies of the brain (cerebral vascular disease, multiple sclerosis, tumour and their psychiatric complications.)

In contrast to these rather specific brain disorders, there are a number of other disorders which affect the brain in a focal fashion or are dispersed throughout it. These conditions have as their characteristic the disruption of cerebral tissue in local regions and produce their psychopathology according to their location and their extent.

Essentially every aspect of cortical or subcortical forms of cognitive psychopathology can be seen within these conditions, including such symptoms as aphasia, apraxia, amnestic syndromes, frontal lobe apathy, and cortical blindness. We will focus on the following issues: (1) the dementia syndromes that can appear in these conditions and their characteristics, (2) the associated emotional disorders that also accompany them, and (3) some of the more unusual neuropsychiatric findings that occur with occasional patients.

Dementia

As these conditions are capable of producing extensive damage to cortical and subcortical regions of the brain, it is not surprising that the psychopathology that is most prominent amongst them is a dementia syndrome. The dementia can be cortical or subcortical in form or a mixture of both, depending upon the location and extent of the lesions. With diffusely scattered lesions, individuals show both the aspects of cortical dementia with symptoms of aphasia and apraxia and as well the apathetic state produced by, and characteristic of, lesions in the subcortical area.

It is usual in these disorders for the patient to have had evidence of motor sensory disorder, essentially from the onset of his condition. In fact for stroke the characteristic is a history of multiple episodes in which a motor sensory loss, transient or persisting, occurs *pari passu* with each decline in intellectual power (Hachinski *et al.*, 1974).

When the pathologies are bilateral in the hemispheres, as with stroke and MS, the patient frequently will show spastic weakness of his bulbar functions. This so-called pseudo-bulbar palsy is not seen in the degenerative disorders of Alzheimer's disease or Parkinsonism. It can be one of the most helpful signs to define the diagnosis of multiple infarct dementia. The presence of pseudo-bulbar palsy is helpful evidence of multi-infarct problems, although its absence does not exclude it (Adams & Victor, 1977).

Patients with MS show the characteristic features of the demyelinative disorder affecting cranial nerves, spinal cord, and brain stem as well as the cerebral hemispheres. The dementia is often a late aspect of their condition since a destruction of over 50 ml of cerebral tissue is probably required before a dementia syndrome begins to appear and much of the early symptoms of MS reflect spinal cord and brain stem injury (Surridge, 1969).

Emotional disturbances

Emotional problems found with these conditions have often been considered understandable responses of the patient to his disabling disorder. Some specific emotional difficulties accompany these conditions, however. These symptoms have specific forms which differentiate them from the demoralization and discouragement of people with chronic illness and it is this feature that prompts the view that they have a specific relationship to the neuropathology.

We begin with the affective condition which is most obviously different in its form from ordinary emotional life, to a degree where neurologists have referred to it as pathological laughing and crying or emotional incontinence (Adams & Victor, 1977). This condition occurs in patients with both stroke and multiple sclerosis if there has been a bilateral corticobulbar tract injury. It is the loss of adequate control of emotional expression. Mildly emotionally-laden events evoke in them extensive and prolonged emotional expressions in the form of either weeping or laughing. Phenomenologically the patients report that they do not feel this emotional state to the degree that they seem to be expressing it. They report that one of their embarrassments is the inability to moderate their emotional expression. The expression of the emotion is exaggerated. The face of the patient assumes a grimace of hilarity or grief. It is very disconcerting, though, to both patients and families. Its association with pseudo-bulbar palsy has led to its being called pseudo-bulbar laughing and crying. Perhaps the term *pathological laughing and crying* is the most useful one since it emphasizes the abnormal form and phenomenology of the condition.

The second condition that is prominent in patients with stroke and particularly patients with cerebral vascular damage to the right hemisphere is a change in their prevailing mood and emotional responsiveness. The patient himself may report such symptoms as feeling depressed and discouraged, but the family sees most prominently a change in the direction or irritability and a loss of pleasure in situations previously enjoyed by the patient (Folstein *et al.*, 1977). Severe depression is seen with lesions toward the frontal pole in the hemisphere (Robinson & Szetela, 1981).

This is a symptom that has to be directly sought and the patient and family questioned about it. It is not usually a symptom that the patient volunteers until it becomes so severe as to be disruptive to the family life. The reasons for this are uncertain but it may relate to the common difficulty in getting people to appreciate a pathological aspect of changes in mood, such changes being so easily explained away as expected states of mind in any impaired person.

Relatively short-lived emotional disruptions are seen in all dementing illnesses including those based on these pathologies (Goldstein, 1975). These *catastrophic reactions* are the rather sudden appearance of emotional distress and anger often associated with the autonomic expression of these emotions that occur in brain-damaged, demented individuals who are faced with tasks that exceed their present capacities. The reaction may be short-lived over a few minutes but if the situation remains unchanged they can continue waxing and waning through longer periods. The crucial recognition though is the association of this emotion with a particular task given the patient. Again, the patient himself may report that he is overcome by his emotions and is surprised by the onset and the exaggeration of their expression.

All of these neurological diseases because of their threatening implications to life and capacity are associated with emotional reactions, many of which are typical of the person and his mode of coping with difficult life situations. Therefore, a reactive and sustained demoralization and depression amongst these patients is not unusual.

An inappropriate good mood or euphoria has occasionally been cited in individuals who are severely afflicted with MS. This euphoria is to be distinguished from pathological laughing which can be seen in other patients. The majority of patients with MS have appropriate and responsive emotional states that relate to the issues of their daily life and the remissions or excerbations of their disorders. The patients who seem indifferent to their situations are rare but are always amongst those individuals who have an extensive disorder and are already showing signs of a dementia that may alter their capacity to recognize their condition and future. A euphoria is found only amongst the demented in MS (Surridge, 1969).

Unique symptoms commonly seen with local pathology and those most common to brain tumours

Tumours can occur anywhere in the brain and produce essentially any kind of neuropsychiatric set of symptoms depending upon their location and their extent. Thus, seizures, progressive disturbances in consciousness leading to coma and death, headache and vomiting, aphasia, apraxia and agnosia, dementia, and delirium all are found in patients with brain tumours and relate to location and extent of lesions in the brain.

There are, though, certain symptom clusters that occur with regularity in relationship to tumours in particular locations. Frontal lobe tumours such as meningioma, but also some forms of glioblastoma restricted to the frontal lobes, can produce symptoms of depression and some cognitive loss that is difficult to differentiate from reactive discouragement and demoralization. The patients and their families often report that the patient has changed in a fashion that is difficult to describe but includes a change in drive and interest in the direction of apathy and negativism. The apathy can affect all aspects of the patient's activity. The eventual appearances of motor symptoms or a dementia syndrome will direct attention to the correct diagnosis (Hunter *et al.*, 1968; Carlson, 1977).

Tumours in the parietal region will provide a variety of psychopathological symptoms depending on whether the dominant or non-dominant hemisphere is affected. These symptoms, though, include the language disorders of the dominant hemisphere (aphasia and alexia) and the special problems of the non-dominant hemisphere (unilateral neglect, apraxia) (Hécaen & Ajuriaguerra, 1956). These issues are discussed elsewhere.

Lesions in the temporal lobe are very prone to produce seizures. Thus, much of their symptomatology is due to the combination of local destruction and mass effects plus seizures. This combination can produce a complicated set of findings. Thus with such lesions there have been reports of hyposexuality, irritability, aggressiveness, and dementia. What is tumour, what is seizure, and what is medication-induced have been difficult to differentiate (Malamud, 1967).

The neoplastic lesions around the third ventricle obstruct the flow of spinal fluid. Such tumours as extensively invasive craniopharyngiomas or colloid cysts of the third ventricle produce a hydrocephalus with all of the symptomatology of the hydrocephalic dementia. A few particular conditions have been reported with lesions in the hypothalamic region. The symptoms relate to this locus rather than to the nature of the pathological process and therefore can occur not only with neoplasms but with such inflammations as sarcoidosis and tuberculosis.

These are changes in the motivated states of the patient. Perhaps the most prominent example is the change in food intake produced in patients with lesions in this region that was first documented by Froehlich at the turn of the century. Individuals with compressive or invasive lesions of the hypothalamus may show a change in food intake and begin to eat ravenously with a steady increase in body weight. Recently a single report by Reeves and Plum (1969) confirmed this in another patient who was not only eating ravenously but had mood changes in the direction of anger, irritability, and explosiveness particularly if food was withheld.

An intriguing feature of these disruptions in feeding is their relative infrequency despite the rather frequent occurrence of neoplastic pathology in this territory. Specifically placed injury that spares some pathways in the network of neuronal connections within the hypothalamus seems required. Most invasive pathologies are too indiscriminate in their destruction.

Many other changes in motivation have been reported in patients with lesions in this area including disturbances in thirst, changes in sexual behaviour, and aggressiveness (Lewin *et al.*, 1972).

Summary

Here we present the neuropsychiatric approach to a group of disorders of the brain. The unifying principle was that all are capable of producing some form of cognitive loss and thus dementia and most of them are complicated by emotional disturbance. The features of these dementias were described and distinguished. Other associated psychopathological symptoms that derive from a variety of neuropathological processes in the brain were discussed.

A neuropsychiatric approach to specific brain disorder brings clinical advantages. Psychiatric symptoms of disordered cognition and mood can be recognized at the bedside, understood, and managed, even though the underlying neuropathological disorder is still incurable and unpreventable. The clinical experience with the psychopathology raises questions for research which attempt to associate specific mental disorders with specific brain disorder.

An assumption of this approach is some familiarity with neurology and clinical medicine – an assumption with implications for the training of all psychiatrists.

Management of neuropsychiatric disorders

Clinical trials of all types of treatment – pharmacological, psychological, and sociological – are needed to place the management of these patients on a firm base. However, in the absence of clinical trials, a practice has developed which is helpful for clinicians caring for these patients. We present some examples of our practice employing pharmacological, psychological, and social measures.

Pharmacological measures seem to help demented patients cooperate with social and psychological interventions. Small doses of neuroleptics (25–50 mg thioridazine) at bedtime are used to promote sleep and reduce irritability. Their care must be minimized however because of the risk of tardive dyskinesia.

Tricyclic antidepressants (amitriptyline 25–50 mg) are useful in promoting sleep and relieving depression. Side effects of cardiac arrhythmias, urinary retention and increased intra-ocular pressure limit dosage.

Sedatives are occasionally required for demented patients (chloral hydrate 500 mg, as necessary). But the most important pharmacological measure is a reduction whenever possible of drugs taken by these patients for other medical disorders. Brain impaired people seem more vulnerable to becoming intoxicated by these drugs.

Psychological management centres on forming habits of behaviour which can be the daily routine of the demented patient and then sustaining these habits. This serves several purposes. Unexpected activities unfamiliar to the patients are avoided, thus reducing the probability of catastrophic reactions. Family members who are caregivers are better able to plan their time, since the patient is on a predictable schedule. Clinicians are able to establish a stable baseline of behaviour on which to base interpretations of response to treatment.

The fate of brain-injured patients is determined to a large extent by his social framework. Thus, clinical attention is required for an analysis of family structure, community supports and occupational rehabilitation.

11
Acute organic reactions

J. CUTTING

Definitions

An acute organic reaction is a short-lasting psychiatric disorder arising in conjunction with a recognized disturbance of cerebral function. The word 'acute' refers to mode of onset, duration, and to some extent the degree of disturbed behaviour. It does not mean that the condition will necessarily resolve, as acute reactions may become chronic and some chronic reactions are reversed by specific treatment. The word 'organic' has two meanings. Its principal sense is to signify that a disturbance of brain function is the overriding aetiological consideration; other factors (e.g. personality) have only a subsidiary role. Secondly, it implies that where such aetiological considerations apply, certain characteristic features may be observed in the mental state. These are broadly referred to as examples of *cognitive impairment*, and include clouding of consciousness, disorientation, poor attention, and memory deficits. Other abnormalities in the mental state may appear, such as mood change or abnormal perceptions and beliefs, but unlike the functional psychoses, where they dominate the clinical picture, in acute organic reactions they are regarded as secondary to cognitive impairment. The word 'reaction' suggests that the cerebral disturbance determines the onset, nature, and course of the clinical picture.

The two meanings attached to the word 'organic' can lead to difficulties in practice, for a disturbance of cerebral function and a mental state with prominent cognitive impairment are not invariably associated. The condition known as alcoholic hallucinosis, where auditory hallucinations appear in clear consciousness in the context of heavy alcohol consumption, can be regarded as *organic* in aetiology but assumes the form of a *functional* psychosis. Conversely, in the course of a severe depressive illness, an *organic* mental state may emerge, resembling for a time that due to cerebral dysfunction and known for this reason as pseudo-dementia. In the first example the lack of correspondence between organic aetiology and organic mental state can be explained by assuming that whilst cerebral dysfunction may be the overriding aetiological consideration in most instances where it occurs, on occasions its influence may be attenuated by genetic, personality, or other factors. Lipowski (1978) proposes a pragmatic classification of the relationship between cerebral dysfunction and psychiatric disorder along these lines. In the second example it is necessary to realize that poor functioning on cognitive tasks may arise from causes other than cerebral dysfunction; these include poor motivation, retardation, and preoccupation with psychotic experiences.

Instead of *acute organic reaction* a number of other terms are used, sometimes interchangeably and sometimes to emphasize a particular clinical picture. The terms *confusion* or *toxic confusional state*, *delirium*, and, more rarely, *twilight state* and *amentia* are encountered. The terms 'twilight state' and 'amentia' have an historical meaning within Bonhoeffer's (1909) scheme of exogenous reactions. He believed that pathogenic factors acting on the brain could produce one of five clinical pictures, including, in addition to these two, 'delirium', 'hallucinosis', and 'epileptiform excitement'. It is doubtful whether this and other detailed classifications of the presentation of acute organic reactions are justified, and so these two terms have no current useful meaning. Lishman (1978) criticizes the use of the terms 'delirium' and 'confusion' when applied to nosological entities and advocates their restricted use for the description of phenomena which appear during an acute organic reaction. 'Confusion', he argues, should be reserved for an 'inability to think with customary clarity and coherence', and 'delirium' for a complex picture 'of impairment of consciousness along with intrusive abnormalities derived from the fields of perception and affect'. The terms *subacute confusional state* and *subacute delirium* are also encountered. They denote an organic reaction whose onset is more gradual,

course more prolonged, or clinical picture less florid than is usual.

Clinical picture

The characteristic features, representative of cognitive impairment, are *clouding of consciousness*, *disorientation*, *poor attention*, and *memory deficits*. Other abnormalities – *disturbed behaviour*, *disordered form of speech and thinking*, *alterations in mood*, *abnormal perceptions*, and *abnormal beliefs* – are common to all psychoses, but when present in acute organic reactions they may have a distinctive pattern. The frequency of these various phenomena, as encountered in a series of 74 acute organic reactions (Cutting, 1980) is shown in table 11.1

Clouding of consciousness

Clouding of consciousness holds a prominent place amongst the features of an acute organic reaction. The detection of this relies principally on the judgement of the clinician, as psychological tests are directed towards the more easily measured deficits in part-function, such as attention. Abnormalities range from slight dulling of one or more faculties through to coma. At the milder end of the continuum the patient appears vague and tends to lose track of conversation. This may be inferred only retrospectively when on a subsequent visit it is apparent that details of the earlier interview have been forgotten or distorted. Moderate clouding may be manifest by a fluctuating awareness of the clinician's presence, with alternations between appropriate behaviour and indifference or preoccupation with extraneous stimuli. At its most severe the patient will be stuporose with little or no response to questioning.

Disorientation

Although not always elicited in milder reactions, disorientation for time and place is easily assessed and for this reason is the best pointer to an organic aetiology (Shapiro, Post, Löfving & Inglis, 1956; Hinton & Withers, 1971). Mistakes in place, year, and month are more significant than failure to give day of week or exact date (Jenkyn, Walsh, Culver & Reeves, 1977). Disorientation for person is rarely seen and is more likely to indicate hysterical mechanisms or an acute functional psychosis.

Poor attention

Inattention, distractibility, and mistakes or slowness in carrying out formal tasks discriminate well between patients with organic reactions and

Table 11.1. *Mental state in acute organic reactions* (% of 74 patients with abnormalities)

	%
Clouding of consciousness	
Total	62
Predominant feature	
Fluctuating stupor	22
Failure to appreciate nature of place (i.e. hospital)	19
Failure to recognize relatives	13
Disturbed nocturnal behaviour	5
Confabulation	3
Disorientation	
Day of week	51
Month	43
Year	36
Name of place (i.e. name of hospital)	34
Poor attention	
Digit span under 6 forwards	41
Memory deficit	
Impaired on-going memorizing	82
Failure to name Prime Minister	62
Abnormality of mood	
Total	85
Predominant feature	
Depression	34
Hostility	18
Elation	16
Lability	8
Anxiety	7
Perplexity	2
Disordered speech and thinking	
Total	23
Irrelevant and rambling replies	10
Incoherence	5
Other	8
Abnormal perceptions	
Total	34
Visual	31
Auditory	15
Somatic	4
Abnormal beliefs	
Total	46
Paranoid	34
Reference	15
Guilt or hypochondriasis	5
Grandiose identity or abilities	3
Influence or primary delusion	3
Other (e.g. concern with imminent death)	12

normal persons (Chedru & Geschwind, 1972). Suitable tasks to elicit these are *serial sevens* (subtracting seven serially from 100 allowing one mistake in one minute) and *digit span* (correct immediate repetition of six or more digits forward and four or more backwards). Unfortunately, for diagnostic purposes, impaired performance is also a feature of functional psychoses (Shapiro et al., 1956; Hinton & Withers, 1971).

Memory deficits

Some degree of memory impairment can nearly always be detected. Most easily tested is *recent* or *on-going* memory, the ability to remember a new piece of information over a given period of time. (Normal persons should make only one mistake with a name and address after five minutes.) A failure of *remote* memory, the inability to recall information acquired before the onset of the condition, is less easily elicited, particularly in milder reactions. Nevertheless, most investigators have found that some questions of general information (e.g. name of prime minister) do discriminate well between functional and organic conditions.

Disturbed behaviour

There may be a reduction of normal activity with apathy and reluctance to carry out habitual tasks. This may go unnoticed unless there is a progression to stupor. A more familiar picture, as it requires intervention from nursing and medical staff, is acute excitement. This may fluctuate and is particularly troublesome at night.

Disordered form of speech and thinking

Speech, reflecting thought processes, may be reduced in quantity, with slowness and poverty in expression and a lack of grasp in comprehension. Qualitative changes include perseveration, incoherence, and, in milder reactions, a vague and rambling form. The disorder of thinking, although difficult to describe, does appear fairly specific to acute organic reactions. Halpern, Darley and Brown (1973) found that an estimate of relevance (i.e. how appropriate a response was to a question) distinguished such patients, who gave irrelevant replies, from those with aphasia, dementia, or speech apraxia. Levin (1956) characterized it as a 'failure to make connections' and gave, as an example, a patient who thought it was Easter because he heard a nurse discussing eggs. Rarely there may be paraphasic errors (Curran & Schilder, 1935; Weinstein & Kahn, 1952), where the word supplied is inappropriate or not even a dictionary item, but its elements bear some connection to the expected answer (e.g. piano-stool for bed-pan, cigaroot for cigarette).

Alterations in mood

Mood change is common. It rarely suggests the aetiology and is often misleading in this respect. The patient may be apathetic, in keeping with a reduction in level of consciousness. The appearance, morbid preoccupations and the content of the abnormal perceptions and beliefs may suggest a depressive illness, and the patient is not infrequently diagnosed and treated as such by the referring physician (Levine, Silberfarb & Lipowski, 1978). Less commonly there is elation. There may be marked anxiety, fear, and excitement, the familiar pattern of the disturbed patient at night. The predominant mood may be one of perplexity: the patient looks puzzled and frightened and gives bizarre replies to questions of orientation. He may be hostile or suspicious. Commonly the mood is labile, fluctuating between all these abnormalities.

Abnormal perceptions

It is often difficult to establish the exact nature of the abnormal experiences. At the time patients may be hostile towards the interviewer; later they may through embarrassment be reluctant to discuss their experiences, may dismiss them as day-dreams or nightmares, or may have complete amnesia for the period of abnormal behaviour and react with surprise on hearing an account of it. However, if the phenomena can be elucidated, almost pathognomonic of an organic aetiology is the close connection with true events in the environment that occurs. In the auditory modality they may misinterpret conversations or background noise and assign some other meaning, usually personal (e.g. presence of spouse on ward) or malign (e.g. medical staff are murdering patients). In the visual modality they may elaborate routine ward scenes into fantastic and terrifying plots or misidentify hospital staff for close relatives. Hallucinations, less influenced by the environment, are characteristically visual, and, in content, brightly coloured, moving or panoramic, distorted in size, and of animals or groups of people.

Abnormal beliefs

As with perceptions, the abnormal beliefs are more transient, more likely to be related to immediate surroundings and less easily categorized than are the delusions of the functional psychoses. Paranoid delusions and delusions of reference are common but it is rare to see the characteristic delusions of the functional psychoses – influence, grandiosity, guilt, or hypochondriasis. Themes of death are not uncommon but unlike those in a depressive illness they express, not a desire for death, but a conviction of its imminence in self or relatives.

Aetiology
General considerations

There are a large number of reported causes of an acute organic reaction. An extensive list, prepared by Lishman (1978), is shown in table 11.2. These conditions are covered elsewhere in this volume, with the exception of infections, which will be given relatively more space in this chapter than their importance in this context deserves. Other conditions will be mentioned only to give their particular association with an acute reaction, emphasizing prevalence and the way in which the diagnosis may be established.

It is also helpful to bear in mind the more likely causes, and for this purpose the contributory and chief conditions in 74 acute organic reactions encountered amongst general hospital in-patients (Cutting, 1980) are shown in table 11.3. The findings were in agreement with those of Peters and Gille (1973), reporting 562 referrals to a neuropsychiatric clinic with 'acute secondary psychosis', where in more than half the cases several factors could have been responsible, and heavy alcohol consumption and intoxication with prescribed drugs were the commonest. Earlier studies (Bonhoeffer, 1917; Wolff & Curran, 1935) are of less interest as the chief causes identified in earlier decades (infections – 52 per cent in Bonhoeffer's series, bromide intoxication and eclampsia – 9 per cent and 4 per cent respectively in Wolff and Curran's series) are now rarely responsible in developed countries.

Factors other than the physical condition itself can affect both the content of the mental state and the risk of occurrence of an acute reaction. Since Bonhoeffer (1909) rejected the idea that each noxious agent gives rise to its own specific mental state, it has been assumed that family history of functional psychosis, personality, background, attitude towards illness, and circumstances of illness influence the content. Wolff and Curran (1935) stressed personality and background. Manfred Bleuler (1951) believed that a depressive or schizophrenic-like picture only

Table 11.2. *Causes of acute organic reactions*

1. Degenerative	Presenile or senile dementias complicated by infection, anoxia, etc.	8. Endocrine	Hyperthyroid crises, myxoedema, Addisonian crises, hypopituitarism, hypo- and hyperparathyroidism, diabetic pre-coma, hypoglycaemia.
2. Space occupying lesions	Cerebral tumour, subdural haematoma, cerebral abscess.	9. Toxic	Alcohol – Wernicke's encephalopathy, delirium tremens.
3. Trauma	'Acute post-traumatic psychosis'.		Drugs – barbiturates (including withdrawal), bromides, salicylate intoxication, marihuana, LSD, prescribed medications (anti-Parkinsonian drugs, scopolamine, tricyclic and MAOI antidepressants, etc.).
4. Infection	Encephalitis, meningitis, subacute meningovascular syphilis. Exanthemata, streptococcal infection, septicaemia, pneumonia, influenza, typhoid, typhus, cerebral malaria, trypanosomiasis, rheumatic chorea.		Others – lead, arsenic, organic mercury compounds, carbon disulphide.
5. Vascular	Acute cerebral thrombosis or embolism, episode in arteriosclerotic dementia, transient cerebral ischaemic attack, subarachnoid haemorrhage, hypertensive encephalopathy, systemic lupus erythematosus.	10. Anoxia	Bronchopneumonia, congestive cardiac failure, cardiac dysrhythmias, silent coronary infarction, silent bleeding, carbon monoxide poisoning, post-anaesthetic.
6. Epileptic	Psychomotor seizures, petit mal status, post-ictal states.	11. Vitamin lack	Thiamine (Wernicke's encephalopathy), nicotinic acid (pellagra, acute nicotinic acid deficiency ancephalopathy), B_{12} and folic acid deficiency.
7. Metabolic	Uraemia, liver disorder, electrolyte disturbances, alkalosis, acidosis, hypercapnia, remote effects of carcinoma, porphyria.		

(Reproduced by kind permission of W. A. Lishman and Blackwell Scientific Publications, Oxford)

appeared in those with a pre-morbid or family history of such. More radical is the idea that some factors may influence not only content but the incidence of a reaction. Increasing age (Titchener *et al.*, 1956; Levine *et al.*, 1978) and a paranoid personality or previous history of depressive illness (Morse & Litin, 1969) have been claimed to act in this way. The quality of the environment can be critical if it leads to sensory or social isolation. Poorly differentiated surroundings, as in a bare side-room of a ward (Wolff & Curran, 1935), an impersonal intensive care ward (Wilson, 1972), and abrupt admission of an old person from well-ordered and familiar surroundings

(Titchener *et al.*, 1956) are considered adverse factors. The post-operative period is a particularly hazardous time as it provides opportunity for physical factors (surgical condition, electrolyte imbalance, anaesthetic risks, unrecognized alcoholism) and these environmental factors to interact and potentiate one another.

The precise way in which the cerebral disturbance produces the clinical picture is not clearly established. The opinion of Engel and Romano (1959), that cerebral insufficiency leads to a lowering of cognitive functions which thus determines the clinical phenomena, is generally accepted. In support of this,

Table 11.3. *Common physical conditions responsible for acute organic reactions (per cent present in a series of 74 patients)*

	Contributory factor	Chief factor
	%	%
Prescribed drugs	27	16
Alcohol	24	19
Carcinoma	24	14
Pneumonia	9	7
Epileptic fit	9	8
Cardiac failure	8	4
Cerebrovascular accident	8	8
Surgical operation	7	0
Electrolyte imbalance	5	3
Head injury	5	5
Parkinson's disease	5	0
Systemic lupus erythematosus	5	3
Dementia	4	0
Diabetes mellitus	4	1
Infections (pulmonary tuberculosis, septicaemia, typhoid fever)	4	3
Uraemia	4	3
Myxoedema	3	3
Cerebral tumour	1	1
Liver disease	1	1
Respiratory failure	1	1

Lipowski (1967) points out that a diminution in the quantity and pattern of sensory input (e.g. sensory deprivation, social isolation, night-time) precipitates, facilitates, or intensifies 'delirium'. This, he argues, is consistent with the idea that an apparatus already impaired by cerebral insufficiency will be further hampered in its job of appreciating and judging the nature of external stimuli when the information that it depends on is reduced. Other authors (Gamper, 1929; Gross *et al.*, 1966) have drawn attention to the similarity between delirious experiences and dreams, and have suggested that a disturbance of sleep function might be responsible.

Specific causes

Cerebral degeneration. There may be an underlying dementia of which the doctor is initially unaware. This becomes apparent when it is discovered that the psychiatric disorder attributed to an acute organic reaction has been present for some time. Alternatively, an intercurrent illness, such as pneumonia, may be responsible for an acute reaction supervening in a previously mild dementia. A careful history from informants will establish the insidious onset.

Space-occupying lesion. Bleuler (1951) gave a figure of 60 per cent for the incidence of an acute organic reaction in 600 cases of brain tumour. Subdural haematoma and cerebral abscess are other possible causes. The diagnosis is suggested by the history of other symptoms – fits, headaches; and by finding localizing neurological signs on examination. It is confirmed by neuroradiological investigations.

Trauma. A transient impairment of consciousness follows all but the mildest head injuries, and an organic reaction of some degree is invariably associated with moderate or severe head injuries, its extent principally determined by the period of unconsciousness which followed the trauma. The diagnosis is usually apparent from the history and physical appearance.

Infections. Although less important than previously as a cause of acute psychiatric disorder in developed countries, infections still contribute largely to psychiatric morbidity in developing countries, and, with increasing international travel, the clinician should be aware of the manifestations of the more common infectious diseases.

Meningitis. Infectious inflammation of the meninges can be *aseptic*, of viral aetiology, chiefly the ECHO viruses; *pyogenic*, where the organism is usually the meningococcus or pneumococcus; or *tuberculous*, where tubercle bacilli are responsible. The aseptic variety rarely gives rise to psychiatric disorder unless there is an accompanying encephalitis. The pyogenic form gives rise to an acute organic reaction in 50 per cent of cases (Pai, 1945). Tuberculous meningitis is the most likely form to be associated with an abnormal mental state (Williams & Smith, 1954), and, as the characteristic meningeal symptoms of headache, photophobia, and neck stiffness are less marked in this form, a psychiatric presentation is common. This may include apathy, irritability, and 'subtle personality changes'. A prolonged amnesia as the delirium subsides is characteristic. The diagnosis in all three varieties is established by lumbar puncture, as the cerebrospinal fluid has a characteristic composition in each, and culture of the organism will be confirmatory.

Encephalitis. Infectious encephalitis is a condition of primary inflammation of the brain resulting from virus infection. It frequently presents as an acute organic reaction, when the diagnosis can be suspected if the clinical picture also includes fever, fits, headache, and vomiting from raised intracranial pressure; photophobia and neck stiffness from associated meningeal involvement; and focal neurological signs. The diagnosis is established by electroencephalography, cerebrospinal fluid examination, the demonstration over time of rising antibody titres in the serum, and, in special cases, brain biopsy.

Cerebral malaria. Malignant malaria, an infection with the protozoon *Plasmodium falciparum*, transmitted by the female anopheles mosquito, is the cause of cerebral malaria. Daroff, Deller, Kastl and Blocker (1967) reported 19 cases amongst 1200 infections with *Plasmodium falciparum*. An acute organic reaction was the presenting feature in 12, in three there was a paranoid psychosis without cognitive impairment, and in four there were focal neurological signs. All recovered with antimalarial treatment. Toro and Roman (1978) reported 19 fatal cases and described the clinical picture as an 'acute or hyperacute onset of alteration in the level of consciousness, with rapid progression to stupor and coma'. The nature of the cerebral pathology is in doubt. Toro and Roman consider that it is a disseminated vasculomyelinopathy, the result of an allergic reaction to plasmodial antigen. The diagnosis should be suspected in those living in endemic areas or recently returned from there. Examination of blood films reveals the characteristic changes in the erythrocytes.

Typhus. Epidemic or louse-borne typhus, an infection by *Rickettsia prowazeki*, and non-epidemic typhus, infections by the remaining members of the rickettsial family, give rise to an acute organic reaction. In epidemic typhus this occurs in the second week of the illness and is preceded by a step-wide rise in temperature and a mulberry rash (Manson-Bahr, 1968). Guttmann (1952) described delirium in 45 per cent of 430 cases of epidemic typhus encountered in Eastern Europe in the Second World War. There is a widespread vasculitis in the cerebrovascular system. The diagnosis is established by demonstrating specific agglutination reactions with the patient's serum.

Other tropical fevers. Typhoid was associated with an acute organic reaction in 57 per cent of 959 cases seen in Nigeria (Osuntokun, Bademosi, Ogunremi & Wright, 1972). *Brucellosis*, by causing a meningo-encephalitis, can give rise to delirium (Roger & Poursines, 1951). *Cholera* characteristically produces apathy during the 'algid phase' (de Wardener, 1946).

Pneumonia. Particularly when supervening in established dementia, pneumonia is a common cause of an acute organic reaction. The diagnosis may only be apparent when a chest X-ray is carried out.

Infectious diseases of childhood. Measles, chickenpox, mumps, and whooping cough may give rise to a transient delirium in children. The incidence of this is unknown, although children are reputedly more susceptible to delirium than adults (Kanner, 1972). Sydenham's chorea, a manifestation of rheumatic fever, is an occasional cause (Diefendorf, 1912).

Septicaemia. The systemic transmission of bacterial infection from a focus on the heart valves, or elsewhere, is a cause. Bademosi, Falase, Jaiyesimi and Bademosi (1976) found 'toxic symptoms' in 13 per cent of 95 patients with infective endocarditis and an acute organic reaction in 2 per cent.

Cysticercosis. Cerebral infestation by the encysted larvae of *Taenia solium*, the pork tapeworm, chiefly results in epilepsy, but an acute organic reaction was present in 8 per cent of 450 cases of systemic infestation (Dixon & Lipscombe, 1961).

Cerebrovascular disease. Fifty per cent of cerebrovascular accidents with hemiplegia, excluding untestable aphasics, were associated with disorientation during the first week (Cutting, 1978). In the presence of focal signs the diagnosis is easily established. After damage to some areas of the brain, particularly right parietal infarction from occlusion of the middle cerebral artery (Mesulam, Waxman, Geschwind & Sabin, 1976), focal signs may be absent and an acute organic reaction the only manifestation.

Epilepsy. Epilepsy and an acute organic reaction may be associated in several ways (Dongier, 1959). The reaction may be ictal, usually a manifestation of petit mal status. It may represent a prolonged post-ictal phase. It may be part of the complex psychotic episodes seen with temporal lobe epilepsy and known as 'twilight states' or 'fugues'. It may result from drug intoxication. Clinical observation, electroencephalography, and estimation of anticonvulsant levels in the blood will help to distinguish these.

Metabolic disturbances. Uraemia, particularly with a urea level above 40 mmol, causes an acute organic reaction in one third of cases (Stenbäck & Haapanen, 1967). The *hepatic encephalopathy* of acute (Williams, 1973) and chronic liver disease (Summerskill, Davidson, Sherlock & Steiner, 1956) presents in this way. *Hyponatraemia, hypokalaemia, acidosis,* and *alkalosis* can precipitate or accentuate a reaction. Levine and colleagues (1978) estimated that one-third of in-patients with *carcinoma* of the lung and a significant proportion of those with cancer in other sites will exhibit an organic reaction. Cerebral metastases are only found in a minority of such patients; metabolic disturbances are probably responsible in the majority. *Porphyria* is a rare cause (Ackner, Cooper, Gray & Kelly, 1962).

Endocrine disease. Myxoedema, thyrotoxicosis, Cushing's disease, and *Addison's disease* are rarely associated with an acute organic reaction. Five per cent of in-patients with *diabetes mellitus* (Ives, 1963) exhibited this, the incidence being higher in those with frequent hyperglycaemic or hypoglycaemic comas. De Jong (1977) points out that predisposition to infection, uraemia, cerebrovascular disease, and encephalopathy also increases the risk. One-third of patients with *hypopituitarism* (Kind, 1958) and the majority of those with *primary hyperparathyroidism* with a serum calcium above 4.0 mmol (Peterson, 1968) will show acute organic reactions; 80 per cent of the hypoglycaemic attacks due to *insulinoma* (Service, Dale, Elveback & Jiang, 1976) will take the form of brief confusional episodes.

Toxic states. Heavy *alcohol* consumption may exert its influence through intoxication, withdrawal (delirium tremens), or associated thiamine deficiency (Wernicke's encephalopathy giving way to Korsakoff's syndrome). It may predispose to liver disease, head injury, or dementia, and increase the risk of a post-operative psychosis (Morse & Litin, 1969). *Illicit drugs* can produce their effect through intoxication (barbiturates, amphetamines, cocaine, marihuana, psychotomimetics – LSD, inhalants – paint, glue), or withdrawal (barbiturates). *Prescribed drugs* in therapeutic doses are one of the commonest causes. Wade

and Beeley (1976) and McClelland (1978) provide helpful accounts of those most commonly incriminated. Anti-Parkinsonian drugs (benzhexol, orphenadrine, levo-dopa, amantidine), antidepressants (amitriptyline, nortriptyline), pentazocine, carbamazepine and nalidixic acid are amongst the commonest causes of 'confusion', 'delirium' and 'visual hallucinations' reported to the Committee on Safety of Medicines (1974). A wider range of drugs is involved in accidental overdose in children or suicide attempt in adults.

Anoxia. Cardiac and *respiratory insufficiency, acute haemorrhage,* and *carbon monoxide poisoning* fall into this category. Smith and Brandon (1970) reported delirium in 20 per cent of non-fatal cases of carbon monoxide poisoning.

Vitamin deficiency. Thiamine, nicotinic acid, folate or B_{12} deficiencies provide rare causes.

Management

The chief considerations in the management of an acute organic reaction are to recognize the clinical picture and to carry out a systematic search for a cause. Treatment is then primarily a matter of alleviating the condition which has been identified. In many cases, however, other considerations apply, either because the underlying condition is not amenable to specific therapy (e.g. inoperable cancer), or because disturbed behaviour threatens to hinder the implementation of treatment or because the patient is a danger to himself or his attendants.

Diagnosis

Awareness of the characteristic features of an acute organic reaction, described earlier, is essential. Particular emphasis can be placed on clouding of consciousness, disorientation, and the character or the abnormal perceptions, as these discriminate best between organic and functional psychoses.

Investigation

Having established or suspected the diagnosis, it is then probably best to consider systematically the commoner conditions listed in table 11.2, progressing to rarer causes in table 11.1 when these possibilities are exhausted. The circumstances at onset, and the age, sex, and background of the patient, will obviously determine priorities. An elderly widow found alone in her flat and a young man brought into a casualty department by friends will suggest different orders of likelihood. A history from a reliable informant should be obtained whenever possible, as pointers to many of the causes may emerge. Dementia, trauma, epilepsy, alcohol, and drug causes may be uncovered in this way. Physical examination may reveal disease of an organ or system and the external appearance may give a clue to one of the fevers or an endocrine disease. Further investigative procedures will be suggested by the information already obtained. Chest X-ray, full blood count, and measurement of electrolytes and urea will probably be required in all cases, even if the cause is obvious, as pneumonia and electrolyte imbalance may complicate and exacerbate established causes, as well as providing a cause in themselves. Electroencephalography is of value. Obrecht, Okhomina and Scott (1979) found it abnormal in 83 of 95 cases, and helpful in distinguishing intracranial from extracranial causes.

Specific treatment

A confident diagnosis of the condition responsible for the organic reaction should be followed by appropriate treatment. A specific therapy and management may relieve the condition (infections, endocrine disease, vitamin deficiency), lead to remission (cerebral tumour, epilepsy, metabolic disturbances, cardiac and respiratory insufficiency), or improve subsequent prognosis (trauma, cerebrovascular disease). Consultation with colleagues in other specialities will be required to determine precise management. In other cases (cerebral degeneration, alcohol, illicit drugs), where the aetiology is already within the psychiatric province, resolution of the acute reaction should be followed by the appropriate management for that condition. Intoxication with prescribed drugs is treated by stopping the suspected drug, or if that is not feasible, substituting another.

General recommendations

Knowledge of the factors which exacerbate the clinical picture can help when advising nurses and general medical staff on management. A certain amount has been learnt from studies of delirium after open-heart surgery, which during the early 1960s had an incidence as high as 70 per cent (Kornfeld, Zimberg & Malm, 1965). Simple remedies, such as nursing in rooms with windows (Wilson, 1972), installing radios beside the bed and making monitoring equipment less intrusive (Kornfeld *et al.*, 1965), conducting pre-operative interviews to explain the forthcoming procedure (Layne & Yudofsky, 1971), and instructing nurses to talk and relate to patients (Lazarus & Hagens, 1968) reduced the incidence significantly. These lessons can be profitably applied to the management of all forms of acute organic reactions.

Symptomatic medication

The administration of sedative drugs should be as sparing as possible. Their use may aggravate the underlying condition, as in liver disease (Williams, 1973). They may exacerbate a reaction already induced by over-medication, as in drug intoxication in the elderly. Nevertheless, the disturbed behaviour, and the hazard which this entails, often make some form of sedation unavoidable. On therapeutic grounds there is no good evidence to recommend a particular drug. The choice is determined, in the main, by the range of side-effects which are most compatible with the underlying condition. For example, phenothiazines should probably be avoided in delirium tremens because they are epileptogenic in a condition which carries a risk of fits. Phenothiazines and other antipsychotic drugs (for example, haloperidol) with marked extrapyramidal side-effects are best avoided in all cases but promazine and thioridazine are useful. Chlormethiazole has acquired a favourable reputation in the management of delirium tremens. Benzodiazepines are relatively safe.

12

The senile and pre-senile dementias*

BARRY J. GURLAND
D. PETER BIRKETT

Concepts of dementia

The word dementia appeared in English in 1845 as a translation of the French *démence* in Esquirol's *Des maladies mentales*. It connoted a general and progressive loss of mental function. The age-specific nature of dementia was later recognized and its occurrence in adolescence, labelled dementia praecox, was separated (Morel, 1860 see 1955) from the senile and pre-senile variety. The notion of a general weakening of the mind was retained but, in senile dementia, the emphasis came to rest on intellectual and memory impairment, probably because these functions are more readily evident and measurable than is emotional impairment.

Alzheimer, in 1898, concluded that senile and arteriosclerotic dementia showed a distinctive progression that distinguished them from other mental conditions of old age. In 1911 he went on to describe the neuropathology associated with a case of progressive dementia occurring in a 50-year-old male, 'Johann F.' The evidence for the identity between the histological changes of senile brain disease, and those of the relatively younger patients with Alzheimer's disease, was reviewed by Simchowicz in 1914.

In 1952, the label organic brain syndrome was introduced into American practice (American Psychiatric Association, 1952) thus recognizing that diagnosis is based usually on symptoms, (impair-

* Work on this paper was partially supported by Administration on Aging grant no. OHD-AOA-90-AT 2155.

ment of orientation, memory, intellectual functions, and judgement, and lability and shallowness of affect), which are attributable to a number of cerebral conditions involving 'diffuse impairment of brain tissue function from whatever cause.' Senile and pre-senile dementias were called chronic organic brain syndromes and were regarded as having a strong tendency to progress, whereas acute brain syndromes were regarded as being reversible if appropriately treated.

As clinical knowledge has increased, there has been greater emphasis on diagnostic terms referring to putatively specific disorders. This trend is reflected in the International Classification of Diseases, Clinical Modification, Ninth Revision (Commission on Professional and Hospital Activities, 1978) and the Diagnostic and Statistical Manual of Mental Disorders, Third Edition (American Psychiatric Association, 1980) in which appear such categories as senile, pre-senile, primary degenerative, and arteriosclerotic or multi-infarct dementia. Some of these terms do however embrace more than one specific disorder and some reflect a view of aetiology that is still subject to debate. Moreover, current diagnostic labels often incorporate defining terms, such as 'with delusional features', that have little to do with the classification of specific mental disorders.

A generally acceptable definition of the term dementia, today, might be that it refers to a cluster of conditions characterized by a widespread loss of intellectual functions after they have matured, a strong tendency towards progressive deterioration, and, usually, distinctive pathological changes in the brain.

Need for treatment
The need for treatment of the conditions which cause dementia can be best understood by considering their frequency and natural history. These conditions are ubiquitous, are concentrated in institutional populations, are very disabling, greatly increase mortality rates, and are disruptive and distressing to the families of victims. The cost to the health and social services of caring for dementing patients in or out of long-term-care facilities is immense, as are the hidden costs which are borne by the families who care for such patients at home. Yet the devastating effect of dementia on the lives of sufferers and their families outweighs even the material consequences.

Dementia of a severity sufficient to impair the capacity of the patients to care for themselves occurs in about 7 per cent of a cross-section of the general population over the age of 65 years; in persons younger than this the prevalence is much lower but in the age group 80 years and over the prevalence may be as high as 20 per cent (Gurland, Dean, Cross & Golden, 1980). In long-term-care facilities, where residents tend to be very elderly, the prevalence rates are often in the region of 50 per cent. When the proportion of the very old in the population increases, as it is projected to do, so may the prevalence of dementia. Another factor likely to increase the prevalence rate of dementia if the incidence remains unaltered is that the better the medical and nursing care these patients receive the longer they tend to live (Gruenberg, 1978).

As the dementia progresses, the disability it causes increases. At first it may affect ability to carry out the instrumental activities of daily living (work performance, shopping, preparation of food, housekeeping, use of public transportation, pathfinding, adherence to medication regimes, communication, or the handling of finances). Later it affects simple tasks such as the basic activities of daily living including bathing, dressing, toileting, transferring, mobility, continence, and feeding, often in that order (Katz & Akpom, 1976). The patient may become distressed as a result of an awareness of diminishing abilities, reduced control over his or her own behaviour and the environment, increasing dependence on others, involuntary relocation, and loss of freedoms and customary gratifications. The family or support personnel may be disturbed by inappropriate behaviours of the patient such as shouting, perseveration, wandering, messy or unkempt manners, incontinence of urine or faeces, hoarding and stealing, destruction of objects, lack of co-operation, and indecencies such as undressing in public places or making inappropriate sexual advances. At times the patient may become dangerous to his or her own life or to the safety of those around; suicidal attempts are not uncommon early on in the course of the illness and at a later stage there may be assaultiveness or incendiary actions, leaving on unlit gas-taps, frequent falling, and so on.

The disabling, disruptive, and dangerous behaviours of dementia may precipitate a decision to admit the patient to a long-term facility. Nevertheless, there are in most regions many more demented patients outside institutions than in them and there is a pressing need for home care services and attention to the supporting family (Gurland, Dean, Gurland & Cook, 1978). The family are often more depressed than the patient. Similarly, in institutions, the staff may need a good deal of encouragement and explanation in order to maintain their morale and the quality of the care they give.

Rational basis of treatment

The two most common associations of dementia are senile and arteriosclerotic changes in the brain; between them they probably account for about 85 per cent of cases of dementia. An understanding of the pathophysiology and presumed causes of these conditions will provide a perspective on the current limitations and possible developments of the treatment of dementia.

Brain changes, associated with impaired function, that occur with ageing and to a greater degree in senile dementia include reduction of brain tissue (with consequent decrease in brain volume and weight, and increase of ventricular and sulcal space) and, at a microscopic level, loss of neurons and dendritic spines with granulovacular changes and accumulation of lipofuscin, amyloid, senile plaques and neurofibrillary tangles (Nandy, 1978). Iqbal and his colleagues (1978) have shown that neurofibrillary tangles have a spiral structure made up of two kinds of protein, which he has called paired helical filaments. The plaques and tangles are particularly increased in quantity in cases of senile dementia, and tend to concentrate in the cerebral cortex and hippocampal region (Malamud, 1972).

It is possible that neuropathological changes interfere with brain function through such mechanisms as disorganization by plaques of the nerve terminals and synapses, or disruption by tangles of the tubular nutrition and cytoplasmic and axonal flow; however, the visible changes may only reflect or accompany the deteriorative processes. It is not clear to what extent the effects of dementia are due to cell loss *per se* (like other post-mitotic cells, the central nervous system neurons are incapable of reproduction so that loss cannot be replaced) or to other neurophysiological changes; or whether the clinical deterioration is due to generalized (mass) changes in the brain or to involvement of specialized centres in the temporal lobe (Wang, 1977); nor is it known whether a transfer of function from damaged to healthy areas of the brain can occur or whether some of the changes in the brain are reversible.

The relationship between number of nerve cell components in the brain and decline in brain weight and intellectual function across the age span is not yet settled (Bowen & Davison, 1980). Loss of neurons after middle age has been reported (Brody, 1955), especially in the hippocampal cortex (Ball, 1977), but not in all areas of the brain (Konigsmark & Murphy, 1970). Comparing age-matched controls, Terry and his colleagues (1977) find no lowering of the total neuron count in Alzheimer's dementia, but, according to Bowen & Davison (1980), there is an increased loss of temporal lobe nerve-cell components. There is perhaps more agreement that dendritic trees show a loss of length and numbers of branches in dementia compared to normal ageing (Buell & Coleman, 1979).

Attention has particularly focused on cholinergic nerve cells because, with their associated acetylcholine neuro-transmitter, they are richly represented in the hippocampus, an area of the limbic system crucially involved in memory functions. The actions of certain drugs in man also point to a cholinergic pathway as being central to memory functions. Scopolamine, which blockades cholinergic brain receptors, interferes with memory storage and the acquisition of new information in man (Petersen, 1977; Drachman & Sahakian, 1979), producing a profile of neuropsychological impairments in young people that resembles that found in the normal aged (Drachman, 1978). Choline, physostigmine and arecoline (a muscarinic agonist) improve certain aspects of learning and remembering in normal elderly persons (Davis *et al.*, 1978; Sitaram *et al.*, 1978).

In Alzheimer's dementia, there is now a considerable volume of evidence that the cholinergic system is affected. Choline acetyltransferase, which is involved in the production of acetylcholine, is reduced in the prefrontal cortex and hippocampus. (Bowen *et al.*, 1976, 1979; Davies & Maloney, 1976; Perry *et al.*, 1977 a, b; Reisine *et al.*, 1978) and there is also a reduction in acetylcholinesterase (Davies & Maloney, 1976; Perry *et al.*, 1978). These changes indicate a degeneration of cholinergic cells or their terminals. The degree of reduction in choline acetyltransferase is correlated with numbers of senile plaques and degree of intellectual deterioration. However, for the most part, muscarinic binding (receptor) sites for acetylcholine appear to be unimpaired (Perry *et al.*, 1977a; Davies & Verth, 1977/78; Bowen *et al.*, 1979).

Changes in the dopamine system and gamma aminobutyric acid neurons have also been reported in Alzheimer's dementia (Bowen *et al.*, 1974; Reisine *et al.*, 1978; Perry *et al.*, 1978). Similarly the noradrenergic system has been implicated; noradrenaline content has been reported as reduced in the putamen and frontal cortex (Adolfson *et al.*, 1979) and locus coeruleus (Mann *et al.*, 1980) of patients with Alzheimer's dementia presumably as a result of a corresponding degeneration of neurons and an impairment of neuro-transmitter metabolism.

An immunological basis for the neuronal degeneration of senile dementia has been suggested by several investigators (Mayer *et al.*, 1976; Ingram *et al.*, 1974; Nandy, 1977; Roseman & Buckley, 1975; Cohen & Eisdorfer, 1977), though findings are not all consistent. Antibrain antibodies in the serum and altered permeability of the blood–brain barrier can lead to neuronal damage according to this causal model. In patients with senile dementia, the presence of the disorder and the severity of intellectual deterioration has been noted to be significantly correlated with altered total circulating immunoglobulin levels, especially IgH (Eisdorfer & Cohen, 1980). However, changes in immunoglobulins may be a reaction to the deteriorating general condition of the dementing person or the prodrome to death. The association between HLA antigens and dementia also has been examined as a possible clue to immunological factors in the causation of this disorder. Conflicting results have been reported (Snowden *et al.*, 1981; Henschke *et al.*, 1978; Cohen *et al.*, 1979; Walford & Hodge, 1980; Renvoize *et al.*, 1979).

The neuropathological hall-marks of senile dementia are found also in Alzheimer's pre-senile dementia (Alzheimer, 1898), which is now considered by most authorities to be the same degenerative process as occurs in senile dementia. An abnormal excess of tangles is also found in certain other dementia syndromes, for example, in the Guam complex, dementia pugilistica, late in Down's syndrome, and in experimental aluminium toxicity; also plaques occur to excess late in Down's syndrome and, occasionally, in Picks disease and Creutzfeld-Jacob disease. A common aetiology to match the similarity in pathological picture has not been as yet established (Drachman, 1978). However, speculative associations with immunological mechanisms, aluminium toxicity, (Crapper *et al.*, 1973) and transmissible viruses have been raised.

A dominant autosomal gene may predispose to the development of senile dementia in certain families but the majority of cases are sporadic. Possibly about 12 per cent of the population carry the gene, with penetrance increasing with age (Larsson, Sjögren & Jacobson, 1963). The risk of dementia developing in first-degree relatives of cases of dementia is about four times greater than for the age-matched general population. Concordance in monozygotic (identical) twins is in the region of 43 per cent, whereas for dizygotic twins it is similar to that expected for first-degree relatives. Genetic distinctions between senile and Alzheimer's dementia are no longer considered valid.

Brain–behaviour relationships

Several studies have placed on a more quantitative level the putative association between the brain changes of dementia and the clinical manifestations. Corsellis (1962) examined the brain in 300 consecutive post-mortems on aged patients in one mental hospital. The patients were divided into an 'organic' group and a 'functional' group. The organic group comprised patients admitted with dementia, confusion, or delirium. The functional group had been admitted with such diagnoses as schizophrenia and affective psychosis. A clear relationship was noted between clinical diagnosis and type of brain pathology, including neuropathological distinctions between the diagnostic subtypes of senile and arteriosclerotic dementia. However, clinical data were obtained retrospectively and, furthermore, as Corsellis pointed out, 'an investigation of this kind, particularly when carried out by one person, must fall short of the ideal, for it is impossible to keep the two sets of information so rigidly apart that all risk of contamination is avoided in every case'.

Blessed, Tomlinson and Roth (1968) in a prospective clinico-pathological study used quantitative and independent measures of both the clinical symptoms and the brain changes. Their sample, not a random one, consisted of patients admitted to a psychiatric hospital, a geriatric hospital, and a number of wards in a general hospital. Included in the sample were eight physically ill subjects without evident psychiatric disorder. The findings referred to 60 patients, in whom neuropathological investigations had revealed 'no more than small amounts of cerebral infarction'. They confirmed the finding of Corsellis that such illnesses as depression and paraphrenia (in other words what is commonly understood by 'functional' cases) did not have any relation to the presence of senile plaques or other senile brain changes. There was a high correlation between plaque counts and the measures of dementia. There appeared to be a critical threshold for the disruption of brain function associated with the plaques and tangles; an increase of the latter beyond a certain quantity was usually reflected in an impairment of intellect and of the subject's performance in the instrumental and basic activities of daily living (Roth, 1971). The authors concluded that 'as far as could be judged with the aid of existing techniques the difference between the senile dements and other subjects reflected a quantitative gradation of a pathological process common in old age rather than qualitative differences'. Most of the limitations of this work are lucidly discussed by the writers themselves. A major problem, as of any study with post-mortem follow-up, is that of selection of the sample.

Although a strong relationship between specific brain changes and syndromes of dementia has been definitively established, this should not be taken to mean that socio-cultural factors have been ruled out as contributing to the causation, precipitation, severity, or course of dementia. This issue has been recently reviewed by Gurland (1980a).

Assessment as a guide to treatment

The usual presentation of the common dementias (senile or arteriosclerotic) is one or other set of symptoms arising from (1) a disorder of memory and orientation; (2) inability to attend, learn, comprehend, solve problems, calculate and make good judgements; (3) a loss of control over emotional reactions, and (4) a decline in previously acquired skills. The symptoms that arise on the basis of these defects include incompetence in the instrumental and basic activities of daily living. Embarrassing and dangerous lapses may occur, such as misidentifying time, place, persons, and self; wandering and becoming lost; leaving the gas on and burning food or lighting unguarded fires; undressing or urinating in public; or screaming and aggressiveness. Restless anxiety may occur, or overactivity at night, depression, suspiciousness, perseverative exclamations and entreaties, stereotypes, and impulsive actions. Alternatively, there may be apathy, withdrawal, and inactivity. These symptoms may occur in combination or as a sequential progression. In addition there may be focal neurological abnormalities such as aphasias, apraxias and agnosias; and involuntary or uncoordinated movements. Superimposed upon this picture may be the symptoms and signs of associated conditions, such as stroke or Parkinsonism, and of the usual concomitant physical conditions that occur in elderly patients.

The basis of accurate differential diagnosis is a tactful, comprehensive, and systematic assessment technique. It is important to take into account the natural anxiety of the patient confronted by symptoms that appear to herald a loss of control over the mind and body; an excessive level of arousal may in and of itself lead to vague and misleading replies and poor performance on tests of intellectual function. The interview should have an unhurried air and tests or probes of mental function should be made gently and interspersed with discussion of physical symptoms or neutral topics (Gurland, 1980b). The Mental Status Questionnaire (Kahn, Goldfarb, Pollack & Peck, 1960), ten questions on orientation and recent memory, offers a clinically feasible way of testing cognitive function; most of these questions can be presented in a non-threatening manner as a routine census-type enquiry. A search for the symptoms of depression or other psychiatric disturbance is just as necessary for the evaluation of a potential case of dementia as are tests of cognitive function or laboratory investigations. Informants close to the patient will often reveal diagnostic information not obtained directly from the patient.

Differential diagnosis

Adequate assessment may prevent some diagnostic problems from arising. However, there may be an overlap of symptoms between diagnostic categories which are nevertheless radically different in their requirements for treatment. Ideas about differential diagnosis in geriatric psychiatry have changed much in recent years. Diagnosis is now to be regarded as an essential prelude to treatment, rather than a futile academic exercise. The general principle remains, to think first of the treatable, rather than the untreatable, and the common rather than the rare. However, notions of what is treatable have been transformed with the advent of physical treatments of the major functional psychoses. Depression and paranoid states are now looked upon as eminently treatable. Advances in medicine and surgery have made it easier to diagnose and treat physical illness underlying a confusional state. The importance of contributory causes has become recognized as well as necessary and sufficient causes. Prevention, particularly of a stroke is emphasized, as well as the prevention of further disability in day hospital, health related facility, skilled nursing facility or mental hospital. Irrevocable incarceration after merely a Wasserman and a thyroid function test, is no longer the order of the day.

Where the presenting symptoms raise the possibility that the diagnosis is dementia, the priority issues to be decided are whether the correct diagnosis is that of a functional rather than an organic brain syndrome, or of an acute rather than a chronic brain syndrome, or of a reversible rather than a progressive type of dementia. These issues have to be continually kept in the forefront because, with respect to the elderly (in whom these symptoms commonly occur), there is a tendency for physicians to regard any suggestive psychiatric symptoms as being definitive evidence of a progressive and irreversible dementia. The distinction between the different types of progressive dementia can be left until the priority issues have been decided.

Acute confusional states due to extracranial disease

A psychiatrist on duty covering an ambulatory care setting, if confronted by an elderly patient who is brought in as a possible case of dementia, is well-advised to ask what his temperature is. If he has a fever, there is the immediate possibility of an acute confusional state, due to infections or toxins. These are commonly regarded as the province of the general physician, and priority is given to medical management of the illness. When the patient is already in a mental hospital, or under psychiatric treatment, then the psychiatrist has greater responsibility to diagnose and initiate treatment.

The term acute, as used in acute confusional state, is usually meant to refer to reversibility rather than sudden onset. It is usual to identify as a separate group all those underlying or causative conditions of cognitive impairment which are potentially reversible, including heart failure, respiratory infections, uraemia, drug reactions, electrolyte imbalance, hypoglycaemia, pernicious anaemia, hypothyroidism, and so forth. Extensive lists of such conditions have been published (Hughes, 1978). Typically these reversible conditions give rise to the clinical picture of acute confusional states which are described more fully in chapter 11; however, the clinical presentation of acute confusional states may sometimes be hard to distinguish from the chronic organic brain syndromes or dementias, especially if the underlying condition is slow in onset.

In the chronic organic brain syndromes the symptoms arise from defect or release effects following death of brain tissue in contrast to the symptoms of dying or dysfunctional tissue that form the basis for the acute states (in both instances the reaction of the patient's personality to the condition may also produce symptoms). Acute states may occur superimposed on a chronic organic brain syndrome; or may precede it where the dementing process has all but removed the margin of reserve in brain function so that additional insults can easily tip the patient into an acute state. If the acute state is not adequately treated the patient may succumb from the underlying cause or may occasionally end up with a chronic (secondary) dementia as the dysfunctional tissue eventually dies.

Seymour et al. (1980) studied 71 patients aged 70 years or older who were admitted as emergencies (acute physical illness) to a general medical unit and found that about 17 per cent had an acute confusional state. This figure compares closely with other reports on the prevalence of acute confusional states in various general hospital settings (Hodkinson 1973; Bergmann & Eastham, 1974).

A thorough physical examination, a review of medications, and a series of laboratory tests form part of the comprehensive approach to assessment of possible causes of dementia. This part of the examination is largely directed at uncovering conditions, usually extracranial, that point to an acute confusional state or to secondary dementia. Lists of the investigations that are useful for this purpose are available (Libow, 1977); they include blood film, serology, urinalysis, electrolytes, enzyme changes, sputum culture, X-ray of chest, ECG, thyroid function, and blood-gas studies.

Acute and chronic organic brain syndromes share many symptoms in common, most notably disorientation for time, place, and person; impairment of recent memory; and functional incapacity and deteriorated behaviour. These syndromes occur most commonly in the elderly and often together. Their treatment requirements are, however, dramatically different in so far as the acute cases generally call for urgent medical intervention while the chronic cases generally need long-term care. An acute rather than chronic condition will be suggested by a recent (few days to few weeks), and relatively sudden, onset, especially if it follows or accompanies a stressful event such as surgery or recognizable disease or new medication regime; by restless and fearful behaviour; a fluctuation in level of alertness and comprehension over a period of hours or days (often worst at nights); and a tendency towards anxious misperception of distracting visual stimuli.

Even in cases of chronic organic brain syndrome the patient's best level of functioning cannot be gauged until possible causes of superimposed acute brain syndrome have been eliminated. In many cases the acute episodes are part and parcel of the usual progressive course of the dementing process, for example when a series of cerebrovascular accidents punctuate the course of arteriosclerotic dementia or when environmental demands periodically overwhelm the failing capacities of the senile dement. However, all the common causes of acute confusional states may at least as commonly occur in patients who are dementing. Some of these superimposed causes may be easily overlooked because they are not a traditional part of the medical model of disease: for example, relocation into an unfamiliar environment, impacted faeces, exhaustion, malnutrition, or darkness or other sensory deprivation (such as occurs after cataract surgery). Other insidious causes of acute or chronic confusional states are physical conditions which are signalled by dramatic symptoms in younger persons but may occur silently or be poorly reported and with few physical signs in the elderly, particularly if they have some intellectual deterioration; for example, myocardial infarction, arrhythmias, lobar pneumonia, or urinary infections. In fact, dementing patients are more likely than the normal elderly with greater cognitive reserves to be precipitated into confusion by a variety of physical causes. Especially likely as causes of acute confusion in dementing patients (but not an intrinsic part of the dementing process) are occult infections, dehydration and electrolyte imbalance, azotaemia secondary to bladder overload in the presence of prostatic obstruction or diuretics, C or B complex vitamin deficiencies, faecal impaction, cardiac failure, or drug toxicity. It is evidently important to maintain vigorously the dementing patient's general health and nutrition and to search for possible physical causes of sudden deterioration.

The drugs often incriminated in cases of toxicity are those with a central anticholinergic effect (e.g. phenothiazines, tricyclic antidepressants, anti-Parkinsonian drugs); those used in the treatment of hypertension, partly because of the side-effect of overcompensatory hypotension; diuretics and steroids which affect the electrolyte balance; hypoglycaemic agents; barbiturates; and digoxin. Indeed, the list of drugs capable of causing confusion is so long that the most useful general principle is to limit drug administration and thus potential side-effects and drug–drug interactions, and to review medications whenever the patient's mental condition deteriorates.

Misdiagnosis of the various alcohol-induced syndromes as senile dementia is most likely to occur in the general hospital setting. The elderly patient's prior history of drinking is often unknown or ignored. After being admitted for medical treatment or surgery the patient may develop delirium tremens, which is very likely to be misdiagnosed as a toxic or post-operative delirium, and, if he survives this, a residual confusion may be misdiagnosed as dementia.

Treatable intracranial conditions

There has been a recent tendency for psychiatrists to neglect their neurological heritage. Every now and then we are brought up abruptly by old-fashioned neurology. Sometimes a positive serological test for syphilis may get buried in the patient's voluminous records while exotic investigations are pursued. It is always worth looking for it in the chart when called into consultation on a case of dementia in a hospital or institution.

The classical pin, feather, and hammer clinical neurological examination has the advantage that it can be repeated many times. In this way one may pick up a subdural haematoma in the back wards, that was missed on the acute medical floor. Testing of sensation, and full cranial nerve testing may, of course, be impossible in the demented patient, but the other elements of the neurological examination should be possible. They are sometimes neglected when the patient is first admitted in a violent or uncooperative state. The initial screening procedures, with automated multiple-channel blood tests that have become routine in many hospitals, will usually be available to indicate the presence of metabolic and blood diseases. However, the special investigations of modern neurology are not yet routine as screening devices. It is only after a space-occupying lesion is first suspected on clinical testing that the special investigations may settle the diagnosis.

Special investigations giving more direct information on brain function include such safe and painless processes as the electroencephalogram, computer assisted tomography (CAT), and non-invasive regional cerebral blood flow studies (Ingvar & Gustafson, 1970). Changes in the EEG, such as slow wave activity in the theta or delta range, or sharp and slow-wave-complexes and disorganization of normal patterns, are regarded by some as reliable indicators of a dementing process although it is admitted that the effects of other physical illnesses or drugs may be identical (Muller, 1978). Estimation of cerebral blood flow by tracking of inhaled radioactive labelled gas (133 Xenon) is a promising method (Caird, 1977) which is not yet widely available for clinical purposes.

In computed tomography (Hounsfield, 1973), patients receive only small X-ray doses. The X-ray attenuation of serial scans of transverse 8 to 13 mm slices of the brain is calculated by computer and used to reconstruct images made up of 1×1 mm area units (pixels). This procedure has virtually rendered obsolete the risky and distressing pneumo-encephalogram. However, there is a general agreement that with the present state of technology the CAT scan must be used with great caution in the diagnosis of Alzheimer's dementia (Wells & Duncan, 1977; Ford & Winter, 1981). Cortical atrophy occurs with normal ageing (Neilsen *et al.*, 1966; Ford & Winter, 1981) and so does ventricular enlargement (Baron *et al.*, 1976). A CAT scan study of 228 normal persons (Yamaura *et al.*, 1980) indicated that the volume percentage of brain to cranial cavity decreased drastically with age after the age of 50 and variability increased. Atrophy on CAT scan has also been reported as occurring in dementia (Fox *et al.*, 1975), but the variability and overlap with normal ranges is great and hence not diagnostic. Moreover, atrophy of the brain as evidenced on CAT scan is not a good guide to the presence of global impairment of intellect or memory (Shraberg, 1980). The use of CAT scanning in senile dementia has been recently reviewed and investigated by Jacoby & Levy (1980). Its main practical usefulness is still in the exclusion of space-occupying lesions as causes of dementia. (In this connection it may be noted that chronic subdural haematoma can be isodense with CSF and not show on CAT). Jacoby and Levy's work indicates that the scans are as yet of limited practical use in such problems as differentiating between dementia and depression. They compared three groups, one of elderly normals, the second of cases of dementia (they excluded patients with definite strokes), and the third of elderly depressed patients. They found that, although there was definitely more ventricular dilatation in the demented group, there was considerable overlap. They also found that radiologists' estimates of ventricular dilatation were about as accurate as more time-consuming quantified methods, such as plani-

metry and measurement of the Evans ratio. Clinical signs and symptoms and a chronological history of the complaints are a more reliable guide to the diagnosis of dementia than is the CAT scan (Kasziak *et al.*, 1978; Wells & Duncan, 1977). Furthermore, the presence of CAT changes should not pre-empt the search for remediable causes of an organic brain syndrome (Ford & Winter, 1981).

Communicating or normotensive hydrocephalus has attracted particular attention because some cases of apparent dementia can be reversed by treatment aimed at relieving the hydrocephalus (Hakim & Adams, 1965). It occurs in about 7 per cent of cases of pre-senile dementia (Harrison & Marsden, 1977). There is no obstruction to the cerebrospinal fluid within the ventricular system and its pressure is normal, but the ventricles are enlarged and there is a slowing of reabsorption of the cerebrospinal fluid into the arachnoid villi. The dementing syndrome associated with normal-pressure hydrocephalus is usually not severe when it first comes to the attention of the physician. It is suggested by the concomitant signs of memory impairment, a shuffling, ataxic gait not due to cerebellar or proprioceptive defect, urinary or faecal incontinence occuring early in the disorder and a predominance of psychomotor retardation (Adams *et. al.*, 1965; Hakim & Adams, 1965; Katzman, 1978). There may be a history of subarachnoid haemorrhage or meningitis but most cases are idiopathic (Symon & Hinzpeter, 1977; Briggs *et al.*, 1981). Possibly the latter variety is due to an asymptomatic low-grade meningeal disease (Adams, 1975). CAT scans may show gross enlargement of the ventricles with normal sulci (Gunasekera & Richardson, 1977), and with the cortex pressed against the skull. A communicating hydrocephalus may also be demonstrated by a variety of other techniques including isotope cisternography. A steep pressure rise on infusion of saline into the lumbar sac may indicate the slowed CSF reabsorption (Katzman & Hussey, 1970) but prolonged monitoring of intracranial pressure may be a more reliable indicator (Crockard *et al.*, 1977). The radiographic signs are mimicked by Alzheimer's disease in a small percentage of the latter cases and the sequence in which the clinical signs develop may thus be an important guide to diagnosis. Since it is possible that shunting procedures may remedy this condition in some cases, it is necessary to distinguish it from the primary dementias.

The treatment of normotensive hydrocephalus is usually by ventriculoperitoneal shunt. The precision of diagnosis and the effectiveness of treatment is in question (Jellinek, 1980). Briggs and his colleagues (1981) report the treatment of three cases with disappointing results (the best case enjoying only 8 months of good-quality life). They point out that the necessary diagnostic tests are expensive and may also be painful or risky, while the treatment success rate is only about 50 per cent and serious complications are in the region of 15 per cent–30 per cent. An alternative approach to treatment may be the repeated removal of CSF either as a predictor of surgical success or as a substitute for surgery (Miller Fisher, 1978).

It is a matter of very fine judgement how vigorously the diagnostic investigations should be pushed in a frail elderly person. Full investigation may be best justified where the symptoms are suggestive, the duration is short (say, less than 6 months), previous mental function was good, and the patient is otherwise strong and healthy (Reichel, 1978).

Overlap between depression and dementia

In practical terms depression is probably the most important treatable entity to bear in mind in the diagnosis and management of dementia. On the one hand, elderly patients with a depressive disorder may give the appearance of intellectual impairment because their inability or lack of motivation to concentrate, or their supra-optimal level of anxiety, may lead them to perform poorly in tests of cognitive function; or they may complain about having a poor memory and being confused even when these functions are not objectively impaired; or their self-neglect and immobility, or the secondary effects on their health, may cause them to look deteriorated, or they may, in a minority of cases, show actual intellectual deterioration (sometimes called pseudo-dementia) which recovers only when their depression is relieved. On the other hand, patients with true dementia may become depressed.

In cases where the distinction between the diagnosis of depression and dementia is in doubt, the former diagnosis is suggested where a history of a previous episode of depression exists, or family members have suffered from an affective disorder, or the depressive symptoms preceded the signs of intellectual impairment, or subjective symptoms overshadow objective signs, or errors on the Mental Status Questionnaire (see above) are less than 30 per cent of the maximum possible, or where the onset is relatively clearcut and of short duration (less than 6 months). Special investigations and extensive psychological testing do not often resolve doubts about these diagnostic distinctions. In some cases of residual doubt it may require serial observations or even a trial of antidepressant treatment in order to make a final diagnosis.

A difficulty may arise in diagnostic–therapeutic trials because of the possible adverse effects of physical treatments. Tricyclic antidepressants may not be clearly effective in small doses. If they are pushed to large doses then the danger arises of an anticholinergic syndrome. With electric shock treatment the problem may be that the patient's general physical condition makes anaesthesia difficult; this may be the case where there has been apathy and withdrawal and prolonged food refusal. In some cases of pseudo-dementia, the results of electric shock or psychotropic treatment are brilliant, though a failure to respond does not rule out pseudo-dementia.

Overlap between paranoid states and dementia

Patients with a functional paranoid state may share some of the features of dementia; for example, patients with paraphrenia may show bizarre behaviour, incoherence, and a deteriorated appearance, or their tendency to accuse others of stealing their belongings may resemble the rationalizations of dementing persons who misplace their possessions. On the other hand, paranoid features may exist on the basis of Alzheimer-type brain disease.

Cerebral arteriosclerosis

Histologically and anatomically, senile dementia and cerebral arteriosclerosis are distinct, although both may co-exist in the same subject.

Cerebral arteriosclerosis is a disease of the blood vessels which supply the brain. Elsewhere in the body, two forms of arteriosclerosis may be distinguished, namely, atherosclerosis and arteriolosclerosis, but in the brain the distinction between these two forms is less sharp. This is because of the absence, in arteries inside the brain, of the muscle coat, hyperplasia of which, in medium size limb arteries, distinguishes arteriolosclerosis. Thus, microscopically evident arteriosclerosis in the brain refers to the presence of thickening of the walls of the small arteries seen under the microscope. The changes seen with the naked eye, in the named branches of the internal carotid and vertebral arteries, is atherosclerosis, the subintimal deposit of plaques of fatty material.

The consequence of these arterial changes is the

development of infarction in the brain tissue; areas of the brain undergo a series of changes, characterized by necrosis, progressing to liquefaction, and then to cavity formation. Although this course of events is identified clinically with cerebral thrombosis, there is a puzzling absence of actual thrombus blocking nearby small vessels. This absence is among the factors that have stimulated support for the idea that extracerebral vessels are the primary disease locus. The suggestion has been made (Hachinski *et al.*, 1974) that 'multi-infarct dementia' is not synonymous with cerebral arteriosclerosis, since multiple small or large cerebral infarcts (usually associated with hypertension), rather than alteration of the cerebral blood flow *per se*, are the mechanisms whereby vascular disease leads to dementia. Using the presence of areas of infarction, rather than cerebral arteriosclerosis itself, as the main criterion of ischaemic damage, a correlation has been confirmed in elderly demented subjects between infarction and the other pathological evidence of cerebral arteriosclerosis (Birkett & Raskin, in press).

The common neurological concomitant of these pathological changes is the condition known as 'stroke', or cerebral thrombosis, and the clinical signs and symptoms of this are well established. More recently, detailed investigation of the natural history has been undertaken by Marquadsen (1969) in Denmark. A major subsequent risk is that of a second stroke. This implies that measures for stroke prevention are important. It is reasonable to suppose that this applies even when the cerebral thrombosis is manifested by mental rather than neurological changes.

Dementia may result not uncommonly (Janota, 1981) from ischaemic changes in the deep white matter of the cerebral hemisphere in the presence of hypertension, a condition known as Binswanger's disease (Binswanger, 1894). The changes result from lesions in the long vessels supplying the white matter together with a relatively poor anastomotic system (Janota, 1981). The attenuation of the white matter may be visible on the CAT scan (Valentine *et al.*, 1980).

The Hachinski Ischaemic Score (Hachinski *et al.*, 1975) is based on a brief inventory of clinical symptoms and signs which can be used to assist the distinction between multi-infarct and Alzheimer dementias. Patients scoring 7 or above are classed as suffering from multi-infarct dementia. Birkett (1972) compared the mental symptoms of two groups of aged mental hospital patients. Ten had senile brain

disease but no brain infarcts. Fourteen had brain infarcts but no positive evidence of senile brain disease. The arteriosclerotic patients were more liable to have preserved the nucleus of their personality, and had a more sudden onset of symptoms. The senile patients were, in general, more severely demented, while maintaining their physical mobility, and had a greater tendency to wander about. Evidence of hemiplegia and a history of stroke was shown also to distinguish cerebral arteriosclerotic dementia. Several cardiovascular changes, including cardiac arrhythmias, electrocardiographic abnormalities, and elevated pulse pressure, were shown to be predictors that cerebral infarcts will be revealed at post-mortem examination in this group. Senile purpura was the only physical change commoner in the senile dementia group.

Degenerative brain disorders of non-Alzheimer type

Diagnostic accuracy within the non-Alzheimer group of dementias is often difficult. Sometimes eponyms have become established on the basis of scanty anecdotal case histories in early and obscure literature. The psychiatric symptomatology has seldom been statistically correlated with the neuropathological findings. Even the neuropathological descriptions may be suspect, since patterns of gliosis and loss of nerve cells may be non-specific and variable.

In any case the distinctions seemed unimportant and academic at one time; until recent evidence of a transmissible virus in some dementias became available it would have been of little importance to issues of treatment to make distinctions between the various pre-senile dementias such as Pick's, Alzheimer's and Creutzfeld-Jacob disease. The latter disorder is now known to be transmissible to subhuman primates with a latent period from about one year to many more and between humans by corneal grafts and similar unusual circumstances (Gadjusek & Gibbs, 1975; Gadjusek, Gibbs, Asher, Brown, Divan, Hoffman, Memo, Rower & White, 1977); its classical presentation is a rapidly progressive dementia, with extrapyramidal signs, muscle wasting and fasciculations and sometimes cortical blindness (Hughes, 1978). Some cases with a clinical picture of Alzheimer's or senile dementia may belong to this category of disorder. It has the pathological features of a spongioform encephalopathy.

Pick's disease is a well established neuropathological entity. In addition to cell loss and gliosis there is a distinctive ballooning of the cortical nerve cells, with the nucleus pushed to one side. Areas of atrophy affect mainly the phylogenetically relatively recent areas thus initially sparing the hippocampus and its memory functions. Its origin is obscure. Clinical criteria for separating Pick's from Alzheimer's disease are sometimes given but the rarity of Pick's disease is probably its main distinguishing point.

A syndrome has been described by Stam and his colleagues (1980), and Suzuki and his colleagues (1971), of pre-senile dementia with forgetfulness, incontinence, and a stiff, unsteady extrapyramidal gait, and a post mortem finding of Lafora bodies (a polysaccharide-protein phosphate complex) in ganglion cells of the cortex and in brainstem nuclei.

Several degenerative diseases of the neurological system may become complicated by dementia. About 20–30 per cent of Parkinsonian patients show evidence also of a dementing process (Lieberman *et al.*, 1979; Pollock & Hornabrook, 1966); possibly indicating a subtype of Parkinson's disease (Serby, 1980). Conversely, Alzheimer cases may show extrapyramidal symptoms. However, the efficacy of levodopa in treating the cognitive deficits in Parkinson's disease is conflicting; at most, temporary improvement may be observed (Drachman & Stahl, 1975; Serby, 1980). Other secondary dementias occur in Huntington's chorea, multiple sclerosis and spinocerebellar degeneration. Chronic and repeated brain insults such as occur in boxers may also end in dementia.

Although differentiation of Alzheimer's presenile dementia and senile dementia has been attempted in the past it is now believed that these conditions are indistinguishable pathologically and clinically. A pathoplastic effect probably occurs such that at younger ages the condition progresses more rapidly and produces more obvious parietal lobe symptoms such as aphasias, apraxias, and agnosias and thus gives the appearance of a distinct disorder.

Neurosyphilis

General paralysis is produced by the presence of spirochaetes in the brain. The onset occurs ten years or more after the primary infection with syphilis. In fact, these days, it is increasingly rare to get any history of the primary infection at all. Impairment of memory and other symptoms suggestive of dementia commonly are found, but any set of mental symptoms may be present (Kraepelin, 1904,

see 1968; Binder & Dickman, 1980). Epileptic seizures are a common early symptom. The physical signs are more characteristic than the mental ones (Kraepelin, 1904, see 1968). They include a dysarthria, described as slurring or 'lalling'. The patient is unable to repeat 'tongue-twisters'. Various tremors may be present, and there may be abnormalities of the lower limb reflexes. Syphilis is amongst the many causes of optic atrophy. Argyll Robertson pupils are especially characteristic.

The serological tests on the blood are more likely to be positive than in any other form of neurological syphilis although a patient with neurosyphilis may yet have negative serological bloodtests. The presence of positive serology in the spinal fluid is definitive proof of the presence of spirochaetes in the brain.

General principles of management

If it is borne in mind that the dementing process does not so much cause disorientation as erode the capacity for orientation, then it will be more readily seen that the emphasis in management should be on making it easier for the patient to cope with the environment rather than on merely restructuring the environment for the protection and restriction of the patient.

The patient who is able to negotiate familiar surroundings reasonably well may reveal a deficit in orientation on relocation to a new setting that demands the learning of topography, rules of conduct, and relationships. Even without relocation, the introduction of unfamiliar elements or routines into the patient's day may be overtaxing and result in confusion. Thus, the environment should be kept as constant as is compatible with the necessity to stimulate and engage the patient; a function of knowing the patient's strengths and limits. If relocation is unavoidable then the patient should be well prepared for it with repeated straightforward explanations of what is intended, visits to the new location and meeting personnel if possible, transfer with familiar possessions, attention to indoctrination and resocialization into the unfamiliar setting, and frequent visiting from the family during the resettlement period. These cautions apply not only to admissions to long-term-care facilities but also to acute hospital admissions since the latter may also be complicated by psychological decompensation and a high rate of accidents through unfamiliarity with the surroundings and the incoordinating effects of stress.

It is easier for a patient to remain in touch with

an environment if it has clear distinguishing characteristics. This is particularly achieved in institutional settings by use of colour, shape, and textural cues to the location of key areas, by provisions of adequate glare-free light, and by routine identification of personnel and activities by name and function. In addition, the dimension of time in the environment can be given identifying structure by a basic schedule of hourly and daily events and a program of weekly events whose content varies sufficiently to reflect the passage of time. In this respect, there might also be a prominent display of current information on newsworthy items, time, and date. All these cues may be reduced in the darkness at night or where perceptual impairment exists and special care will be required in those circumstances to maintain environmental cues by, for example, a night-light, spectacles, a hearing aid, removal of wax from the ear, or the removal of cataracts.

The patient's own identity and relationship to the environment may be enhanced by addressing patients by name and keeping them informed on all occasions about where they are going and what they will do there, and by their gossiping with friends and visitors, being involved in group activities, and being surrounded by personal memorabilia.

Placement on the continuum of care

Although most elderly persons are able to care for themselves, the majority of those with chronic organic brain syndrome are dependent on another person for assistance in the basic or instrumental activities of daily living. The informal social network, usually the family, is not always able to provide the required services and consequently a variety of formal medical, nursing, and social services have evolved for the purpose of supporting the disabled old person.

There are certain frontier posts in the land of senile dementia, where behaviour becomes so intolerable that the patient cannot be maintained at home (Isaacs, 1977). At this extreme, long-term-care institutions, such as the geriatric hospital or skilled nursing facility, will provide total care of the severely disabled person, including extensive personal assistance for the bed- or chair-bound patient or for specific disabilities such as transferring, dressing, walking, bathing, toileting, or feeding. At the other extreme, an 'outreach' program may offer a variety of limited services such as shopping for essential supplies, which may be all that is required by a person able to

manage duties inside the household. Between these extremes lies a continuum of care which may be more or less complete and systematized and, if ideal, with a single point of entry and referral to a co-ordinated network of services. In actual practice, the range, packaging, and availability of services offered will vary from one region to another, as will eligibility and mode of entry.

In a fully developed continuum of care the patient will be placed in that setting which affords the least change and restriction in life-style that is compatible with the reasonably economic provision of the care and support the patient needs to maximize health, comfort, and social pursuits. Between the extremes already mentioned there exist institutions to care for the relatively healthy but confused and demented elderly; to provide a modest amount of personal and medical services (health-related facilities and local authority old age homes); sheltered or enriched apartments and housing with a resident warden and readily available home-care services; day hospital and day-care centres, with the former emphasizing medical rehabilitation, and the latter, social activities. Besides the services already described there are visiting nurses, health visitors and home-helps; respite admissions and sitting services to give relief to the families of the dependent elderly; telephone checking services and other means to reassure the vulnerable person that someone will be alert to a need for emergency intervention; transportation, especially important as an adjunct to centralized services; carpentry to provide ramps and other mechanical aids in the home; a laundry service; meals-on-wheels or centralized luncheon clubs; and many other innovative approaches.

Judgement is required to determine how much of the available array of services to muster on behalf of a patient and at what point in the course of the illness. At best, intervention will be early enough to prevent unnecessary deterioration in the patient's physical condition and morale and before the informal support members are themselves overstressed; but not so as to make the patient feel even more helpless and dependent or to displace the sense of involved responsibility that family or friends may have. The high rate of depression among the family members of the dependent elderly calls for special efforts to provide psychological and social relief services for them.

Barnes *et al.* (1981) found that families of Alzheimer patients frequently disclose in support-group discussions that they do not receive enough help or information from physicians and thus do not properly understand the nature and course of the disease. They become isolated as friends drop away and are often overwhelmed by the patient's behaviour, such as wandering at night or belligerence, and the great demands upon their time. These relatives were found to be helped through group discussions which made them feel less guilty about the deterioration in the patient and their response to the patient's behaviour, and enhanced their ability to deal with the practical problems of caring and with legal issues, as well as to take better care of themselves.

Psychotherapy

Psychotherapists are often reluctant to treat the elderly and, even more so, those elderly who are dementing. This reluctance may stem from the therapist's fear of confronting the ageing declines in him- or herself, from mixed feelings about relationships with someone old enough to be a parent, from the therapist's desire to withdraw from a dying patient, or, most likely, from a sense that the dementing patient cannot respond to the interpersonal and insightful elements in therapy. However, advocates of psychotherapy for the dementing elderly person claim that behaviour problems and anxiety can be reduced in such patients by suitably modified forms of psychotherapy (Steury & Blank, 1977).

The goals of treatment in these circumstances must be limited mainly to improving morale and social behaviour, rather than changing personality. The therapist plays a much more active role than with younger, more alert and intellectually intact patients; this includes discussions with the family or institutional staff to increase their understanding and tolerance of the patient's behaviour, or giving advice and sympathetic encouragement to the patient. Some therapists believe that touching the patient is important as a means of giving reassurance. Therapeutic sessions are best given for 5–15 minutes at a time (or longer if the patient appears to have a sufficient span of attention), with widely spaced intervals and flexibly synchronized with the time of day at which the patient is most alert. The course of therapy rarely has a planned termination date, but rather may be intermittent or continue until the death of the patient. The latter event is particularly difficult to manage for therapists who feel defeated by such limitations on their effectiveness as healers.

Therapists with extensive experience of the elderly in institutions have emphasized the covert feelings of fear and rage experienced by disabled patients who are aware of their increasing helplessness and loss of control over gratifying relationships (Goldfarb, 1956). A vicious circle may ensue in which the patient believes his or her angry feelings are perceived by the therapist who, so the patient thinks, will respond with rejection of the patient, thus increasing the latter's sense of powerlessness and loss. Reassurance by the therapist may not be credible to the patient and may simply raise the patient's level of guilt and intensify a sense of worthlessness. The patient's search for aid may take the form of persistent complaining, excessive demands, restless attention-seeking, or domineering aggression, with a gathering of momentum as relationships deteriorate. This negative progression may be interrupted by so arranging the sequence of interactions in the interview that the patient is able to assume that the therapist's respect, affection, and acquiescence has been won by the patient rather than freely granted by the therapist. The patient comes to feel more in control of this crucial source of authority and emotional support and feels more confident that the therapist will be accessible when the patient decides to call upon his services. Critics of this approach may object to its contrived nature or question its effectiveness. However, it is at least a feasible and economical method for coping with dementing persons; it takes into account the real increase of dependent needs in these persons and allows for their lack of insight. Since there is no attempt to lower the defences of the patient it is unlikely that his anxieties will be increased or his self-esteem damaged, while much good may be accomplished.

Remotivation therapy

It has been claimed that some, if not many, of the symptoms shown by patients in long-term-care facilities are caused by the effects of a prolonged stay in an institutional environment. Such symptoms include apathy, social disengagement, and inactivity as well as a diminution in an appreciation of one's own identity, limits, and strengths. Remotivation therapy is designed to revitalize and resocialize such persons and to sharpen and improve their self-image. This type of therapy was developed for mental hospital patients, mostly young, and its application to geriatric patients in various long-term-care settings has met with variable success (Dennis, 1978; Birkett & Boltuch, 1973; Moody, Baron & Monk, 1970).

Therapeutic sessions are conducted by a trained worker, who may or may not be a psychologist, nurse, or other health care professional, a few times a week for about twelve sessions. Some recognition is given to the need to make the clients feel part of a group process but the major focus is on discussion and vivid concrete illustration of preselected topics which are chosen to draw the attention of the patient away from the sick role and towards shared experience of the non-institutional world. The participation of the clients in the group discussions and their presentation of their relevant personal history is said to allow the assumption of healthy roles and the acquisition of a more accurate self-image, as well as to increase motivation to take part in other rehabilitative programs.

The time limit for remotivation therapy lends itself to objective evaluations of the treatment. A controlled trial of remotivation therapy versus conventional group therapy in 39 ambulant geriatric inpatients showed some advantage for remotivation therapy, but the difference was not statistically significant (Birkett & Boltuch, 1973).

The effects on staff morale of remotivation therapy, of the feeling that something is being done with apparently hopeless patients who are under custodial care, is not to be ignored. However, these effects are more complicated and ambivalent than some of the enthusiasts suggest. On introducing this therapy to a psychogeriatric unit, there may be some initial resistance from the nursing aides who are asked to use it. One impression is that some aides may feel self-conscious about the public speaking that is involved. Perhaps also they may resent the failure to recognize that their non-verbal skills are of value. The material emphasizes the merits of talking with patients. Violent, dirty, incontinent patients demand degrees of skill in their management, aside from verbal communication, and recognition of this may be good for the morale of in-patient unit staff.

Reality orientation

One of the most striking symptoms of the chronic organic brain syndrome is disorientation. It is therefore not surprising that a good deal of attention has been given to a treatment, reality orientation, that is intended specifically to relieve the symptom of disorientation by increasing the patient's awareness of the relationship between the self and the current and changing environment (Taulbee & Folsom, 1966; Taulbee, 1976; Taulbee, 1978).

The treatment is usually but not necessarily given in an institutional setting. It comprises both a consistent style of interaction with patient and a regular daily series of relatively brief small group meetings of patients led usually by a non-physician.

All members of the staff take pains to jog and encourage the patient's memory about time, place, and person whenever in contact with the patient and through environmental cues ('twenty-four-hour' orientation). They also correct the patient's confused or misperceived beliefs after careful enquiry as to the reasons for apparently irrational behaviour. The group meetings are viewed as educating the patient, first at a very simple level covering basic orienting information and, later, at a more advanced level with mental exercises to develop attention and recall. For the better preserved patients, the scope of reality orientation can be stretched to include general education or training in coping with a variety of situations from shopping to overcoming physical handicaps. Patients who do not improve within about two months after starting the basic classes should be given a rest from treatment.

Much of the value of this treatment may derive from its common-sense adherence to the principles of keeping patients mentally active within the limits of their capacity, and promoting good communication and rapport with patients, and therapeutic optimism among the staff. In home-care programmes the family may be given a sense of direction by involvement in administering the orienting information to the patient.

Reality orientation (RO) is widely practised in long-term-care facilities in the US (Scarborough, 1979), but quantitative findings on the effectiveness of reality orientation in senile dementia have not given evidence of dramatic benefits (MacDonald & Settin, 1978; Voelkel, 1978), though some studies have reported modest gains. Classroom RO has been reported as effective in enhancing orientation information as verbally expressed (Harris & Ivory, 1976; Citrin & Dixon, 1977); however, behavioural changes indicating a better sense of orientation after RO are infrequently reported (Brook *et al.*, 1975).

A controlled comparison of 24-hour reality orientation (including classroom sessions) over a one-year period (Zepelin *et al.*, 1981) was conducted with 22 elderly subjects and 14 controls with varying degrees of cognitive impairment. A plateau of improvement was obtained by RO in about 3 months of treatment but the benefits were slight and restricted to tests of orientation with no effects evident on levels of independence or on social responsiveness.

Classroom reality orientation (Drummond *et al.*, 1978) was compared with a twenty-four hour orientation training programme in the ward in a controlled study of 57 elderly residents with dementia in an old age home (Hanley *et al*, 1981). The twenty-four hour programme included training sessions in identifying key locations on the ward through practice and reinforcement. The classroom RO improved verbal, but not behavioural or other cognitive, improvements. The ward training sessions were, by contrast, relatively dramatic in improving behaviours.

Brook, Degun and Mather (1975) carried out a controlled study of reality orientation, with particular attention to the possibility that any benefit might be a non-specific effect of change of environment. Their subjects were eighteen hospital patients with diagnoses of dementia. They found that very deteriorated patients did not appear to benefit, but noticed a subgroup in which significant improvement took place. This group started off with relatively little impairment in intellectual and social functioning. Simply taking patients out of their ward environment was a major factor producing improvement in the first few weeks of the experiment, but this did not in itself seem adequate to maintain improvement. Possibly RO does improve social and interpersonal activity but these changes are not dramatic or are hard to measure (Zepelin *et al.*, 1981; Hellebrandt, 1978; Voelkel, 1978).

Carroll and Gray (1981), have described a Memory Development technique suitable for the elderly in long-term-care facilities, which is claimed to be less confrontational than reality orientation and more responsive to current theory regarding learning, performance, and memory. Cues to assist memory are provided through arrangement of the environment (e.g. seasonal decorations), and are keyed by the nursing staff to the patient's personal and cultural background. The strength of this technique lies in the detailed guide-lines to its implementation: how to make cues visible and audible to the elderly; when to vary and when to keep cues consistent over time; specific cues for recognition memory and remote memory; the inadvertent inaccuracies in cues that may confuse the elderly person; how to achieve optimal conditions for learning by the elderly (e.g. by verbal rehearsal of visual tasks, by a slow pace, and by limiting distractions); and what factors motivate the elderly person to learn (e.g. avoiding over-arousal,

choice of meaningful material, providing a set to recall rather than reliance on incidental learning). This approach is plausible but not yet demonstrated to be effective.

Behavioural treatment

Apathy and withdrawal is a problem commonly observed in the elderly in long-term-care facilities. Burton (1980) noted in a psychogeriatric ward in which nearly all residents suffered from dementia that there was relatively little stimulation of the residents by staff, environmental events or entertainment; and that the most deteriorated patients received the least stimulation. A variety of behavioural techniques have been described for increasing the engagement in occupational and interpersonal activities of elderly residents. Reinforcement of selected behaviours can increase participation in self-care activities (MacDonald & Butler, 1974; Baltes & Zerbe, 1976) or social functions (Mueller & Atlas, 1972). Manipulation of the environment, such as by organizing social occasions or increasing availability of recreational materials, may accomplish the same ends (Miller, 1977; Jenkins *et al.*, 1977; Powell *et al.*, 1979). Occupational therapists can be trained to cue patients to the use of appropriate materials and to reward desirable behaviours (Burton, 1980).

Other applications of behavioural techniques to improve the social behaviour of elderly nursing-home residents are reported by Sachs (1975) and Blackman and colleagues (1976).

Symptomatic treatment

The distressing, disabling, and disturbing symptoms which are rooted in the dementing process can be reduced to levels which are tolerable to the patient and family or supporting personnel by attention to certain principles of management and, where all else fails, the judicious exhibition of medications. Although these approaches do not arrest the dementing process they may allow the patient to remain relatively comfortable and independent for some length of time, and may make a great deal of difference in postponing the need for admission to an institution, or relocation to a more intensive and restrictive type of care. Common symptoms requiring such symptomatic treatment include sleep disturbance, difficulty with locomotion, incontinence, agitation, wandering, noisiness, aggressive outbursts, apathy, and self-neglect.

For sleep disturbance or noisiness or wandering at night, sedation may sometimes be obtained by increasing daytime activities, providing a hot milk drink at bed-time and leaving a night-light on. If simple measures fail then it may be useful to give chloral hydrate (Noctec), 500 mg h.s.; or flurazepam (Dalmane), 15 mg h.s. Insomnia is a very common complaint in the elderly. Most practitioners would admit to occasionally prescribing a benzodiazepine on a short-term basis. This practice is probably harmless (Goldstein *et al.*, 1978), although heavy habitual use of hypnotics may accelerate the rate of intellectual decline in dementia. Barbiturates should be avoided.

Difficulty in ambulation may develop as a direct result of the dementing process, but also because of concomitant physical conditions, because of a failing ability to cope with handicaps and the management of mechanical aids, or because of oversedation and inadequate activity. A vicious cycle may be entered when these factors lead to the patient spending lengthy periods of time in a geriatric chair or in bed where further loss of mobility may follow and even wasting and flexion contractures may develop. Maintenance of ambulatory activity is essential and it is evident that this will require limiting sedation or other drugs that affect energy, balance and co-ordination, giving rehabilitation to aid coping skills with mechanical aids to ambulation, and encouragement and assistance to allow involvement in physical activities. The more energetic the efforts at preventing immobility the less will this state appear an inevitable part of the dementing process.

Similarly, the frequency of incontinence may be reduced in dementia by preventive steps or careful investigation. Medications which have an anticholinergic effect, low residue diets, or painful fissures and haemorrhoids may be associated with constipation, faecal impaction, and secondary faecal incontinence. The symptoms of impaction may not be reported by the somewhat confused old person and the only suggestions of this condition may be restlessness and vomiting or other evidence of abdominal discomfort such as doubling up; a rectal examination should be routine in cases of incontinence. One should also consider the possibility that the patient is incontinent because of an inability to adopt a regular defaecation schedule, sometimes resulting from confusion about the location and availability of toilets and sometimes from insufficient awareness of bowel sensations. It can be helpful under these circumstances to identify toilets clearly, and to programme for the patient a schedule of visits to the toilet either timed to anticipate the pattern of incontinent bowel actions or simply at regular intervals.

Agitation, pacing, anxious perseveration, irritable aggressiveness, excessive suspiciousness, and misperceptions may need symptomatic control, although the possibility of an underlying depressive disorder or confusional state should first be ruled out. Reassurance, resolution of interpersonal tensions, or the introduction of structured activities sometimes helps. As a last resort, drugs may be required.

The major antipsychotic drugs are probably the most useful general agents in pharmacological treatment of behaviour disturbance associated with dementia in the aged (Yesavage, 1979). In prescribing them, it must be borne in mind that the patient may be taking other drugs. The risk of adverse drug reactions in the elderly is more often associated with this type of drug than any other, especially when anticholinergic and sedative drugs are prescribed concurrently (Segal *et al.*, 1979).

Side-effects include drowsiness, unsteadiness, falling, and constipation. Tremor is common. A safe technique of dosage adjustment is to start with a small night-time single dose, such as 25 mg of chlorpromazine, and record standing morning blood pressures, increasing the dosage if there is no postural hypotension. Higher dosage levels up to 200 mg of chlorpromazine can be built up over several weeks (Birkett & Boltuch, 1972).

Claims to particular geriatric application have been made on behalf of thioridazine, haloperidol, and thiothixene. Comparisons between these drugs in psychogeriatric patients have revealed no significant difference in their psychotropic efficacy (Tsuang *et al.*, 1971). None of these drugs is especially low in side-effects (Birkett & Boltuch, 1971; Birkett, Hirschfield & Simpson, 1972). The practitioner is well advised to use the major antipsychotic drug with which he is most familiar, although the individual preference of patients, families, and nurses may prevail.

Specific physical treatments

Many physical treatments have been devised for the prevention or alleviation of chronic organic brain syndrome. The range of treatments proposed has been reviewed by Murray Jarvik (1973) and includes attempts to prevent atherosclerosis (e.g. diets, clofibrate, antioxidants); to improve oxygen flow to the brain (e.g. hyperbaric oxygen, vasodilators); anticoagulants; nutritional supplements (particularly vitamins of the B complex and choline); and substances intended to increase RNA synthesis, facilitate neurotransmission (e.g. glutamic acid, choline) enhance neuronal repair and ganglion function (e.g. procaine amide, hydergine) or alter arousal levels (e.g. amphetamines, metrazol). However, most of these once promising leads have proved disappointing when carefully tested. Jarvik concludes that 'it can be fairly stated that at this stage in history no treatment has been unequivocally shown to improve the mental status of the aged'. Nevertheless, some of the agents in contemporary use are described below.

Dihydroergotoxine (hydergine). There have been several controlled studies in which hydergine has been shown to improve mood, intellectual function, initiative, sociability, and self-care capacity in cases of mild to moderate dementia (Gerin, 1969; Ditch & Resnick, 1971; Roubicek, Geige & Abt, 1972; Bazo, 1973; Abramowicz, 1976). However, findings in these studies have been inconsistent and the improvements noted have not been substantial. Suggestions have been made that this drug improves the cerebral blood flow or works directly on glial or nerve cells. It can be given sublingually in doses of 1 mg t.i.d. for a period of at least 3–4 weeks. There may be some local and gastric irritation but there are no serious side-effects.

Central nervous system stimulants. Central nervous system stimulants such as methylphenidate, and pentylenetetrazol, which have amphetamine-like effects, are often prescribed for the elderly (Crook, 1979). Crook has reviewed the literature and concludes that such drugs do not produce any useful improvement in memory or mental function. Their multiple adverse effects seem to argue against their use in aged patients.

Cholinergic substances. The evidence previously cited that receptor sites for acetylcholine appear to remain intact in dementia, whereas the cholinergic neurons and acetylcholine synthesis are affected (Bowen & Davison, 1980), has led to the development of approaches to treating dementia based upon methods which enhance acetylcholine production or retard its breakdown. The number of dendritic cell processes is reduced in senile dementia, and so, presumably, is the number and functional capacity of interneuronal synapses. The possibility exists that inadequate synaptic function could be restored by a quantitative increase in the humoral juices which transmit messages from cell to cell. Such logic has borne fruit in the treatment of Parkinson's disease, where the introduction of levo-dopa as a treatment method arose directly from neurochemical observations that dopamine was deficient in the Parkinsonian brain. Success has been claimed in treating Parkinsonian dementia with anti-Parkinsonian drugs, such as amantidine (Chierichetti *et al.*, 1977). A difficulty in assessing such claims is that depression, dementia, and Parkinson's disease often go hand in hand. Improvement in one of the triad may affect judgement of improvement of the others (Asnis, 1977). Attempts to improve cholinergic neurotransmission in Alzheimer's dementia have been made with dietary supplements of choline in egg yolks, fish and beans, more concentrated sources of choline such as lecithin (Cohen & Wurtman, 1975), or by injecting anticholinesterases to retard the breakdown of acetylcholine (Perry, Perry & Tomlinson, 1977c). However, so far, this speculation has not been vindicated by actual clinical application (Boyd *et al.*, 1977).

Trials of the administration in dementia of choline chloride, lecithin physostigmine, or arecoline have not been promising (Boyd *et al.*, 1977; Smith & Swash, 1978; Signoret *et al.*, 1978; Christie *et al.*, 1981) though there is some modest evidence that the less severely demented patients may be improved (Etienne *et al.*, 1978; Christie *et al.*, 1979). The possibility that if patients were more precisely selected then more favourable results of treatment would be observed has led to the testing of the acute administration of physostigmine and arecoline as a predictor of response to prolonged choline treatment. Eleven pre-senile Alzheimer cases in a relatively early stage of the disease were studied in a controlled randomized double-blind design (Christie *et al.*, 1981). A significant improvement in cognitive functions similar to that obtained in normal subjects was observed but this was only slight and not of an order that would be clinically useful. Possibly, the therapeutic model is incomplete in failing to take account of other possible impairments of neuronal metabolism (Geinisman *et al.*, 1977) and dysfunctions in other neurotransmitter systems.

Aluminium toxicity. The hope that the allegedly high aluminium content of neurofibrillary tangles would lead to therapeutic measures based on treatment of aluminium toxicity has not been fulfilled. McDermott, and colleagues, (1977) have provided evidence suggesting that increased aluminium is a nonspecific ageing change.

Gerovital (GH-3). Ostfeld, Smith and Stotsky (1977) reviewed 285 papers on this controversial drug which has been claimed to reverse or retard many of the changes of ageing including those of intellectual decline. Gerovital is a 2 per cent solution of procaine and is usually given by intramuscular injection several times a week in a series of courses each lasting a month. Increased potency has been claimed for various modified solutions of procaine but there is little evidence to support such claims. According to Ostfeld and colleagues, almost all the better-controlled studies have been negative or at best equivocal with respect to reversing the effects of dementia or of atherosclerosis. It seems likely that procaine is a mild antidepressant (a monoamine oxidase inhibitor) and that improvement in the patient's mood may be added to a placebo effect to induce better performance on the part of some patients without in any way affecting the dementing process.

Cyclandelate (cyclospasmol) and meclofenoxate (lucidril.) These drugs have been claimed to produce small but significant improvement in several mental functions; however, results have been conflicting (Soukupová, Vojtechovsky & Safratová, 1970; Oliver and Restell, 1967; Fine *et al.*, 1970; Aderman, Giardina & Koreniowski, 1972,; Rao *et al.*, 1978). For example, in a controlled trial of cyclandelate (Rao *et al.*, 1978) there was no significant improvement in the cyclandelate group as compared with the placebo group on any score at the end of four weeks on the study, but, significant improvement as compared with placebo was evident at the end of twelve weeks. However, personal neatness was found to be significantly improved in a placebo group as compared with the cyclandelate group.

Hyperbaric oxygen. In this treatment the patient is exposed to 100 per cent oxygen at 2.5 atmospheres twice daily in 90-minute sessions for 15 days. Jacobs and colleagues (1969) obtained positive results with an experimental group (N–13) and a control group breathing 10 per cent oxygen in nitrogen. However, Raskin and colleagues (1978), in a much larger study, found no significant differences between an experimental and a control group.

A note on the effectiveness of treating dementia in relation to the distinction between the arteriosclerotic and other types of dementia

There are several drugs in current use which purport to dilate arteries. It is doubtful whether they can do so at all, even more doubtful whether they can do so in the brain, and, more doubtful again, whether doing so has any beneficial effect in dementia.

McAlpine and her colleagues (1981) investigated cerebral blood flow using the xenon-133 inhalation method (Wyper *et al.*, 1976) in 54 elderly persons (90 years or older) ranging from normal to moderately demented. Cerebral blood flow level was significantly lowered by old age (compared with normal young adult controls) but not additionally by dementia.

Although treatments of dementia aimed at improving the blood supply to the brain have been generally disappointing in their effects, it might be argued that results would be better if the arteriosclerotic dementias could be singled out from all the rest. With this in mind, Birkett (1971), developed an Arteriosclerotic Rating Scale intended to identify cases most likely to be arteriosclerotic in type. Items were grouped into cardiovascular and neurological findings. Cardiovascular items included the presence or absence of thickened radial arteries, locomotor brachialis, kinked carotid arteries, temporal artery pulsation, poor peripheral pulses in the legs, retinal artery changes, hypertension, cardiac enlargement on chest X-ray, aortic changes on chest X-ray, and electrocardiographic abnormalities. Neurological items included the presence or absence of a paralysis of sudden onset, a history of epileptic fits or convulsions after the age of 50, signs of unilateral spasticity or weakness with bilateral Babinskis, and pseudobulbar palsy or any of the classical syndromes of individual artery obstruction (e.g. posterior inferior cerebellar artery syndrome).

The Arteriosclerotic Rating Scale was used in a single blind study of cyclandelate in 24 psychogeriatric patients (Birkett, 1971). Response to the drug was evaluated by means of the Brief Psychiatric Rating Scale, Crichton Rating Scale, and a physician's global estimate. Patients were divided into good responders and bad responders. Clinical evidence of arteriosclerosis was not a useful predictive factor. None of the items on the Arteriosclerotic Rating Scale had any predictive value.

A further trial of the Arteriosclerotic Rating Scale was made in the course of the study by Raskin

& his colleagues (1978) of the effects of hyperbaric oxygen on the elderly with cognitive impairment. As previously related, this study showed negative findings: furthermore, a group of patients identified by the Arteriosclerotic Rating Scale as likely to have the arteriosclerotic type of dementia did no better (or worse) than the remainder of the patients.

Thus, at the moment, it would have to be said that differentiating cerebral arterial sclerosis as a separate entity in dementia has not borne direct fruits in the shape of a treatment, specifically directed toward arterial disease.

Several measures are employed in general medical neurological practice for the prevention of recurrences of stroke and also for the reduction of hypoxia during the actual stage of acute onset. These have recently been reviewed (Sahs, Hartman & Aronson, 1976). While it is to be assumed that this would have some bearing on the prevention and treatment of dementia, no direct connection has yet been made. For example, evidence from the Framingham study (Kannel, 1966) suggests that control of blood pressure can reduce the incidence of neurologically evident strokes, but it has not yet been directly shown that this will affect the incidence or progress of dementia.

The chain of events involved in cerebral haemorrhage is not considered here, since this is a commonly fatal condition, not usually leaving a residuum of survivors with mental impairment.

The treatment of neurosyphilis

The treatment of this condition must often follow official rules. Guidelines are suggested in such publications as those of the US Public Health Service (1968). There has been little recent opportunity to test and modify methods of treatment which were established when case material was more plentiful. Oral penicillin is not recommended. Penicillin G is given by intramuscular injection, twelve million units being given over twenty days. Spinal fluid examination is recommended (but often not done) every three months for a year, and then every six months for a second year. If the patient is allergic to penicillin then a tetracycline or erythromycin may be substituted, in a total dose of 30–40 g. Treatment should be given four times daily in equally divided doses, and should extend over ten to fifteen days.

Concluding remarks

Over the past decade, interest in the scientific and clinical study of the dementias has quickened. The major models of enquiry and care that grace the field of psychiatry have now been brought to bear upon dementia. A preoccupation with decay of brain tissue has given way to lively debate and investigation regarding the psychology and neurophysiology of disorders of memory. Emphasis on custodial modes of care has been expanded to include ameliorative approaches that draw impetus from the mainstreams of psychotherapy, developmental psychology, learning theory and psychopharmacology. In some ways the clinical studies of dementia are even outstripping the rest of psychiatry. For example, in the integration of the skills of medicine and neurology with psychiatry, and in the application of advances in diagnostic high technology.

The intellectual challenges and clinical problems posed by dementias have attracted a response from some of the best minds in a variety of disciplines. This response comes, perhaps, none too soon, given the projected epidemic of dementia, occasioned by the increased expectation of living to the age of greatest risk for dementia, which threatens to overwhelm the health care system. Equally important is that the victims of this most terrible of disorders are coming to be accepted as patients, like any other. Thus the quality of care for such patients is slowly improving, their families are being supported more sympathetically and the hope of eventually discovering a means of prevention or a cure for this disorder, though still remote, has strengthened.

13
Epilepsy
GEORGE W. FENTON

Introduction

Epilepsy, derived from the Greek word meaning 'to take hold of', is a disorder of the brain characterized by recurring clinical seizures. The essence of an epileptic seizure is an abnormal and excessive discharge of nerve cells within the brain. The clinical manifestation of seizures depends on the number and location of discharging neurones. When relatively few motor cortex neurones discharge, there may be only jerking of a contralateral limb, without loss of consciousness (a simple partial seizure). When millions of neurones throughout the cerebral cortex discharge, loss of consciousness is accompanied by a tonic–clonic convulsion often followed by post-ictal confusion as consciousness gradually returns (major or grand mal attack). Between these two extremes are many different types of generalized or partial (focal) epileptic seizure; complex partial seizures due to temporal lobe discharge and the petit mal absences caused by generalized spike and wave complexes are the commonest.

Basic seizure mechanisms

Virtually all we know about basic seizure mechanisms is derived from animal models of epilepsy. The epileptic neurone has been intensively studied in cortical foci. The major abnormality is a tendency to recurrent high-frequency bursts of action potentials. Ouabain has been shown to inhibit active transport of ions through neuronal membranes, causing depolarization with membrane instability, repetitive, paroxysmal discharges, and seizures. Hence it is probable that the final common set of mechanisms responsible for epilepsy involves changes in cell membrane stability and excitability (Tower, 1974).

There is also a highly significant relationship between the number of epileptogenic neurones in a focus and the frequency of epileptic attacks. These findings suggest that the attack frequency in focal epilepsy is directly related to the amount of epileptic tissue present. It is this abnormal tissue which recruits normal neurones, leading to propagation and ultimately to clinical attacks, when a sufficiently large pool of neurones is involved to disrupt the subject's behaviour.

The generalized seizures elicited by photic stimulation in the Papio papio baboon have been extensively studied (Meldrum, 1978). Drugs such as bicuculline and picrotoxin which block the inhibitory action of gamma aminobutyric acid (GABA) induce generalized seizures with a short latency. Allyglycine has a similar effect on seizure activity, though it acts by inhibiting the enzyme glutamate decarboxylase and thus impairs the synthesis of GABA. Neurochemical changes which increase excitatory processes can also cause fits. Anticholinesterases interfere with the breakdown of acetyl choline, a putative excitatory neuro-transmitter, and cause an accumulation of this excitatory substance, which leads to increased neuronal firing and generalized seizures.

In contrast, an anti-epileptic effect is seen after the administration of drugs which raise brain 5-hydroxy tryptamine (5-HT) levels, while dopamine agonists also have an anticonvulsant action. These findings may have clinical and therapeutic relevance since the major CSF metabolites of 5-HT (5-hydroxy-indoleacetic acid) and dopamine (homovanillic acid) are significantly raised by effective anticonvulsant medication (Chadwick et al., 1975).

Experimental seizure models are also beginning to further our understanding of the effects of seizures themselves. Although clinicians have long thought that chronic, frequent, generalized tonic–clonic seizures with attendant anoxia may cause permanent damage to brain cells, new evidence suggests that the developing brain may be especially vulnerable to the metabolic consequences of seizures that would leave the mature brain unaffected (Wasterlain & Plum 1973). This finding has important

therapeutic implications since epilepsy so often begins in childhood. Another animal model of clinical relevance is the 'kindling' phenomenon, where periodic electrical stimulation too mild for behavioural or electrographic effects may eventually result in spontaneously occurring seizures. Apart from outlining a potential hazard of frequent ECT, the observations on kindling suggest that certain types of seizure foci may be self-perpetuating. A lesion which tends to fire repeatedly may worsen simply because of the effect of frequent abnormal discharge on the cells in and around the focus (Pinel & Van Oot, 1976).

Classification of epilepsy

Following the introduction of electroencephalography to the investigation of epilepsy and the pioneering work of Penfield and Jasper (1954), it has become usual to classify epilepsy according to the presumed site of origin in the brain of the seizure discharge. To achieve uniformity of terminology, in 1964 the International League Against Epilepsy prepared a classification which was recommended by the International League Against Epilepsy, World Federation of Neurology, the World Federation of Neurosurgical Societies, and the International Federation of Societies for Electroencephalography and Clinical Neurophysiology. The revised version (Gastaut, 1969) has now achieved international recognition, though a further revision is currently being undertaken by a Commission of the International League Against Epilepsy. The classification reads as follows:

I. Generalized epilepsies

These are epilepsies, in which the seizures are generalized from onset. They occur bilaterally and begin without local onset. The clinical signs are not referable to an anatomical or functional system localized in one hemisphere. Sudden unconsciousness is the usual initial feature of seizure onset with or without motor phenomena. No aura is reported, since an aura is a manifestation of the local area of brain where the seizure discharge commences to spread and precedes generalization.

The common types of generalized attack are the tonic–clonic convulsion and the petit-mal absence. Photosensitive seizures and myoclonic attacks also occur. Myoclonus, sudden involuntary jerking of a muscle or group of muscles, is an exception to the rule that there is initial unconsciousness in generalized seizures. Myoclonic jerks occur in clear consciousness due to descending activation of the spinal cord anterior horn cells. Occasionally prolonged absence seizures lead to automatic behaviour, the petit-mal automatism.

Between attacks the EEG records generalized, bilaterally synchronous, spike and wave complexes at 2–4Hz. Penfield and Jasper (1954), in order to account for the process of seizure generalization, presented the hypothesis that the activity of both hemispheres is integrated by a system of neurones located in the midline of the upper brain stem, including the interlaminar thalamic nuclei and diencephalic reticular system. This centrencephalic system projects diffusely to all areas of the cerebral cortex of both hemispheres and downwards to the anterior horn cells. When the seizure discharge activates the centrencephalic system, either by descending spread from a local cortical focus (partial seizure) or primary onset in the centrencephalon itself rapid generalization occurs as a result of ascending spread via the nonspecific thalamo-cortical pathways and diffuse and synchronous involvement of the cortex of both hemispheres. Epileptic attacks of primary onset in the centrencephalon were known as centrencephalic seizures (generalized seizures in modern terminology). However, Penfield and Jasper's centrencephalic model has been challenged during the past decade. Present evidence appears to support the idea that the thalamic and midbrain structures are intimately involved in the processes concerned with maintaining, spreading, and inhibiting seizure discharges. It seems that the thalamus becomes engaged early in the development of sustained cortical seizure discharges and that both inhibitory and facilitatory functions come into play. Cortical and subcortical structures clearly operate together in nearly all sustained epileptic processes but evidence is not convincing that the thalamus is the initiator of either primarily unilateral or generalized seizures (Goldensohn & Ward 1975).

Gloor (1978) has recently presented a new hypothesis for the mechanism of generalized spike and wave discharge in human generalized epilepsy based on the findings obtained in feline generalized penicillin epilepsy. It is postulated that in generalized epilepsy there is a diffuse and relatively mild state of cortical hyperexcitability which increases the responsiveness of cortical neurones. This leads to spike and wave discharges developing in the cortex in response to the afferent thalamo-cortical volleys normally involved in the genesis of spindles and recruiting responses.

The generalized epilepsies are subdivided into primary and secondary generalized epilepsies. The former are not a result of cerebral disease, genetic factors being dominant in the aetiology. The secondary generalized epilepsies are associated with acquired brain disease, usually diffuse but occasionally secondary to a cortical focus, usually located in the mesial surface or orbito-frontal areas of one or other hemisphere.

II. Partial (or focal) epilepsies

In the partial epilepsies, the epileptic attacks known as partial seizures originate in a local area of cerebral cortex or related subcortical structures. Most are considered to have an acquired cause leading to focal brain damage and a local epileptogenic lesion manifested by focal EEG spike and sharp wave interictal discharges. When the abnormal neuronal discharge remains localized and involves only one hemisphere, it may elicit a conscious sensation or series of sensations which the patient learns to recognize as a warning or aura. The character of the aura is determined by the function of the neuronal systems involved. It is thus not a warning but the initial event of the seizure. Motor phenomena can also occur as the initial events of a partial seizure. Such attacks may spread bilaterally and develop into generalized seizures (secondary generalization). The generalization may occur so rapidly that focal features are unobservable and no aura will be experienced. Partial seizures with onset in 'silent' areas of cortex like the frontal lobe usually have no aura and one in five patients with temporal lobe epilepsy present with major convulsions without aura.

Partial seizures are subdivided into the following two groups according to the type of clinical phenomena manifest.

(a) partial seizures with elementary symptomatology (simple partial seizures): attacks without impairment of consciousness accompanied by simple sensory or motor symptoms due to activation of one or more primary cortical or special sense areas of one hemisphere. Such seizure manifestations reflect the functional representation of the areas involved, for example motor Jacksonian attacks, somatosensory seizures, and so forth.

(b) partial seizures with complex symptomatology (complex partial seizures): attacks with disturbance of highest level function of one or more cortical areas often with impairment of consciousness, for example seizures with purely intellectual (dysmnesic ideational), psychosensory (illusions and hallucinations), psychomotor (automatism), and affective (especially ictal fear) symptoms.

Definition and diagnosis of the epileptic seizure

Epileptic attacks may be defined as repetitive, stereotyped, and transient disturbances of consciousness, behaviour, sensation, affect, or cognitive function, primarily cerebral in origin, due to excessive and disorderly discharge of neurones. Hence, for a diagnosis of epilepsy to be made, the transient episodes of altered consciousness or behaviour should fulfil the following criteria:

(1) Clinical pattern of attacks: the clinical description of the attacks should be compatible with one or more of the well established epileptic seizure patterns, for example generalized convulsions, petit-mal attacks, partial seizures. Recurrent episodes of disturbed behaviour with amnesia but not conforming to classical seizure patterns should be investigated carefully and critically before being accepted as having an epileptic basis, especially if the behaviour during the attack seems well co-ordinated and structured.

(2) Neurophysiological origin of the attacks: the attacks should be associated with excessive and disorderly cerebral neuronal discharge. This association can usually only be presumed, since, in ordinary clinical practice, it is rare to have an EEG recording of one or more of the patient's seizures. This presumed evidence of primary cerebral neuronal dysfunction excludes attacks of hysterical dissociation of consciousness. Such hysterical pseudo-seizures often present with dramatic behavioural manifestations, never associated with abnormal neuronal discharge.

Equally, the diagnosis of epilepsy should not be dependent on EEG findings alone, since EEG paroxysmal activity of the type associated with epilepsy (spike-wave complexes, focal spikes and sharp waves) can be recorded from people not suffering from epileptic attacks. These paroxysmal abnormalities can arise from focal cerebral lesions e.g. meningiomata (focal spike and sharp waves), in patients with extensive or diffuse bilateral brain disease (generalized atypical spike and wave complexes) and even from quite healthy persons (generalized fast spike-wave complexes). The latter can occur in up to 3 per cent of normal people. It is presumed that such fast spike-wave phenomena in healthy subjects reflect a greater risk of having isolated seizures in response to

states which lower their convulsive threshold further, for example sleep deprivation, withdrawal states in alcohol and drug abusers, sudden withdrawal of barbiturates or benzodiazepines, epileptogenic drug effects, especially tricyclic antidepressants and phenothiazine drugs and hypoglycaemia (Fenton, 1974, Fenton & King, 1979).

On the other hand, a normal EEG can never exclude epilepsy completely. A routine clinical EEG recording samples only a few minutes of the subject's ongoing cerebral activity. The time of day chosen for the recording, the short length of the sampling period or the patient's state of arousal may all reduce the probability of recording paroxysmal abnormalities. The frequency of occurrence of the latter varies widely with time of day and occurrence of clinical seizures and is also affected by the patient's level of awareness during the recording session. EEG activation by sleep or prolonged recording using an ambulatory monitoring technique with a portable tape recorder may be necessary. Further, since the scalp EEG only picks up electrical potential changes that are due to synchronous involvement of a large area of cortex (6 square cm), an abnormal electrical discharge confined to a small area of superficial cortex, the deeper cortical layers, or the mesial temporal lobe structures may not cause any scalp EEG change and yet result in a minor clinical seizure because of activation of those structures. Hence brief temporal lobe or even focal motor or sensory seizures may occur in the presence of a normal EEG. On the other hand, a generalized convulsion is always associated with EEG changes both during the seizure and the recovery phase.

(3) Recurrent and chronic nature of the seizure disorder: the attacks must be recurrent. Isolated seizures may occur as the result of intracerebral pathology or from more benign causes such as fever in children between the ages of 6 months and 3 years, the epileptogenic effect of psychotropic drugs, drug or alcohol withdrawal, and so forth. Only patients who experience more than two epileptic seizures at intermittent intervals should be diagnosed as suffering from epilepsy. Febrile convulsions are relatively common between the ages of 6 months and 3 years, 30 to 60 per 1000 population having one or more such fits, generally precipitated by fever. These convulsions are nearly always benign and more than 90 per cent grow out of them by the age of 5. Only 5 per cent later develop chronic epilepsy. Mislabelling and treating a child as a chronic epileptic because of febrile

convulsions could have a serious effect on the child's development. Indeed the diagnosis of epilepsy should not be made lightly since it implies long-term treatment with potentially toxic anticonvulsant drugs and has serious social consequences.

Aetiology of epilepsy

The causes of epilepsy are as complex as their manifestations. In the past, epilepsy has been divided into two broad categories; symptomatic epilepsy, where the condition results from a demonstrable brain lesion, such as damage from an infection, and idiopathic epilepsy where there is no demonstrable underlying brain lesion associated with the condition. However the validity of the concept of idiopathic epilepsy is increasingly questioned as each advance in knowledge explains more and more epilepsies, hitherto classified as idiopathic, in terms of known causes. There are three main groups of causative factors. First is the individual predisposition, which is inherited. The second is the presence of an epileptogenic lesion in the brain. The third factor is the local or generalized biochemical or electrical change playing on the epileptogenic lesion which precipitates an attack. The more powerful the influence of one of these factors is, the less is required of the others to produce a seizure.

The patient with a strong genetic tendency towards epilepsy may readily have seizures precipitated by fever, flickering lights, television, or sleep deprivation. The person who has developed an epileptogenic lesion in the brain is more likely to have seizures if there is a strong genetic background. The age of the patient or the degree of maturation of the brain is another factor in determining the tendency to seizures as well as the type of seizure. Statistical studies indicate that the possibility of seizures decreases as the infant grows through childhood to adulthood. An exception is around puberty when many endocrine changes are taking place in the body. Infantile massive spasms are found to be associated with many different types of cerebral pathology, either focal or diffuse, and are seen only in infants. Typical absence (petit-mal) attacks occur mainly in children, either where the only known aetiological factor is genetic or in the presence of diffuse brain pathology. As the child grows older, the absence attacks tend to disappear and are often replaced by generalized tonic–clonic seizures. Seizures with automatism and psychical phenomena such as change in affect, illusions, or hallucinations tend to appear

in the teens and later and are usually due to a variety of lesions in the temporal lobe.

The site of the lesions in the brain is also important in determining whether epilepsy will develop as a complication. Lesions involving the cerebral cortex are more likely to result in epilepsy than those in the subcortical areas. For example, epilepsy is much more common with supratentorial than with infratentorial tumours and is rare in extrapyramidal disease. Within the cerebral hemispheres, focal lesions involving the temporal lobe structures are most likely to cause epilepsy. The next most likely are lesions of the sensorimotor cortex and the frontal lobe. Occipital lesions are only rarely accompanied by epilepsy. The rate of progress of the underlying lesion is also important, epilepsy being more likely to develop in response to a benign or slowly progressive pathological process, e.g. an oligodendroglioma. Very malignant cerebral tumours are rarely accompanied by recurrent fits.

The known causes of epilepsy can be summarized under the following headings:

(1) Genetic factors which increase the risk of 'idiopathic' epilepsy and to a lesser extent, susceptibility to symptomatic epilepsy (Metrakos & Metrakos, 1974).

(2) Heredofamilial diseases of the brain such as tuberose sclerosis, the leucodystrophies, the lipoidoses, Lafora disease and phenylketonuria are frequently accompanied by recurrent fits.

(3) Antenatal and birth factors, including congenital abnormalities, can lead to brain dysfunction which manifests itself in recurrent epileptic fits. Maternal bleeding, infections, and toxaemia are suspected of causal involvement in the early epilepsies. Prematurity, prolonged labour, forceps delivery, neonatal hypoxia, and low birth weight have all been mentioned as possible perinatal aetiological factors. Controlled studies have demonstrated associations between transient metabolic disturbances such as hypocalcaemia and hypoglycaemia, and neonatal seizures.

(4) Acute infections of the CNS: convulsions may accompany an acute infection of the central nervous system, or epilepsy may be a later consequence of damage done to the brain by the infection. Damage can be localized as in a brain abscess or diffuse as in virus encephalitis.

(5) Damage to the hippocampus, amygdala, parahippocampal and fusiform gyri (mesial tem-

poral sclerosis) resulting from prolonged febrile convulsions or status epilepticus in children has been claimed to be a common cause of temporal lobe epilepsy. This lesion has been found in about half of patients treated by unilateral temporal lobectomy (Falconer *et al.*, 1964). However, other temporal lobectomy series have not confirmed this association (Jensen & Klinken, 1976). An association between febrile convulsions and temporal lobe epilepsy was not found in the 1958 British national birth cohort (Neugebauer and Susser, 1979).

(6) Toxic factors can also precipitate convulsions, as in the case of alcohol, or lead to residual epilepsy, as in the case of lead poisoning.

(7) Accidents involving cerebral injury constitute one of the primary causes of symptomatic epilepsy. The risks are related to whether the dura is penetrated or not. Thus in missile wounds to the head the incidence of fits may be as high as 40 per cent while 5 per cent of those with non-missile injuries develop seizures (Jennett, 1965). Trauma is more likely to cause partial epilepsy than generalized epilepsy but may be responsible for fits in about 5–15 per cent of all cases of epilepsy.

(8) Metabolic and endocrine disorder can frequently cause seizures, e.g. pyridoxine deficiency in infants, hyponatraemia, hypernatraemia, magnesium depletion, hypokalaemia, hypoglycaemia, phenylketonuria.

(9) Finally cerebrovascular disorders, neoplasms, and degenerative diseases can be responsible for brain lesions leading to epilepsy.

In addition, there are a number of known precipitating factors which may bring on an attack in susceptible people, for example high fever, anoxia, low blood sugar, lack of sleep, overbreathing, emotional stress, and the specific stimuli of the reflex epilepsies. The reflex epilepsies occur in some 1–6 per cent of people with epilepsy. The most common modality of sensory precipitation is visual: 20–40 per cent of epileptics show abnormal EEG responses to flickering light, and in 2–4 per cent seizures can be induced by the laboratory stroboscope or – more importantly – in daily living by sunlight on water, television, discotheques, escalators, and so on. Occasionally children with photosensitive fits learn to induce minor attacks by self-stimulation: by staring into the light and moving their fingers rhythmically in front of their eyes at the appropriate flicker

rate. Their motives are usually difficult to determine. Sometimes attention-seeking and manipulative factors are important. The process of induction of the fit itself may be pleasurable to the child. In some children it seems to be merely a habit. Often no satisfactory explanation can be given. Frequently there is a history of mental retardation. Rarer sensory precipitants include sound, touch, proprioception, and possibly visceral, olfactory, or vestibular stimuli. Less commonly seizures are triggered by a particular mental activity; hearing or performing music, reading, writing, specific visual or auditory imagery, mathematical calculation, and sequential decision-making under stress. The reflex epilepsies are reviewed by Merlis (1974).

At present, between 70 per cent and 75 per cent of patients with seizures identified in population studies do not have evidence of an underlying pathological lesion. Of the remainder, whose epilepsy can be related to definite or presumed cerebral pathology, the reported nature of the acquired lesions varies widely in different surveys; doubtless a reflection of the amount of detailed case-record information available and variability in diagnostic criteria used. However, the prevalence studies in Rochester, Minnesota, between 1935 and 1967 are noteworthy for the thoroughness of case ascertainment and length of follow-up (Hauser & Kurland, 1975). It is therefore of interest to draw the reader's attention to their findings, which are as follows: 23 per cent of their sample of 516 patients had epilepsy of known cause; 2 per cent birth injury, 4 per cent congenital anomalies, 4 per cent post-natal head injuries, 3 per cent infections, 5 per cent vascular, 4 per cent cerebral tumours, 0.6 per cent degenerative disorders.

Prevalence and natural history

Prevalence rates for epilepsy in the general population range widely from 1.50 per 1000 in Japan to 20 per 1000 among the Wapogoro tribe in Tanzania (Neugebauer & Susser, 1979). Even in England, prevalence rates have varied from 3.33 per 1000 to 7.9 per 1000. Such differences clearly result from differing criteria in the diagnosis of epilepsy and the thoroughness of case identification. For example, the inclusion of febrile convulsions and isolated fits can artificially inflate the rate whereas the use of hospital records only may reduce substantially the number of cases identified in any population. Nevertheless, in Europe and North America the prevalence rates in most surveys lie between 4 and 6 per thousand (Hauser & Kurland, 1975; Neugebauer & Susser, 1979). If the latter figure is accepted, the total number of people with epilepsy in England and Wales is about 290 000.

Probably one person in 20 has a fit of some sort in the course of a lifetime. However, only one in eight of those who have had an isolated fit will develop chronic epilepsy, that is, a continuing liability to fits. In these patients, the onset of epilepsy occurs before the age of five in nearly a quarter and before school-leaving age in more than half. In the majority, the epileptic seizures are likely to recur intermittently over the years. Only just over a third will have prolonged seizure-free periods. The probability of remission is greatest in those patients who are normal in all other respects apart from the seizures, especially if they have grand-mal attacks only. Patients whose EEG is normal or normalizes with treatment, can likewise expect a good outcome. The prognosis becomes poor with an early age of onset, long duration of illness, a combination of different seizure types, a frequent seizure occurrence, and evidence of widespread brain damage (Rodin, 1968, 1972; Kiørboe, 1974). Fortunately, however, a substantial proportion of those with chronic epilepsy have comparatively infrequent major attacks. For example, Pond, Bidwell, and Stein (1960) in their survey of 14 general practices, found that only 40 per cent had fits more often than monthly, while Gudmundsson (1966) reported an essentially similar finding for major seizure frequency in his survey of epilepsy in Iceland. Minor attacks were common, however; 80 per cent of patients experienced some form of minor seizure more than once a month.

About three-quarters of all epilepsy commences before the age of 20, 10 per cent to 20 per cent between the ages of 20 and 29 years, and between 2 per cent and 8 per cent over the age of 50 years (Merlis, 1972; Hauser & Kurland, 1975). The annual incidence rate lies between 30 and 54 per 100 000. It is highest in the pre-school period, especially in the first year of life, about 150 per 100 000. Then the rate falls rapidly to between 20 and 40 in the second decade of life. Similar incidence rates persist throughout adult life, though the Rochester study reports an increase in the over-sixties to about 80.

Types of handicap.

After this brief outline of the extent of the problem caused by the epilepsies, it is now necessary to describe the types of handicap with which the person with epilepsy has to cope. The fits themselves, usually unpredictable in occurrence, with sudden loss of consciousness, convulsive movements, or other inappropriate and often embarrassing behaviour beyond the person's control, expose the person to risk of injury or even death. For example, the life expectancy of people with epilepsy is considerably less than that of the general population (Rodin, 1968, 1972). The risk of injury to self or others places severe restrictions on choice of work, vehicle driving may be prohibited and in the severe case there may be serious limitation of ability to leave home and travel by public transport because of the risks of having seizures crossing busy roads or while using public transport.

The ancient fears and prejudices concerning epilepsy have been by no means dispelled by twentieth-century enlightenment. Although few still regard the epileptic seizure as the result of possession by spirits or as divine retribution for wickedness, the occurrence of fits still arouses much anxiety, fear, and prejudice amongst the general population. These negative feelings contribute to discrimination against the epileptic employee and lead to difficulties in making friends outside the immediate family circle. Prejudice against people with epilepsy appears to have much in common with racial prejudice and it seems that social acceptance of epilepsy is even lower than that of mental illness (Bagley, 1972).

In patients with symptomatic epilepsy, cerebral dysfunction due to the lesion that causes the fits may lead to impaired intellectual and learning abilities. The depressant effect on the brain of the various drugs used for the treatment of epilepsy can also cause cognitive impairment (Trimble, 1979). These effects of the underlying lesion and/or the drug treatment may result in a low IQ, psychomotor slowing, impaired learning ability, and poor educational achievement. Educational progress may be further retarded by poor concentration and attention span which are due to the occurrence of frequent minor seizures in the classroom. These may be so brief as to escape the teacher's notice. Similar concentration and attention difficulties are a common finding in epileptic children with conduct disorder, even in the absence of frank fits (Rutter *et al.*, 1970).

Parents of a child handicapped by epilepsy are not unnaturally concerned to protect their child from coming to harm as a result of the fits. Over-protective attitudes readily develop as a result of parental anxiety. The inevitable but usually minor restrictions as regards swimming, cycling and similar activities, may be exaggerated to an unnecessary degree. Usually parental over-protective attitudes appear to arise from natural concern for their child's well-being. Less often, more negative feelings such as anger and rejection may be present and are defended against by ever increasing watchfulness. Although appropriate for the younger child, parental over-protectiveness in the long term may encourage the development of life-long passive, dependent attitudes and impair the capacity to establish normal peer relationships. In adult life such passive, dependent attitudes may lead to difficulties in relating to heterosexual partners and in making and keeping friends generally. During and after adolescence parents often find it difficult to give their epileptic offspring the freedom required to permit maturation to independence. Hence the usual adolescent independence conflicts are often heightened in the person with epilepsy. The individual's bid for independence often clashes with the parents' need to maintain close supervision. Emotional difficulties and frank behaviour disorder may follow.

A discrepancy between the individual's vocational aspirations and ability to fulfil these aspirations is sometimes a problem, especially in middle-class, professional families. The epileptic child may acquire the aspirations and expectations prevalent in the family but may not have the necessary intellectual equipment to carry them out, because of brain damage due to the epileptogenic lesion or the depressant effects of anti-convulsant drugs. This can lead to much frustration and disappointment as well as failure to accept a work role more compatible with his intellectual ability. More often parental expectations are lower than those held for their non-epileptic offspring. Long and Moore (1979) found that parents were less optimistic about their epileptic child's future achievements. These findings were linked with greater restrictiveness on the parents' part, and the epileptic child's lower self-esteem and academic achievement.

Employment

The person with epilepsy suffers from a three-fold handicap in employment. First, the fits restrict the range of employment open to the individual, although this is rarely a cause of unemployability in itself. Secondly, psychiatric and behavioural problems which may be associated with epilepsy may create employment difficulties and these difficulties can reinforce existing psychiatric problems when the individual finds himself unable to fulfil this work role satisfactorily. Thirdly, there remains prejudice and discrimination against the epileptic employee. Hence there is a reluctance on the part of people with epilepsy to disclose their disability, because of the consequence this may have on their employment prospects. Various studies have set the proportion experiencing job problems as between one-quarter and three-quarters of epileptics of work age. Of those working in industrial plants, one-half to two-thirds will have to change their jobs within the factories for safety reasons. As well as the issue of safety, a major epileptic attack in a crowded, busy work environment can cause considerable disturbance and interference with production, the effects of which may outlast the duration of the attack. Fear, suspicion, and ignorance on the part of the employee's work-mates may not only reinforce similar feelings amongst management but also provide a pressing, non-economic reason why epileptics subject to fits should be employed separately from these persons. This has the effect of placing them in jobs which are menial, uninteresting, and poorly paid. None the less, surveys have shown that three-quarters or more of all epileptics are employed in virtually the full range of occupations. A study covering almost 150 000 employed people in the north-west of England has shown that a substantial number work in heavy industry, doing a wide range of jobs and having an average (lost time) accident frequency-rate of 0.06 per cent, which compares favourably with healthy industrial workers (MacIntyre, 1974). There is evidence that employer attitudes tend to be a function of the individual employer's favourable experiences with epileptic persons who display good work adjustment.

Chronic unemployment or serious difficulty over holding down jobs tends to be associated with IQs at the lower end of the normal range or below, organic mental changes, evidence of diffuse brain damage, the presence of temporal lobe pathology, and/or personality disorder. A general personality trait of social competence or the ability to cope effectively with the interpersonal demands of different social situations, seems to be an important factor in the successful adjustment to work of the epileptic persons. The social and family environment of the patient may play a crucial role. Over-protective family attitudes may reinforce the patient's own feelings of passivity and dependence and impair motivation for work. When epilepsy first develops in adult life, lack of specialized training before the epilepsy began predisposes to difficulties afterwards. Goodglass and colleagues (1963) in a study of veterans with late-onset epilepsy found that pre-morbidly unskilled had a 37 per cent chance of being totally umemployed after the onset of seizures. On the other hand, workers with manual or other skills tended to retain occupational level after the onset of fits. Surprisingly enough, most studies have found that seizure frequency is less important in causing job difficulty than intellectual impairment, psychosocial difficulty, and factors related to motivation. When these factors are excluded and only patients of normal intelligence and stable personality are considered, unemployment is high only in the most severely affected, that is, with daily minor attacks and several major seizures each month, For example, Goodglass and colleagues (1963) reported that their sample of 119 epileptic veterans split into a small, severely affected group of 24 persons for whom the unemployment rate was 50 per cent, and a larger number (95 out of 119) for whom the unemployment rate was only 11 per cent. When the former group of severe epileptics was excluded no significant relationship between severity of seizure frequency and rates of complete unemployment could be observed. However a substantial number experienced a decline in earning power after the development of the epilepsy. Even those rated as being suitable for work in ordinary office or shop conditions and having only several seizures a year showed almost a 50 per cent decline in one or more of the indices of occupational adjustment, namely regularity of employment, job changes, and occupational status. The neurological, psychological, and social factors related to employability of people with epilepsy are discussed by Fenton (1976).

Epilepsy and intellectual functioning

A number of variables can influence the cognitive function of the patient with epilepsy: namely, the site and extent of the brain lesion underlying the fits, the disruptive effect of the seizure discharges on brain function, the sedative effects of anticonvulsant medication, and the motivation of the patient, which will be affected by personality, social, and psychological factors. Those who have been institutionalized have lower IQs, while epileptics living in the community have a distribution of intelligence similar to that of the general population. Those with fits due to brain damage have lower IQs than people who

have fits of unknown aetiology. The earlier the age of onset of the seizures, the greater is the chance of cognitive impairment. Those with major seizures tend to show more impairment than patients with temporal lobe attacks. However careful studies carried out by a group of workers at the University of Wisconsin have demonstrated that even persons with seizures of unknown aetiology show some degree of cognitive impairment compared with well-matched healthy controls. These changes may well be the result of the anticonvulsant medication. Trimble (1979) has recently reviewed the literature on the cognitive effects of anticonvulsant drugs.

Transient impairment of cerebral function occurs as the result of brief spike-wave discharges, even in the absence of a clinical seizure (Mirsky *et al.*, 1960; Porter *et al.*, 1973; Goode *et al.*, 1970). These transient but continued interruptions in performance can be crucial to education. The reading retardation demonstrated by Rutter and colleagues (1970) in one-fifth of children may well have been due to subclinical epileptic discharges, though lower parental expectations may play a part. Another factor, demonstrated by Stores and Hart (1976), is the presence of left-hemisphere epileptogenic lesions. These workers also found that reading skills were significantly worse in boys and in children on long-term phenytoin medication.

Left-sided temporal lobe lesions have been associated with impairment of verbal reasoning and learning functions and right-sided ones with impairment of discrimination and appreciation of temporal and spatial patterns. However, these cognitive changes have been most consistently demonstrated following temporal lobe excision. Though complaints of poor memory and difficulties in recalling names are common in temporal lobe epilepsy, lateralized memory deficits in TLE patients who have not had temporal lobectomy are not invariably present. Indeed a recent study suggests that the interictal memory impairment may be due to a dysphasic disturbance, an anomia. The circumlocution and circumstantiality of speech often observed may compensate for this anomia (Mayeux *et al.*, 1980).

Finally, it is not clear how often intellectual deterioration occurs in people with epilepsy. Often, apparent 'deterioration' is demonstrated to be the result of overmedication, social and psychological withdrawal. If definite evidence of intellectual decline can be demonstrated by formal testing, the following causes should be looked for; (1) chronic anticonvulsant intoxication, (2) frequent subclinical seizures, (3) anoxic damage due to recent status epilepticus or uncontrolled and frequent convulsive attacks, (4) progression of underlying brain disease, (5) the occurrence of psychosis, (6) the onset of bilateral temporal lobe involvement due to a mirror focus developing in patients with a previously unilateral temporal lobe epileptogenic lesion. The cognitive aspects of epilepsy have been reviewed in detail by Reitan (1974).

Epilepsy and psychiatric disorder
A historical review

For centuries people with epilepsy have been said to be abnormal in personality. Aretaeus (Guerrant *et al.*, 1962), in the second century AD, described epileptics as 'languid, spiritless, stupid, unsociable. . . . . slow to learn from torpidity of the understanding and of the senses (and with) utterances indistinct and bewildered either from the nature of the disease or from the wounds during the attacks.' Thus, eighteen hundred years ago not only was it asserted that people with epilepsy were of abnormal personality but also the question was raised as to whether the abnormalities were an essential part of the disease process or a consequence of it. This question still awaits a definitive answer. The thinking on this subject has shown a number of clear trends over the past hundred years. Gowers, in his textbook of epilepsy published in 1881, in common with other writers of that period, suggested that patients with epilepsy underwent personality deterioration and that this was directly related to their fits. The changes were thought to be mainly intellectual in nature and the rate of progress in direct proportion to the number and severity of the seizures. Frank psychosis was regarded as rare and the physical appearance of people with epilepsy received little attention, any alterations being considered the result of damage caused by the seizures.

At the turn of the century opinions changed and the belief that epilepsy was a constitutional disorder with specific personality changes as well as seizures became prevalent. People with epilepsy were considered to be rarely, if ever, normal mentally. Profound disturbances of mood, attitudes, and behaviour followed by inevitable intellectual deterioration were the rule. The character changes were so characteristic that a diagnosis of epilepsy could be made in the absence of fits providing a family history was present. The whole syndrome was thought to have a congenital, constitutional basis rather like that of dementia praecox. The constitutional defect was also reflected in the physical characteristics of the face; an 'epileptic facies – characterised by a broad forehead, broad and flattened nose, prognathism, thick lips and staring eyes with wide pupils' (Kraepelin, 1904). This concept evolved as a result of observations made on patients in institutions, where bromism was common and the reason for admission often was disturbed behaviour. No doubt the teachings of Kraepelin, which dominated psychiatry at that time, were highly influential. His main contribution was the description of clear-cut psychiatric syndromes such as dementia praecox, genetically determined, with characteristic symptoms and a deteriorating progress to an inevitable end-state. The epileptic personality fits perfectly into this model and is described graphically in the works of Alden Turner (1907), Kraepelin (1904), Bleuler (1924) and Pierce Clark (1931).

The development of more effective methods of neurological investigation and the consequent realization that epilepsy is not a disease entity but a symptom of a variety of cerebral disorders, many of which may cause mental changes, led to a change in thinking about the middle of this century. Lennox, in 1944, reviewed the literature about the personality of epileptics. He commented that the majority of patients he saw did not show the classical personality traits and pointed out the difficulties in distinguishing between the complex effects of heredity, brain damage, drug intoxication and the reactions to the psychological and social problems that the person with epilepsy has to face. It became recognized that many epileptics were well-adjusted people and that structural brain disease, chronic drug overdosage, uncontrolled seizures, and the psychological problems associated with being an epileptic made a contribution to the genesis of psychiatric disorder in those who were mentally disturbed. As Lennox put it, much of the difficulty in assessing the mental state in epilepsy is due to the fact that 'the clear stream of essential epilepsy has been modified by a symptomatic tributary'. The change of climate in psychiatry with the development of a more dynamic approach may have also played an important role in this change in attitude.

In the late forties and early fifties the intensive application of clinical electroencephalography to the study of the epilepsies, especially the work of Penfield and his colleagues in Montreal, led to the identification of the syndrome of temporal lobe epilepsy.

Surveys of large numbers of patients with epilepsy by Gibbs and others reported an unduly high prevalence of functional psychiatric disorder in patients with temporal lobe epilepsy. The psychiatric symptomatology was not specific in any way, a wide spectrum of neurotic, psychotic, and behavioural symptoms being present. In parallel with these clinical observations, the work of Papez, Maclean, and others on the physiology of the limbic system and its possible role in the control of affect, the temporal lobe ablation studies of Kluver and Bucy, and the electrical stimulation studies carried out by Penfield and associates during operations for the relief of epilepsy, drew attention to the relation between temporal lobe function and emotion. No doubt these experimental observations have also had a profound influence on current thinking about psychological disorder and temporal lobe dysfunction. The view that temporal lobe dysfunction predisposes the epileptic patient to a high risk of psychiatric breakdown and personality change is currently the most popular one, though it is by no means universally accepted.

Classification of the psychiatric disorders of epilepsy

Pond (1957) classified the psychiatric disorders of epilepsy into three main groups. These are as follows:

(1) Disorders due to the brain disease causing the fits

(2) Disorders directly related to the seizures

(3) Those disorders whose occurrence is unrelated in time to seizure occurrence: namely, the inter-ictal disorders.

I shall briefly discuss each of these groups separately.

(1) The disorders due to the brain disease causing the fits. These can be subdivided again into those cases with diffuse cerebral dysfunction and those with focal cerebral lesions. The diffuse cerebral dysfunction category includes the dementias, mental handicap, where about one in three patients have fits, the specific epileptic syndromes, for example West's syndrome, Unverricht-Lundborg disease, tuberous sclerosis, the Lennox-Gastaut syndrome, subacute sclerosing leucoencephalitis, and behaviour and personality change due to generalized brain damage. In such cases it is always difficult to know how much the initial brain disease contributes to the causation and how much is the result of the interaction of such factors as the repeated anoxic effects of recurrent sei-

zures, the psychological and social consequences of being an epileptic and the depressant effects of anticonvulsant medication on the brain. Cerebrovascular disease is a common cause of both fits and dementia in the elderly, and the pre-senile dementias, especially Alzheimer's, may present with fits. The focal brain disease category includes brain tumours, 50 per cent of which are accompanied by mental and seizure manifestations, though it is only the more chronic, benign tumours that really are of interest, when dealing with patients with chronic epilepsy. Other localized brain lesions may also cause focal brain syndromes, involving the frontal, temporal, and parietal lobes. These can cause disorders of behaviour, personality, and cognitive function. I suppose it is reasonable to include also the HHE syndrome (hemiconvulsion–hemiplegia–epilepsy). This is a syndrome consisting of a unilateral convulsive seizure or a unilateral convulsive condition in early childhood, followed by transient or permanent hemiplegia and, after a variable free interval, by the subsequent development of epilepsy, usually partial in nature. This is frequently associated with some degree of mental handicap and behaviour disorder is common. As well as these focal brain syndromes, one needs to include the specific focal cognitive deficits, which are often subclinical and only detected by psychometric testing: for example, the memory, verbal, and non-verbal learning deficits associated with temporal lobe lesions. These organic psychosyndromes are discussed in detail by Lishman (1978).

(2) Disorders related in time to seizure occurrence. These can be divided into prodromal (pre-ictal), ictal, and post-ictal events. Prodromal symptoms during the few days or hours immediately preceding the occurrence of a fit are often reported, particularly in institutionalized epileptics; irritability and dysphoria seem the most commonly found. This type of behaviour or mood change usually improves following seizures. Psychiatric disturbances directly due to seizure discharge include complex partial seizures, petit mal, and psychomotor status. Complex partial seizures occur when the seizure onset is localized to one part of the brain and the initial seizure manifestations involve higher-level mental processes. The other two ictal psychiatric disorders are petit mal and psychomotor status. Both are states of clouding of consciousness resulting from continuing generalized spike and wave complexes or local temporal-lobe discharges respectively. Post-ictal disorders are those which immedi-

ately follow one or more seizures, usually generalized convulsions. The common feature is clouding of consciousness due to post-seizure depression of cortical function and hence the EEG is usually dominated by diffusely slow frequencies within the theta and delta range, little or no normal activity being present. Such patients usually manifest behaviour associated with confusional states (clouded states, twilight states, fugue states) or automatic behaviour.

(3) *Interictal disorders unrelated in time to the seizures.* In this group the psychiatric symptomatology is present between seizures. It is not triggered by the occurrence of clinical seizures, though the intensity may be influenced by the frequency of seizure occurrence. It is assumed, however, that the epilepsy and/or the cerebral epileptogenic lesions have played a role in the genesis of the psychiatric disorder. These disorders resemble in form the functional psychiatric syndromes. They consist of the neurotic, conduct, and mixed disorders in children. In adults personality change, personality behaviour, and neurotic disorder, sexual dysfunctions, and psychoses can occur. By personality change is meant a change in personality developing in adult life out of a previously 'normal' personality profile following the onset of fits, and contrasts with personality disorder which refers to lifelong deviations from 'normal'. The psychoses are functional in form and occur in a setting of clear consciousness with affective, schizoaffective, or schizophrenia-like symptoms.

Paroxysmal psychological disturbances of ictal origin

Epileptic attacks may take the form of recurrent transient episodes of psychological disturbances. These are usually accompanied by a seizure discharge in the electroencephalogram and can often be induced by direct electrical stimulation of the cortex or by the intravenous injection of a convulsant drug such as Metrazol. Paroxysmal psychiatric symptoms observed as ictal phenomena include 'force thinking', hallucinations, illusions, disturbances of mood, and automatic behaviour. These vary in complexity and duration from a mere momentary alteration in perception of colour or depth to prolonged and vivid auditory and visual hallucinations. These phenomena may occur by themselves or as aurae for a major attack and are now known as complex partial sei-

zures. With the exception of 'forced thinking', the epileptic discharge, which produces these symptoms, usually originates in the temporal lobes (Mulder, 1953).

Brain (1962) has classified temporal lobe epileptic disturbances as follows:

(1) Disordered awareness of the body, manifested in its simplest form by a sensory aura consisting of a peculiar sensation, often in the epigastrium and rising to the head; or the body or some part of it may feel abnormal in size and shape. A feeling of depersonalization may be regarded as a disordered awareness of the relationship between the body and the self.

(2) Impaired awareness of the external world may take the form of illusions involving the size, shape or distance of objects seen. Corresponding to depersonalization is derealization, in which the external world seems unreal.

(3) Hallucinations may occur, involving the senses of smell, taste, sight or hearing. More complex hallucinations may consist of remembered scenes or scenes which are believed to be the revival of experienced events.

(4) Such hallucinations merge into disorders of memory. The *déjà vu* phenomenon, a false sense of familiarity applied to current experience, is a common symptom. The revival in vivid form of long tracts of memory does occur but is less frequent.

(5) Emotional disturbances may result from a discharging lesion in the temporal lobe. The most common ictal affect is fear. Williams (1956) found, among 2000 cases of epilepsy, 165 patients with complex feelings as ictal symptoms, which in 100 cases could be described as emotion. Of these, 61 (3.1 per cent of the total series) experienced fear. In 35 the EEG focus was localized to the anterior part, and in 17 to the middle part of the temporal lobe. He also noted that ictal fear was an emotion inappropriate to the circumstances of the patient at the time and was not related to the impending fit. In 50 per cent of cases it was associated with visceral sensory symptoms, for example, epigastric sensation, flushing, sweating, palpitation. Others have reported similar findings. Ictal anger is less common, being found by Williams in 18 out of his 2000 cases. He found depression to be an ictal manifestation in 21 cases (1 per cent) while feelings of pleasure were even less common (0.5 per cent). This symptom tended to be related to the posterior part of the temporal lobe, while in depression the lesion was diffuse or unlocalized. Laughter is rare

as an epileptic phenomenon but can sometimes result from a discharging temporal lobe lesion (Weil, 1959).

(6) What has been said shows that the content of consciousness may be grossly disturbed by discharging lesions of the temporal lobe. Perceptual experiences may be distorted, leading to illusions, or may correspond to no external stimulus – hallucinations. Such experiences tend in themselves to impair attention and awareness. Hence the patient, though he may still be to some extent aware of what is going on, is less completely conscious of it than normally. Such a state may also occur in the absence of the perceptual disorders mentioned. In fact, all degrees of impairment of consciousness ranging to complete unconsciousness may occur as a result of discharging lesions of the temporal lobe.

(7) In association with such impairment of awareness, the patient may behave abnormally, carrying out simple or more complex movements without being aware of what he is doing. Such actions are known as automatisms. Behavioural automatism can occur either as a direct result of a seizure discharge or as a post-ictal event following any type of fit, especially a generalized one. The area most commonly involved in the initiation of an ictal automatism appears to be the periamygdaloid region. This includes the uncus, the amygdaloid nucleus, the central claustrum, and the temporo-insular cortex deep in the anterior part of the sylvian fissure. However, Jasper (1964) has pointed out that stimulation of these structures will only produce automatic behaviour in about 50 per cent of cases. Automatism will not occur while the afterdischarge remains confined to the amygdala or hippocampus. There is always bilateral involvement of the amygdaloid–hippocampal structures with invariable spread to the mesial diencephalon and the temporoparietal cortex. In many cases the frontal and central areas will be involved as well. Indeed automatic behaviour in some patients results from lesions at sites other than the mesial temporal structures, namely the frontal, orbitofrontal, and parietal regions or the mesial surfaces of the hemispheres. Presumably, the discharging focus causes secondary activation of the periamygdaloid–hippocampal structures with rapid spread to the mesial diencephalon and subsequent projection back to the neocortex via the diffuse projection system of the upper brain stem. Ictal automatism can occasionally result from prolonged generalized spike-wave discharge (petit-mal automatism) or generalized frontotemporal theta or delta rhythms initiated by primary activation of the diencephalon (Jasper, 1964).

Behaviour during epileptic automatism varies greatly from patient to patient and in the same individual on different occasions. The person's actions have a quasi-purposeful quality but are often inappropriate to the environmental situation. There is usually impairment of awareness and lack of responsiveness to the environment. Brief attacks lasting 10 seconds or less merely cause cessation of activity. More prolonged episodes of 20 to 30 seconds' duration display stereotyped repetitive movements, for example chewing, swallowing, clenching fists. Attacks which last several minutes are associated with more complex, variable, but quasi-purposeful behaviour, for example undressing, wandering away, which involves interplay with the environment and gradually merges into normal behaviour. The earlier stereotyped phenomena are a direct manifestation of the ictal discharge, while the later complex behaviour continues during the post-ictal phase of the attack. The majority of automatisms are brief, five minutes or less in 80 per cent and never over an hour. Violence during epileptic automatisms is rare. The relation between epilepsy and automatisms has been reviewed in detail by Fenton (1972, 1980).

An exception to the rule that most complex partial seizure phenomena are of the temporal lobe origin is 'forced thinking', an ideational seizure phenomenon, where a recurring compulsive thought or thoughts enter the mind to the exclusion of other thoughts. This is associated with epileptogenic foci in the posterior part of the frontal lobe. Further, though ictal dysphasias, speech automatisms, and other language disorder are often a feature of temporal epilepsy, ictal dysphasia can occur with discharging lesions elsewhere in the dominant hemisphere, especially in the inferior frontal and parietal areas.

Many of the phenomena I have described, such as *déjà vu*, depersonalization, hallucinations, occur in the functional psychiatric illnesses but can be distinguished because when they occur as ictal events there is a sudden onset and a relatively rapid resolution, the duration is transient, lasting minutes rather than hours, days, or weeks. They are recurrent and the attacks have a stereotyped quality, each one being essentially similar to the previous ones. Further, careful observation and questioning will usually reveal some degree of alteration of consciousness during the attacks, while consciousness is clear in the functional psychiatric syndromes.

Non-psychotic psychiatric disorder in patients with epilepsy

Prevalence: Reliable estimates of the prevalence of psychiatric symptoms in people with epilepsy are difficult to obtain. Surveys have shown that between 4 per cent and 5 per cent of patients resident in mental hospitals have epilepsy (Liddell, 1953; Betts, 1974). The prevalence of chronic epilepsy in the general population can be assumed to be around 6 per 1000. Therefore the number of epileptics under inpatient psychiatric care is around 7 to 8 times greater than the number expected by chance. Further, amongst epileptic patients living in the community, 7 per cent will have been admitted to a psychiatric hospital at some time in their lives (Pond & Bidwell, 1960).

The prevalence of overt psychiatric disorder in patients with seizures attending general hospital clinics or consulting their general practitioners, is surprisingly high, as many as 1 in 3; they comprise mainly conduct disorders in children and adolescents and mild affective disorders in adults (Pond & Bidwell, 1960; Stevens, 1966; Standage & Fenton, 1975).

It is probable that the relatively high prevalence of psychiatric symptoms and conduct disorders in epileptics attending general hospitals reflects a tendency for patients with psychiatric complications to be referred for specialist investigation. Pond and Bidwell (1960) have shown that psychological difficulty is twice as common in patients referred to hospital by their GP as in those who are not. Hence hospital-based studies will have an undue loading of subjects with psychological problems. In any event, only half of the general-practice patients in the Pond and Bidwell survey were actually attending hospital for management of their seizure disorder. Hence, community studies are necessary in order to obtain unbiased estimates of the distribution of psychiatric symptoms in epileptics.

The findings of Rutter and colleagues (1970) obtained by a survey of Isle of Wight school children are of special interest because of the careful sampling method and detailed psychiatric, physical, and cognitive assessments carried out. The prevalence rate for psychiatric disorder in a random control group was 6.6 per cent. The rate was slightly higher (11.5 per cent) for children with physical handicaps not involving the brain, and about four times greater (28.6 per cent) for epilepsy uncomplicated by brain disease. The prevalence rates for psychiatric disorder

rose to 37.5 per cent in children with lesions above the brain stem without fits. The maximum prevalence, more than eight times that of the controls, occurred in those children with epilepsy complicated by lesions above the brain stem (58.3 per cent).

Psychiatric disorder in children

Hence, children with uncomplicated fits are much more likely to develop psychiatric complications than those with physical handicaps in the absence of epilepsy. Damage to the cerebral cortex and higher CNS areas further increases the risk. Factors significantly associated with psychiatric disorder were the presence of psychomotor attacks, evidence of emotional disturbance in the mother, and parental social class. Psychiatric disability was less common in children whose fathers had non-manual occupations. This study demonstrated clearly that multiple factors interact to produce psychiatric disorder in epilepsy as in other child psychiatric syndromes. Organic brain dysfunction, temporal lobe disorder as manifest by the psychomotor fits, and adverse familial influences all predispose to psychiatric breakdown. The symptom clusters displayed by the epileptic children did not differ from the controls nor from other patients.

However, when disturbed children with epilepsy are selected by EEG criteria, the site of origin of the epileptogenic process does appear to influence symptom profile. Nuffield (1961) demonstrated that children with temporal lobe spikes had higher aggression and low neuroticism ratings while those with generalized spike-wave complexes showed the reverse trend: low aggression and high neurotic ratings.

Stores (1978), in a series of studies in which the behaviour of epileptic and non-epileptic children was compared, found that those with seizure disorders were significantly more anxious, inattentive, overactive, and socially isolated as well as dependent on their mothers mainly for their emotional needs. However, the most important finding in these studies was that these characteristics did not apply generally. Boys with epilepsy and epileptic children of either sex with left temporal-lobe abnormalities appeared to be particularly predisposed to this range of behaviour problems.

Neurotic disorder in adults

The adult studies of non-psychotic epileptics with psychiatric disorder are less satisfactory.

Nevertheless, the study by Pond and Bidwell (1960) of epileptic patients of fourteen general practices specially selected to be representative of the population of the country (England and Wales) as a whole is worthy of note. They identified 245 epileptic patients. Nearly one-third (29 per cent) had psychiatric problems, mainly neuroses in adults and conduct disorders in children. Only 4 per cent showed features of the 'epileptic personality'. Seven per cent of the total sample had been patients in psychiatric hospitals; half of the latter having temporal lobe epilepsy. In fact, temporal lobe epilepsy, low intelligence, and adverse environmental difficulties were the factors which seemed to predispose to psychiatric breakdown. As in children, no specific symptom profiles could be identified.

The first detailed, quantitative assessment of the mental state of non-psychotic, adult epileptic patients was carried out by Standage and Fenton (1975), using the Present State Examination technique (PSE): a reliable, semi-structured clinical interview method providing a symptom profile of the patients' current mental state. Examination of a series of patients attending a general hospital neurological clinic revealed a high prevalence of neurotic symptoms; mainly mild depression, anxiety, irritability, and low self-esteem. These symptoms were present in 40 per cent to 60 per cent of patients.

However, the symptom profiles were similar in type and prevalence to those recorded from a control group of patients, matched for age, sex, and duration of illness and attending the same general hospital complex with chronic locomotor disorders. When the epilepsy group was divided into those with temporal lobe epilepsy and those with other types, there was no marked difference.

As well as neurotic disorders manifested by anxiety and depression, hysterical pseudo-seizures sometimes occur as a complication of genuine epilepsy. Pseudo-seizures tend to be found in patients of low IQ and/or diffuse brain damage with personality and social problems. Their epileptic attacks are usually well controlled. An increased prevalence of family history of psychiatric disorder, and of past history of psychiatric illness, attempted suicide, and sexual maladjustment has been reported in those with a double diagnosis of epilepsy and hysteria. Depressed mood is also common (Roy, 1977, 1979). The pseudo-seizures develop as a response to emotional stress or conflict arising from a difficult life situation. The previous experience of true epilepsy no

doubt determines the choice of attacks of alteration of consciousness as the hysterical symptom. Such attacks tend to occur in the presence of other people, rarely result in injury, tongue biting, or incontinence of urine, and never occur during sleep. They may be ushered in by hyperventilation. The clinical pattern of the pseudo-seizures is variable. Muscular rigidity with random violent struggling or thrashing movements of the limbs, trunk, and head are common. This pattern is a marked contrast to the stereotyped tonic/clonic convulsions of the grand-mal fit. The level of consciousness may fluctuate during this phase, so that the patient may be able to recall afterwards some or all of the events of the fit. The pseudo-seizure frequency is sometimes very great, attacks recurring many times a day. Such a frequency of occurrence is rare in true epilepsy, with the obvious exceptions of status epilepticus and petit-mal attacks.

Neither during nor immediately after pseudo-seizures does the EEG show paroxysmal abnormalities, though EEG background activity changes due to underlying brain damage may be recorded then as well as in the intervals between attacks.

It should also be emphasized that pseudo-seizures can sometimes take a much less dramatic form, presenting with transient episodes of unconsciousness associated with pallor and slumping to the ground without 'convulsive' movements. In some attacks, transient dissociation of consciousness occurs with preservation of posture; sometimes accompanied by adversion of the head. Twitching of the facial muscles or jerking of the limbs may accompany these brief attacks, which are difficult to distinguish from minor temporal lobe seizures. A further confusing observation is that, on rare occasions, incontinence of urine and tongue biting are observed during hysterical pseudo-seizures (Scott 1978a). The occurrence of persistent and frequent attacks despite adequate doses of anticonvulsant drugs and serum concentrations well within the therapeutic range should raise the suspicion of hysterical pseudo-seizures. It also should be borne in mind that hysterical pseudo-seizures can develop in the epileptic patient as a consequence of drug intoxication.

On rare occasions, phobic states occur in patients with epilepsy and centre on the dread of having an attack. Although fears of having a fit, especially in public places, are common, frank phobic symptoms or morbid fears are surprisingly infrequent. Pinto (1972) describes a man with reflex epilepsy, who developed an agoraphobia. His attacks began at the age of 7 and were triggered reflexly by sudden voluntary, bodily movements. At 16 years he became phobic of going out because of fears of having fits in public. The phobic symptoms responded well to behaviour therapy, using a flooding technique. One of my own patients with musicogenic epilepsy presented with a music phobia. This was acquired at a time when she was in a stressful life situation and having frequent fits. The phobia persisted for a number of years, after complete control of the epilepsy. However, the symptom disappeared after a programme of systematic desensitization. Marks (1969) describes a 51-year-old lady with right-sided temporal lobe epilepsy, who had multiple phobias only during a 10-day period following each of her temporal lobe attacks. The onset of the phobic disorder dated from an emotionally traumatic experience shortly after a seizure. It would appear that she may have been unusually vulnerable to the acquisition of a new neurotic pattern of disability during the period immediately following her attacks, possibly because of temporal lobe dysfunction occurring at that time.

Epilepsy and personality disorder

Among the prejudices which have surrounded epilepsy and coloured public attitudes towards the disorder is the concept that people share specific personality characteristics.

Descriptions of traits specific to the 'epileptic personality' include the adjectives 'pedantic', 'circumstantial', 'religiose', 'egocentric', 'suspicious', 'touchy' and 'quarrelsome'. Speech is slow and perseverative and thought processes stereotyped and concrete. In both thought and emotions, the patients were described as 'adhesive', 'sticky' or 'viscous'.

It does appear that a small number of epileptic patients, usually with a chronic disorder and often institutionalized for many years, display many of these traits (4 per cent in Pond and Bidwell's general practice survey). However their development almost certainly results from multiple handicaps, both personal and environmental. Brain damage, childhood deprivation, the chronic effects of heavy anticonvulsant therapy, and difficulties with schooling, employment, accommodation, and interpersonal relationships may all contribute.

Assessment of personality disorders associated with epilepsy presents considerable methodological problems (Tizard, 1962). First, there are selection factors; observations made on patients in institutions

do not generalize to patients in the community. Secondly, allowance has to be made for the different types of epilepsy and for the presence, location and extent of brain lesions or damage. Tizard points out that most studies in which personality tests have been employed have not taken into consideration the intelligence of the patients or possible effects of medication. Like most recent authors (Betts *et al.*, 1976; Lishman, 1978; Scott, 1978a) she concludes that there is no specific personality disorder associated with epilepsy.

The prevalence of personality disorder in people with epilepsy in the community is unknown. However, as one would predict, personality difficulties are common in patients presenting at specialized epilepsy clinics and psychiatric units. For example, of 80 consecutive admissions to the Maudsley Hospital with epilepsy and psychiatric disorder, 60 per cent had a primary diagnosis of personality disorder. Though no specific category of abnormal personality predominated, immature and passive dependent traits were common (Pahla *et al.*, 1983). Clearly, such a high prevalence of personality disorder reflects the specialized nature of the hospital. Also, it is not known whether the categories of abnormal personality amongst the epileptic group differ from those of non-epileptic patients referred to the same hospital.

The hypothesis by Gibbs (1951), Gastaut (1954), and others that behaviour and personality disorder in epilepsy can be related to the presence of long-standing seizure discharges in the mesial temporal lobe structures, has led to the view that a specific temporal lobe syndrome exists (Geschwind 1979). According to this view, the syndrome consists of an excessive tendency to adhere to each thought, feeling, and action (hypometamorphosis or viscosity); irritability and deepened emotionality (hyperemotionality); decreased sexual interest and arousal (hyposexuality) and represents a partial inverse-Kluver-Bucy syndrome. In the latter syndrome, bilateral temporal lobe ablation causes hypometamorphosis, hypoemotionality and hyposexuality. Bear and Fedio (1977) have developed a questionnaire to rate eighteen personality traits in patients with temporal lobe epilepsy. They report differences between temporal lobe patients and controls and differing behavioural profiles in patients with right and left foci.

The temporal lobe epileptic patients displayed a distinctive pattern of traits, namely humourless sobriety, dependence, circumstantiality, obsessionality, undue preoccupation with religious and philosophic concerns, emotionality, and irritability. Bear and Fedio point out that there is now extensive evidence that lesions within the temporal lobes of primates may act to disconnect emotion mediating limbic structures such as the amygdaloid complex and hippocampus from the sensory association cortices of the visual and auditory system, resulting in the loss of learned emotional associations. Surgical disconnection appears both to disrupt old emotional bonds and to inhibit formation of new stimulus-reinforcement linkages. The authors speculate that in temporal lobe epilepsy, similar limbic-system structures and adjacent cortex are stimulated by the epileptogenic process. This leads to enhanced affective association to previously neutral stimuli, events, or concepts. Thus, experiencing objects and events with an unduly intense affective colouring engenders a mystically religious view of the world. If the patient's immediate actions and thoughts are so coloured, the result is an augmented sense of personal destiny. Sensing emotional importance in even the smallest acts may lead to these being performed ritualistically and repetitively, with lengthy circumstantial speech or writing. The right-temporal patients were seen as more overtly or externally emotive (sadness, irritability, emotionality, periods of elation); patients with left temporal foci displayed an internal, ideational (verbal) pattern of traits (religiosity, philosophical interest, an augmented sense of personal destiny, hypergraphia). Bear and Fedio tentatively use these results to suggest that each hemisphere has the capacity to develop (or overdevelop) emotional associations utilizing its own characteristic style of cognitive processing.

Though the patients were drawn from five general epilepsy clinics, the numbers in each sample were small. The controls were healthy adults or patients with neuromuscular diseases. Epileptics without temporal lobe involvement were not studied. Hence the authors claim that these behavioural profiles are a specific feature of temporal lobe epilepsy is not valid. Nevertheless, their quantitative approach is interesting and could easily be applied to relatively large numbers of patients identified during a community prevalence survey. Indeed the concept of a specific temporal lobe syndrome faces the same methodological problems as the 'epileptic' personality. The association with temporal lobe epilepsy may be a consequence of sample bias and lack of regard for the validity and reliability of behavioural assessments. The problem can be resolved only by an epidemiological investigation of epileptic patients living in the community, with the use of quantitative ratings of personality and behaviour.

Aggression and epilepsy. The possibility that dangerous violence can occur during a period of epileptic automatism has been known for many years. Delasiauve (1854) in his textbook on epilepsy devoted a chapter to the legal responsibility of the epileptic and cited a number of instances in which an individual had committed a crime of violence during or after an attack. Maudsley (1874) stated: 'Whenever we meet with isolated acts of violence, outrages on persons, homicide, suicide, arson, which nothing seems to have instigated, and when, upon attentive examination and thorough enquiry, we find a loss of memory after the perpetration of the act with a periodicity in the recurrence of the same act, and, a brief duration, we may diagnose ''larval'' epilepsy'. Nevertheless violent behaviour in relation to seizures is rare, the evidence in favour of such an association being confined to occasional case reports (Gunn, 1979).

Knox (1968), in the first systematic study of the relationship between epileptic automatism and violence, found only one patient who had acted in an extremely aggressive and violent fashion during an epileptic automatism out of a total of 434 epileptic outpatients. Surveys of more deviant populations have confirmed these findings. Although a survey of epileptic offenders in prisons and borstal institutions in England and Wales has indicated that the prevalence of epilepsy in these institutions is significantly higher than in the general population, there were only two persons out of a total of 158 whose crime was probably committed during or following a seizure: one during the post-ictal phase and the other in a possible ictal automatism. A parallel electroclinical study of the epileptic population of Broadmoor Hospital, one of the special hospitals in England and Wales for psychiatric offenders and patients displaying dangerously antisocial behaviour, revealed a prevalence of epilepsy similar to that of a conventional mental hospital. Of the 29 male patients who had committed offences, in only two could a definite relationship be established between their crimes and the occurrence of seizures: both behaved violently during a post-ictal confusional state (Gunn & Fenton 1969, 1971).

Explosive aggressiveness, moodiness, and irritability unrelated in time to the occurrence of fits have long been considered features of the 'epileptic personality'. During the last few decades, interictal aggressive behaviour has come to be regarded as a specific manifestation of temporal lobe epilepsy. The published studies on the relation between aggression and temporal lobe epilepsy have used a variety of definitions. Some authors have restricted their attention to outright physical assault, while others have included verbal abuse, bullying, stubbornness, and assertiveness.

Kligman and Goldberg (1975) have carried out a comprehensive review of the possible connections between temporal lobe epilepsy (TLE) and aggression. They critically reviewed the 8 published controlled studies. All the studies were open to question because of sampling bias and only two produced definite evidence of a positive association between TLE and aggression. Only the study by Nuffield (1961) on children was regarded as being methodologically sound. Though this study did offer some support for the association in children, Kligman and Goldberg feel that it will be necessary to have Nuffield's study replicated and applied to adults before a conclusion can be reached. They conclude that TLE is too heterogeneous and ill-defined and human aggression too complex to allow definite interpretations of correlations between them at present.

Aggressiveness has been a not uncommon finding in those temporal lobe patients referred for anterior temporal lobectomy. About one-third of a large series of TLE patients operated on by Murray Falconer were noted to have displayed overtly aggressive behaviour (Serafetinides, 1965; Falconer, 1973). This behaviour was much more common in males, especially those in their teens. It tended to be associated with left-sided lesions, a pathological diagnosis of mesial temporal sclerosis, and a favourable outcome in terms of successful rehabilitation after the operation and a cessation of fits.

It may well be that temporal-lobe epileptic patients with drug-resistant fits complicated by aggressive behaviour are more likely to be referred and selected for surgical treatment because the presence of the aggressiveness undoubtedly causes greater management and social adjustment problems. Indeed comparison of temporal-lobe epileptic patients treated medically with those treated surgically indicates that the latter have an early age of onset (the majority within the first 15 years) and a much higher prevalence of disturbances of personality and behaviour

(Currie et al., 1971). This early age of onset within the first decade of life tends to be associated with mesial temporal sclerosis (MTS) and may account for the relation between TLE, aggression, and MTS in the surgically treated patients.

As discussed previously, the occurrence of frequent fits throughout childhood may have adverse effects on parental and peer-group attitudes, the processes of social learning, and personality maturation. A cluster of other environmental factors that may produce a coincidental correlation between TLE and aggression by leading to a high incidence of both in the same people includes low socioeconomic status, parental psychopathology, and child abuse. Antisocial children are more likely to have a low socioeconomic background than neurotic children. The same background may expose children to poor parental and medical care with greater risks of acquiring brain damage as a result of poor obstetric care, head injuries caused by parental neglect or abuse, or infections which may provoke febrile convulsions and consequent mesial temporal lobe sclerosis. Unfortunately, little attention has been paid to controlling for socio-economic status in many of the studies of TLE and aggression. Indeed such criticisms can be applied to most investigations of the relation between epilepsy and behaviour.

Pathogenesis of personality, neurotic and behaviour disorder in patients with epilepsy

As discussed above, epilepsy with onset in early childhood and frequent fits throughout the growing-up period is quite likely to have adverse effects on parental and peer-group attitudes, the learning of social skills, and academic achievement, and to put severe restrictions on the patient's activities and life style. These influences may interfere with personality maturation and the development of personal competence. Taylor (1972a) presents an interesting model to explain the effect of seizures on the various stages of personality maturation based on a modified version of Erikson's schematic view of personality development.

Seizures are likely to be further aggravated by the existence of parental psychopathology and poor socio-economic conditions, which indeed may have created the milieu for the development of both the epilepsy and behaviour problems. It has been demonstrated clearly by Grunberg and Pond (1957) and Rutter and colleagues (1970) that adverse family and environmental factors play a major role in the genesis of psychiatric disorder in epileptic children.

Temporal lobe dysfunction acquired at an early age is likely to have a particularly serious effect on personality development because of the role of the temporal lobes in the processes of learning, memory and ego development. Early, acquired diffuse cortical damage will have similar adverse effects on the individual's potential for personal growth. As well as its influence on general intelligence and learning capacity, the irritability, impulsiveness, and psychomotor slowing associated with diffuse loss of cortical neurones will accentuate the difficulties.

The depressant effects of anticonvulsant drugs on cognitive function and emotional control are a further complication in patients both with and without acquired cerebral lesions. In particular, phenobarbitone may have a paradoxical exciting effect with a consequent increase in irritability and hyperkinetic behaviour. Phenytoin induced hirsutism is a special problem for the female patient.

The influence of seizure pattern on psychiatric morbidity has not been examined in detail. In common sense terms, the experience of complex, frightening aurae might be expected to arouse anxiety. Frequent major convulsions with threat to life and limb will lead to greater restriction of activity and dislocation of social and vocational opportunities. The potential risk of loss of consciousness and self-control during automatisms would seem to be an especially potent threat to the individual's well being. Yet, one's clinical impression is that such factors do not play a significant role in the onset of psychiatric morbidity.

Finally, the potentially precarious adjustment of the person with epilepsy may be undermined by difficulties in obtaining work because of the inevitable restrictions of choice applied as a result of having fits, often reinforced by the prejudices of both employers and employees. The inability to have a driving licence is particularly frustrating for the male adolescent, who sees his friends happily riding motor cycles at the age of 16 years. The loss of a licence in an adult with late-onset epilepsy may also have serious consequences both in terms of employment prospects and leisure pursuits.

Personality difficulties acquired by having epilepsy, especially the dependency, general lack of social skills, and low self-esteem, combined with parental overprotectiveness and popular prejudice, will cause problems in findings friends of both sexes as well as work. This, in turn, will lead to social isolation, feelings of rejection, frustration, and despondency.

Hence, the personality, neurotic, and behaviour difficulties in people with epilepsy are caused by an interaction of many factors, both organic, psychological and social. The relative importance of any particular causative factor will vary from individual to individual. It is a general rule that the early onset of epilepsy in the developing child especially in the presence of either temporal lobe dysfunction or diffuse cortical damage is particularly likely to result in psychiatric morbidity, conduct disorder being the most common manifestation. In the adult, where the personality maturation is complete and the person's life-style stable, the onset of fits has less serious psychological consequences and the prospects of successful adjustment are much better. In this situation, personality change or behaviour disorder is rarely seen, unless, as the result of focal brain disease causing the fits or of overmedication. Nevertheless, mild depressive or anxiety symptoms with lowered self-esteem are common, though no more so than in other chronic illnesses. It would seem that these affective symptoms are a response to the stresses induced by living with a chronic illness and its social consequences, possibly complicated in some people by the effects of long-term drug treatment on mental or bodily function.

Sexual dysfunction in epilepsy. The same problems arise in the relationship between sexual behaviour and temporal lobe epilepsy as exist between TLE and aggression. This subject is reviewed by Scott (1978b). There is no doubt that partial seizures with a focal onset on the medial surface of a hemisphere in the central region can have contralateral genital sensations as part of the initial seizure phenomena. The patient's behaviour both during and after epileptic automatism may rather crudely simulate sexual behaviour (Currier *et al.*, 1971, Hooshmand & Brawley, 1969). Hooshmand and Brawley described three patients who showed exhibitionist behaviour as a result of undressing during epileptic automatisms. In at least one patient (Hoenig & Hamilton, 1960) with temporal lobe epilepsy, partial seizures were triggered by orgasm. Occasionally seizures, usually occurring in the female partner, occur early during coitus and terminate the act. In such cases their occurrence seems to reflect difficulties in the relationship between the two partners (Scott 1978b). The temporal lobe has been implicated in those cases where an association between sexual deviation and epilepsy has been reported. Fetishism and transvestism have been described. The abnormal sexual behaviour in both cases was abolished by successful temporal lobectomy. The case of fetishism is particularly interesting: a 38-year-old man derived sexual satisfaction from staring at a safety pin, following which activity he would have a partial seizure. An active left-temporal-lobe focus was seen in the EEG and an attack, while he was viewing a safety pin, was monitored. A temporal lobectomy was performed, and this resulted in control of both his seizures and his fetish. In the second patient transvestism was abolished after operation. It is tempting to speculate about a relationship between the sexual abnormalities and limbic system dysfunction, but it is difficult to draw any firm conclusions from such a small number of patients. In any event temporal lobe dysfunction is rare among sexual deviants.

Much more common in patients with epilepsy are complaints of reduced libido and impotence. As with other associations between epilepsy and behaviour, the relationships are complex. In many cases, the poor sexual skills are a reflection of poor social skills in persons of immature and dependent personality. However, there is no doubt that the chronic effects of anticonvulsant medication play an important role. Toone and colleagues (1980) have recently carried out a pilot study of the relationship between sexual function, sex hormone levels, and medication. Estimates of free testosterone circulating in the serum were low in a group of chronic epileptics. There was a positive correlation between low free testosterone levels and increased serum gamma-glutamic-transaminase-concentrations. The latter is a measure of increased liver enzyme induction. Hence it would seem that the chronic medication leads to rapid metabolism of testosterone by liver enzymes induced by anticonvulsant drug action. Further, a low serum-free testosterone level correlated with ratings of low sex drive and activity. If these findings are replicated in a larger series of patients, the case for sex-hormone replacement therapy in patients on chronic anticonvulsant medication will have to be considered. Whether the reduced sex drive and impotence can also be related to limbic system dysfunction in patients with temporal lobe epilepsy, as is often

claimed, remains an open question and awaits further control studies of less biased samples of patients.

Epilepsy and psychosis

The little available data about the prevalence of psychosis in patients with epilepsy must be interpreted with caution, since it is obvious that epileptic patients who develop psychosis will be referred to psychiatric services and hence over-represented amongst patients under psychiatric care and under-represented in general hospital samples. Nevertheless, Standage and Fenton (1975) in a small sample of 27 epileptic subjects attending a neurological clinic, found that 8 per cent had a previous history of psychosis. In more selected groups of patients, the prevalence of psychosis is higher. A survey of 80 successive admissions of patients with epilepsy to the Maudsley Hospital, where a special unit for the investigation and treatment of the epilepsies has existed for many years (Pahla, Fenton, Driver & Fenwick, in preparation), found that 17 per cent had a diagnosis of psychosis. In two series of 100 patients treated by temporal lobectomy for intractable temporal lobe epilepsy, the prevalence of psychosis was 12 per cent and 16 per cent respectively (Falconer, 1973). However, this high figure may merely result from a tendency for patients disabled by both epilepsy and psychoses to be referred for specialist investigation and considered as candidates for surgical treatment should a unilateral temporal-lobe epileptogenic focus be confirmed.

An interesting review paper by Stevens (1980) challenges these views. She claims that, though epileptic patients are four or five times more likely to be admitted to psychiatric hospitals than would be expected by chance, the prevalence of functional psychoses, especially schizophrenia, is less than a third of that amongst non-epileptic admissions, support in her view for Von Meduna's early observation of a biological antagonism between epilepsy and schizophrenia. However, the reasons for admitting patients with epilepsy and psychiatric disorder for in-patient treatment may differ significantly from those leading to the admission of non-epileptic patients.

Classification and clinical features. The psychoses of epilepsy can be classified as follows:

(1) *Psychoses directly related to the occurrence of seizure activity.* These present as epileptic clouded or

twilight states which are the direct result of ictal or post-ictal cerebral events. Clouding of consciousness of varying degrees is the dominant feature of the mental state.

(a) Clouded states of *ictal* origin: the more common is petit mal status (absence status). Petit mal status is a well-defined clinical syndrome occurring usually in subjects suffering from generalized epilepsy with typical absences. However, it sometimes occurs in epileptic subjects who have never had absences or even in those without a prior history of epilepsy. The former usually have other types of generalized seizure, especially grand mal attacks.. Petit mal status occurs before the age of 20 years in three-quarters of cases but can appear *de novo* in the middle-aged, when it may stimulate the clinical picture of pre-senile dementia (Schwartz & Scott, 1971). The incidence in patients with generalized epilepsy is 6 per cent (Dalby, 1969).

Continuous EEG spike and wave complexes of generalized origin occur and cause the clouding of consciousness. This varies in degree from slight (about one-fifth of cases), with simple slowing of ideation and expression, to marked (about two-thirds), with disorientation, short attention span, impaired grasp of what is happening in the environment, and automatic behaviour. Somnolence, marked psychomotor retardation, or stupor occurs in about 14 per cent. Myoclonus of variable location occurs in about 50 per cent, being usually bilateral, involving especially the eyelids and arms. Occasionally the jerks may be so localized as to suggest a partial (focal) status. The onset is gradual without precipitating cause in most cases and the duration varies from a few hours to several days. The condition ends gradually within 12 hours in the great majority of patients, either spontaneously or in response to treatment. In some cases petit mal status terminates with a grand mal seizure (Dongier, 1959; Roger *et al.*, 1974).

A rare event is the occurrence of psychomotor complex partial status, a clouded state due to continuous temporal lobe discharges (Betts, 1974; Roger *et al.*, 1974; Blumer, 1977).*

(b) Clouded states of *post-ictal* origin: These are acute organic psychoses characterized by clouding of consciousness with disorientation, narrowing of attention span, impaired grasp of environmental events, perceptual illusions, hallucinations, and poorly systematized delusions, usually of a paranoid nature. Although clouding of consciousness dominates the

clinical picture, excitement is not uncommon. These psychoses can occur in any class of epilepsy, either generalized or partial. They almost invariably follow one or more generalized convulsions, mostly within 24 hours but very occasionally as long as 2 to 7 days afterwards (Levin, 1952; Dongier, 1959). Clouded states often follow a series of fits and are especially common after an episode of major status epilepticus. Nevertheless they do sometimes develop after a single grand-mal seizure and have even been reported in 2 patients following their first known major epileptic attack. Post-ictal clouded states tend to be more common in males (in over two-thirds of cases) and in patients whose fit frequency is more than one major attack a week.

The clouding of consciousness is a direct result of diffuse inhibition of neuronal function, which invariably follows the intense, generalized seizure discharge associated with a grand-mal attack. This inhibition of neuronal function is manifested by diffuse slowing of the predominant EEG rhythms. Such changes are similar to those developing immediately on cessation of an isolated grand-mal attack but are more prolonged with gradual resolution as clear consciousness becomes maintained. The duration of these post-ictal clouded states varies from a few days to several weeks, the majority clearing up within 7 days.

(2) *Interictal psychoses.* Such psychotic states are not directly related in time to the occurrence of clinical epileptic attacks nor ictal discharges within the brain. It is therefore possible that in many such patients the two disorders are independent of each other, occurring together in the individual by chance. This null hypothesis still requires to be satisfactorily rejected. Nevertheless, it is considered that the changes in brain function and organization brought about by the continuing, subclinical epileptogenic activity in affected brain structures and/or the underlying brain lesions causing the epilepsy have contributed to the development of the psychoses. These psychotic states also differ from the clouded states in always occurring in clear consciousness. They can be divided into the following two main groups:

(a) Psychoses with *primary mood disorder*: these psychoses are also of longer duration than the clouded states, lasting weeks or months rather than hours or days (Dongier, 1959). The most common clinical picture is that of classical depressive illness. For example, in his study of mental hospital admissions in

---

* Hallucinations and/or affective change in clear consciousness may occur.

Birmingham, Betts (1974) found that 31 per cent of the patients with epilepsy were suffering from depressive illness. Pahla, Fenton, Driver and Fenwick (in preparation) found 6 patients with affective psychoses out of a total of 14 psychotic patients in a sample of 80 consecutive admissions of epileptic patients to the Maudsley Hospital. A further 5 had schizo-affective disorder. Hence, 11 out of 14 had affective or schizo-affective psychoses. No cases of pathological elation were observed. Hypomania and manic-depressive mood swings do occur in the epileptic psychoses but are rare (Dongier, 1959). As well as being characterized by a primary disturbance of mood, these psychoses run a course similar to that of typical affective illness lasting weeks or months only. Complete remission is usual but, as in classical depressive illness, relapses and further episodes are not uncommon. In the Maudsley series recovery had occurred in more than 50 per cent within 3 months.

In contrast to the clouded states, the onset of the psychotic state is rarely heralded by clinical seizures, but is occasionally terminated by a generalized convulsion (Dongier, 1959). Betts (1974), in his series of 72 epileptic admissions found a significant association between a 50 per cent reduction in seizure frequency before admission in patients admitted with depressive illness, while an increase in seizure frequency was common in those admitted with either acute behaviour disturbance or clouded states. Hence a reduction of seizure frequency may contribute to the pathogenesis of the affective psychoses of epilepsy. The phenomenon of an inverse relationship between mental state and seizure frequency in some but not all patients with epilepsy has been observed by many clinicians over the years (Flor-Henry, 1976). Another difference is the clear relationship to temporal lobe epileptogenic lesions (Dongier, 1959; Pahla, Fenton, Driver and Fenwick, in preparation). Furthermore, there is some evidence of a lateralization effect, non-dominant lobe involvement being associated with affective psychoses and dominant temporal lobe involvement with schizophreniform states. This will be discussed in detail later.

(b) *Schizophrenia-like* psychoses: the mutual antagonism theory that epilepsy protected against schizophrenia led to the introduction of convulsive therapy to psychiatric practice. However, this hypothesis has not stood the test of time. Over subsequent years, it has become apparent that a schizophrenia-like psychosis occurs more often than can be accounted for by chance in patients with epilepsy.

Although this association with epilepsy had been noted by a number of authors over the past half century, including Gruhle (1936) and Clark and Lesco (1939–40), it was Denis Hill (1953) who first drew attention to its special relationship to temporal lobe epilepsy. He described a paranoid, hallucinatory psychosis resembling paranoid schizophrenia developing gradually in the third and fourth decades of life at a time when the seizures were diminishing in frequency. The syndrome was described in more detail by Pond (1957), who further confirmed the association with temporal lobe epilepsy. He reported the psychotic states as closely resembling schizophrenia, with paranoid ideas which might become systematized, ideas of influence, auditory hallucinations often with a menacing quality, and occasional frank thought-disorder with neologisms, condensed words, and inconsequential sentences. All the patients had epilepsy arising from the temporal lobe region with complex aurae; occasional major seizures occurred in sleep only. The epilepsy began some years before the onset of the psychosis, usually in the late teens or twenties, the psychosis often seemed to develop when the seizure frequency had declined, either as a result of drug treatment or natural remission. Pond considered temporal lobe epileptics to be particularly prone to this illness, because the repeated stereotyped and involuntary intrusion into consciousness of abnormal ideas and emotions formed the psychological *Anlage* of a subsequent psychosis. Both Hill (1953) and Pond (1957) commented that these psychoses could be distinguished from typical schizophrenia. Their affect tended to remain warm and appropriate. Personality deterioration was unusual. The paranoid delusions often had a religiose colouring.

Slater and colleagues (1963) published the first detailed study of the schizophrenia-like psychoses of epilepsy. They examined 69 patients with a diagnosis of both schizophrenia and epilepsy, 31 at the National Hospital for Nervous Diseases and 38 at the Maudsley Hospital, London. The following four groups of patients were identified:

(1) 11 patients whose chronic psychosis had been preceded by repeated occurrence of short-lived confusional episodes

(2) 46% patients whose psychoses were highly typical of a paranoid schizophrenia

(3) 8 patients with a picture of hebephrenic schizophrenia

(4) 4 patients with chronic schizophrenia associated with petit mal attacks due to generalized spike and wave discharges

These 69 patients were generally similar in profile to non-epileptic schizophrenics. There were a number of differences. Paranoid states were unduly common. Mystical delusional experiences were especially frequent, the patients feeling in communication with God or endowed with supernatural powers or experiencing passivity phenomena with a mystical content. Often delusional states would begin with a single abnormal experience, which is delusionally interpreted. This might be forgotten but a further abnormal experience would occur, again misinterpreted so that a progressive insidious systematization might develop. Often the delusional state fluctuated, remissions or intermissions frequently being related to changes in seizure frequency.

Auditory hallucinations were predominant. However, visual hallucinations were more common than in typical schizophrenia, being often experienced during dream-like states in the absence of confusion. Again, a mystical content to the hallucinations was common.

The patient's affect was better retained. Flattening was less frequent and slower in developing. The patients tended to be irritable but not unfriendly. Their social adjustment was better, over half having adequate personal relationships and 45 per cent being in some sort of paid employment. The progress of the disorder also differed from typical schizophrenia. The onset was insidious in about half, but 11 out of the 69 had an acute onset while 20 had a number of acute episodes before the development of a chronic psychotic state.

Follow-up one to three years after first hospital admission (2 to 25 years after the onset of the psychosis) indicated a less progressive disorder. Remissions in one-third and improvement in another third were observed. On the other hand, psycho-organic sequelae such as perseveration, dullness, retardation, circumstantiality, and impairment of memory had become prominent in 40 per cent of patients.

There was no genetic loading for schizophrenia nor any excess of schizoid pre-morbid traits amongst the patients.

Just over two-thirds had clinical and EEG evidence of temporal lobe epileptogenic activity, bilateral in slightly less than half, unilateral in the rest; right- and left-sided unilateral involvement being equally common.

A past history of acquired brain damage was elicited in slightly less than half the patients. In the 56 patients who had air encephalography, 37 had atrophic lesions. Tumours were rare, being found in two patients.

The mean age of onset of epilepsy was at puberty (15.7 years), 70 per cent were under 25 years, while the mean age of onset for the psychoses was 29.8 years. The psychosis developed on average 14.1 years after the fits. There was a positive correlation between the ages of onset of the epilepsy and psychosis (correlation coefficient= +0.6). In all cases epileptic fits persisted up to the onset of the psychosis. In the majority there was no relation between seizure frequency and onset of mental illness. In 2, an increase of seizures occurred shortly before the appearance of psychotic symptoms while in a further 15 patients, there was a suggestion of an inverse relationship, i.e. psychotic symptoms first appearing when the fit frequency was falling. The quantity of medication had no effect nor had the severity of the epilepsy.

In summary then, Slater and colleagues (1963) demonstrated that a schizophrenia-like psychosis in patients with epilepsy cannot be coincidental. The schizophrenic picture differs somewhat from non-epileptic schizophrenia in not infrequently being episodic or having a fluctuating onset, in producing a clinical syndrome in which the warmth of the personality is well preserved and paranoid delusions are unduly common. Progress is towards an organic type of personality impairment rather than a typical schizophrenic end-state. Over two-thirds have temporal lobe dysfunction. A long duration of epilepsy is the rule and is regarded by Slater and colleagues (1963) to be of causative importance. There is no definite relation between severity of epilepsy, seizure frequency, nor amount of medication.

The authors calculated that the expectation of a person developing first epilepsy and then schizophrenia is 0.00003. Taking account of the age distribution of onset of the disorder, 20 new cases would be expected each year in England and Wales, i.e. 4 to 5 per annum in the Greater London area – the area where the majority of patients referred to the Maudsley and National Hospitals reside.

It was therefore argued that a chance occurrence of epilepsy and schizophrenia leading to an incidence of only 4 or 5 a year in Greater London could hardly account for the large pool of 69 new cases collected at only two of the many hospitals in the Greater London area.

The lack of a genetic predisposition to schizophrenia, relative absence of schizoid pre-morbid traits and the slight but definite qualitative differences in psychotic symptomatology made the authors reject the alternative hypothesis that the epilepsy had merely acted as a precipitating factor in persons already genetically vulnerable to schizophrenia. A third hypothesis that schizophrenia-like illness was an epileptic psychosis, directly due to the temporal lobe epilepsy was taken as the most acceptable one. The aetiological relationship between the epilepsy and psychosis was considered to result from limbic system dysfunction caused by the temporal lobe epileptogenic activity. Two possible mechanisms were postulated.

(1) The limbic system is closely connected with the emotional life of the individual, and when it is disturbed he is liable to experience affects and perceptual disturbances of a compelling and disquieting kind not connected with external reality, for example pathological fear, *déjà vu*, depersonalization, derealization. Over time these transient but recurrent abnormal experiences of physiological origin become totally integrated into the psychic life of the individual as a psychodynamic process. For the development of a complex and lasting paranoid psychosis out of recurrent abnormal experiences a number of other conditions are probably necessary. Thus the experience itself should have a strong reality value, so that at the time it occurs the patient does not easily recognize it as hallucinatory, but puts it down as a real event. It should be accompanied by a strong affect so that it impresses the mind, and once remembered is not easily forgotten. It should occur in such a state of consciousness that it is not subsequently obliterated by an amnesic gap. It should not be easily dismissed by the patient as of trivial importance, nor seen through on reflection by subsequent use of powers of insight.

The complex seizures of temporal lobe epilepsy can fulfil most of these criteria, whereas the simple visual hallucinations triggered by a discharging lesion of the occipital cortex do not. The authors regard this hypothesis as unsatisfactory. Although it provides a plausible explanation of the paranoid symptomatology it cannot explain the other schizophrenic features. Furthermore, in this author's experience, the abnormal psychic phenomena of complex temporal lobe seizures are usually experienced by the patient as discrete events which are short-lived and foreign to his ego state. They rarely become incorporated in his psychic reality. Schizophrenia-like psychoses can also develop in temporal lobe epilepsy whose only manifestation is generalized convulsions without aura, neither during wakefulness nor sleep. About one-fifth of patients with temporal lobe epileptogenic lesions present in this way (Penfield & Kristiansen, 1951).

(2) The disorderly and excessive discharge of temporal lobe epileptogenic neurones involves neuronal circuits concerned with the physiological basis of the psychological disorder we call schizophrenia (Symonds 1962). Hence, not only do the ictal discharges cause recurrent seizures, but years of subclinical disruption of function by continual interictal irregular and excessive neuronal firing lead to the appearance of psychosis. Slater and colleagues (1963) favour this hypothesis. They regard the illness as a symptomatic schizophrenia due to temporal lobe dysfunction analogous to the paranoid schizophrenia-like states found in amphetamine abuse. In this view they differ from Hill (1953) and Pond (1957), who regard the illness as a paranoid, hallucinatory psychosis due to temporal lobe dysfunction but clinically distinct from schizophrenia.

Slater and colleagues (1963) also consider that an important predisposing factor is the temporal lobe atrophic process frequently demonstrated by pneumoencephalography. This gradual cell loss could account for the late development of the psychosis and the tendency for the psychotic symptoms in time to resolve and be replaced by an organic deficit. However, it must be pointed out that the authors' diagnosis of the organic changes depended largely on notoriously unreliable subjective and objective mental state observations. No systematic psychometric data is available to confirm the clinical observations. No attempt was made during the follow-up study 1 to 3 years after the initial hospital assessment to search for the electrophysiological and psychometric changes associated with progressive organic deterioration (Slater *et al.*, 1963). Hence the evidence for a progressive atrophic process involving one or both temporal lobes in these patients is not substantial.

Since the classic study of Slater and his colleagues, Asuni and Pillutla (1967) in Western Nigeria have reported schizophrenia-like psychoses in 11 out of 42 mental hospital epileptics. Standage (1973) in a survey of 53 long-stay epileptic patients at Bexley Hospital, a London psychiatric hospital, found 6 patients, 5 males. None had temporal lobe epilepsy. Kristensen and Sindrup (1978 a,b) in Denmark have reported a study of 96 patients with temporal lobe epilepsy and paranoid/hallucinatory psychoses in clear consciousness compared with 96 non-psychotic, temporal lobe epileptic patients. Finally, Toone (1980) at the Maudsley Hospital is at present completing a follow-up study of 57 epileptic patients with psychosis. Just over one-third are schizophrenic and a fifth are affective in nature; 12 per cent had paranoid psychosis. In nearly one-fifth episodes of more than one diagnostic category occurred at different times in patients with recurrent psychoses.

Pathogenesis. Like most psychiatric disorders, it is probable that the psychoses of epilepsy result from a complex interaction of multiple causative factors; biological, psychological, and social; the relative importance of any one factor varies from individual to individual. Hence, in each patient, psychosis will develop as a consequence of an interplay of pathogenic factors unique to that individual. In the evaluation of the individual patient the following factors should be taken into account:

(1) *Cerebral epileptogenic activity.* (a) Global cerebral dysfunction: a diffuse disruption of cortical function is invariable in patients presenting with post-ictal confusional states following one or more seizures. This is due to post-ictal cortical neuronal exhaustion or inhibition, manifested by clouding of consciousness and diffuse slowing of the dominant EEG frequencies. A similar disturbance of cortical function results from the continuous generalized spike and wave discharges of petit mal status. In both these cases, the disruption of cortical function as a consequence of abnormal physiological activity is the major cause of the psychosis, which is organic in form. Alteration of consciousness is the dominant clinical feature. However, it should not be assumed that these abnormal cerebral mechanisms have not been influenced by environmental factors. For example, the episode of status epilepticus or serial epilepsy precipitating the clouded state may have resulted from the changes in the patient's physical state, for example a febrile illness, or sleep deprivation, or the omission of medication, which sometimes is caused by a complex of social and/or psychological factors unique to that individual. In addition, some patients' seizure frequency is surprisingly vulnerable to the impact of stressful life-events, such as bereavement, loss of job, changes in family psychopathology. Such adverse stressful events may trigger status or a series of fits.

(b) The location of the cerebral epileptogenic activity: apart from the rare cases of psychomotor status, temporal lobe dysfunction is associated with psychoses in clear consciousness. The apparent specific relationship between temporal lobe epilepsy and psychosis was first emphasized by Gibbs (1951). In an analysis of 275 epileptic patients with sharply localized EEG spike foci, he found that 59 per cent had anterior temporal foci. Psychosis occurred in 17 per cent of these patients and was extremely rare (2 per cent) in patients with foci elsewhere in the cerebral cortex.

Gibbs postulated that the prime function of the anterior temporal lobe structures is the evaluation and interpretation of afferent input already received and initially processed by the sensory receiving areas and postero-lateral temporal regions. This integrative function of the temporal lobe, bringing together the information necessary to maintain the essential self, that 'I am', has also been pointed out more recently by Denis Williams (1968). Gibbs (1951) hypothesized that if the anterior temporal disturbance of integrative function results in the individual evaluating his total experience as unpleasant and undesirable, depressive illness develops. On the other hand, such misevaluation of subjective experience may bring projective mechanisms into operation and encourage the development of paranoid psychosis. Since then many other workers, including Slater and colleagues (1963), Glaser (1964), Flor-Henry (1969, 1972, 1974), Davison and Bagley (1969), Taylor (1971, 1972b, 1975, 1977), Toone (1980) and Pahla and colleagues (in preparation) have reported significant associations between temporal lobe epilepsy and the functional psychoses.

This work has been extensively reviewed by Flor-Henry (1976). He points out that a number of studies have failed to find an association between psychosis and temporal lobe epilepsy (Small *et al.*, 1962, 1966; Stevens, 1966; Small & Small, 1967). They may well be an artefact of the referral practices at the hospitals concerned. Few psychotic patients will be referred to general hospital neurological clinics. The incidence of schizophrenia in temporal lobe epilepsy is of the order of 2 per cent. Most of the negative studies have dealt with at most 100 epileptic patients and hence may be expected to contain not more than two patients with schizophrenia-like psychoses; a number likely to be dismissed as a chance finding.

Nevertheless a note of caution must be maintained. Although global cerebral dysfunction following generalized convulsions or due to petit mal status is almost invariably followed by clouding of consciousness, functional psychosis in clear consciousness is a relatively rare association of temporal lobe epilepsy. For example, Currie and colleagues (1971), in a study of 666 unselected patients with temporal lobe epilepsy, found psychosis in only 16 (2 per cent), schizophrenia in 12 and severe depressive states in 4. Furthermore, although temporal lobe tumours appear to be more commonly associated with psychosis than tumours elsewhere in the cerebral cortex, the occurrence of psychosis is relatively rare, being between 1 and 4 per cent (Davison & Bagley, 1969). Hence temporal lobe dysfunction alone cannot account for psychosis in the temporal lobe epileptic.

A more plausible hypothesis accounting for the relatively small number of index cases, is that the temporal-lobe epileptogenic activity, by disrupting limbic system 'circuitry', increases vulnerability to psychotic breakdown. Hence florid psychotic illness develops only when the person is exposed in addition to a number of other pathogenic factors, both predisposing and precipitating, which interact with the temporal lobe dysfunction to disrupt the person's capacity to deal with the environment.

(c) The nature of the underlying pathological lesion: a further problem, which requires examination, is the question whether the abnormal electrical activity localized to the temporo-limbic structures in the absence of structural pathology can cause sufficient disruption of function to increase vulnerability to psychosis. The observation that frequency of focal paroxysmal discharges can be related to psychosis certainly suggests the former.

Nevertheless, the nature of the underlying pathological process is obviously important in the schizophrenia-like psychoses of temporal lobe epilepsy (Falconer, 1973; Taylor 1975, 1977). Mesial temporal sclerosis is rarely associated with schizophrenia-like psychosis (2 out of 41 cases). On the other hand, small, 'cryptic' tumours, hamartomata or alien tissue (AT) lesions are commonly accompanied by schizophrenia-like psychoses (11 out of 47 cases). Jensen and Larsen (1979) report similar findings.

The alien tissue pathology is a developmental lesion arising early during embryogenesis. In contrast, mesial temporal sclerosis is a post-natal insult. The age of onset of fits is earlier in the MTS cases, usually within the first decade of life, while the majority of AT patients first develop fits after the age of 10 years. Those who develop psychosis tend to have an onset of epilepsy around puberty (Taylor, 1971, 1975, 1977). The disruptive effect of epilepsy that develops during such a crucial developmental stage as adolescence and interacts with the underlying temporal lobe dysfunction and its potential effect on the individual's 'I am' state may be more important than the nature of the pathological process causing the epilepsy. Hence the AT lesion may only act through its tendency to trigger the first fits at puberty.

(d) Temporal lobe epileptogenic foci and their relation to cerebral dominance: Flor-Henry (1969), in a controlled study of 50 patients with temporal lobe epilepsy and psychosis, was the first to report a significant association between psychosis and dominant (left-sided) temporal lobe involvement. The relationship applied particularly to those patients with schizophrenic psychoses. Similar laterality effects have been reported by Gregoriades and colleagues (1971) in abstract form and by Taylor (1975), who found a trend for dominant lobe involvement to be associated with schizophrenia-like psychosis, in Murray Falconer's temporal lobectomy series. This, however, did not reach statistical significance. Toone's present investigation using both the EEG and CT scanning also provides some confirmation of Flor-Henry's findings (Toone, 1980). A significant excess of left-sided lesions has been found in the psychotic patients. Flor-Henry (1969) also related affective psychoses to non-dominant temporal lobe involvement. This observation was made on a small number of patients and has not been confirmed by either Jensen and Larsen (1979) or Toone (1980).

These findings contrast with those of Slater and colleagues (1963) and Kristensen and Sindrup (1978b) who report an excess of bilateral foci. The latter also observed that, in the psychotic group, sphenoidal lead spike foci were significantly more common than spike discharges arising from the temporal lobe convexity or neocortex. They took this to mean that dysfunction specifically involving the deep temporal lobe structures, namely the uncus, amygdala, hippocampus, and related limbic system areas is important in the pathogenesis of psychosis. Kristensen and Sindrup (1978b) also regarded the extent of the epileptogenic lesion to be important as a causative factor; the finding of a significant higher frequency of bilateral and multiple spike foci and diffuse background activity indicated more extensive and severe epileptogenic lesions in the psychotic patients.

It is difficult to reconcile these differing observations and interpretations. It may be that either epileptogenic dysfunction localized to the dominant temporal lobe or extensive bilateral damage to the deep limbic system structures can independently make patients vulnerable to psychotic break-down. Certainly, extensive and possibly bilateral limbic-system damage aggravated by surgery is a plausible explanation of the mechanism of onset of psychosis in patients whose seizures have been relieved by temporal lobectomy. Such an event occurs in 7 per cent to 15 per cent of patients after temporal lobectomy (Stevens, 1980). The increased proportion of left-handers amongst epileptics with psychosis may also be a reflection of either dominant lobe dysfunction or impaired lateralization of hemisphere function due to bilateral organic pathology (Taylor, 1975; Kristensen & Sindrup, 1978a; Toone, 1980).

Another problem is that the various series of temporal lobe epileptic patients may contain subsets of persons, whose psychotic processes are fundamentally different, being provoked by an interplay of widely differing pathogenic factors acting upon different physiological substrates. For example, Flor-Henry's 50 psychotic subjects with temporal lobe epilepsy contained a mixture of schizophrenia-like, schizo-affective and affective psychoses and included a few clouded states. His control group of non-psychotic temporal lobe epileptics was heterogeneous, comprising 25 patients referred to a neurosurgeon for temporal lobectomy and 25 patients attending an epilepsy unit in a psychiatric hospital. The series of Slater and colleagues (1963) consisted of 4 distinct subgroups of patients. In the latter 2, the hebephrenics and the chronic schizophrenics with petit mal attacks, the occurrence of schizophrenia and epilepsy was probably fortuitous. Clearly, further study of more homogeneous and better-controlled patient samples with well-defined symptom and neurophysiological profiles is indicated. These should include CT scan investigations in order to determine location and extent of structural pathology.

(e) Temporal occurrence of seizure activity: both the frequency of occurrence of seizure activity and clinical pattern of attack appear important.

(1) Increase in major seizure frequency of at least 50 per cent appears to relate significantly with psycho-organic syndromes associated with clouding of consciousness or behaviour disorder (Betts, 1975). The increase in seizure activity presumably causes a global disruption of cortical function, with the consequent development of clouded states or disinhibition of behaviour.

(2) A decline in major seizure frequency has been reported in a variable proportion of psychotic states occurring in clear consciousness, an inverse relationship between epilepsy and mental state being observed.

For example, Slater and colleagues (1963) reported an inverse relationship between psychosis and major seizure frequency in 22 per cent of their 69 patients with schizophrenia-like psychoses of epilepsy, mainly in those whose illness had an episodic course with relapses and remissions. Betts (1974) found a 50 per cent reduction in occurrence of grand mal attacks in 9 out of 15 epileptics admitted to hospital for treatment of endogenous depression, a finding significant at the 0.001 level.

Flor-Henry (1969, 1976) emphasizes the importance of type of seizure. In his 1969 study of 50 temporal lobe epileptics with psychosis, the incidence of psychomotor and complex psychosensory seizures was greatly reduced in those patients with schizophrenia-like psychoses. No difference in generalized seizure frequency was noted. Kristensen and Sindrup (1978) report similar findings in their longer series. Since complex partial seizures are the result of activation of the frontotemporal limbic system, Flor-Henry (1976) considers that the reduced frequency of such seizures in psychotic patients is a manifestation of under-activity of this neuronal system. Stevens (1980) relates this to a local inhibitory effect of the catecholamine receptors on paroxysmal neuronal discharge. Though the inverse relationship between complex partial seizures and schizophrenia-like psychoses of epilepsy has now been well documented, other workers have not been impressed by the frequency with which the phenomenon occurs. In fact Toone (1980) found the reverse to be more common; namely the psychosis being heralded by an exacerbation in seizure frequency.

Apparent normalization of the EEG during psychotic episodes, both in confusional states associated with generalized epilepsy and the schizophrenia-like psychoses of temporal lobe epilepsy, has also been described by Landolt (1958), and confirmed by Bruens (1971) in 25 per cent of 19 epileptic patients with psychotic symptoms. In the schizophrenia-like psychoses the temporal lobe spiking may disappear for the duration of the psychotic episode and in the confusional psychoses or twilight states associated with primary generalized epilepsy the generalized spike and wave discharge might subside or disappear with subsequent return on termination of the psychosis. This phenomenon is known as 'forced normalization'. Although such changes can be explained as an epiphenomenon of the mental state, the increased arousal of the psychotic process inhibiting the epileptic discharges, Landolt (1958) regards these EEG changes as having a causative relationship to the psychoses. He quotes in support the observation that the efficacy of ECT is related to the amount of EEG abnormality induced (Fink & Kahn, 1957). However, Landolt refers to psychoses which are episodic in type. Also the inverse relation between epilepsy and psychosis is observed in a minority of cases only. Therefore such mechanisms may only operate in a small subgroup of the epileptic psychosis; possibly when the psychotic states are episodic and occurring in a setting of clear consciousness.

This problem can only be resolved by the longitudinal study of epileptic patients with psychotic states which remit and relapse. The cross-sectional, statistical approach used by Flor-Henry and others, comparing seizure frequency in psychotics and controls, is open to error because of selection factors. Non-psychotic control patients may have a higher seizure frequency because the problem requiring hospital admission is uncontrolled epilepsy. On the other hand, psychotic epileptics will be taken into hospital because of their psychotic mental states, not on account of seizure control.

To summarize and interpret the conflicting observations about seizure frequency and psychosis is difficult. However, it may well be that changes in seizure frequency in either direction cause brain dysfunction by different mechanisms, each of which can contribute to psychotic breakdown. Frequent major convulsions or complex partial seizures may respectively cause generalized impairment of cortical function or disrupt limbic system processes as a result of neuronal metabolic changes caused by the intense and repetitive epileptic excitation of the cerebral neurones. On the other hand, reduced seizure frequency and psychosis may both be a manifestation of inhibition induced by changes in neuro-transmitter concentration. One last observation worthy of comment is as follows. When the inverse relationship between fits and psychosis does exist, it seems to be confined to complex partial seizures in patients with schizophrenia-like psychoses and to major convulsions in the affective psychoses. It is probable that these seizures involve activation of two different brain systems: respectively from temporal limbic area and the mesial frontal–dorsomedial thalamic–mesencephalic reticular system. It is tempting to speculate with Flor-Henry (1976) that dysfunction in these two systems provides the neural substrate for the schizophrenia-like and affective psychoses respectively.

(2) *Neurochemical 'bridges' between epilepsy and psychosis.* (a) Lamprecht (1973) has argued that a disturbance in the feedback control of the mesolimbic dopaminergic neurones might provide a common neurochemical mechanism underlying the epileptic attacks and schizophrenia. The dopaminergic drug, amphetamine, which can cause a schizophrenia-like psychosis, has a powerful anticonvulsant action. The dopamine precursor, dopa, raises the convulsive threshold. Diphenylhydantoin, the anticonvulsant drug, inhibits dopamine uptake, making more available for postsynaptic membranes. Hence dopaminergic mechanisms may be involved reciprocally in the control of epilepsy and schizophrenia. Lamprecht proposes a dysfunction of the regulatory circuit of central dopamine synapses: insufficient inhibitory feedback evokes an increased number of occupied post-synaptic dopamine receptors, which in turn induces both psychosis and elevation of the convulsive threshold; the converse, excessive inhibitory feedback, leads to a decreased number of occupied post-synaptic receptors, a lowering of the convulsive threshold and the occurrence of epilepsy rather than psychosis.

Trimble (1977) presents a similar dopamine hypothesis, pointing out that stimulation of dopamine activity appears to be anti-epileptic and schizophrenogenic, whereas diminution of such activity decreases the seizure threshold but has a therapeutic effect in schizophrenia. Sato and colleagues (1979) have recently demonstrated the importance of dopaminergic receptor sensitivity in inhibition of amygdaloid seizure development.

Stevens (1980) points out that the amygdala and hippocampus have the lowest threshold for epileptic discharge of any region of the brain. The perpetuation by natural selection of such a low threshold confined to these areas must have important benefits for the survival of the individual or the species. This phenomenon may be related to the intense physiological paroxysmal discharge which occurs in several limbic nuclei during sexual activity, pulsatile release of neuroendocrine factors and ovulation. The low threshold for epileptic discharge of the amygdala and hippocampus requires a potent 'wall' of inhibition to prevent spread of the physiological paroxysmal discharges to systems subserving consciousness and motor behaviour. The schizophrenia-like psychoses associated with epilepsy may represent over-development of the physiological inhibitory protection against seizure propagation, which the catecholamine systems normally provide. The excess inhibition may be manifest in a reduction in complex partial seizure frequency. The seizures themselves may prevent psychosis by desensitizing supersensitive catecholamine receptors.

(b) Other amine systems may be involved. For example, 5-hydroxytryptophan, a precursor of serotonin (5HT), has a powerful though transient anticonvulsant effect (Chadwick *et al.*, 1975; Meldrum, 1978), while reserpine, which depletes the brain of 5HT and causes depression, lowers the convulsive threshold. Hence deficient serotonergic mechanisms may form the neurochemical substrate for some patients with both epilepsy and depression.

(c) Anticonvulsants, especially diphenylhydantoin, lower serum, red cell, and CSF folate levels. Reynolds (1967) suggested that this antifolate effect may provoke schizophrenia-like symptoms. Folate coenzymes are involved in the synthesis of labile methyl groups essential for the transmethylation processes which detoxify metabolic compounds produced during the catabolism of biogenic amines. Levi and Waxman (1975) suggest that in epileptic patients low folate levels due to medication may prevent the donation of enough labile methyl groups to S-adenosylhomocysteine for the formation of S-adenosylmethionine (SAMe). SAMe is the only compound involved directly in the methylation of biogenic amines. Failure of the transmethylation processes may prevent the breakdown of toxic amine metabolites with consequent development of a schizophrenia-like psychosis. However, there is no convincing evidence that folate replacement therapy improves the mental state of patients with low serum folate levels.

(3) *Anticonvulsant drug intoxication.* Anticonvulsant drug intoxication is a rare cause of psychiatric hospital admission (4 per cent in Betts' Birmingham series). This usually presents as an organic psychosyndrome with drowsiness, dysarthria, ataxia,

and sometimes mild clouding of consciousness. Occasionally poorly systematized paranoid ideas may be present. This drug-induced confusional state is readily distinguished from post-ictal clouded states by the presence of nystagmus, dysarthria, and ataxia. Nevertheless, these pathognomonic signs may be minimal in the subnormal and it is always wise in cases when drug intoxication is suspected to estimate serum anticonvulsant levels. The toxic patient shows diffuse slowing of the predominant EEG frequencies indicating a drug-induced global impairment of cortical neuronal function. Drug intoxication should also be borne in mind as a possible factor contributing to the inverse relationship between seizure frequency and mental state.

(4) *Age of onset of epilepsy and its relation to psychosis.* Slater and colleagues (1963) place considerable emphasis on their finding of a correlation coefficient of +0.6 between the ages of onset of epilepsy and of psychosis as indicating that duration of epilepsy is an aetiological factor in the psychosis. However, as Davison and Bagley (1969) point out, the correlation may be a statistical artefact produced by the absence of cases in which psychosis precedes epilepsy. It cannot be assumed that the latter situation never occurs, particularly if the view that the psychosis is related to the cerebral lesion rather than the fits is accepted.

More important are the observations of Taylor (1971) that schizophrenia-like psychoses tend to occur in those patients whose epilepsy begins at puberty, a phase of rapid somatic growth and crisis in psychological maturation. The onset of fits at such a critical stage of development is potentially a powerful disruptive influence on consequent psychic development, especially if the abnormal electrical activity involves the temporal lobes. Hence the epileptogenic activity may interfere with the integrative functions of the temporal lobe structures in bringing together the information to maintain the essential self, the 'I am' (Williams, 1968).

In females, puberty occurs relatively early. As demonstrated by Taylor (1971), those who later develop schizophrenia-like psychoses of epilepsy have a peak onset of fits earlier in puberty than males. The first occurrence of seizures at a younger and possibly more vulnerable phase in pubertal development may have a greater potential to disrupt personality development. This may account for the greater preponderance of females amongst epileptic patients with schizophrenic-like psychoses. Epilepsy is more common in males but the sex ratio for the epileptic psychoses is approximately equal in the combined series of Falconer, Flor-Henry, Slater, and Beard. Furthermore the onset of psychosis tended to occur sooner in females. In the series of Slater and colleagues (1963) more than one-third of females and only 2 out of 24 males had become psychotic before the age of 20 years. However, a sex difference in prevalence of psychosis has not been found by Kristensen and Sindrup (1978) and Jensen and Larsen (1979).

(5) *Genetic influences.* Although Slater and colleagues (1963) found only 2 out of their 19 cases of schizophrenia-like psychoses of epilepsy with evidence of genetic predisposition, it is premature to regard these negative results as the definitive rejection of the role of genetic influences in predisposing epileptic patients to the risk of psychosis. Pahla and colleagues (in preparation) found a history of psychosis in first-degree relatives in about one-third of their small series of epileptic psychoses, predominantly affective or schizo-affective in nature. Jensen and Larsen (1979) also reported a positive family history for major psychiatric illness in two-thirds of their patients with temporal lobe epilepsy and psychosis.

(6) *Social and environmental influences.* Despite the fact that it is well known that emotional stress can increase seizure frequency in some patients (Mattson *et al.*, 1970) and adverse life-events such as bereavement can be followed by late-onset epilepsy (Dominian *et al.*, 1963), there has been no systematic work on the role of adverse life-events in precipitating psychosis in epileptic patients. Nevertheless, one's clinical impression is that life-events are as important in provoking psychosis in the epileptic as they are in the non-epileptic patient (Birley & Brown, 1970; Brown *et al.*, 1977).

Conclusions. In summary then, the psychoses of epilepsy can be subdivided into the following 2 groups:
(1) Those directly related to the seizure discharge; namely, the epileptic clouded or twilight states. These include the following syndromes: petit mal or absence status, complex partial status and post-ictal clouded states. All these conditions are due to direct and widespread interference of cortical function by the ictal discharge.
(2) The interictal psychoses: psychotic states not directly related to the ictal discharge.
None the less it is assumed that involvement of the limbic system structures by abnormal electrical activity and/or the lesion causing the fits and/or the effect of drug treatment on cerebral neuronal systems alter brain function and organization and hence have contributed in varying degrees to the development of psychoses. These occur in clear consciousness and consist of either (i) brief psychotic episodes lasting weeks or months with recovery; predominately affective or schizo-affective in nature, or (ii) chronic schizophrenia-like illnesses. Both appear related to specific temporal lobe dysfunction. The influence of lateralization remains in dispute at present. Both bilateral damage to the mesial temporal limbic structures and dominant temporal lobe dysfunction appear to predispose to psychosis. Change in seizure frequency in either direction is important; increased seizure activity causes dysfunction through intense neuronal activation; the phenomenon of lower fit-frequency and psychosis may reflect underlying neuro-transmitter changes. In contrast to the psychoses directly related to the ictal events, the interictal psychoses result from a more complex interaction of causative factors; biological, psychological, and social. The cerebral disorder caused by the epilepsy merely acts as one of a number of vulnerability or provoking factors.

Investigation and management

The investigation of a patient with seizures and psychiatric disorder requires a multidisciplinary approach. The neurological, psychological, psychiatric, and social aspects of the problem must be considered separately during the initial assessment. However the final diagnostic formulation will take account of the interaction between these various influences, all of which may contribute to the genesis of the person's problems. Of course, the relative importance of each of these groups of factors will vary from individual to individual.

Investigation of the seizures

It will be necessary to establish the type of epilepsy (whether generalized, partial, or unclassifiable) and attempt to identify the nature of the underlying pathology, if any. The clinical examination should include a complete family and medical history along with a thorough medical and neurological examination. Descriptions of the seizures should be obtained, not only from the patient but also from relatives, friends, or colleagues who have observed the fits.

Attention is directed towards those subjective and objective events occurring at the onset of the attack. The aura is not a warning but an initial seizure phenomenon, which may be the only clinical clue to indicate its partial or focal nature. The patient is often unaware of events at the onset, but a careful history from his family may reveal early or continued focal features. The symmetry or otherwise of the convulsive movements should be enquired about, since lateralization of onset or asymmetry of the convulsion may be yet another clue to a partial onset. The duration and mode of cessation of minor attacks are also important. Petit mal absences usually last 10 seconds or less and cease abruptly with immediate return to clear consciousness and resumption of normal behaviour. Complex partial (temporal lobe) seizures may present with transient episodes of unconsciousness without aura or other lateralizing features and hence be mistaken for petit mal absences due to generalized spike and wave discharges. However, the complex partial seizures are of longer duration, a minute or more, and recovery to clear consciousness is gradual with a brief period of confusion being common. Seizure frequency is also of diagnostic importance. Petit mal absences often occur many times a day. Complex partial seizures tend to be less frequent and it is rare for major convulsions to occur more than once or twice a day. Frequently recurring major attacks throughout the day should raise the suspicion of hysterical pseudo-seizures.

Post-ictal events should be thoroughly investigated. Post-ictal confusion is not uncommon after grand mal convulsions or complex partial seizures. It may be the only event during the attack which the patient can recall. Its presence may be useful in reaching a diagnosis of epilepsy in the absence of eye-witness accounts of the fits. A history of incontinence of urine and tongue biting is also helpful in the same way, though, on rare occasions, both these events have been described in patients with hysterical pseudo-seizures. Post-ictal focal neurological signs such as hemiparesis (Todd's paralysis), dysphasia, or a transient visual field defect should be enquired about. Such residual phenomena indicate a focal epileptogenic lesion. If a fit occurs in the consulting room or ward, a careful search for such focal signs should be performed during the post-ictal phase.

The relationship between possible provoking or precipitating causes should be explored. The following should be enquired about: stimuli which precipitate reflex seizures, for example music, flickering light, sudden voluntary movement, hyperventilation, the menstrual cycle especially the premenstrual phase, sleep, sleep deprivation, emotional upsets, alcohol consumption, sudden withdrawal of narcotic or sedative drugs or alcohol in patients dependent on such substances, non-compliance with anticonvulsant medication, the prescription of potentially epileptogenic drugs such as phenothiazines and tricyclic antidepressants.

Every patient should receive a systematic enquiry to search for other evidence of organic brain dysfunction, especially in those patients with late-onset fits and where the seizures present with focal features. The past history must be searched for possible causative factors: for example, perinatal trauma, previous head injuries, infections or vascular lesions involving the CNS, severe episodes of infantile convulsions. Genetic histories, especially of first-degree relatives, should be carefully obtained.

On neurological examination, classical CNS signs are relatively rare but soft or minimal signs are often useful in lateralizing the epileptogenic lesion. Left-handedness, in the absence of family history, raises the possibility that the left hand may be used preferentially because an early or minimal defect in the left hemisphere function impaired the use of the right hand. Early acquired lesions of one cerebral hemisphere may lead to a reduction in somatic growth on the opposite side of the body. This will result in slightly shorter and smaller limbs on the contralateral side. There may also be clumsiness or ungainliness in skilled acts or in play activities, in writing, or bouncing a ball on the affected side. The skull may be asymmetrical; smaller on the side of an early acquired atrophic lesion. A lower facial weakness for emotional expression is useful as a lateralizing sign for a contralateral temporal lobe lesion. Routine auscultation of the skull will occasionally be rewarded by hearing a bruit due to a vascular malformation.

On rare occasions, certain abnormalities on general examination will indicate the specific cause of the seizures. The port wine stain involving the skin of the 5th nerve distribution represents a cutaneous angioma due to the Sturge-Weber syndrome. It is part of a congenital ectodermal defect. The brain is affected with intracranial calcification in the second and third layers of the cortex, usually in the occipital lobe. The butterfly rash on the face (adenoma sebaceum), *café au lait* spots, shagreen patches and vitiligo are characteristic of tuberose sclerosis.

Routine examination of the ocular fundi is essential; to exclude evidence of increased intracranial pressure and to look for other potentially significant abnormalities such as vascular malformations, the scars of toxoplasmosis, the infiltrations of tuberose sclerosis and the macular cherry-red spots of Tay–Sacks disease.

Laboratory investigations should include routine serological tests for syphilis. Though neurosyphilis is now very rare, the occasional case can still be missed. If the patient is already on chronic anticonvulsant medication, full blood picture, serum folate and B_{12} estimations should be carried out since drug-induced bone marrow megaloblastic change is common. Similarly serum calcium and alkaline phosphatase levels should be checked because of the risk of anticonvulsant induced osteomalacia. Finally, serum anticonvulsant drug concentrations should be estimated if toxicity or non-compliance is suspected or if seizure control is a problem.

EEG investigation should be carried out as a routine. This contributes to the differential diagnosis between epileptic attacks, hysterical pseudo-seizures, transient ischaemic attacks, and transient episodes of sudden unconsciousness from other causes. It will help to classify the type of epilepsy. Correct classification is important since this process identifies those patients with primary generalized epilepsy, who require no further neurological investigation, and those with the partial epilepsies, where more intensive investigation may be indicated in order to exclude a progressive focal brain lesion. The classification also enables rough guidelines as to choice of anticonvulsant medication to be used and will almost certainly contribute to the understanding of the relation between the epilepsy and the patient's mental state. In drug-resistant cases of partial epilepsy, especially those involving the temporal lobe, the EEG studies will help to lateralize and localize the site of the epileptogenic lesion. Finally, the presence of diffusely slow dominant background EEG frequencies in the absence of recent fits will raise the suspicion of anticonvulsant drug intoxication.

A standard waking EEG of 20 minutes' duration including 3 minutes' hyperventilation and 1–2 minutes of photic stimulation is the usual initial EEG investigation procedure. This is a short time in the daily life of a person and may not be long enough to sample the epileptic abnormalities. These may occur at infrequent intervals. Further, the novelty of the procedure may induce arousal and anxiety, which often tend to inhibit focal epileptic activity. Finally, patients with temporal lobe foci may show no EEG change during the waking state, the temporal lobe spikes only appearing during light sleep. Hence, a single standard EEG recording often makes little contribution to the diagnosis and management of the seizures.

A sleep EEG is required if temporal lobe epilepsy is suspected. In the EEG laboratory, sleep is usually induced by oral quinalbarbitone. A study of the symmetry of the barbiturate fast rhythm, the result of a direct action on the cortex, is a useful, but not always consistent or reliable, aid to lateralization. Relative reduction of amplitude or quantity of the fast rhythm response of a local area of cortex suggests structural pathology at that site. Insertion of sphenoidal electrodes and induction of barbiturate narcosis by an intravenous injection of 2.5 per cent thiopentone or 1 per cent methohexitone may be required to obtain precise localization of spikes of temporal lobe origin. Those originating in the mesial structures (uncal–amygdaloid–hippocampal complex) will show phase reversal at the sphenoidal electrodes. All-night sleep recording may be helpful in the study of nocturnal attacks or when day time sleep EEGs have proved negative. If surgical treatment is being considered, recording of the patient's partial seizures simultaneously by EEG and on videotape is useful. The fits can be induced by slow intravenous injection of 5 per cent metrazol or may be recorded spontaneously during long-term monitoring by telemetry. Sphenoidal electrodes are usually in site during these procedures though implanted electrodes in the mesial structures of both temporal lobes may be used. The special EEG techniques involved in the investigation of epilepsy have been reviewed by Driver and MacGillivray (1976). Continuous ambulatory EEG monitoring using a portable cassette tape recorder is now commonly applied to patients with fits. Such a procedure is now technically feasible because of the development of suitable miniature EEG pre-amplifiers attached to the scalp and a rapid replay system, that permits scrutiny of the recorded data in 20 to 60 times real time. Such ambulatory monitoring throughout the 24 hours enables the patients to be studied in their home environment. It has been successful in the differential diagnosis of hysterical pseudo-seizures from epilepsy and in providing a detailed and accurate measure of the effect of medication on petit mal absences.

A plain X-ray of the skull should always be carried out. Raised intracranial pressure often produces characteristic changes. A shift of a calcified pineal gland from the midline raises the suspicion of a space-occupying lesion. Bone erosion, sclerosis, or hyperostosis of the vault occurs with meningiomata and there may be enlarged vascular channels in the vault. Bone changes also occur with cerebral metastases. Pathological calcification occurs in 10 per cent to 15 per cent of meningiomata, 10 per cent of gliomata especially the more benign ones, temporal lobe glial hamartomata (4 per cent), and 15 per cent of arteriovenous malformations including Sturge-Weber's syndrome, and nodular, curvilinear calcification adjacent to the ventricular system and in the basal ganglia is seen in tuberose sclerosis. Atrophic temporal lobe lesions are indicated by a small middle fossa area floor, a relatively high petrous ridge due to the shallow fossa and thickening of the temporal part of the vault. More widespread thickening of the hemicranium, with flattening of the vault, elevation of the base with enlargement of the air cavities in the sinuses or mastoids on the affected side, occurs with unilateral hemisphere atrophy (hemiatrophy) of early onset. Calcified cysts in skeletal muscles are found in cysticercosis. Hence, soft tissue films of the thighs should be carried out if the patient has lived in the tropics.

If a diagnosis of partial epilepsy is made on clinical and/or EEG grounds, computerized transverse axial tomography should be carried out, if possible. A recent review of the use of CT scanning in epilepsy has demonstrated that 11 per cent of patients of all ages have tumours (16 per cent in those over 20 years). If only partial epilepsies are considered, 22 per cent have tumours. Fifty per cent of all patients have evidence of cerebral lesions, around 60 per cent in the partial and secondary generalized epilepsies. CT scan abnormality is found in 10 per cent or less of patients with primary generalized epilepsy. Of all those patients with epilepsy, in whom CT scanning reveals a lesion, the pathology is atrophic in nature in 56 per cent (Gastaut & Gastaut 1976, Gastaut 1976). Should access to CT scanner be difficult it may be necessary to select for referral those patients with partial epilepsy who have one or more of the following features: (1) recent onset of epilepsy in adult life or late adolescence, (2) if there are clinical, radiological, or EEG grounds to suspect a space-occupying lesion, (3) drug-resistant epilepsy with clinical and/or EEG evidence of a unilateral epileptogenic lesion being considered for surgical excision.

Assessment of the relationship between the epilepsy and the psychiatric disorder

A conventional psychiatric diagnostic formulation should first be carried out. This will include diagnosis of the presenting psychiatric syndrome and an evaluation of the relative importance of genetic, organic, environmental, personality factors, and current situational problems in the genesis of the illness. Then the following sequence of questions concerning the interaction between the fits and mental state, which relate to the time relation between seizure occurrence and mental state disturbance, must be considered.

(a) If there is a direct relationship, then the mental state changes are a direct reflection of the cortical and subcortical dysfunction caused by the epileptogenic discharges.

pre-ictal – usually dysphoric symptoms

ictal – complex partial seizures, petit mal, or psychomotor status

post-ictal – automatisms or confusional states

(b) If there is no direct relationship in time to the fits, the phenomenology of the consequent interictal disorder is likely to resemble that of a functional psychiatric illness and the causation will be multifactorial. The respective roles of the following factors must be considered:

(i) the influence of the underlying epileptogenic lesion on the person's cognitive function, behaviour and emotional state because of its extent (diffuse), location (temporal lobe) or occurrence of frequent subclinical seizure discharges

(ii) the relation between seizure type and frequency and the mental state disturbance

(iii) the respective effects of the anticonvulsant medication on the individual's behaviour, mental processes, and neurological, metabolic, and haematological status

(iv) the effects of having fits and being labelled epileptic on the person's emotional development and acquisition of social, academic, and vocational skills. The impact of all these personal and social factors on the development of the individual's social competence and capacity to cope with current life events should be evaluated. The person's individual style of reacting to the problems of living with a chronic handicap should also be noted, for example the use of the sick role, aggressive acting out behaviour, the ego defence mechanisms of projection, reaction formation.

Of course, all the factors which influence the

development of the interictal disorders may also play a role in determining the psychosocial adjustment of the person who presents with a mental disturbance directly related to seizure occurrence.

Principles of management

After the neuropsychiatric assessment is complete, the psychiatric disorder should be treated and a satisfactory suppressant anticonvulsant drug regime established, care being taken not to further impair the patient's level of functioning by overmedication with consequent psychomotor slowing, lack of alertness, ataxia, and perhaps irritability.

Anticonvulsant medication. The ideal of the drug therapy of epilepsy is to stop all the fits without producing unwanted effects. Unfortunately it is often possible only to decrease their frequency or severity and frequently the therapist must strive to reach a balance between maximal control of fits and the presence of excessive side-effects. Nevertheless it has been estimated that current drugs now completely control seizures in more than half of patients with epilepsy, though not without mild side-effects (Coatsworth, 1971). Another 30 per cent to 40 per cent gain a varying degree of improvement. The treatment usually has to continue for many years because anticonvulsant medication merely raises the seizure threshold and does not cure the disease. Indeed, up to 50 per cent of those controlled on therapy relapse within 5 years when treatment is stopped. The indications for cessation of medication are 3 years of freedom from attacks on treatment. Even then, the presence of abnormal EEG paroxysmal activity such as spikes or spike-wave complexes makes relapse so likely that such a finding is a strong contra-indication to withdrawal of medication. Further, because of the high relapse rate, cessation should not be considered if having a seizure will imperil the patient's wellbeing, for example, if the inevitable loss of a driving licence because of a recent fit will threaten his livelihood. Fortunately, even after a relapse owing to drug withdrawal, control is quickly re-established by resuming the previous doses of medication.

The principles to consider in supervising anticonvulsant medication include patient compliance (at least 40 per cent to 50 per cent of epileptic outpatients do not take the pills as prescribed), drug absorption, distribution, and elimination. All antiepileptic drugs are of small molecular weight and also cross lipid membranes with relative ease, allowing almost total absorption in most cases. On rare occasions, a specific absorption defect in some patients may interfere with the bio-availability of the drug. Further, the rate of absorption will vary with different drug preparations. Drugs taken when the stomach is empty may be absorbed much more rapidly than those taken after a meal. Anticonvulsants, whose lipid solubility is generally high, are distributed to all body tissues in various proportions. The brain concentration is, in most cases, equal to or greater than that of other body tissues. The brain and blood concentrations are usually proportional. Hence, the blood concentrations can be used as an important guide to therapy. Optimum ranges of blood concentration have been formulated for most of the commonly used drugs. Toxic effects are likely if these levels are exceeded.

Knowledge of the elimination half-life of each drug is important clinically. The half-life refers to the time required to remove half of the active drug from the body and influences the following aspects of therapy: (1) frequency of administration. Drugs with longer half-lives (phenytoin, phenobarbitone, and ethosuximide) can be administered once a day without large fluctuations in their concentrations in the blood. Drugs such as carbamazepine and sodium valproate have much shorter half-lives and require to be given two or three times a day; (2) time to reach a steady state. Drugs with long half-lives may require many days to reach a steady state at a new dose level, the time being approximately five times the drug's half-life. However, it must be noted that phenytoin shows peculiar pharmacokinetic characteristics. It undergoes what is called 'saturable metabolism', so that as the dose increases the plasma level rises to much greater levels than would be expected. Hence within the therapeutic range of plasma concentrations the relationship between dose and serum level is such that an increment in dose of less than 100 mg will raise the plasma level from subtherapeutic to toxic levels. Dosage increments of 25 mg with careful monitoring of serum levels are necessary when the serum phenytoin level is in or near the therapeutic range. It should also be noted that some anticonvulsants have active metabolites, which may have much longer half-lives than the parent compounds. Primidone is rapidly converted to phenobarbitone and phenylethylmalonamide. The primidone dosage must be adjusted by monitoring the serum phenobarbitone levels.

Details of the commonly used drugs are dis-

Table 13.1 *Pharmacological properties of six common anticonvulsant drugs*

Drug	Daily dose (mg)	Timing of administration	Therapeutic range (μg)	Serum half-life (hours)	Days to achieve steady state	Toxic level (μg)
Phenytoin	300	Once daily	10–20	24	5–10	20
Phenobarbitone	120	Once daily	15–40	96	14–21	40
Primidone	750–1500	Twice daily	5–15	12	4–7	12
Carbamazepine	1200	Twice daily	4–10	12	2–4	8
Sodium valproate	1000	Twice daily	60–100	short	2–4	100
Ethosuximide	1000	Twice daily	40–80	35	5–8	100

Adapted from Penry, J. K. & Newmark, M. E. (1979) The use of anti-epileptic drugs. *Ann. intern Med.*, **90**, 207–10

played in table 13.1. The drug should be chosen on the basis of type of seizure and EEG findings. Generalized tonic–clonic seizures respond best to phenytoin or carbamazepine. In resistant cases both can be used together. If control is still not possible with these drugs, it will be necessary to resort to phenobarbitone or primidone. The current view is that these latter two drugs are no longer drugs of first choice because they can cause an unacceptable degree of cognitive impairment. Phenobarbitone can also cause irritability and restlessness and aggravate behaviour problems especially in children.

Partial seizures also tend to respond to the same drugs used for generalized seizures, though carbamazepine is now regarded as the drug of first choice for the treatment of temporal lobe epilepsy, which is one of the most difficult types of epilepsy to treat. Carbamazepine does not have the sedative effects of the barbiturates. Indeed it may have a psychotropic effect. However, there is still debate whether this psychotropic action is a primary effect or the result of withdrawal of more sedative compounds. It is certainly equal in anticonvulsant efficacy to phenytoin and phenobarbitone, and may be preferred to phenytoin especially in females because it does not cause hirsutism, coarsen the face, or induce gum hypertrophy, common complications of phenytoin therapy.

If the sole type of seizure is absence attacks, the patient should be treated with ethosuximide or sodium valproate. Atypical absence seizures due to secondary generalized epilepsy and the myoclonic epilepsies are difficult to treat. Sodium valproate and the benzodiazepine drug, clonazepam, are the drugs of choice. Clonazepam is sedative in therapeutic doses

and may aggravate behaviour. Hence sodium valproate is to be preferred. Infantile spasms should be treated by nitrazepam, clonazepam, sodium valproate, or ACTH, the latter being the most effective.

Sulthiame has little value as a primary anticonvulsant agent, though it potentiates the action of phenytoin, phenobarbitone and primidone by inhibiting their metabolism. There is some evidence to suggest that it may improve the behaviour of mentally handicapped patients, possibly because of a sedative effect. Beclamide, another weak anticonvulsant drug, may also have a similar beneficial effect on the behaviour of subnormal patients.

In previously untreated patients, it is best to begin with a small dose of a single drug, given once at night for the first week. The dose should be increased at weekly intervals until control is achieved, unwanted side-effects develop, or the serum level is at the upper end of the therapeutic range. It should be noted that some patients become well-controlled with low serum concentrations. The addition of a second drug should be considered only if fits continue despite adequate serum concentrations. If the fits cease after the introduction of the second drug, the first one should be slowly withdrawn, as the second drug alone may be adequate. When fits continue, the tendency is to add more and newer drugs. Monotherapy is to be preferred because drug interactions are common with many anti-epileptic drugs, usually because of liver enzyme induction or protein binding. The more important drug interactions are summarized in table 13.2. Indeed, studies have shown that the majority of newly diagnosed adult patients with epilepsy can be controlled by the administra-

Table 13.2. *Some important drug interactions involving anti-epileptic drugs*

Drug causing interaction	Result
Interactions between anti-epileptic drugs	
Sulthiame Pheneturide	Increase plasma levels of phenytoin with risk of intoxication
Carbamazepine Phenytoin	Reduce plasma levels of each other diminishing their effects
Sodium valproate	Increases plasma levels of phenobarbitone causing sedation
Interactions with other drugs Isoniazid Chloramphenicol Coumarin anticoagulants Phenothiazines Tricyclic antidepressants Chlorpheniramine	Increase plasma levels of phenytoin with risk of intoxication
Phenytoin Phenobarbitone Primidone Carbamazepine Pheneturide	Cause hepatic enzyme induction, increasing rate of metabolism and therefore reducing effectiveness of many drugs, e.g. oral anticoagulants, corticosteroids, contraceptive pill, tricyclic antidepressants, phenothiazines, benzodiazepines

From Richens, A. (1977) Interactions with anti-epileptic drugs. *Drugs*. 1977, **13,** 266–75

tion of a single drug, carbamazepine or phenytoin, the dosage being adjusted to keep the serum levels within the therapeutic range.

Chronic patients who have long been taking many drugs concurrently are difficult to manage; only a few are likely to be free both of fits and unwanted side effects. Such patients are frequently amongst those presenting with psychiatric problems. Their anticonvulsant drug regime should be reviewed. If their serum folate levels are low, replacement therapy should be given. The earlier fears that folic acid therapy causes an exacerbation of fits have not been realized. A slow reduction in the number of drugs or the dose over a period of several months should be undertaken. This may reduce unwanted effects without worsening control. Indeed there may be an improvement because of increased alertness. Drug-induced drowsiness tends to activate seizure activity. A concomitant psychotropic effect is also often observed with drug reduction. An increase in fit frequency means that the withdrawal was too rapid or that the existing drug regime was having a suppressant effect on the seizures. Another problem with drug withdrawal is that some patients feel safer when taking more than one drug and are reluctant to reduce the number, especially if the multiple drug combination has contributed to seizure control in the past. If polytherapy continues to be necessary to maintain optimum seizure control, it is worth while attempting to replace the drug with the most sedative action, for example, phenobarbitone, by carbamazepine. Further, the combination of drugs with similar actions, for example, phenobarbitone and primidone, should be avoided. Combined preparations should also be avoided as they make it impossible to adjust the dose of each anticonvulsant individually. However, in patients on stable regimes they may allow the total number of tablets to be reduced. The drug treatment of epilepsy is reviewed in detail by Richens (1976) and the chronic side effects by Reynolds (1975).

Surgical treatment of epilepsy. The presence of a focal cortical lesion raises the possibility of excision of the local area of epileptogenic cortex. Surgical excision is considered if the following criteria are fulfilled: (1) the patient is seriously handicapped by frequent seizures, (2) an adequate trial of anticonvulsant medication over 3 to 5 years has failed, (3) clinical and EEG evidence that the attacks arise from a consistently lateralized and localized area of cortex, which can be excised without producing significant neurological deficit or without significantly increasing one that is already present. Rasmussen (1975) reviewed the work of Penfield and his colleagues at the Montreal Neurological Institute. A total of 1267 patients had local cortical excisions between 1928 and 1972 with a median follow-up period of 10 years. Of these 36 per cent became seizure free and 28 per cent were markedly improved. Slightly more than 50 per cent of the patients had temporal lobectomies performed, of whom 39 per cent became fit free and a further 32 per cent had rare or infrequent attacks after surgery. Excisions involving the frontal lobe had a somewhat lower success rate (23 per cent seizure free, 32 per cent marked improvement). Parietal, central, and occipital lobe resections and those for large destructive lesions had outcomes similar to those of the temporal lobectomy patients. The outcome of other temporal lobectomy series have been reviewed by Rodin (1968) with essentially similar results.

Aggressiveness in young men with temporal lobe seizures due to unilateral temporal lobe pathology (more often left-sided and due to mesial temporal sclerosis) frequently responds to temporal lobectomy, though only if there is also control of the seizures. However, it should be stressed that interictal aggressive behaviour in the absence of frequent seizures is not an indication for surgery (Falconer, 1973). Psychoses are not influenced by temporal lobectomy, apart from post-ictal confusional states, which also clear up if the seizures respond to surgery. Hemispherectomy in patients with hemiatrophy, fits, and behaviour disorder often results in relief of seizures and improvement in behaviour. Unfortunately there is a high late mortality and morbidity rate in almost a third due to intracranial haemorrhage into the empty hemicranium (Wilson, 1970).

More recently Cooper (1973) has introduced chronic cerebellar stimulation via implanted electrodes as a treatment for epilepsy and has reported impressive results in quite a large series of patients (Cooper, 1978). Results from other centres using the same technique on small numbers of intractable cases have been disappointing (Fenton, 1979) and we must await the outcome of controlled studies.

Management of the psychiatric disorder. The management of the psychiatric disorder in the person with epilepsy is essentially similar to that of non-epileptics presenting with the same syndrome, with the exception of such ictal events as complex partial seizures, petit mal, and psychomotor status, which require energetic anticonvulsant treatment. Post-ictal confusional states, if prolonged, require a short hospital admission and treatment with adequate doses of chlorpromazine if the patient's behaviour requires sedation.

The schizophrenia-like psychoses also respond well to phenothiazine medication. Depot injections of fluphenazine decanoate or flupenthixol are as useful in controlling chronic psychotic symptoms as they are in the non-epileptic schizophrenic patients. Occasionally, the epileptogenic effects of the phenothiazine drugs can cause an increase in fits. However, this is rarely a problem, providing adequate anticonvulsant medication is prescribed. If such a problem does occur the anticonvulsant drug dosage can be adjusted accordingly or a small dose of diazepam (5mg three times a day) can be added. Depressive psychoses in the person with epilepsy should be treated with antidepressant drugs. Though the tricyclic antidepressants have an epileptogenic action, the same principles of management can be adopted as for the phenothiazine drugs. However nomifensine, which differs from the tricyclic and other antidepressants in that it is a strong inhibitor of dopamine re-uptake at central synapses, has been demonstrated to be one of the few antidepressant drugs which does not alter seizure threshold (Trimble *et al.*, 1977, Nawishy *et al.*, 1980). Hence, in divided daily doses of 50 to 150 mg, it would seem to be the drug of choice, though it does increase serum phenytoin levels during the first week of treatment. In the seriously depressed epileptic patient, who does not respond to an adequate trial of antidepressant medication, there is no contra-indication to the use of ECT. When the florid psychotic symptoms are controlled, the usual principles of management of a depressed or schizophrenic patient should be applied.

In the neuroses and personality disorders associated with epilepsy, anxiety and depressive symptoms, if troublesome to the patient, can be treated by appropriate anxiolytic and antidepressant drugs. The benzodiazepine group, especially diazepam, is useful because of their anticonvulsant action.

A psychotherapeutic approach is also necessary. During the initial few interviews devoted to detailed history taking, rapport will be established with the patient. This will facilitate the process of clarification and non-directive discussion of the patient's symptoms, emotional difficulties, current life problems, and their inter-relationship. Provided that the patient's intelligence level is appropriate and motivation for self-examination present, the exploratory psychotherapy can progress to an in-depth examination of the psychological meaning for the patient of the illness and his habitual defence mechanisms against anxiety. Such an approach will tend to focus on an examination of the relationship between the therapist and patient and how this reflects relationships in his formative years and problems in his current life. The number of sessions of such focal psychotherapy will depend on the amount of available therapeutic time and the therapist's assessment of the patient's capacity to benefit. If this dynamic approach is inappropriate, a more supportive psychotherapeutic role is likely to help by permitting abreaction, reducing emotional distress, providing encouragement and guidance, support of the necessary neurotic defences, and manipulation of the current life situation. In the adolescent or child with behaviour problems associated with epilepsy, work with the parents will be necessary. This will include simple explanation, provision of support, encouragement to ventilate anxiety and other feelings about the patient and his behaviour, discussion and exploration of parental attitudes towards the epilepsy, and attempts at modification of those that are abnormal such as over-protectiveness, unduly high or low expectations of the patient's academic or vocational achievement, and so on. Family or marital psychotherapy may occasionally be indicated if serious family or marital problems are evident. It should be stressed that the selection criteria for admission to psychotherapy of the person with epilepsy should not differ from those applied to non-epileptic patients with neurotic, personality, or psychosomatic disorders.

Because of their very socially restricted and over-protected upbringing, many young people with epilepsy are grossly deficient not only in social skills but also in the basic skills of looking after themselves, for example basic cooking, washing clothes, shopping, and the general aspects of self-care necessary for an independent existence. A ward milieu and occupational therapy programme to improve basic self-care skills and capacity for social interaction can do much to enhance the person's self-esteem and ability to function independently. Formal social skills training can also be helpful. Participation in a ward or out-patient group can help those with deficient interpersonal skills. Such group involvement may be encouraged by participation in the local Action for Epilepsy branch organized by the British Epilepsy Association, a voluntary organization devoted to the welfare of people with epilepsy and their relatives. Active involvement in the local activities of the Association will provide a source of advice and guidance about the problems of living with epilepsy, cater for the needs of those who are socially isolated, and add to the restricted range of their leisure activities. For some, it will provide the setting for the development of hidden talents in organization, administration, persuasion, and various types of handicraft.

Concerning vocational guidance and occupational rehabilitation, collaboration between the social worker and Disablement Resettlement Officer is vital. Skilled counselling may help someone with epilepsy who is looking for a job to take a realistic view of his prospects and to present his disability to a prospective employer in an acceptable way. Admission for assessment to an industrial rehabilitation unit can be arranged with consequent training in a skilled occupation in suitable cases at a government training centre or residential training college. People with epilepsy should be encouraged to enter skilled trades and professions. Such skills as well as making them more viable in the open employment market, will help to dispel some of the stigma which attaches to people with the disease by associating them only with poorly paid or unskilled work.

One hiatus in the system exists between the protected atmosphere of home or school, in which an adolescent with epilepsy may grow up and socially mature, and the vocational and industrial rehabilitation services which are intended to prepare for employment people who have already achieved social maturity. There is a need for much more hostel and other residential accommodation where the immature, dependent person with epilepsy can be encouraged to develop independent attitudes under a degree of supervision which can be tailored to meet his needs.

Once established in a place of work the help of the Industrial Medical Officer is invaluable to ensure that the work is suitable, to inform the person's supervisors and immediate colleagues about what action to take in the event of a fit, and to deal with any other crisis which may occur from time to time. Designers of new industrial equipment may help by making as much equipment as possible safe (by guards, inertia switches, and so on) so that a loss of consciousness by the operator (whether he has epilepsy or not) should not cause injury. Perhaps there should be government grants for the development of such equipment safeguards, to be tried out initially in sheltered workshops.

For the minority of epileptics handicapped so severely as not to be viable in the open employment market, the possibility of sheltered employment must be taken up. For the unemployed epileptic there is no easy transition from life in an institution or at home, with no set occupation except what may be offered at a day centre or in a colony, to full-time employment whether sheltered or not. For some people with epilepsy the early morning is the most dif-

ficult part of the day, and opportunities for a short working day with a late start might remove the risk of regression resulting from the sudden stress of full-time employment. It may be that as day centres for the handicapped develop and take in outside work on a near industrial basis they will enable people with epilepsy to get the feel of a situation progressively approaching that of open industry. Such work-orientated day centres will provide an opportunity for those epileptics incapable of ever sustaining a full-time job because of their handicaps to derive self-esteem and satisfaction from doing productive work and being useful. The successful development of such a centre in Stockholm has been described by Gustaffsson and Prave (1972).

Once the initial diagnosis has been made, treatment commenced, and any necessary social rehabilitation measures put under way, the patient should be reviewed at regular intervals to make sure that he is taking his drugs and that they are effective; to sustain him in handling his life while his fits continue; to minimize the side effects and toxic effects of the drugs; and to ensure that he benefits from advances in treatment.

PART III
Drug-induced disorders

14
Mental disorders due to alcoholism

MAURICE VICTOR

Alcoholism has been defined as both a chronic disease and a disorder of behaviour, characterized in either context by repeated episodes of intoxication or sustained heavy drinking, to the point where it interferes with the drinker's health or his effectiveness on the job, at home, or in the community. Reduced to pharmacological terms, alcoholism is a form of addiction. The need to ingest progressively larger quantities of alcohol in order to obtain the effects of previously smaller doses (tolerance), and the development of distinctive symptoms and signs when alcohol is withdrawn after a period of chronic intoxication (physical dependence), are the major pharmacological criteria of the addictive state. *Alcoholics* are individuals who satisfy these medical, social, and pharmacological criteria.

Virtually every organ system may be adversely affected in the course of alcoholism, but the most common and serious effects are on the nervous system. Some of these effects are attributable to the direct action of alcohol on cerebral neurons, i.e., alcoholic intoxication, and others to the withdrawal of alcohol, following a period of chronic intoxication. Still other effects, such as a loss or impairment of retentive memory (Korsakoff's psychosis), are due not to alcohol *per se*, but to an associated nutritional deficiency. In a similar vein, alcohol may act primarily to cause cirrhosis of the liver, which in turn deranges cerebral function (hepatic encephalopathy). Recently it has been established that alcohol is a relatively uncom-

Table 14.1. *Mental disorders due to alcoholism*

1. Alcoholic intoxication (including 'pathological intoxication', and 'blackouts')
2. The abstinence or withdrawal syndrome (tremulousness, hallucinosis, 'rum-fits,' delirium tremens, atypical confusional–hallucinatory–delusional states)
3. Nutritional diseases of the nervous system, secondary to alcoholism:
   The Wernicke–Korsakoff syndrome
   Pellagra (including 'nicotinic acid-deficiency encephalopathy')
4. Hepatic encephalopathy
5. Foetal alcohol syndrome
6. Alcoholic disorders of uncertain pathogenesis:
   Marchiafava–Bignami disease
   Alcoholic deteriorated state
   'Cerebral atrophy'
   Alcoholic paranoia and jealousy

mon but important cause of mental retardation, the result of the damaging effects of maternal alcoholism on the foetal brain. Finally, there are several neuropsychiatric disorders which are practically confined to alcoholics but in which the pathogenetic role of alcohol is not understood.

Table 14.1 lists the diverse alcohol-induced mental disorders, according to the presumed mechanisms by which alcohol produces its effects.

Alcoholic intoxication
Clinical features

These are so familiar as to require little elaboration. Varying degrees of exhilaration and excitement, loss of restraint, irregularities of behaviour, loquacity, slurred speech, incoordination of movement and gait, irritability, combativeness, drowsiness, stupor, and coma are the usual manifestations.

In a small number of drinkers alcohol has an excitatory rather than a sedative effect. This reaction has been referred to as *pathological* or *complicated intoxication*, and as *acute alcoholic paranoid state*. Since all forms of intoxication are pathological, 'atypical intoxication' would be a more appropriate designation. Nevertheless, pathological intoxication is the term that has survived. The boundaries of this syndrome have never been clearly drawn. In the past, variant forms of delirium tremens and epileptic phenomena as well as psychopathic and criminal behaviour were indiscriminately included under this title (see Banay, 1944, for review of early writings and nosology). Now the term is generally used to designate an outburst of blind fury with assaultive and destructive behaviour. Often the patient is subdued only with difficulty. The attack terminates with deep sleep, which occurs spontaneously or in response to sedation, and on awakening the patient has no memory of the episode. We have not observed the reflex fixity of the pupils which has been said to characterize this syndrome and to outlast the mental symptoms (Bowman & Jellinek, 1941). Nor do we subscribe to the statement that such a reaction may follow the ingestion of a small amount of alcohol; in our experience the amount has always been substantial.

Pathological intoxication has been ascribed to many factors, the most common being constitutional differences in the susceptibility to alcohol, craniocerebral trauma, and an underlying 'hysterical or epileptoid temperament' (Bowman & Jellinek, 1941; Chafetz, 1975). There are no meaningful data to support any of these beliefs. An analogy may be drawn between pathological intoxication and the paradoxical reaction that occasionally follows the administration of barbiturates.

The diagnosis of pathological intoxication may have important legal implications. A person suffering from alcoholism or the usual forms of drunkenness is considered responsible for his actions, whereas a person with pathological intoxication is considered insane at the time and therefore not responsible. The main disorders that need to be distinguished from pathological intoxication are temporal lobe seizures that occasionally take the form of an outburst of rage and violence, and the explosive episodes of violence that characterize the behaviour of certain sociopaths. The diagnosis in these cases may be difficult and depends on eliciting the other manifestations of temporal lobe epilepsy or sociopathy.

'Blackouts', in the language of alcoholics, refer to transient episodes of amnesia which accompany severe degrees of intoxication. After the patient becomes sober, he cannot recall events that had occurred during the drinking episode, even though the state of consciousness (as observed by others) was not grossly altered during that time. The nature and significance of such episodes are unclear. Some psychiatrists deny that a loss of memory has occurred and view the blackout as a form of malingering; others speak of 'repression', which prevents conscious awareness of painful memories. These views are purely speculative. Since 1952, when Jellinek introduced his concept of a step-like development of alcoholism, it has been widely held that the occurrence of blackouts is an early and serious prognostic sign of this disease. On the other hand, the observations of Goodwin, Crane and Guze (1969a, 1969b) indicate that blackouts more often begin at an advanced stage of alcoholism and, more importantly, that this phenomenon may occur in relation to isolated episodes of drinking in persons who never become alcoholics.

It has been proposed that blackouts are related to the deleterious effect of alcohol on short-term memory function (Goodwin *et al.*, 1970; Tamerin *et al.*, 1971). This notion has been discredited by Mello (1973) who showed that tests of short-term memory (up to 6 minutes) were performed equally well by alcoholics with a history of blackouts and those without such a history, at blood alcohol levels above 200 mg per 100 ml; furthermore, there was little difference in the accuracy of performance during periods of intoxication and sobriety.

Pathogenesis

The symptoms of alcoholic intoxication are the result of the depressant action of alcohol on neurons of the central nervous system. Some of the early symptoms, such as garrulousness, aggressive behaviour, and increased electric excitability of the cerebral cortex, suggest an excitatory effect but are probably due to the depression of the high brainstem reticular formation, which ordinarily modulates (inhibits) cerebral cortical activity (Kalant, 1975). Similarly, the initial hyperactivity of tendon reflexes probably represents a transitory escape of spinal motor neurons from higher inhibitory control. As the alcohol concentration rises, the depressant action spreads to involve the cerebral cortical neurons directly, as well as other cerebral and spinal neurons. In these respects, alcohol acts like the inhalation anaesthetics. Unlike the latter agents, the margin between the dose of alcohol that produces surgical anaesthesia and that which dangerously depresses respiration is very narrow. This fact adds an element of urgency to the diagnosis and treatment of alcoholic narcosis.

Treatment

The usual manifestations of alcoholic intoxication require no special treatment. Certain time-honoured remedies such as a warm shower followed by a cold one, strong coffee, forced activity, or induction of vomiting may temporarily reduce the intensity of alcoholic intoxication, but there is no evidence that any of these methods or any of the 'sobering-up' medicines have any lasting effects or significantly influence the rate of disappearance of alcohol from the blood. *Pathological intoxication* may require the use of restraints and the parenteral administration of phenobarbitone 200 mg subcutaneously, or amylobarbitone 500 mg intramuscularly, or corresponding doses of parenteral phenothiazines.

Coma due to alcoholic intoxication represents a medical emergency. Treatment should be carried out in an intensive care unit since the main object is to tide the patient over the crisis in respiration. One must make certain that the patient has a clear airway, by insertion of an endotracheal tube. At the same time, an intravenous infusion of 5 per cent glucose in water should be started, and other causes of coma, particularly those to which the alcoholic is vulnerable – subdural haematoma, pneumonia, meningitis, hepatic failure, and gastrointestinal bleeding – must be systematically excluded. Roentgenograms of the chest and skull, lumbar puncture, and examination of the blood for alcohol, barbiturates, and bromides are routine procedures in these circumstances. If repeated suctioning fails to control the accumulation of secretions, a tracheostomy is required, and an automatic positive-pressure respirator should be available in case of respiratory paralysis. If shock supervenes, immediate treatment with vasopressor drugs and steroids must be instituted.

The use of haemodialysis or peritoneal dialysis has not been fully tested in patients with alcoholic coma, but should be considered in those with extremely high blood alcohol concentrations, particularly if accompanied by acidosis, and in those who have concurrently ingested methanol or ethylene glycol, or some other dialysable drug.

The alcohol withdrawal syndrome

Included under this title is the symptom complex of tremulousness, hallucinations, seizures, and delirium. Each of these major manifestations of alcoholism may occur in more or less pure form and will be so described, but usually they occur in various combinations. The most important and the one indispensable factor in their genesis is a period of relative or absolute abstinence from alcohol, following a period of chronic excessive drinking. For this reason they may collectively be referred to as the abstinence or withdrawal syndrome.

Clinical features

Alcoholic tremulousness. By far the most common manifestation of the abstinence syndrome is tremulousness ('shakes', 'jitters'), combined with general irritability and gastrointestinal symptoms, particularly nausea and vomiting. These symptoms appear after a few consecutive days of drinking, in the morning, after a night's abstinence. The patient 'quiets his nerves' by taking a few drinks, and then he is able to drink for the remainder of the day without distress. This cycle repeats itself for weeks or even months on end; most sprees that result in admission to the hospital last about two weeks. Drinking is usually terminated because of increasing severity of the recurring tremor and vomiting, but for many other reasons as well, such as general weakness, intercurrent injury or infection, or simply a lack of funds or the desire to stop drinking. The symptoms then become greatly augmented, reaching their peak of intensity in 24 to 36 hours after complete cessation of drinking.

The clinical picture is distinctive. The face is flushed, the conjunctivae are injected, and the patient startles easily. Anorexia, nausea, retching, general muscular weakness, mild tachycardia, and insomnia are usual features. The patient may be mildly disoriented and unable to reconstruct the events of the final days of the drinking spree, but he shows no significant confusion, being aware of his surroundings and the nature of his illness.

Generalized tremor is a prominent feature. It is of fast frequency (6 to 8 oscillations per second), slightly irregular and variable in severity, tending to diminish when the patient is in quiet surroundings and attempting no activity and to increase with motor activity or emotional stress. The tremor may be so violent that the patient cannot stand without help, speak clearly, or feed himself. Sometimes there is only fine rapid tremor of the outstretched hands, or there may be little objective evidence of tremor, and the patient complains only of being 'shaky inside'.

Within a few days, the florid appearance, anorexia, weakness, tachycardia, and tremor subside to a large extent, but the tendency to startle easily, jerkiness of movement, sleeplessness, and general feeling of uneasiness may not leave the patient completely for 10 to 14 days.

Alcoholic hallucinosis. Symptoms of disordered perception occur in about 25 per cent of the tremulous patients. The patient may complain of 'bad dreams' – nightmarish episodes associated with disturbed sleep – which he finds difficult to separate from real experience. Sounds and shadows may be misinterpreted, or familiar objects may appear distorted. These are not hallucinations in the strict sense of the term but represent the commonest forms of disordered perception in the alcoholic.

In patients who experience true hallucinations, mixed visual–auditory ones are the most frequent; less often, the hallucinations are purely visual or auditory. Tactile and olfactory hallucinations are relatively infrequent and almost always combined with visual and auditory ones. Visual hallucinations are more often animate than inanimate; persons or animals may appear singly or in panoramas, shrunken or enlarged, natural and not unpleasant or hideous and frightening. There is little evidence to support the popular belief that certain visual hallucinations (bugs, 'pink elephants') are particular to alcoholism. Auditory hallucinations are described below.

Acute and chronic auditory hallucinosis. A special type of alcoholic psychosis, consisting essentially of an auditory hallucinosis, has been recognized for many years. This disorder was referred to by Kraepelin (1946) as the *hallucinatory insanity of drunkards* or alcoholic mania, and by Wernicke (1900) as the *acute hallucinosis of drunkards.* Kraepelin believed that auditory hallucinosis was related to delirium tremens, but Bleuler (1930), who named this condition *alcoholic hallucinosis,* stated that in such cases he could 'demonstrate with certainty or greater probability that besides the alcoholism a long-standing schizophrenia was present'. Subsequent writings have tended to support one or other of these contentions. The literature on this subject has been reviewed by Victor and Hope (1958), who also described the clinical features of 76 personally-studied patients with this disorder.

The central feature of the illness is the occurrence of auditory hallucinations in an otherwise clear sensorium. The hallucinations may take the form of unstructured sounds such as shots, clicking, and so forth (the elementary hallucinations of Bleuler), or they may have a musical quality, taking the form of a low-pitched hum or chant. Buzzing and ringing in the ears or other forms of tinnitus are reported by more than a third of the patients with auditory hallucinations (Sabot *et al.*, 1968). But the most common type of hallucination, occurring in practically every patient with this disorder, is vocal. The voices may address the patient directly, or, more frequently, discuss him in the third person and are attributed by the patient to family members, friends, or neighbours, and rarely to God, the devil, or radar. The voices are intensely real and tend to be exteriorized; that is, they come from behind the door, from the corridor or floor below, or through the wall, and the patient's response to them is appropriate (this is true of visual hallucinations as well). Most often the voices are maligning and threatening in nature and the patient may call the police for protection or barricade himself against invaders; he may even attempt suicide to avoid what the voices threaten. Less often the hallucinations are concerned with casual items and are unrelated or undirected to the patient, in which case there may be little or no objective evidence of their presence.

Some patients report the occurrence of hallucinations 'while drinking', presumably in relation to a decrease in the blood alcohol level, and in this circumstance the hallucinations can be suppressed by a few drinks or a large dose of paraldehyde or other sedative medication. More often the hallucinations become apparent only after complete cessation of drinking and are most prominent in the following 24 to 48 hours. The hallucinations vary from fleeting and fragmentary experiences to an elaborate, more or less continuous series of events. The total duration of the illness is usually brief, 6 days or less in 85 per cent of our cases (Victor & Hope, 1958). While hallucinating, patients are rarely aware of the unreality of their sensory experience; most gain insight only when the hallucinations have ceased. Characteristically the patient begins to doubt the reality of his hallucinations and is reluctant to talk about them, and he may even question his sanity. Full recovery is marked by the realization that the voices were imaginary and by the ability of the patient to recall, often with remarkable clarity, the content of the psychotic episode.

A unique feature of this disease is the evolution, in a small proportion of patients, of a state of *chronic auditory hallucinosis*. The chronic disorder begins like the acute one, but after a short period, perhaps a week, the symptomatology begins to change. The patient becomes quiet and resigned, despite the fact that the hallucinations remain threatening and derogatory. Ideas of reference and influence and other poorly systematized delusions become

Table 14.2. *Analysis of 266 consecutive patients admitted with complications of alcohol abuse to the Boston City Hospital*[a]

	Number	%
Acute intoxication	56	21
Stupor or coma (27 patients)		
Combative state (15 patients)		
Acute alcoholic tremulousness	92	34.6
Tremor and transitory hallucinations	30	11.3
Auditory hallucinosis	6	2.3
Typical delirium tremens	14	5.3
'Atypical' delirious–hallucinatory states	11	4.1
Nutritional diseases of the nervous system	8	3.0
Others[b]	49	18.4
Rum fits[c]	32	12

[a] Source: Victor, M. & Adams, R. D. (1953)
[b] Patients who could not be categorized precisely because of severe head injury or medical or surgical disease.
[c] The figure for rum-fits means that seizures complicated the various alcohol withdrawal states in 12 per cent of cases.

prominent. At this stage, the illness may be mistaken for schizophrenia, and indeed has been so identified by Bleuler (1930). There are, however, important differences between the two disorders: the alcoholic illness develops in close temporal relationship to a drinking bout and at a considerably later age than schizophrenia, and the past history rarely reveals schizoid personality traits. Alcoholic patients with hallucinosis are not distinguished by a high incidence of schizophrenia within their families (Schuckit & Winokur, 1971; Scott, 1967). Also, such patients who were studied long after their acute attack did not show an increased incidence of schizophrenia (Victor and Hope, 1958; Benedetti, 1952).

Delirium tremens. This is the most dramatic and serious form of the alcohol withdrawal syndrome. It is characterized by profound confusion, the presence of vivid hallucinations and delusions, tremor, agitation, and sleeplessness, as well as by signs of increased autonomic nervous system activity. Defined in this way, delirium tremens is a relatively rare disease (table 14.2). At the Boston City Hospital the diagnosis of delirium tremens was made in only 5 per cent of alcoholic admissions (Victor & Adams,

1953), and at the Bellevue Psychiatric Hospital, in 2.6 per cent (Wortis, 1940).

Delirium tremens develops in one of several settings. The patient, practically always one who has been drinking excessively for many years, may have been admitted to the hospital for an unrelated infectious illness, accident, or operation. More frequently the problem is clearly one of alcoholism from the beginning; following a protracted drinking spree, the patient may already have experienced varying degrees of tremulousness, hallucinosis, and/or seizures. Or he may even be recovering from these symptoms when those of delirium tremens assert themselves.

The clinical picture, in severe cases, is one of the most colourful in all of medicine. The patient is constantly agitated, disarranging the bedclothes, or tugging at his restraints. More complex restless movements are usually related to some delusion or hallucination; characteristic are the turning of the head and eyes toward some imaginary person, persistent searching movements in which the patient ransacks his bedclothes for some object which he supposes to be concealed there, and re-enacting of habitual acts having to do with the patient's occupation. Some of the patient's incessant activity may be explained by the misbelief that he is in some way being retained against his will; he strives to escape, and although he may momentarily be persuaded to return to bed, he is soon attempting to get up again.

A coarse, irregular tremor affecting the extremities, face, and tongue is a universal feature. The tremor tends to increase with any sustained action, and it may be so violent as to render the simplest voluntary movement impossible. Picking and fumbling movements are also typical. The patient's speech may be slurred and garbled, to the point of unintelligibility. He may shout and scream for hours on end, or his speech may be reduced to an almost inaudible muttering. At times he falters over words, or he may speak in neologisms, indicating the presence of a mild dysphasia as well as a disturbance of articulation. Signs of over-activity of the autonomic nervous system are characteristic of delirium tremens and serve, more than any other feature, to distinguish it from nonalcoholic forms of delirium. Dilated pupils, tachycardia, fever, and hyperhidrosis are the usual manifestations; excessive pilomotor responses, pallor or flushing, nausea, constipation, and diarrhoea may also be present.

Invariably there is an impairment of those faculties which enable the patient to place himself properly in time and place and to grasp the meaning of his surroundings. The patient may not know, for example, whether he is standing or lying, what clothing he is wearing, and whether he is indoors or out. Also impaired are the power of attention and ability to concentrate. At times the patient cannot be distracted from a preoccupation with some abnormal activity or thought process; at other times he seems to be overly alert and is distracted by the slightest stimulus. A new stimulus may make only a momentary impression, or it may become the focal point for a new preoccupation from which it is again difficult to turn the patient's attention. If one can gain the patient's attention for a moment, flashes of clear insight and accurate responses may be obtained. He may even recall material that he was asked to remember at a previous examination and which left him seemingly unimpressed at that time. These observations indicate that the patient's confusion is largely due to inattention and inaccurate interpretation of sensory experiences, rather than to a primary defect in retentive memory.

The perceptual disturbance in delirium tremens most often consists of the false interpretation of sensory impressions (illusions). The patient misidentifies people and misinterprets the meaning of what he sees and hears. Or the perceptual disorder may have no apparent basis in reality (hallucinations). The disorder in perception is further characterized by the patient's ready response to suggestion. He may, for example, be provoked to go through the motions of opening and drinking down a bottle of beer or lighting a cigar simply by handing him such imaginary objects. Poorly systematized delusions may be prominent and frequently have a paranoid colouring – the patient believes that he is being imprisoned, stalked or pursued and that he is in imminent danger of being shot, poisoned, or castrated.

The mood and affect in delirium tremens are marked by their lability. The patient may appear elated, detached, or perplexed, with a tendency to be facetious. Or, at any moment, the patient's attitude may be transformed to one of suspicion or truculence. Vague apprehension and fear are the rule; when threatened by imaginary danger the patient not only reacts by visible concern or terror, but displays the physiological concomitants of fear as well.

In the majority of cases, delirium tremens is of short duration and ends abruptly with deep sleep. Less often the delirium subsides gradually; more

Table 14.3. *Course and duration of 101 cases of delirium tremens*[a]

	No. of Cases		
Nonfatal outcome		86	
Single episode		76	
Abrupt termination	49		
Gradual termination	27		
Recurrent episodes (3–31 days)		10	
Fatal outcome		15	

Duration of 69 single episodes of delirium tremens Hours	No. of Cases	%
24 hr or less	10	*(14.5)*
25–48 hr	17	*(24.6)*
49–72 hr	30	*(43.5)*
73–96	6	*(8.7)*
>4 days	6	*(8.7)*

[a] Source: Victor & Adams (1953)

rarely still there may be one or more relapses, several episodes of delirium of varying severity being separated by intervals of relative or complete lucidity, the entire process lasting for several days, or exceptionally, for several weeks. The course and outcome of delirium tremens, as observed in 101 patients, are summarized in table 14.3. Noteworthy in this series is the mortality of 15 per cent. In some of these patients death was attributable to associated infection or injury. Other patients died of inexplicable hyperthermia or peripheral circulatory collapse. In still others, death came so suddenly that the terminal events could not be discerned and the cause of death remained obscure even after post-mortem examination. With optimal treatment the mortality from delirium tremens has been reduced considerably (Tavel, Davidson & Batterton, 1961). However, reports of a negligible mortality in delirium tremens can usually be attributed to a failure to distinguish between delirium tremens, as defined above, and the minor withdrawal syndrome, which is far more common and almost invariably benign.

Atypical delirious–hallucinatory states. Reference is made here to variant forms of delirium tremens in which one facet of the symptom complex assumes prominence to the practical exclusion of the others. There may be a transient state of quiet confusion,

agitation, or violent behaviour. Other cases are characterized by a vivid delusional state, in which the patient relates some loosely-connected and implausible tale. In still others, hallucinations are prominent or several of these symptoms may be combined. These 'atypical' states are about as common as typical delirium tremens (table 14.2) and resemble the latter in their duration and in the relatively long interval that separates their onset from the cessation of drinking. Unlike typical delirium tremens, they present as a circumscribed episode without recurrences, are only rarely preceded by epilepsy, and do not end fatally. This may simply mean that we are dealing with a partial or less severe form of delirium tremens.

The pathological basis of delirium tremens and related disorders has not been determined. The most frequently described abnormalities are cerebral oedema or 'wet brain', pial congestion, thickening of the meninges, and diffuse pyknosis and 'acute swelling' of cerebral neurons (Courville, 1955; Marchand, 1932). These changes are of questionable significance. Pial congestion and meningeal thickening are ubiquitous neuropathological findings and by no means typical of delirium tremens, and the neuronal changes are probably artefactual. Pathological examination of our own material has been singularly unrevealing, as one might expect of a disease that is essentially reversible. Brain swelling and oedema have been absent except where shock or anoxia had occurred terminally, and even in these latter instances the changes have been mild in degree. Nor have there been any significant microscopic changes in the brain.

Pathogenesis of the tremulous–hallucinatory– convulsive–delirious states

As has been indicated, the most important and the one indispensable factor in the genesis of delirium tremens and kindred disorders is the relative or absolute withdrawal of alcohol after a period of chronic intoxication. Although this idea is hardly new, it only gained general acceptance in relatively recent years. As long ago as 1852, Magnus Huss (quoted by Jellinek, 1943) drew a distinction between convulsions in epileptics who drank and convulsions brought about by the cessation of drinking. This latter relationship was also commented upon by other writers in the last century (Bratz, 1899; Féré, 1892). In 1901, Bonhoeffer stated that the sudden withdrawal of alcohol was an important factor in the precipitation of delirium tremens, and this concept was subsequently reaffirmed by others (Hare, 1915; Osler,

1928; Lambert, 1934; Kalinowsky, 1942). For reasons that are difficult to understand, this point of view failed to prevail. In the 1930s, statements that denied the causative role of alcohol withdrawal came to carry as much weight as those which affirmed it. One notion in particular gained credence, namely that 'abstinence is in itself an expression of the beginning of delirium'. Originally stated by Bumke and Kant (1936), this view was elaborated by Noyes (1939), and by Bowman and his colleagues (1939). The latter authors regarded 'disgust for alcohol', as well as nausea and vomiting consequent on gastritis and hepatitis, as the initial symptoms of delirium tremens, rather than possible precipitating factors. Some authors rejected the withdrawal theory on the ground that only a small proportion of their alcoholic patients developed delirium tremens after being jailed or admitted to the hospital (Bostock, 1939; Bowman et al., 1939). A study that was often quoted to discredit the withdrawal theory was that of Piker (1937), who stated, after questioning 275 patients with 'delirium tremens', that 74.5 per cent had the onset of their symptoms while still drinking; implicit in Piker's statement was the view that delirium tremens was but an extreme form of alcoholic intoxication. It was evidence such as this which led to the rejection of the alcohol withdrawal theory and enabled Bowman and Jellinek to write, in 1941, that the alcohol withdrawal theory had been virtually discarded in the United States. In Europe, also, the role of alcohol in the causation of delirium tremens was relegated into obsolescence, judging from the writings of Bumke and Kant (1936) and of Bleuler (1951).

The arguments that denied the role of alcohol withdrawal in the genesis of delirium tremens were supported neither by logic nor meaningful evidence. Piker's data (1937) were based solely on patients' statements, without corroboration from independent sources; like other authors of his period, he failed to consider the possible effects of relative abstinence or a falling blood alcohol level in the genesis of symptoms. And Bowman and colleagues (1939) simply overlooked the facts that delirium tremens need not develop in a setting of nausea, vomiting, and disgust for alcohol and that these disorders occurred frequently in other settings, viz., following the abrupt imposition of abstinence by injury, infection, admission to the hospital for elective surgery, lack of funds, or other factors.

The idea that delirium tremens and related disorders simply represent the extreme effects of alcoholic intoxication is untenable for several reasons. The symptoms of toxicity (slurred speech, staggering, drowsiness, stupor, and so on) are in themselves distinctive and quite different from the symptom complex of tremor, hallucinosis, fits, and delirium. The former symptoms are invariably associated with an elevated blood alcohol level and the latter with a *reduction* in the blood alcohol from a previously higher level (Freund, 1969; Isbell et al., 1955; Mendelson & LaDou, 1964). Finally, the symptoms of intoxication worsen with the continued ingestion of alcohol, whereas the administration of alcohol may nullify tremor and hallucinations and even delirium tremens may subside in an ordinary manner when the patient is being given a pint or more of whiskey daily (Victor & Adams, 1961).

Our clinical observations, which were made on open medical wards of a large general hospital, strongly supported the withdrawal theory (Victor & Adams, 1953). We found that the mildest withdrawal symptoms, such as tremulousness and morning nausea, appeared after only a few days of drinking and after a relatively short period (several hours) of abstinence. The most severe symptoms, those of delirium tremens, required a background of many weeks or months of chronic intoxication and became manifest only after several days of abstinence (peak incidence between 72 and 96 hours). These conclusions were confirmed by Isbell and co-workers (1955) and later by Mendelson and LaDou (1964), who studied the effects of alcoholic intoxication and withdrawal in human volunteers under controlled conditions. Ultimate corroboration of the withdrawal theory came with the production of unmistakable alcohol abstinence phenomena, consisting of tremor, over-activity, and convulsions, in several animal species – in mice (Freund, 1969; Goldstein, 1972a; Goldstein, 1972b; Goldstein & Pal, 1971; Griffiths, Littleton & Ortiz, 1973), in rats (French & Morris, 1972; Lieber & DeCarli, 1973) and in rhesus monkeys (Ellis & Pick, 1970). The animal models of alcoholism which fulfil the pharmacological criteria of tolerance and physical dependence have been reviewed in detail by Mello (1976).

The precise mechanisms that are involved in the production of withdrawal symptoms are not fully understood. Nutritional deficiency is probably not a factor, since withdrawal symptoms may occur in patients who are adequately nourished (Isbell et al., 1955; Mendelson & LaDou, 1964; Victor & Adams, 1961) and have been observed to subside uneventfully in patients denied all food and vitamins (Victor & Adams, 1961). The claim by Smith (1950), that exhaustion of the adrenal cortex, the result of stimulation of ACTH secretion by alcohol, is a factor, has not been substantiated by other workers (Czaja & Kalant, 1961; Krusius, Vartia & Forsander, 1958).

Low serum concentrations of potassium, sodium, and calcium are observed inconsistently in patients with chronic alcoholism. These electrolyte abnormalities may be found during intoxication as well as withdrawal and probably reflect the poor nutritional state of many alcoholics. Hypomagnesaemia is regularly associated with the withdrawal syndrome, at least its early stages (Flink *et al.*, 1954; Heaton *et al.*, 1962; Mendelson *et al.*, 1959; Randall, Rossmeisl & Bleifer, 1959; Suter & Klingman, 1955; Wacker & Vallee, 1958; Wolfe & Victor, 1969). The fact that the serum magnesium level may return to normal by the time the patient develops delirium tremens indicates that hypomagnesaemia cannot be incriminated in the genesis of the latter syndrome (Wacker & Vallee, 1958; Wolfe & Victor, 1969).

Probably of greater significance than hypomagnesaemia is the rise in arterial pH that accompanies the withdrawal state (Sereny, Rapoport, & Husdon, 1966; Wolfe & Victor, 1969). This alkalosis has proved to be respiratory in nature, the result of tachypnoea and increased depth of respiration (Wolfe *et al.*, 1969). On the basis of a series of clinical-experimental studies, we have proposed that the compounded effects of acute hypomagnesaemia and respiratory alkalosis, each of which is known to be associated with hyperexcitability of the nervous system, are responsible for the symptoms of the early withdrawal period (Victor & Wolfe, 1973).

Treatment of the withdrawal syndrome

The following remarks deal primarily with the treatment of delirium tremens, but the same principles are applicable to the minor forms of the withdrawal syndrome.

Treatment begins with a careful search for an associated injury or infection, particularly cerebral laceration, subdural haematoma, pneumonia, and meningitis. Skull and chest films and lumbar puncture should therefore be obtained routinely, and liver function should be assessed. The noisy and agitated patient has to be placed in a separate room; if he is extremely active, a locked room, a screened window, and a low bed or mattress on the floor should be arranged. If an attendant or family member can be

with the patient, it is preferable to allow the patient to move about the room rather than to tie him in bed.

The most important aspect of treatment is the correction of fluid and electrolyte imbalance. Tavel and colleagues (1961) analysed the clinical records of 39 patients who had died of delirium tremens and estimated that only 10 of them had received adequate fluids. Severe degrees of agitation and perspiration require the administration of 4 to 10 litres of fluid daily, of which one-quarter should be normal saline. Other electrolytes are added as indicated by the laboratory examinations. Occasionally, the withdrawal syndrome is characterized by hypoglycaemia which calls for the administration of glucose (Field *et al.*, 1963; Freinkel *et al.*, 1963). Because the intravenous use of glucose in nutritionally-depleted alcoholics may precipitate Wernicke's disease, B vitamins should be added to the parenteral fluid. The occurrence of peripheral circulatory collapse requires the use of whole-blood transfusions and vasopressor drugs, and hyperthermia should be managed with ice packs or a cooling mattress, in addition to specific drugs for any infection that may be present.

Finally, one must not neglect the many small measures that may allay the patient's fears and suspicion and reduce the tendency to hallucinations. The room should be kept well lighted and the patient should be moved as little as possible. Every procedure should be explained in detail, even such simple ones as taking the blood pressure or temperature. The presence of a member of the family may help the patient to maintain contact with reality.

The use of drugs in the treatment of delirium tremens and related disorders. This is the subject of a vast literature, much of which is uncritical and misleading. Extravagant claims, unsupported by meaningful data, have been made for innumerable drugs. Another shortcoming of this literature is the failure, on the part of many authors, to define what is being treated, no distinction being made between alcohol dependency, alcoholic intoxication, withdrawal symptoms, and even Korsakoff's psychosis and polyneuropathy. In so far as the pathogenesis of each of these disorders is different, it is hardly logical to treat them as one disease. Furthermore, many authors fail to distinguish between the early and relatively mild syndrome, from which the patient almost invariably recovers, and delirium tremens, which occurs later in the withdrawal period and is potentially lethal. The former or 'minor' withdrawal syndrome responds to treatment with virtually any sedative-hypnotic drug; in fact, it responds in a comparable manner without the use of any drugs (Whitfield *et al.*, 1978). In contrast, the symptoms of delirium tremens ('major' withdrawal syndrome) are relatively resistant to all forms of drug therapy.

These caveats notwithstanding, the medical literature, particularly of the last two decades, does contain a number of careful studies of the value of drugs in the treatment of the alcohol withdrawal syndromes. These have been reviewed fully by Victor (1966) and more recently by Gessner (1979). It is evident that many drugs, in addition to paraldehyde and the barbiturates, have the capacity to alleviate the symptoms of alcohol withdrawal. A partial list includes prochlorperazine (Compazine), chlorpromazine (Thorazine), promazine (Sparine), promethazine (Phenergan), meprobamate, reserpine, chlordiazepoxide (Librium), diazepam (Valium), benactyzine, haloperidol and perhaps propranolol. Chlormethiazole has achieved considerable popularity in Europe, but is not available in the United States. Also, it appears that some of these drugs are more effective than others. Chlorpromazine and promazine are essentially indistinguishable in performance (Laties *et al.*, 1958) but both are superior to reserpine and meprobamate (Godfrey, Kissen & Downs, 1958), and promethazine is superior to promazine (Shea, Schultz, Lewis & Fazekas, 1958). Sereny and Kalant (1965) found little difference in the effects of chlordiazepoxide and promazine, and both of these drugs proved to be only slightly more effective than a placebo.

Although all of the above-mentioned drugs are effective to some degree in controlling minor withdrawal symptoms, there is little convincing evidence that any of them can prevent delirium tremens or shorten the duration or reduce the mortality of the latter disorder (Rosenfeld & Bizzoco, 1961; Fazekas, Shea & Rea, 1955; Gruenwald, Hanlon, Wachsler & Kurland, 1960). The study of Kaim, Klett and Rothfeld (1969) would indicate that chlordiazepoxide is more effective than chlorpromazine in preventing alcohol withdrawal seizures and delirium tremens, but neither of these drugs was compared with paraldehyde. In fact, in the management of severe forms of the withdrawal syndrome, there is evidence that paraldehyde or a combination of paraldehyde and chloral are superior to both the major and minor tranquillizers (Friedhoff & Zitrin, 1959; Ewing, 1960; Hart, 1961; Thomas & Freedman, 1964; Golbert, Sanz,

Rose & Leitschuh, 1967; Muller, 1969). Recently, Thompson and co-workers (1975) reported that patients with delirium tremens who were treated with diazepam (10 mg initially, then 5 mg intravenously every 5 minutes) became calm in a shorter period of time than patients treated with paraldehyde (10 ml in 2 volumes of cottonseed oil rectally every 30 minutes). However, the mode of paraldehyde administration in this study does not permit the assessment of the comparative value of the two drugs (Gessner, 1979).

Phenothiazines are to be avoided in the treatment of the alcohol withdrawal syndrome, because they reduce the threshold to seizures and patients treated with these drugs have a higher mortality than those treated with other sedatives and hypnotics (Golbert *et al.*, 1967; Thomas & Freedman, 1964). ACTH and cortisone have no place in the treatment of the withdrawal syndrome. The startling original claims for this form of treatment (Smith, 1950) have not been borne out by subsequent studies (Berman, 1956; Owen, 1954; Tavel *et al.*, 1961; Victor & Adams, 1953; Wexler *et al.*, 1958). In addition, these hormones have several serious disadvantages, namely, the masking of infection, a deleterious effect on tuberculosis and peptic ulcer, and a tendency to produce a negative nitrogen balance and excessive excretion of potassium. All of these complications are of more than theoretical interest in the alcoholic patient.

Finally, it should be emphasized that the object of drug therapy in delirium tremens is not the absolute suppression of agitation and tremor; to accomplish this requires an amount of drug that might seriously depress respiration. The purpose of medication is to blunt the agitation and prevent exhaustion and to facilitate nursing care and the administration of parenteral fluids. It would appear that the safest and most effective drugs for this purpose are paraldehyde given orally and diazepam or chlordiazepoxide, when parenteral administration is necessary.

The Wernicke-Korsakoff syndrome

In deference to conventional practice, the clinical features of Wernicke's disease and Korsakoff's psychosis will be described separately. In alcoholics, however, the two disorders usually occur together. For this reason, and others to be elaborated later, Wernicke's disease and Korsakoff's psychosis should be regarded as two aspects of the same disease. Stated in another way, Korsakoff's psychosis is the chronic mental component of Wernicke's disease.

Unless otherwise stated, the following description of the Wernicke-Korsakoff syndrome is based on the personal study of 245 patients with this disorder, many of whom were followed for 10 years or longer and 82 of whom had complete post-mortem examinations (Victor, Adams & Collins, 1971). The reader is referred to this study for a more complete account than can possibly be given here.

Wernicke's disease (Wernicke's encephalopathy; polioencephalitis haemorrhagia superioris)

In 1881, Carl Wernicke described an illness of sudden onset characterized by paralysis of eye movements, ataxic gait, and mental confusion. His observations were based on the study of three patients, two of whom were alcoholics and one a young woman who had developed persistent vomiting after the ingestion of sulphuric acid. In all three, there was progressive drowsiness, stupor, and death. Wernicke also described petechial haemorrhages in the grey matter around the third and fourth ventricles and aqueduct of Sylvius. He regarded these lesions as inflammatory in nature and named the disease 'polioencephalitis haemorrhagica superioris'.

The clinical triad of ophthalmoplegia, ataxia, and mental disturbance is still diagnostically useful, but Wernicke's designation is no longer appropriate. The neuropathological changes are neither inflammatory nor limited to the grey matter or upper brain-stem; haemorrhages occur in only a minority of cases, and when present they usually do not constitute the most significant pathologic change.

Incidence, sex distribution and age of onset

Precise information about the incidence of the Wernicke-Korsakoff syndrome is not available. At the Boston City Hospital, in a two-year period (1950–51), this syndrome accounted for 0.13 per cent of all admissions and about 3 per cent of the alcoholic admissions. At the Massachusetts General Hospital, which drew its patients from a much wider territory, the incidence was roughly 0.05 per cent of all admissions. The incidence, as judged from post-mortem material, is much higher. At the Cleveland Metropolitan General Hospital, in a series of 3548 consecutive autopsies in adults, the lesions of the Wernicke-Korsakoff syndrome were found in 77 cases, or 2.2

per cent (Victor & Laureno, 1978). At the Royal Perth Hospital, in Western Australia, such lesions were found in 1.7 per cent of all necropsies (Harper, 1979). In our series, males were affected slightly more often than females (3:2); since the incidence of alcoholism is much higher in men than in women (Keller & Gurioli, 1976) the incidence of the Wernicke-Korsakoff is disproportionately high in female alcoholics, a feature that characterizes other alcoholic-nutritional disorders as well. The disease had its highest incidence in the fifth and sixth decades (range 30 to 70 years).

The ocular abnormalities are the most consistent clinical manifestations and the diagnosis of the illness, at least at its onset, can hardly be made in their absence. The usual ocular abnormalities are horizontal and vertical nystagmus, abducens palsies, and palsies of conjugate gaze. Each of these may represent the only ocular abnormality, but usually they occur together. The pupils are usually normal but may become small and non-reactive in the most advanced stages of the disease. Funduscopic examination rarely discloses small retinal haemorrhages, but we have never observed papilloedema in this disease. Pallor of the optic disc, also a rare finding, is usually attributable to an associated optic neuropathy ('tobacco–alcohol amblyopia').

Ataxia is the second major abnormality. In its most severe form the patient cannot stand or walk without support. Less severe forms are characterized by a wide-based stance and a slow, short-stepped, unsteady gait. The mildest degree of ataxia can be demonstrated only by heel-to-toe walking.

Signs of *peripheral neuropathy* are found in more than 80 per cent of cases. Usually the polyneuropathy is mild in degree and does not account for the gait disorder, but in a small proportion of patients the neuropathy is so severe that stance and gait cannot be tested.

Mental disturbances. All but 10 per cent of patients who present with Wernicke's disease show some derangement of mental function. Most often this takes the form of a profound confusional state, compounded of apathy and an incapacity to sustain physical and mental activity, impairment of awareness and responsiveness, disorientation, inattention, and derangement of perceptual and memory functions. Coma is uncommon as a presenting feature. In these circumstances, adequate assessment of memory function is not possible. Some patients, however, are alert and responsive from the time they are first seen, and in them it can be recognized that memory function is disproportionately affected. In fact, an amnesic (Korsakoff's) psychosis may be the only manifestation of the syndrome, ocular signs and ataxia being absent.

Course of the illness

The manifestations of Wernicke's disease respond to specific treatment (administration of thiamine) in a fairly uniform manner. Recovery of the *ocular abnormalities* often begins within hours after the administration of thiamine. The sixth-nerve palsies recover completely, within a week in most cases. Ptosis and gaze palsies also recover completely but somewhat more slowly. In 60 per cent of cases, a fine horizontal nystagmus remains as a permanent sequela. A failure of the ocular palsies to respond in this manner should raise doubt about the diagnosis.

In comparison to the ocular signs, the response of *ataxia* to the administration of thiamine is somewhat delayed. Furthermore, in about half of the cases recovery is incomplete and the patient is left with a slow, shuffling, wide-based gait and inability to walk tandem. The residual disturbance of gait, like horizontal nystagmus, provides a means of identifying obscure and chronic cases of dementia as alcoholic–nutritional in origin.

The global confusional state improves also under the influence of thiamine, but the mode of recovery is variable. In about 15 per cent of patients the confusion recedes rapidly and completely, in a matter of a week or two, and the patient then remains mentally clear. In the remainder, the confusional state improves more slowly and, as it recedes, the defects in memory and learning (Korsakoff's psychosis) stand out more clearly. The memory disorder, once it becomes established, improves in only a small proportion of patients, as indicated in the following section.

Korsakoff's psychosis (Korsakoff's syndrome; amnesic or amnestic-confabulatory psychosis; psychosis polyneuritica)

These terms refer to a unique mental disorder in which retentive memory is impaired out of all proportion to other cognitive functions, in an otherwise alert and responsive patient. Although a number of early writers, beginning with Magnus Huss, in 1852, made casual reference to a disturbance of memory in the course of chronic alcoholism, the first compre-

hensive account of this disorder was given by S. S. Korsakoff, in a series of articles published between 1887 and 1891 [for English translation and commentary, see Victor & Yakovlev (1955)]. Korsakoff's original report (1887), based on observations of 20 alcoholic patients, stressed the relationship between polyneuritis and the disorder of memory, which, he proposed, represented 'two facets of the same disease' (*psychosis polyneuritica*). In later articles he made the points, generally disregarded by subsequent authors, that the mental disorder may complicate a variety of nonalcoholic illnesses and that it need not be accompanied by affection of the peripheral nerves (Korsakoff, 1889a & 1889b).

Clinical features

Korsakoff's psychosis is characterized by two fundamental abnormalities: (1) an impaired ability to recall information that had been acquired over a period of years before the onset of the illness (*retrograde amnesia*); and (2) an impaired ability to acquire new information, i.e., to learn or to memorize (*anterograde amnesia*). Confabulation, an ill-defined symptom which has come to be regarded as a specific feature of Korsakoff's psychosis, is neither consistently present nor is it a requisite for the diagnosis. Other cognitive functions are impaired to a relatively minor degree. As a rule, patients have only limited insight into their disability and tend to be apathetic and inert, and indifferent to persons and events around them.

The definition of Korsakoff's psychosis also requires that certain aspects of mental function be intact. The patient must be alert and responsive, aware of his surroundings, and capable of understanding the meaning of what is said to him, of making proper deductions from given premises, and of solving such problems as can be concluded within his forward memory span. These intact aspects of mental function distinguish Korsakoff's amnesic psychosis from other behavioural and mental disorders which have their basis not in a primary defect of retentive memory but in some other psychological abnormality, such as drowsiness and stupor, delirium, depression, inattention, and so forth.

The amnesic disorder. Invariably there is a permanent gap in the patient's memory for the acute phase of the illness, attributable no doubt to the perceptual disorder and clouding of consciousness which are so prominent during that period. In addition, there is a defect in memorization (anterograde amnesia), which is never complete but usually severe in degree. The patient may be incapable, for example, of learning three simple facts (such as the examiner's name, date and time of day) despite countless attempts; he can repeat each fact as it is presented, indicating that he understands what is wanted of him and that 'registration' or 'immediate memory' is more or less intact, but by the time the third fact is repeated, the first may have been forgotten. This defect applies to all aspects of new learning, whether it be names of people or objects, nonsense syllables, a line of poetry, or some non-verbal task, such as a new card game. Since the adaptation to every new situation requires the formation of new memories and their integration with past experience, it is this defect that renders the patient helpless in society and capable of performing only the most habitual tasks.

Wechsler (1917) and later Barbizet (1963) singled out the inability to memorize as the fundamental psychological abnormality in Korsakow's psychosis, and attempted to explain the other abnormalities in behaviour and mental function on this basis. Certain aspects of confabulation could possibly be explained in this way: the patient, unable to make appropriate associations, responds with the readiest one derived from his stock of old memories. However, a defect in memorization can hardly explain the inability to recall information that had been acquired many years before the onset of the illness.

The defect in past memory is quite variable in extent and degree of completeness. In most patients it embraces a period that antedates the onset of the illness by several years, and the point which separates it from earlier intact memories cannot be identified. The retrograde amnesia is rarely complete; the patient retains isolated bits of information with varying degrees of accuracy and relates these to one another without regard to the gaps which separate them or to their proper temporal sequence. Usually the patient 'telescopes' events, at times the opposite. This defect becomes prominent after the acute stage of the illness has passed and remains a dominant feature in all but the few patients who make a complete recovery. The inability to correlate experiences in terms of time relationships accounts for certain instances of confabulation and for the characteristic manner in which patients retell stories (see below).

The statement that memories of the recent past are more severely impaired than those of the remote past is probably correct, but requires qualification. Clinically, remote memory is more difficult to assess than recent memory and the two are therefore difficult to compare. It is our impression that memories of the distant past are impaired in practically all cases of Korsakoff's psychosis and seriously impaired in most of them. Nor has this matter been resolved by formal psychological testing. Sanders and Warrington (1971) have presented evidence that alcoholic Korsakoff patients have as much difficulty in retrieving remote events as recent ones, whereas the studies of Albert and co-workers (1979) and of others indicate that temporal gradients in the retrograde memory deficits do exist.

We have not been able to discern the factors which govern what is forgotten and what is remembered. This aspect of the memory disorder seems to follow no distinctive or consistent pattern. Patients may show gaps in their past memory for seemingly important and 'emotionally-charged' events and yet be able to recall casual items or ones in which they were not personally involved. A similar paradox pertains to the formation of new memories.

Other cognitive and behaviour abnormalities. All the manifestations of Korsakoff's psychosis cannot be explained on the basis of memory defect alone (Victor, Herman & White, 1959; Victor, Talland & Adams, 1959). Formal psychological testing, using the Wechsler Adult Intelligence Scale consistently discloses failures with digit–symbol test and, to a lesser degree, with arithmetic and block design. Applying the usual interpretations to these subtests, the patients show defects in concentration, in verbal and visual abstraction, and in the ability to shift from one mental set to another. In other words, the patient has an impaired capacity to reason with data immediately before him, that is, circumstances in which memory function is not the major factor.

Talland (1965) found that the Korsakoff patient shows no deficit in tasks which depend on immediate apprehension, but is handicapped if the task is changed and a new mental set required, especially while the first task is continued. It seems that the patient is excessively dependent upon the immediate sensory input, in the sense of being unable to detach himself from it by imagery or to change his orientation toward it, and this prevents him from assimilating a diversity of newly-presented material. In addition, the patients can construct only the simplest concepts, and the criteria for the classification of a series of newly-presented material are much more vague than those of control subjects. Usually the

Korsakoff patient is incapable of discovering the unfamiliar criteria necessary for categorization, and the concepts once acquired are not effectively applied in the formation of sequential concepts. Talland (1965) has suggested that the inability to adopt new attitudes of orientation to a situation may be the basic abnormality in both the perceptual and conceptual deficits. The foregoing observations of the psychological deficits in alcoholic Korsakoff subjects have been amply confirmed and elaborated in the last 15 years. The recent studies have been reviewed by Butters (1979) and by Butters and Cermak (1980), to which the reader is referred for a far more detailed account than can possibly be provided here. These studies have greatly enhanced our understanding of certain manifestations of the amnesic state, but an all-embracing theory – one which explains all of the symptoms of Korsakoff's psychosis and their relationship to the observed clinical and pathological findings – remains to be formulated.

Confabulation. This is generally considered to be an invariable manifestation of Korsakoff's psychosis. The validity of this view depends to some extent on how one defines confabulation but some patients simply do not confabulate, no matter how broad the definition. In the initial phase of Korsakoff's psychosis, confabulation probably has its origin in a gross perceptual disorder, that is, in the misidentifications and misinterpretations that characterize this stage of the illness. As the general confusional state recedes the nature of the confabulation changes. It is rarely spontaneous but has to be elicited by questioning the patient and the response often depends upon how the examiner intonates his question. Thus, the same question may provoke confabulation on one occasion and not on the next. If one is aware of the patient's past activities, it is apparent that many of the events which are described by the patient and which may sound implausible, did indeed occur. However, they are remembered imperfectly; events that were separated by long intervals are juxtaposed or related out of sequence, so that the narrative has a fictional aspect. Whether one regards this disorder as confabulation or as a particular kind of retentive memory defect is academic. In the chronic stable stage of the disease confabulation is rarely observed.

The statement is often made that the Korsakoff patient fills the gaps in his memory with confabulation. In so far as the patient has gaps in his memory and whatever he supplies in place of the correct

answers fills these gaps, the statement is incontrovertible. It is hardly explanatory, however. The implication that confabulation is a deliberate attempt to hide the memory defect, out of embarrassment or for other reasons, is probably not correct. In fact, as the patient improves and becomes more aware of his memory defect, the tendency to confabulate becomes less.

Prognosis. Once Korsakoff's psychosis is established, a significant degree of recovery occurs in only a small proportion of patients (less than 20 per cent in our series). Some improvement does occur in most patients, so that they can find their way to their room or dining hall or can carry out routine tasks under supervision. Improvement usually begins within a few weeks after the amnesia is recognized and treated, but is sometimes delayed beyond this point, and the maximal degree of recovery may not be attained for a year or longer.

The unity of Wernicke's disease and Korsakoff's psychosis in the alcoholic patient

It is of interest that the relationship between these two disorders was appreciated neither by Wernicke nor by Korsakoff. Wernicke's 1900 edition of *Grundriss der Psychiatrie* contains four well-described examples of Korsakoff's psychosis, but the presence of brainstem signs is not mentioned. Korsakoff (1887) mentioned the presence of nystagmus and ophthalmoplegia in some of his patients, but nothing more was said about them. Other early case reports also mentioned that in some patients the signs of both Wernicke's disease and Korsakoff's psychosis were present, but their concurrence provoked no comment (Boedeker, 1892; Hurd, 1905; Jelliffe, 1908; Stanley, 1909–10).

Murawieff (1897) appears to have been the first to appreciate the close relationship between Wernicke's disease and 'polyneuritic psychosis'. He postulated that a single cause was responsible for both the cerebral and peripheral nerve affection. This opinion was supported by Raimann (1900, 1901) and by Elzholz (1900), who noted that the ocular muscles were frequently paralysed in patients with Korsakoff's psychosis but only rarely in those with delirium tremens. They deduced from these observations that there was a basic difference between Korsakoff's psychosis and delirium tremens. This contradicted the prevailing view of that time (and one that persisted long thereafter) which held that Korsakoff's psychosis and delirium tremens were the same disease, differing only in degree of acuteness and severity (Bonhoeffer, 1901; Jolly, 1897). The intimate clinical relationship between Wernicke's disease and Korsakoff's psychosis was established by Bonhoeffer (1904) who stated that in all cases of the former he found neuritis and an amnesic psychosis. Confirmation of this relationship on pathological grounds came much later (Campbell & Russell, 1941; Gamper, 1928; Girard, Devic & Garde, 1956; Kant, 1932; Malamud & Skillicorn, 1956; Victor *et al.*, 1971).

It is apparent from the foregoing account that Wernicke's disease and Korsakoff's psychosis are not separate diseases but that the changing ocular and ataxic signs and the transformation of the global confusional state into an amnesic syndrome are successive stages in the recovery of a single disease process. Of 186 patients in our series who presented with Wernicke's disease and survived the acute illness, 157 (84 per cent) showed this sequence of recovery. As a corollary, a survey of Korsakoff patients in a state mental hospital disclosed that in most of them the illness had begun with acute Wernicke's disease and that most still showed the ocular and/or cerebellar stigmata of Wernicke's disease many years after the onset. As indicated below, the lesions in the brain are very much the same, whether the patient dies in the acute stage of Wernicke's disease or in the chronic phase of the disease when the ocular palsies have cleared and the amnesic symptoms are prominent. For these reasons *this symptom complex should be called Wernicke's disease with or without Korsakoff's psychosis, or the Wernicke-Korsakoff syndrome, if both components are present.*

Finally, it is important to repeat that Korsakoff's psychosis may become manifest in alcoholic patients in whom the signs of Wernicke's disease are not apparent. About 10 per cent of our patients with Korsakoff's psychosis fall into this category. In this connection the observations of Ryan and his associates (1980) are of interest. These authors subjected a group of seemingly 'intact' chronic alcoholics (50–59 years of age) to a series of complex and difficult cognitive tests and found a significant degree of impairment in learning and memory functions. Since a younger group of alcoholics (34–49 years of age) who were examined by Ryan and his associates did not show such cognitive abnormality, the impaired performance of the older patients was attributed to premature aging of the brain, induced by alcohol. Equally logical, however, is the suggestion that the highly

sensitive tests simply uncovered very mild forms of Korsakoff's psychosis, of a degree that could not be detected by the standard clinical examination of memory function.

Neuropathological findings and clinical–pathological correlation

The lesions take the form of varying degrees of necrosis of parenchymal structures, symmetrically distributed in the paraventricular regions of the thalamus and hypothalamus; in the mammillary bodies, peri-aqueductal region of the midbrain, and floor of the fourth ventricle, particularly in the regions of the dorsal motor nuclei of the vagus and vestibular nuclei; and in the superior vermis. The lesions are consistently found in the mammillary bodies, less consistently in other areas. Within the areas of necrosis there is a varying degree of nerve cell loss; some of the remaining neurons are damaged but others are intact. These changes result in prominence of the blood vessels, although in some cases there is a true endothelial proliferation. In the areas of parenchymal damage there is a density of cells, representing astrocytic and microglial proliferation. These alterations are most intense in the centre of the lesion, shading off toward the periphery. Discrete haemorrhages, usually petechial, were found in only 20 per cent of our cases and many of them appeared to be agonal in nature. Occasionally the haemorrhages are large or even confluent (Rosenblum & Feigin, 1965; Tashiro & Nelson, 1972). The cerebellar changes consist of a degeneration of all layers of the cortex, but particularly of Purkinje cells; usually this lesion is confined to the superior parts of the vermis, but in advanced cases the cortex of the anterior parts of the anterior lobes and the flocculonodular lobe are involved as well.

The ocular muscle and gaze palsies are attributable to lesions of the sixth and third nerve nuclei and adjacent tegmentum, and the nystagmus to lesions in the regions of the vestibular nuclei. The latter are also responsible for the loss of caloric responses ('vestibular paresis') and probably for the gross disturbance of equilibrium that characterizes the initial stages of the disease (Ghez, 1969). The lack of significant nerve cell loss in these lesions would account for the rapid recovery of oculomotor and vestibular functions. The persistent ataxia of stance and gait is attributable to the loss of neurons in the superior vermis of the cerebellum, and ataxia of individual movements of the legs to an extension of the lesion into the anterior parts of the anterior lobes.

As has been indicated, the neuropathologic changes in patients with Korsakoff's psychosis are much the same as the acute changes in Wernicke's disease. Apart from the expected differences with respect to the age of the glial and vascular reactions, the only important difference is in the involvement of the medial-dorsal nucleus of the thalamus and perhaps of the pulvinar. These latter structures were consistently involved in our patients who had shown Korsakoff's psychosis; patients with Wernicke's disease but without amnesia did not show thalamic lesions, although the mammillary bodies were always involved. These observations would indicate that the lesions of the medial thalamic nuclei, rather than those of the mammillary bodies, are responsible for the amnesic syndrome. The role of medial thalamic lesions in the production of an amnesic state has been critically discussed by Horel (1978).

Recently McEntee and Mair (1978) have pointed out that the paraventricular and brainstem lesions which characterize the Wernicke-Korsakoff syndrome correspond with the regions of the brain that contain the highest concentration of ascending projections of monamine-containing neurons. These authors examined the cerebrospinal fluid of a group of alcoholic Korsakoff patients and found an abnormally low concentration of 3-methoxy-4-hydroxyphenyl glycol (MHPG), the primary brain metabolite of norepinephrine. In a later study (1980) they reported that the administration of clonidine (a norepinephrine agonist) in alcoholic Korsakoff patients resulted in a significant improvement in tests measuring recall of recently presented information. These observations have raised a number of interesting questions about the relationships of central norepinephrine systems to the symptoms of Korsakoff's psychosis, which are now being actively studied.

Aetiology

For many years Wernicke's disease was attributed to the toxic effects of alcohol. The notion that this disease might be nutritional in origin originated with the observations that it sometimes complicated hyperemesis gravidarum (Henderson, 1914; Wagener & Weir, 1937), and gastric carcinoma and other disturbances of the alimentary tract (Ecker & Woltman, 1939; Wagener & Weir, 1937; Neuburger, 1936, 1937). Shortly after the appearance of these reports, Alexander, Pijoan, and Myerson (1938) drew attention to the similarity between the neuropatho-

logical changes in vitamin-B-deprived pigeons and those in Wernicke's disease. It then became evident that the lesions in many thiamine-deficient mammalian species also bore such a resemblance (Dreyfus & Victor, 1961; Evans, Carlson & Green, 1942; Jubb, Saunders & Coates, 1956; Kalm, Luckner & Magun, 1952; Prickett, 1934; Rinehart, Friedman & Greenberg, 1949).

The specific nutritional factor responsible for most, if not all the symptomatology of Wernicke's disease is thiamine. As has been indicated, ophthalmoplegia, nystagmus, and ataxia can be reversed by the administration of thiamine alone, although horizontal nystagmus and ataxia may persist in mild form for months or years after their onset (Phillips, Victor, Adams & Davidson, 1952; Victor & Adams, 1961; Wortis, Bueding, Stein & Jolliffe, 1942). The marked sensitivity of the ocular palsies to the administration of thiamine accounts for the rapid disappearance of these abnormalities after a meal or two and the quality of prompt reversibility suggests that the symptoms are due more to a biochemical abnormality than to structural change.

Many of the initial mental symptoms – apathy and fatigue, drowsiness, inattentiveness, and so forth – clear rapidly under the influence of thiamine alone (Phillips *et al.*, 1952; Victor & Adams, 1961); it is likely therefore, that these symptoms are due to thiamine deficiency. With respect to memory defect, the role of thiamine is less certain. The amnesic symptoms tend to recover slowly and incompletely, and the rate of recovery is much the same in patients who are given a full diet and all vitamins from the onset and in those who receive a deficient diet, supplemented only with thiamine (Victor & Adams, 1961). These observations suggest that the lesions responsible for the memory loss are structural rather than biochemical in nature.

The recent observations of Blass and Gibson (1977) suggest that a hereditary factor may be operative in the pathogenesis of the Wernicke-Korsakoff syndrome. They found a defect in transketolase, a thiamine-dependent enzyme, in fibroblasts cultured from patients with this syndrome. The defect, which consisted of a diminished binding of the coenzyme thiamine pyrophosphate to the apoenzyme, persisted through serial passages of tissue-cultured cells in medium containing an excess of thiamine and no alcohol. These observations, if confirmed, would indicate that some patients have a constitutional predisposition to the Wernicke-Korsakoff syndrome and might explain why only a small proportion of-nutritionally-depleted alcoholics develop the disease.

Treatment of the Wernicke-Korsakoff syndrome

The recognition of Wernicke's disease constitutes a medical emergency and demands the prompt administration of thiamine. This prevents progression of the disease and reverses those lesions that have not progressed to the point of structural change. In patients who show only ocular signs and ataxia, the administration of thiamine will prevent the development of an amnesic psychosis. Although 2 to 3 mg of thiamine may be sufficient to modify the ocular signs, much larger doses are usually employed – 50 mg intravenously and 50 mg intramuscularly, the latter dose being repeated each day until the patient resumes a normal diet.

It is good practice to give B vitamins to all alcoholic patients, particularly those being treated with parenteral glucose. Characteristically, the alcoholic subsists on a diet low in thiamine and disproportionately high in carbohydrate and often gastroenteritis and diarrhoea are associated. His reserves of thiamine may be seriously depleted by the time he is hospitalized and the administration of glucose in these circumstances precipitates Wernicke's disease or causes an early form of the disease to deteriorate rapidly.

Pellagra

In the early part of this century, pellagra attained epidemic proportions in the southern United States and in the alcoholic population of large urban centres. Now pellagra is a rarity. At the Cleveland Metropolitan General Hospital we have observed only two clinical examples in the past 16 years. The virtual eradication of this disease, attributable no doubt to the widespread practice of enriching bread with niacin, carries the important implication that other alcoholic and nutritionally-determined mental disorders are also preventable.

In its fully-developed form, pellagra affects the skin, the alimentary tract, and the haematopoietic and nervous systems. The most important manifestations are the cerebral ones. In the early stages the symptoms may be mistaken for those of psychoneurosis. Insomnia, fatigue, nervousness, irritability, and feelings of depression are common complaints and examination may disclose mental dullness, apathy, and impairment of memory. Sometimes an acute

confusional psychosis dominates the clinical picture. Pellagra may not only produce insanity but occasionally may result from it, by virtue of the anorexia and refusal of food that accompanies certain mental illnesses. The spinal cord may also be involved but the clinical manifestations have not been clearly delineated, perhaps because the patient's mental state often precludes accurate testing; in general the signs are referable to both the posterior and lateral columns, predominantly the former. Signs of peripheral nerve affection are relatively less common and are indistinguishable from those of beriberi.

Under the title of *nicotinic acid deficiency encephalopathy*, Jolliffe, Bowman, Rosenblum & Fein (1940) described an acute encephalopathy in alcoholic patients, consisting of clouding of consciousness progressing to coma, extrapyramidal rigidity and tremors ('cogwheel' rigidity) of the extremities, and uncontrollable grasping and sucking reflexes. Most of their patients showed overt manifestations of nutritional deficiency, such as Wernicke's disease, pellagra, scurvy, and polyneuropathy. These authors believed that the encephalopathy represented an acute form of nicotinic acid deficiency, since most of their patients recovered when treated with a diet of low vitamin B content supplemented by large doses of nicotinic acid. Cleckley, Sydenstricker and Geeslin (1939) had previously reported the salutary effects of nicotinic acid on the unresponsive state of elderly undernourished patients, and Spillane (1947) described a similar syndrome and response to nicotinic acid in the indigent Arab population of the Middle East.

The status of this syndrome and its relation to pellagra are uncertain. The clinical and pathological features never were delineated precisely. Nor is it likely that new information will be forthcoming, for this syndrome seems to have disappeared. Virtually nothing new has been written about it in the past 30 years and during this time we have been unable to find any convincing examples, despite the systematic examination of large numbers of undernourished patients in the alcoholic populations of Boston and Cleveland.

Pathological changes

These are most readily discerned in the large cells of the motor cortex, the cells of Betz, although the same changes are seen to a lesser extent in the smaller pyramidal cells of the cortex, the large cells of the basal ganglia, the cells of the cranial motor and dentate nuclei, and the anterior horn cells of the spinal cord. The affected cells appear swollen and rounded, with eccentric nuclei and loss of the Nissl particles. These changes were originally designated by Adolf Meyer (1901) as 'central neuritis' and are frequently referred to as 'axonal reaction' because of their similarity to the changes which occur in the anterior horn cells when their axons are severed. It has never been decided whether the 'central neuritis' of pellagra is dependent on injury to the axons of the Betz cells, or represents a primary cytolytic degeneration of the motor cell.

The spinal cord lesions in pellagra take the form of a symmetrical degeneration of the dorsal columns, especially the column of Goll, and to a lesser extent of the corticospinal tracts. The few studies that have been made of the peripheral nerves have disclosed changes like those of alcoholic–nutritional neuropathy.

Aetiology

It has been known since 1937, when Elvehjem and his coworkers showed that nicotinic acid cured black tongue (a pellagra-like disease in dogs), that this vitamin is effective in the treatment of pellagra. Many years before, Goldberger had demonstrated the curative effects of dietary protein and proposed that pellagra was caused by a lack of specific aminoacids. Now it is known that pellagra may result from a deficiency of either nicotinic acid or of tryptophan, the aminoacid precursor of nicotinic acid (Goldsmith, Sarrett, Register & Gibbens, 1952). This explains the frequent occurrence of pellagra in persons who subsist mainly on corn, which contains only small amounts of tryptophan and of niacin, some of the niacin being in bound form and unavailable to the organism. There is evidence that the lingual and cutaneous manifestations of pellagra may also be produced by a deficiency of pyridoxine (Vilter *et al.*, 1953) and that the neuropathologic changes may be due to pyridoxine deficiency as well (Victor & Adams, 1956).

Hepatic encephalopathy

Subsumed under this title are the cerebral abnormalities consequent upon advanced hepatocellular disease and portal-systemic shunting of blood. All forms of liver disease may give rise to hepatic encephalopathy, but the most common is portal cirrhosis. In a series of 3548 consecutive autopsies in adults, we found the lesions of hepatic encephalopathy in 273 (7.7 per cent), in 70 per cent of whom the liver disease proved to be of the alcoholic or portal cirrhosis type (Victor & Laureno, 1978).

Clinically, two characteristic and overlapping forms of hepatic encephalopathy can be recognized: (1) a relatively acute neurological syndrome that complicates or fatally terminates liver failure (hepatic coma); and (2) a chronic and irreversible form of hepatocerebral degeneration.

Acute hepatic encephalopathy (hepatic stupor or coma; portal-systemic encephalopathy)

The clinical syndrome, as delineated originally by Adams and Foley (1953), is characterized by an impairment of consciousness, presenting first as mental confusion with increased or decreased psychomotor activity, followed by progressive drowsiness, stupor, and coma. The confusional state is frequently combined with a characteristic intermittence of sustained muscle contraction, imparting an irregular, 'flapping' movement to the outstretched hands (asterixis). The electroencephalogram (EEG) becomes abnormal during the earliest phases of the disordered mental state. The usual EEG abnormality consists of paroxysms of bilaterally synchronous slow waves, in the delta range, which at first are interspersed with alpha activity and later, as the coma deepens, displace all normal activity. Some patients show only random high voltage asynchronous slow waves. The variable occurrence of a fluctuating rigidity of the trunk and limbs, grimacing, suck and grasp reflexes, exaggeration or asymmetry of tendon reflexes, Babinski signs, decerebrate or decorticate postures, and focal or generalized seizures rounds out the clinical picture. This state evolves over a period of days to weeks and often terminates fatally; or, after reaching a certain stage, it may regress completely.

Sherlock and her colleagues have described a form of hepatic encephalopathy in which the disorder of mood, personality, and intellect is prolonged for months or even years (Sherlock, Summerskill, White & Phear, 1954; Summerskill, Davidson, Sherlock & Steiner, 1956). These symptoms fluctuate widely in severity or are intermittent in nature and are essentially reversible if proper therapeutic measures are instituted. For this reason, this chronic syndrome accords more closely with hepatic coma in its many variations than with the chronic hepatocerebral syndrome described below.

The chronic, acquired (non-Wilsonian) form of hepatocerebral degeneration

Patients who survive an episode of hepatic coma are occasionally left with residual impairment of neurological and intellectual functions and these abnormalities may worsen with repeated episodes of coma. The fully-developed syndrome consists of dementia of variable severity, dysarthria, ataxia, intention tremor, choreo-athetosis that is most prominent in the cranial musculature, cortico-spinal tract signs, and EEG abnormalities. Other less frequent signs are muscular rigidity, grasp reflexes, tremor in repose, nystagmus, and asterixis. In essence, each of the neurological abnormalities that occurs in hepatic stupor or coma may also be observed in patients with chronic hepatocerebral degeneration, the only difference being that the abnormalities are transient (or terminal) in the former and chronic and fixed in the latter.

The pathological changes take two forms, corresponding to the clinical syndromes outlined above: (1) In patients who die in hepatic coma, post-mortem examination shows a diffuse increase in the number and size of protoplasmic astrocytes in the deep layers of the cerebral cortex, thalamus, basal ganglia, and brainstem and dentate nuclei, with little or no visible alteration in the nerve cells or other parenchymal elements. Many of the astrocytic nuclei contain periodic acid-Schiff(PAS)-positive inclusions, consisting mainly of glycogen. (2) Patients with the chronic fixed neurological syndrome show, in addition to the astrocytic changes, a patchy but diffuse cortical laminar or pseudolaminar necrosis and polymicrocavitation at the corticomedullary junction, in the striatum (particularly in the superior pole of the putamen), and in the cerebellar white matter.

The pathogenesis of hepatic encephalopathy has not been established with certainty, but most of the evidence indicates that it is due to the neurotoxic effects of nitrogenous substances (ammonium or other amines). These substances, which are absorbed from the intestine, fail to be metabolized by the diseased liver and make their way into the systemic circulation, either through naturally-formed or surgically-created portal-systemic shunts. A full account of this subject can be found in the review by Fischer and Baldessarini (1976). (See also chap. 2.)

The foetal alcohol syndrome (FAS)

That parental alcoholism may have an adverse effect on the offspring has been a recurrent theme in medical lore. The documented occurrence of such a relationship was lacking, however, until the turn of the century, when Sullivan (1899) reported that the mortality among the children of drunken mothers was almost two and one-half times greater than among children of non-drinking women of 'similar stock'. The increased mortality was attributed by Sullivan and later by Haggard and Jellinek (1942) to post-natal influences such as poor nutrition and chaotic home environment rather than to the intra-uterine effects of alcohol. Following Sullivan's studies there appeared isolated clinical reports in which damage to the foetus was ascribed to alcoholism in the mother (for historical surveys see Jones & Smith, 1973; Warner & Rosett, 1975), but in general this idea was rejected and relegated to the category of superstitions about alcoholism. Thus, as late as 1959, Keller wrote: 'the old notions about children of drunken parents being born defective can be cast aside, together with the idea that alcohol can directly irritate and injure the sex glands'.

In the past decade, the effects of alcohol abuse on the foetus have been rediscovered, so to speak. Lemoine, Harrousseau, Borteyru & Menuet (1968), Ulleland (1972), and Jones and Smith (1973) have described a distinctive pattern of abnormalities in infants born of severely alcoholic mothers. The affected infants are small in length in comparison to weight and most of them fall below the third percentile for head circumference. They are distinguished also by the presence of short palpebral fissures (probably a reflection of microphthalmia) and epicanthal folds; maxillary hypoplasia, micrognathia, and cleft palate; dislocations of the hips, flexion deformities of the fingers and a limited range of motion of other joints; cardiac anomalies (usually spontaneously-closing septal defects); anomalous external genitalia; and capillary haemangiomata. The newborn infants suck and sleep poorly and many of them are irritable, hyperactive, and tremulous; the latter symptoms resemble those of alcohol withdrawal, except that they persist. In one series of such infants there was a neonatal mortality of 17 (Jones, Smith, Streissguth and Myrianthopoulos, 1974). Seriously-affected infants who survive the neonatal period fail to achieve normal weight, length, and head circumference and remain backward mentally to a varying degree, even under optimal environmental conditions. The early descriptions of this syndrome have been confirmed by subsequent studies (Hanson, Jones & Smith, 1976; Mulvihill & Yeager, 1976).

The anatomical basis of this syndrome is unknown. To date, the neuropathological findings have been described in only one newborn infant (Jones & Smith, 1973). The brain in this case weighed only 140 g and histological examination disclosed numerous abnormalities of neuronal migration, lack of cortical sulcation (lissencephaly) and agenesis of the corpus callosum – findings which indicate that the developmental abnormality occurred in the first few months of foetal life. Whether these changes are representative of the FAS will only be determined by the examination of more cases.

Although the relationship of this syndrome to severe maternal alcoholism seems undoubted, the mechanism by which alcohol produces its effects is not fully understood. It is noteworthy that infants born to non-alcoholic mothers who had been subjected to severe dietary deprivation during pregnancy were small and often premature, but these infants did not show the pattern of malformations that characterizes the FAS (Smith, 1947; Cravioto, Delicardie & Birch, 1966). Alcohol readily crosses the placenta in man and animals. In the mouse, alcohol has both embryotoxic and teratogenic effects; foetuses of mothers maintained on alcohol throughout gestation showed skeletal, cardiac, and cerebral abnormalities (Chernoff, 1975). Similar effects have been demonstrated in rat and chick embryos (Randall, Taylor & Walker, 1977). Thus, the limited evidence to date favours a toxic effect of alcohol or perhaps one of its metabolites or contaminants, for example, lead (Sneed, 1977), rather than a nutritional or genetic factor.

The critical degree of maternal alcoholism that is necessary to produce the FAS and the critical stage in gestation during which it occurs are not known. Cases observed to date have occurred only in children born to severely alcoholic mothers who continued to drink heavily throughout their pregnancy – an average of 6 ounces of absolute alcohol (or 12 ounces of 86° proof whisky) daily, according to Rosett, Ouellette & Weiner (1976). Preliminary data, derived from the collaborative study being sponsored by the National Institutes of Health, indicate that about one-third of the offspring of such women have the FAS (Jones & Smith, 1973). Prospective studies of these problems, and of the effects on the foetus of lesser degrees of maternal alcoholism are in progress.

Alcoholic disorders of uncertain pathogenesis

Included under this heading is a diverse group of neuropsychiatric disorders, the common feature of which is their frequent association with alcoholism. One of them, Marchiafava-Bignami disease, probably has a metabolic or nutritional cause, but this remains to be defined. So-called alcoholic deteriorated state and alcoholic cerebral atrophy are not acceptable clinical or pathological entities, but they are still mentioned repeatedly in medical writings and should be discussed for this reason. The same can be said for 'alcoholic jealousy'. Although the disorders in this category are designated as 'alcoholic', all of them occur in non-alcoholics as well, so that one can be certain that alcohol is not fundamental in their causation.

Marchiafava-Bignami disease (primary degeneration of the corpus callosum)

This disorder is best defined in terms of its pathological anatomy because the latter stands as its most certain feature. The principal alteration, as has been emphasized since the original descriptions by Marchiafava and Bignami (1903), is a clearly demarcated zone of demyelination in the middle portion of the corpus callosum; less consistently, lesions of a similar nature are found in the central portions of the anterior and posterior commissures, cerebral hemispheres, cerebellar peduncles and columns of Goll (King & Meehan, 1936).

Clinical features

Marchiafava-Bignami disease is decidedly rare. In our autopsy material, comprising 3548 adult brains, there were only 2 cases. The disease affects persons in middle and late adult life. Except for the patient of Giannelli (quoted by Mingazzini, 1922) and the one of Schwob and his colleagues (1953), all of the reported cases have been in males, and with equally few exceptions, all have been severe chronic alcoholics.

In other respects, the clinical features are quite variable and a clear-cut syndrome has not emerged. Some of the reported patients have presented in a state of terminal stupor or coma, which precluded detailed neuropsychiatric assessment. In others, the clinical picture was dominated by the manifestations of chronic inebriation and withdrawal, and in yet other patients, a progressive dementia has been described, evolving slowly over several years. Emotional disorders, leading to acts of violence, or marked apathy, moral perversions, and sexual misdemeanours have been noted frequently. Dysarthria, slowing and unsteadiness of movement, transient sphincteric incontinence, hemipareses, and apractic or aphasic disorders were superimposed. An impressive feature of these neuropsychiatric deficits has been their tendency to remission. The last stage of the disease is characterized by physical decline, seizures, stupor, and coma.

It is generally believed that Marchiafava-Bignami disease is invariably fatal, but we have observed reversible instances, as have others (Leventhal, Baringer, Arnason & Fisher, 1965). In two such cases that have come to our attention, the clinical manifestations were essentially those of bilateral frontal lobe disorder – motor and mental slowness, apathy, prominent grasping and sucking, *Gegenhalten*, incontinence, and a slow, hesitant, wide-based gait. In both of these patients, the neurological abnormalities evolved over several months and both recovered within a few weeks of hospitalization. Death occurred several years later, as a result of liver disease and subdural haematoma, respectively. In each case, autopsy disclosed a healed lesion of Marchiafava-Bignami disease, confined to the central portion of the corpus callosum.

In view of the variability of the clinical picture, and the obscuration in many patients of subtle mental and neurological abnormalities by the effects of chronic inebriation, the *diagnosis* of Marchiafava-Bignami disease is understandably difficult, and, in fact, is rarely made during life. The occurrence, in a chronic alcoholic, of a frontal lobe syndrome or a symptom complex that points to a diagnosis of Alzheimer's disease or frontal or corpus callosum-tumour, but in whom the symptoms remit, should suggest the diagnosis of Marchiafava-Bignami disease. Computerized tomography (CT) scan may prove to be helpful in diagnosis.

Pathogenesis and aetiology

Originally, Marchiafava-Bignami disease was attributed to the toxic effects of alcohol, but this is an unlikely explanation, in view of the prevalence of alcoholism and the rarity of the corpus callosum lesion. Nor has the distinctive callosal lesion been observed with other neurotoxins. As has been indicated, rare but undoubted examples of Marchiafava-Bignami disease have occurred in abstainers, so that alcohol is not an indispensable causative factor. Nutritional factors may be important in the pathogenesis, in view of the specificity of localization of the lesion and its bilateral symmetry – attributes that characterize diseases of known nutritional aetiology. However, the nutritional factor or factors, if they are causative, have never been defined. 'Oedema damage' and a 'vasocirculatory defect' have been invoked

to explain the selective necrosis of particular areas of white matter, but there is no firm basis for these theoretical concepts.

Alcoholic deteriorated state (alcoholic dementia)

The syndrome designated as alcoholic dementia or deteriorated state has never been delineated satisfactorily, either clinically or pathologically. In the *Comprehensive Textbook of Psychiatry* this state is defined as 'a gradual disintegration of personality structure, with emotional lability, loss of control and dementia' (Chafetz, 1975). To other psychiatrists (Strecker, Ebaugh & Ewalt, 1951) the alcoholic deteriorated states denotes 'the common end reaction of all chronic alcoholics who do not recover from their alcoholism or do not die of some accident or intercurrent episode'. Judging from the illustrative case reports presented by these authors, the manifestations of this syndrome are remarkably diverse and include jealousy and suspiciousness; blunting of moral fibre and other personality and behavioural disorders associated with chronic inebriation; deterioration of work performance, personal care, and living habits; disorientation; impaired judgement and defects of intellectual function, particularly of memory. Some authors (Keller & McCormick, 1968) have even included certain physical symptoms in the definition, such as dilatation of facial capillaries, a 'bloated look', flabby muscles, chronic gastritis, tremors and recurrent seizures. Earlier authors were apparently impressed with similarities between the deteriorated state of alcoholics and that of general paresis, hence the term 'alcoholic pseudoparesis'. Mercifully the latter term no longer appears in medical writings.

Recently, Seltzer and Sherwin (1978) have attempted to sharpen the definition of alcoholic dementia. They made a clinical evaluation of 80 patients who had been given a diagnosis of 'organic' or 'chronic brain syndrome'. In ten of these patients there was a definite history of alcoholism, coupled with dementia. The dementia in these patients was said to be characterized by a stable course and an absence of language abnormality (thus distinguishing it from senile dementia) and by prominent constructional and behavioural disturbances, in addition to amnesia, distinguishing it from Korsakoff's psychosis. In none of the patients designated as alcoholic dementia by Seltzer and Sherwin was the nervous system examined pathologically.

Courville (1955) described a series of pathological changes which he considered to be the basis of the 'alcoholic deteriorated state' and 'alcoholic pseudoparesis': progressive atrophy of the cortex of the frontal lobes, associated with opacity and thickening of the overlying meninges and enlargement of the lateral ventricles; swelling, pyknosis, and 'pigmentary atrophy' of nerve cells; irregular loss of the smaller pyramidal cells of the superficial and intermediate laminae; and secondary degeneration and loss of nerve fibres. In Courville's view, these changes were the result of the toxic effects of alcohol.

The neuropathological changes described by Courville and his interpretation of these changes are simply not acceptable, despite the fact that they are quoted widely and have seemingly been accepted without question by psychiatrists (Kolb, 1968; Kessel & Walton, 1965; Horvath, 1975; Ron, 1977), and even by pathologists (Lynch, 1960). Many of the abnormalities described by Courville are not specific. Opacity of the meninges and moderate dilatation of the lateral ventricles, for example, are observed both in alcoholics and non-alcoholics as well as in persons who had betrayed no neurological or psychiatric abnormalities during life. Some of the cellular changes noted by Courville probably reflect a terminal state of hepatic or anoxic encephalopathy or of chronic hepatocerebral degeneration, and other changes reflect nothing more than the effects of aging or artefacts of tissue fixation and staining. Lacking in Courville's account are any systematic clinical observations in patients who eventually were labelled 'alcoholic deteriorated state' on pathological grounds. Nor is there any information about the presence or frequency of the aforementioned pathological changes in alcoholics without deterioration. Much the same criticisms apply to Lynch's (1960) notions about the brain changes in chronic alcoholism, attributed by him to such unverified factors as 'interference with capillary blood supply' and 'repeated episodes of hepatogenic fat embolism'.

In our experience, the majority of cases that come to autopsy with the label of alcoholic dementia or deteriorated state prove to have the lesions of the Wernicke-Korsakoff syndrome, the clinical features of which had not been recognized during life. Traumatic lesions of varying degrees of severity are commonly added. Other cases show the lesions of anoxic encephalopathy, acute or chronic hepatic encephalopathy, communicating hydrocephalus, Alzheimer's disease, ischaemic infarction or some other disease quite unrelated to alcoholism. Practically always, in our material, the clinical state can be accounted for by one or a combination of these disease processes, and there has been no need to invoke a hypothetical toxic effect of alcohol on the brain.

'Cerebral atrophy' in chronic alcoholics

This disorder, like the 'alcoholic deteriorated state', does not constitute a clinical–pathological-entity. To some authors, for example, Courville (1955), (see above) the concept of 'alcoholic cerebral atrophy' is a pathological one, but in most writings on this subject the diagnosis of alcoholic cerebral atrophy has been made on the basis of radiological abnormalities, namely, a symmetrical enlargement of the lateral ventricles and a widening of the sulci, mainly of the frontal lobes. Originally these abnormalities were disclosed by air studies (Brewer & Perrett, 1971; Haug, 1968); more recently, similar findings have been reported in chronic alcoholics examined by computerized tomography (CT) scans (Carlen *et al.*, 1978; Epstein, Pisani & Fawcett, 1977; Fox, Ramsey, Huckman & Proske, 1976; Cala, Jones, Mastaglia & Wiley, 1978).

The clinical and pathological states which underlie the 'cerebral atrophy' of alcoholics are far from uniform. In some patients the dilated ventricles and widened sulci are associated with the Wernicke-Korsakoff syndrome (we found these changes in about one-quarter of our autopsied patients). In other patients there had been a history of recurrent seizures, or evidence of liver disease, cerebral trauma, or some other event that might have resulted in ventricular enlargement. But in some alcoholic individuals the finding of large ventricles comes as a surprise, no symptoms or signs of neuropsychiatric disease having been recorded, and the cause may remain obscure, even after post-mortem examination (Giove & Viani, 1965).

Some of the problems relating to the 'cerebral atrophy of alcoholics' and the hazard of assessing the presence and degree of atrophy by radiological means are illustrated by the study of Carlen and co-workers (1978). These authors examined eight chronic alcoholics at varying intervals after admission to the hospital, using a battery of psychological tests and CT scans. Four patients improved clinically and showed a reduction in the size of the ventricles as well as in the width of the sulci, as judged by the CT scans. Such reversibility is hardly consistent with the concept of cerebral atrophy, which implies a progressive, irreversible neuronal decay. In two of the patients described by Carlen and co-workers (1978) there was improvement of the clinical state and psychological test performance but little or no change in the CT scans. The remaining two patients continued to drink and showed no change in either their clinical state or CT scans.

We have observed several mentally-intact alcoholic patients whose CT scans showed dilatation of the ventricular system and widening of the cerebral and cerebellar sulci. These patients died from non-alcoholic causes, after varying periods of abstinence, and at autopsy no ventricular dilatation or sulcal widening could be discerned. Reversibility of ventricular dilatation and of widened sulci, as revealed by the CT scan, has also been shown to occur in patients with Cushing's syndrome, anorexia nervosa, and in patients with the Lennox-Gastaut syndrome who had been treated with ACTH. In view of these observations, one cannot assume that dilatation of ventricles and sulci, observed in a single CT scan, represents an irreversible tissue loss. The reversibility of the CT picture suggests that a major shift of fluids had occurred within the brain. Until this matter has been settled it would be preferable to refer to the asymptomatic ventricular enlargement in alcoholics as such, rather than as 'cerebral atrophy'.

It is apparent that the meaning of ventricular dilatation and sulcal widening in alcoholics, loosely referred to as 'cerebral atrophy', remains unclear. An obvious need in relation to this problem (and to alcoholic dementia) is a discerning neuropathological study of patients whose neuropsychiatric state had been rigorously evaluated clinically and of suitable controls (unimpaired alcoholics).

Alcoholic paranoia and jealousy

These are outmoded terms that were used in the past to designate what was thought to be a special type of paranoid reaction in chronic alcoholics, in which the patient, usually a male, developed ideas of infidelity on the part of his wife. The delusions of jealousy that might occur acutely in the course of alcoholic intoxication or withdrawal or chronically, as part of the 'alcoholic deteriorated state', were generally not included under this rubric.

The notion that pathological jealousy merits classification as a distinctive complication of alcoholism is not warranted. Several comprehensive studies have made it clear that pathological jealousy which develops in alcoholics differs in no essential from the morbid jealousy in non-alcoholics (Langfeldt, 1961; Shepherd, 1961; Johanson, 1964; Mooney, 1965). Nevertheless, among individuals with the syndrome of morbid jealousy, chronic alcoholism may be an important associated factor (11 of 66 cases reported by Langfeldt, 1961). Among the alcoholic patients, the delusions of jealousy may at first be evident only in relation to episodes of acute intoxication, but later they evolve, through a stage of constant suspicion and efforts to detect infidelity, into definite morbid beliefs which persist during periods of sobriety (Bowman & Jellinek, 1941). The subject of morbid jealousy is considered in volume 1, chapter 3, and volume 3, chapter 5.

15
Drug dependence and intoxication

A. HAMID GHODSE

The difficulties of defining the essential characteristics of drug dependence are exemplified by the changes that have taken place since 1957 when drug addiction and drug habituation were regarded as separate entities; since 1964 new definitions have been formulated by the WHO (World Health Organization, 1957, 1964, 1974; Eddy *et al.*, 1965):

Drug: 'any substance that, when taken into the living organism, may modify one or more of its functions'.

Drug dependence: a state, psychic, and sometimes also physical, resulting from the interaction between a living organism and a drug, characterized by behavioural and other responses that always include a compulsion to take the drug on a continuous or periodic basis in order to experience psychic effects, and sometimes to avoid the discomfort of its absence. Tolerance may or may not be present.

Psychic dependence: a condition in which a drug produces 'a feeling of satisfaction and a psychic drive that requires periodic or continuous administration of the drug to provide pleasure or to avoid discomfort'.

Physical dependence: an adaptive state that manifests itself by intense physical disturbances when the administration of the drug is suspended. These disturbances, that is, the withdrawal or abstinence syndrome, are made up of a specific array of symptoms and signs of a psychic and physical nature that are characteristic for each drug type.

Physical dependence capacity: the ability of a drug to act as a substitute for another upon which an organism has been made physically dependent, that is, to suppress abstinence phenomena that would otherwise develop after abrupt withdrawal of the original dependence-producing drug.

Drug abuse: persistent or sporadic excessive drug use inconsistent with or unrelated to acceptable medical practice.

Drug dependence and intoxication

Although the use and abuse of psycho-active substances dates back to antiquity the associated problems used to be culturally controlled and geographically contained. Social and economic changes at local, national, and international levels coupled with the development of rapid international communication have resulted in the relaxation of these traditional constraints and many drugs are now abused on a world-wide scale. Drug abuse and dependence have thus become a major human problem throughout the world, involving many different social and health-caring agencies. The complexity of drug-seeking behaviour and the resulting morbidity and mortality has attracted great resources and the interest of psychologists, psychiatrists, sociologists, and politicians. Indeed the spectrum of research into these problems ranges from the study of individual brain cells to that of anthropology.

In this chapter some general aspects of drug dependence are considered including the mechanisms of tolerance, theories of dependence and epidemiological aspects. In particular the currently important problems of multiple drug abuse and of the effects of maternal drug abuse on the foetus and neonate are discussed. The nature of dependence on specific groups of drugs (e.g. opiates, analgesics, cannabis) is also described although this systematic but convenient approach to the study of drug-dependence risks diverting attention from the more general and fundamental aspects of the subject.

Tolerance

Tolerance is the state of decreased responsiveness of the system to the pharmacological action of the drug resulting from prior exposure of the system

to that drug (Hug, 1972). In other words, the dose of a drug to which tolerance has developed has to be increased to maintain the drug effect. Tolerance is not totally drug-specific as cross-tolerance also occurs – that is, the decreased response of the organism to one drug induced by the development of tolerance to another drug of similar or dissimilar chemical structure or pharamacological activity. Tolerance does not necessarily develop equally to, or at the same rate as, all of the effects of a drug.

Mechanisms of tolerance

At least three types of mechanism may be involved in the development of tolerance:

Altered biological disposition. Changes in absorption, metabolism, distribution, and excretion may theoretically affect the serum concentration of the drug and consequently its effect on target cells.

Cellular mechanisms. Theories about cellular mechanisms of tolerance are based on knowledge about the release of endogenous neuro-transmitters and their reaction with specific synaptic receptors. For example, Paton (1969) proposed a 'surfeit' theory for opiate dependence which could theoretically apply to other drugs too. According to this theory, the amount of neuro-transmitter released by each nerve impulse is reduced by opiates so that more neuro-transmitter therefore remains within the axon terminal. This increasing concentration of neuro-transmitter means that more is available for release by subsequent nerve impulse, and that the effect of the drug is progressively reduced. On drug withdrawal a high concentration of neuro-transmitter is available and produces the characteristic withdrawal syndrome. Sharpless and Jaffe (1969), while agreeing that opiates interfere with neuro-transmitter release, believe that this results in a sort of pharmacological denervation hypersensitivity of the post-synaptic receptors. This would account for the development of tolerance, as the reduced amount of neuro-transmitters available would then have an enhanced effect; the persistence of hypersensitive receptors in the presence of normal concentrations of neuro-transmitter after drug withdrawal would account for the phenomena of the abstinence syndrome.

Alternatively, if a drug produces its effect by a reaction with a specific receptor on the post-synaptic membrane, anything that reduces the number of these available receptors, or perhaps the rate of drug-receptor reaction or even the proportion of occupied to unoccupied receptors, might serve to reduce the effect of the drug – that is, tolerance would be induced.

All of these mechanisms can be grouped together as *adaptive responses* of the neurone to oppose the action of the drug.

Homoeostatic mechanisms. It has been suggested that there may be more than one neural pathway for any physiological function and that if one pathway is depressed by a drug, another will hypertrophy in compensation so that tolerance to the drug develops (Martin, 1968). An elaboration of this theory has been suggested by Sapira and Cherubin (1975) who proposed that in a non-tolerant individual most of the receptors for a particular drug are vacant; when the drug is administered, it will 'fire' these receptors, larger doses reacting with more receptors than smaller doses. If the drug is administered on a chronic basis, a relatively constant state of receptor occupancy is maintained and the CNS adapts to this new steady state by 'endogenous compensation' – by the activation of secondary internal compensatory systems, so that tolerance appears. On drug withdrawal the compensatory systems will be unopposed by the drug-fired receptors for the first time and their activity accounts for the abstinence syndrome.

Before leaving these highly theoretical models of tolerance, it is interesting to consider the parallels that have been drawn between tolerance and learning or memory. Learning has been defined as a relatively permanent change in behaviour on repeated presentation of a stimulus; similarly, in order to develop tolerance it is necessary to subject an organism to a new stimulus (i.e., a drug) and this procedure results in an altered response when the same stimulus occurs again. Presented in this way the analogy is clear and suggests that there may be similar physiological mechanisms underlying both tolerance and memory. There is some experimental evidence to support this idea as tolerance to morphine can be inhibited by the administration of drugs such as actinomycin D or other inhibitors of protein synthesis which also appear to interfere with the consolidation or expression of memory (Kumar & Stolerman, 1977).

Relationship between tolerance and dependence

The nature of the relationship between tolerance and physical dependence is not clear. It has been suggested that a common mechanism is responsible for both phenomena but it should be remembered that the drugs which have most frequently been the subject of investigation are morphine and its derivatives – drugs to which tolerance develops rapidly and on which physical dependence is clear-cut and easily recognizable. Similarly tolerance develops to some of the effects of alcohol, barbiturates, and other sedatives, and physical dependence upon these drugs is again well known. Although for all of these drugs tolerance and physical dependence appear to develop in parallel this does not mean that the two phenomena are fundamentally related. Certainly for other drugs their relationship is less clear cut. Tolerance develops very rapidly, for example to the effects of LSD, but physical dependence upon it does not occur. It is probably true to say that tolerance develops to some of the actions of all drugs that produce physical dependence, but further statements about the nature of this relationship can only be conjectural.

Dependence

It is generally accepted that drug-related behaviour is the interaction between drug, personality and environment and that there is no single causative factor responsible for drug dependence. Indeed it is impossible to imagine that any single factor or theory could account for the wide range of dependence behaviour that exists, for example, in the young person who abuses a wide range of drugs, the middle-aged woman dependent on barbiturates or amphetamines, the adolescent sniffing glue and the Middle Eastern opium smoker. Indeed such is the range of theories on the aetiology of dependence that it is difficult to remember that they are all dealing with the same phenomenon.

Physiological theories

Physiological theories about dependence deal with those drugs that cause physical dependence. As tolerance develops simultaneously to at least some of the effects of the drugs and as many observers believe that the two phenomena are inextricably related, it is perhaps not surprising that theories about physical dependence resemble those about tolerance very closely.

An important observation about the state of physical dependence is that there is little, if any, objective or subjective evidence of the presence of the drug in the body; in fact, it appears as if this state is one of physiological adaptation to the drug. However, when drug administration ceases, the withdrawal or abstinence syndrome develops with an array of symptoms and signs characteristic of the drug or group of drugs upon which the patient is dependent, and which are often opposite in nature to the effects of the drug when acutely administered. The significance of this very basic observation is not known, but attempts to explain it are fundamental to all theories of physical dependence, some of which are outlined below (Wikler, 1972).

Disuse supersensitivity. Dependence-producing drugs are said to reduce the amount of synaptic activity, either by reducing the amount of neural activity or by pharmacological blockade. On drug withdrawal, normal neuro-transmitter activity acts on receptors rendered hypersensitive by their earlier, functional denervation and this accounts for the rebound hyperexcitability of the abstinence syndrome.

Enzyme expansion. By inhibiting the action of a rate-limiting enzyme that synthesizes neuro-transmitters or other important substances, dependence-producing drugs can reduce the concentration of these substances. Increased synthesis of the enzyme then occurs, to restore the status quo, but on drug withdrawal the excessive amount of enzyme produces an increased amount of neuro-transmitter, thereby causing the rebound effects of the abstinence syndrome.

'New receptors' theory. According to this theory, dependence-producing drugs induce the formation of new, post-synaptic receptors for an endogenous neuro-transmitter. Some of these receptors may be occupied by the drug and the drug-receptor combination may be 'silent' or 'active'. The phenomena of the abstinence syndrome are accounted for by the excessive number of receptors in the presence of normal concentrations of neuro-transmitter.

It can be seen that the 'enzyme expansion' and 'new receptor' theories differ only in the proposed site of action of the drug of dependence. In the former the action is pre-synaptic, with increased formation of transmitter-synthesizing enzyme, while in the latter the action is post-synaptic with increased formation of 'receptor-synthesizing enzyme'.

However, none of these physiological theories can satisfactorily account for the initiation of drug abuse and the possible role of genetic factors should not be ignored. As yet this has only been explored in relation to alcohol-dependence and it is clearly difficult to evaluate the relative importance of environmental and inherited factors.

Psychological theories of dependence
Personality theories. Many attempts have been made to define and describe an addiction-prone personality, and most studies have compared drug-dependent with non-dependent individuals. However, any observable personality differences may be the result of dependence on drugs rather than a cause. It is difficult and unreliable to assess personality retrospectively, before dependence on drugs occurred, and unfortunately prospective investigation is not feasible. Another problem is that any one study usually concentrates on a particular subgroup of drug-dependent individuals, for example, those in prison or hospital; not only are these highly selected groups and probably not representative, but institutionalization may affect the result obtained.

Bearing these limitations and criticisms in mind the conclusion of many investigators is that drug-dependent individuals have 'personality disorders in excess of that found in the general population', although many base their conclusions more on personal impressions than on the results of objective tests.

Learning theory. Although the occurrence of an abstinence syndrome is an integral part of physical dependence and could be one of the reasons why a dependent individual continues to take a drug, this is not necessarily always the case and other mechanisms underlying the maintenance of drug-taking should be considered. Different groups of drugs have been examined to see if, apart from causing an abstinence syndrome, they can serve as reinforcers in their own right – in other words, if behaviour resulting in administration of the drug increases. It must be emphasized that a reinforcing drug does not necessarily produce a pleasurable state and, if it does, it is not necessarily the pleasurable state that leads to drug-seeking behaviour.

Animal experiments have shown that some stimulants of the central nervous system, especially amphetamines and cocaine, can be primary reinforcers of drug-seeking behaviour. The same can be said of opiate drugs and of some sedative-hypnotic drugs, including alcohol, although the latter group are less powerful reinforcers than stimulants or opiates; the evidence for reinforcing properties of hallucinogens including cannabis is, at present, very weak. It is interesting that drug-directed responses, previously reinforced by morphine, continue to occur for as long as a year after morphine withdrawal. This behaviour, which does not occur after stimulant withdrawal, is of particular interest in view of the high relapse rate of opiate-dependent individuals even after long periods of enforced abstinence.

In addition to the primary reinforcing properties of drugs, the role of secondary reinforcers may also assume importance in the maintenance of drug-taking behaviour. For example, it is possible that the syringe and needle assume secondary reinforcing properties through their association with the rewards of the drug itself, and measures aimed at extinguishing such secondary reinforcers might be an important contribution to the treatment of dependence on opiates.

It can of course be argued, according to learning theory, that, for those drugs with marked abstinence syndromes, drug-taking is under the control of aversive stimuli – in other words, that drug-taking is continued to avoid the unpleasant experience of withdrawal symptoms. In fact there is little evidence in support of this theory, although many opiate-dependent individuals do claim that they take drugs for this reason (Kumar & Stolerman, 1977).

Sociological theories

The main sociological theory attempting to explain dependence is that of *anomie* (Merton, 1957). This describes the 'goals' of a culture, the 'norms' that can be used to achieve these goals and the 'institutionalised means' which is the distribution of opportunities available for achieving these goals. 'Socially structured strain' arises if there is marked disjunction between these factors, and this strain can be dealt with in several ways. One way is to reject the goals and means and to 'retreat' by joining a deviant, drug-taking subculture. This is not, however, an appropriate explanation, for example, for the behaviour of a successfully employed doctor addict, or even for a young urban addict, who appear to have many goals in common with those of conventional society. Variations on this theory suggest that alternative ways to deal with socially-structured strain or 'dissonance' include attacking the dissonance directly by escapist behaviour, such as taking alcohol or amphetamines. Alternatively, while accepting society's goals, an individual may despair of ever being able to achieve them because of his own personality and may take

hallucinogenic drugs, for example, to change his perception of himself even if only temporarily (Oppenheim, 1976).

In conclusion, many factors may play a part in causing dependence and may assume a different importance in different cases. It is certainly possible that apparently different physical and psychological factors share common or at least communicating pathways within the brain, perhaps, conjecturally, in the hypothalamus so that argument over their relative importance is irrelevant and unnecessary as both are different manifestations of the same 'malfunctioning' of the nervous system.

Epidemiology

From 1920, when the first Dangerous Drugs Act was introduced, right up until about 1950 the pattern of drug dependence in Britain was very stable as far as the number of people involved and the drugs of dependence were concerned. At any one time there were never more than a few hundred addicts of whom a high proportion were members of the medical or nursing professions or those who had become addicted during the course of an illness (so-called therapeutic addicts). There was also a very small group of non-therapeutic addicts in London in the pre-war years; these patients received their prescriptions for heroin or morphine from ordinary physicians because, according to the Rolleston Report of 1926 (Departmental Committee, 1926), those to whom heroin and morphine could be prescribed included 'persons for whom . . . after every effort has been made for the cure of addiction, the drug cannot be completely withdrawn, either because (i) complete withdrawal produces serious symptoms which cannot be satisfactorily treated under the ordinary conditions of private (general) practice; or (ii) the patient, while capable of leading a useful and fairly normal life, so long as he takes a certain non-progressive quantity, usually small, of the drug of addiction, ceases to be able to do so when the regular allowance is withdrawn'.

With the Rolleston Report arose the so-called 'British system' for dealing with narcotic addiction. A 'system' was never planned or even visualized but the idea that addicts were patients, not criminals, and could receive drugs on prescription contrasted sharply with the way that addicts were dealt with in the USA, and probably because of these differences, over the years, the British way of handling the problem was promoted, in trans-Atlantic terminology at first, into a 'system'. As a result of enquiries made in 1958–59, the Brain Committee's first report into the problem of drug addiction (Interdepartmental Committee, 1961) came to the conclusion that the problem was static and that no special measures need be taken. Soon afterwards there was a marked rise in the number of known heroin addicts, from 68 in 1959 to 94 in 1960. It would seem that an important factor accounting for this increase was over-prescribing by a few notorious doctors who thereby gave addicts surplus heroin to peddle in the black market. By 1962 it was clear that the problem of drug addiction needed re-assessment and the Brain Committee was reconvened. Its second report, in 1965 (Interdepartmental Committee, 1965), came to definite conclusions which formed the basis of the Dangerous Drugs Act of 1967. The most important features of this Act were the compulsory notification of addicts to the Home Office, the limitation of the right to prescribe heroin and cocaine to addicts to those doctors holding a special licence from the Home Office and the setting up of special clinics to treat drug-dependent patients. Addictive drugs covered by the Act included methadone, morphine, heroin and cocaine.

Central to the recommendations of the second Brain Committee Report, and therefore to the 1967 Act, was the belief that it was the 'British system' of legal prescription of the drugs to addicts that had been responsible for a relatively low and static addiction rate, and that undercutting the illegal supplier had prevented the development of an organized criminal black market.

In retrospect this interpretation of events was probably too simple. It is far more likely that from 1920 to 1960 Britain, because of prevailing social conditions, had only a small addiction problem without an organized black market, and therefore it was possible to deal with it by legal prescribing. However, by the late 1950s and early 1960s the accumulated social changes of 40 years left the country open for a drug problem and because of the 'British system' unscrupulous doctors were able to respond to the demand for drugs (Edwards, 1978).

The changes in the pattern of drug abuse and dependence that occurred in the late 1960s led to further changes in the law and after some delay the Misuse of Drugs Act 1971 came into operation in 1973, replacing earlier legislation. Briefly the principal innovations of the Act were to divide controlled drugs into three categories according to their harmfulness, and to relate penalties for offences involving these drugs to these categories, making a distinction between unlawful possession of drugs and trafficking. Recognizing that the favoured drugs of dependence and misuse are constantly changing, the new Act introduced a new flexibility and gave the Government power to bring new substances under control when necessary, without having to pass another Act of Parliament.

Opiates

Opium is obtained from the milky exudate of the incised unripe seed capsule of the poppy. The exudate is allowed to dry and becomes a brown, gummy mass which is scraped by hand from the plant, allowed to dry further and then powdered. This powder is crude opium which contains a number of alkaloids of which the most important is morphine. All of the clinically valuable opiate analgesics share similar structural characteristics and are remarkable, more for their general similarity of action rather than for the differences between them, which tend to be differences of degree rather than of nature.

Effects of opiates

Morphine has two main sites of action – on the central nervous system and on smooth muscle. The analgesic effect of morphine is probably due not only to its direct action at one or more sites within the nervous system, but also to the way in which it makes pain seem more tolerable. Other depressant actions in the nervous system include respiratory depression, depression of the cough reflex, drowsiness, inability to concentrate, and sleep. Higher doses cause increasing respiratory depression, unconsciousness, and death. Some excitation of the nervous system may also occur, resulting in miosis, vomiting and, in some species, gross excitation and hyperthermia. A euphoric mood change is common, although dysphoria sometimes occurs. The action of morphine on the hypothalamus and the hypothalamo-pituitary axis has also been studied. Release of antidiuretic hormone (ADH) results from morphine administration and other effects on growth hormone (GH), adrenocorticotrophic hormone (ACTH), follicle-stimulating hormone (FSH) and luteinizing hormone (LH) have also been reported (Reed & Ghodse, 1973; Jaffe, 1975). The most important site of action of morphine on smooth muscle is in the gastro-intestinal tract, where there is increased contraction, producing increased segmentation, rather than increased peristalsis. There is biliary tract spasm, and the muscles of the bronchi, ureters and bladder are affected too. In addition morphine administration, perhaps by causing histamine release, may produce pruritus and sweating. Unfortunately, when morphine is administered regularly, tolerance to its effects occurs and there is marked physical and psychological dependence on it.

Tolerance

Tolerance develops rapidly to many of the effects of morphine. High-grade tolerance develops to analgesia, euphoria or dysphoria, mental clouding, sedation and sleep, respiratory depression, and vomiting whereas little or no tolerance develops to miosis, constipation and convulsions (Hug, 1972).

Although it has been suggested that even a single dose of morphine can induce tolerance to some of its effects, tolerance is usually promoted and maintained by large, frequently administered doses. Any period of abstinence leads to a loss of tolerance so that a regular opiate user may become markedly intoxicated by a dose which, before abstinence, was well tolerated. However, it has been suggested that tolerance to some of the effects of morphine can persist for six months or more. If this is true, relapse to opiate use after prolonged abstinence could be due to physiological causes instead of, or as well as, psychological causes (Fraser & Isbell, 1952; Cochin & Kornetsky, 1964). Morphine-tolerant animals, including man, also show cross-tolerance to other morphine derivatives and morphine-like analgesics, regardless of their chemical type. In practical terms, significant cross-tolerance to analgesics occurs among all opiate analgesics when they are given in equi-analgesic doses.

Opiate receptors

The high degree of specificity of opiate action has been demonstrated by research over the past 50 years and during the last few years, new theories about the mechanism of action of opiates have been proposed, based on the discovery within the brain of specific opiate receptors. These have been found in the central grey matter and in the central thalamus, in pathways thought to be concerned with the transmission of the dull, chronic, poorly localized pain which is effectively relieved by opiates. High concentrates of opiate receptors are also found in the limbic system which is concerned with emotional behaviour and which may, therefore, be involved with the emotional component of pain and the euphoric effects of opiates. In the spinal cord opiate receptors have been identified in the substantia gelatinosa, another tract involved in the perception of pain. The identification of opiate receptors implies the presence within the brain of endogenous morphine-like substances which might act as neurotransmitters. These substances were searched for diligently, and were first isolated in 1975 by Hughes and Kosterlitz (Hughes 1975, Hughes & Kosterlitz 1977) from the brains of pigs. They were found to consist of two pentapeptides, identical except for one amino-acid. These substances were named enkephalins, and there is now good evidence that they are indeed neuro-transmitters, mediating information about pain and emotional behaviour and located like other neuro-transmitters, in nerve endings rather than cell-bodies. Outside the brain, enkephalin has been found in the gastro-intestinal tract of several species.

Within the brain, enkephalin appears to act as an inhibitory neuro-transmitter, probably at a pre-synaptic site, by reacting with opiate receptors on the terminal axon of an excitatory cell. By means of its inhibitory effect the amount of excitatory neuro-transmitter released is reduced. Morphine, which binds to unoccupied opiate receptors, potentiates the analgesic effects of the enkephalin system but with the sustained administration of morphine, the receptors become overloaded. By means of a hypothetical feedback mechanism, the enkephalin neurone stops firing, and in the presence of a reduced concentration of enkephalin, a higher dose of morphine can be tolerated. If morphine is withdrawn suddenly, with only a small quantity of enkephalin available, the phenomena of the abstinence syndrome occur. Obviously, much of this is conjectural, although supportive evidence comes from the observation that in morphine-dependent rats, with endogenous enkephalin release inhibited, there is an increase in brain concentration of enkephalin which returns to normal on drug withdrawal.

It is interesting that enkephalins appear to have very little analgesic activity, but this is probably due to the speed of their degradation, as chemical modification of the molecule to resist degradation increases its analgesic potency. In addition to enkephalins, other substances with opiate-like activity have been found in the brain and given the name of endorphins (endogenous morphine). The term endorphin is used to mean any morphine-like peptide. At present, the role and function of the endorphins is not known, although it has been suggested that they may have a hormonal role within the pituitary or as blood borne hormones. One specific endorphin, isolated from the pituitary gland, has 31 amino-acids and is known as beta-endorphin. The role of enkephalins, if any, in 'endogenous analgesia' is also not known. The observation that prolonged exposure of opiate receptors *in vivo* to enkephalin and endorphin can lead to typical opiate tolerance and dependence suggests that attempts to separate the analgesic and dependence-producing properties of opiates, even if they are based on endogenous compounds, are unlikely to be successful (Snyder, 1977). The role of endorphins in opiate addiction is not yet understood but it has been suggested that when opiate receptors are repeatedly or continuously exposed to heroin or other opiates, the natural production of opiates might be reduced. The withdrawal syndrome could be due, in part to endorphin deficiency when the heroin is taken away and it is possible that the symptoms and signs of the protracted abstinence syndrome could be due to the endorphin system taking a long time to return to normal (Goldstein, 1979).

Epidemiology

Since the opening of the drug-dependence treatment clinics in 1968, the number of opiate addicts known to the Home Office has been increasing, albeit less dramatically than formerly. At the end of 1970, for example, there were 1426 addicts and by 1980 this number had doubled to 2849. In 1980 the number of addicts notified for the first time was 1606, the average rate of increase in the number of first notifications for the decade 1970–80 being about 9 per cent a year. The total number of addicts coming to notice during the course of each year has also been increasing progressively and between 1977 and 1978 there was a 22 per cent increase in the number of addicts notified for the first time from 1108 in 1977 to 1352 in 1978. It is perhaps somewhat encouraging that the proportion of notified addicts under the age of 20 years is falling and that the doses of opiate (predominantly methadone) prescribed by the clinics are much lower than previously. However, there is considerable evidence of an increasing dependence on another opiate, dipipanone, which although manufactured for oral use, is frequently injected. Many addicts obtain this drug legitimately from a sympathetic medical practitioner, as it is not subject to the same legal restriction as heroin or cocaine. However, illicit methods of obtaining both dipipanone and other opiates are also used and in recent years there has been a big increase in the quantity of heroin seized by H.M. Customs and Excise.

The reliability of the Home Office figures and the validity of the index as an epidemiological monitor are always questionable. For example, Blumberg and colleagues (1974) found that half of the patients approaching a drug dependence treatment clinic had been injecting opiates daily for at least two years before approaching the clinic and that half of their friends, who also injected, had never been to a clinic either. Similarly, Ghodse (1977) found that a substantial proportion of narcotic addicts attending an accident and emergency department in London as a result of a drug-related problem were not known to the Home Office, and that 41 per cent of 134 addicts who died in Greater London during a five-year period were also not known (Ghodse *et al.*, 1978). The Home Office figures are inaccurate, partly because addicts do not attend drug-dependence treatment clinics until relatively late in their drug-taking career and also because many doctors fail to fulfil the statutory obligation to notify the Home Office of any addict (or suspected addict) whom they attend.

Opiate addicts in the UK are predominantly male and in their twenties. Their socio-economic background does not differ significantly from the general population norm and unlike US addicts, poverty and minority-group status are not particular features of addiction in the UK. However addicts frequently leave school at younger ages or else withdraw from further training and underachievement is characteristic. Most are born in the UK or Eire and are white. There is a marked association between opiate dependence and delinquency in notified addicts; about 50 per cent of addicts have criminal records that pre-date their drug use and do not involve the use of drugs (Bewley, James & Mahon, 1972; Hawks, 1974).

In the USA methadone maintenance treatment or treatment in a residential setting is followed by a significant reduction in the crime rate (Dole, Nyswander & Warner, 1968; De Leon, Holland & Rosenthal, 1972). In the UK, however, treatment at a drug dependence clinic appears to have no effect on the overall crime rate, although the pattern of offences during the treatment stage is different with a significant increase in the proportion of drug offences (d'Orban, 1975; Gordon, 1978; Wiepert, d'Orban & Bewley, 1979).

Morbidity

There is no clear evidence that chemically pure opiates themselves cause any direct physical damage even with a long period of administration, and the high morbidity and mortality rate of opiate addicts is caused more by the life-style of the addict and the method of drug administration, rather than by any direct effect of opiates. Factors such as dirty injection techniques, the injection of drugs not manufactured for parenteral use (for example, dipipanone tablets), and the contamination of illegal drugs with adulterants are all important in accounting for the formidable list of complications associated with opiate use (Bewley & Ben Arie, 1968).

Despite the high incidence of abnormal liver function tests in opiate addicts and the high incidence of hepatitis, opiates themselves do not seem to be directly hepatotoxic as experimental dependence does not produce signs or symptoms of liver disease. Interestingly, although hepatitis used to be a useful indicator of heroin dependence (de Alarcon & Rathod, 1968) it has been a less successful indicator more recently, as jaundice, hepatitis, and gross abnormalities of liver function seem to occur less frequently now (Reed & Ghodse, 1973). Whether this change, if it exists, is due to a decline in injecting activity or to a true improvement in injecting techniques is not clear.

Two main pulmonary conditions may occur in opiate users – acute pulmonary oedema and angiothrombotic pulmonary hypertension, which is caused by the embolization to the lungs of the inert filler material in capsules and tablets when they are administered intravenously.

Drug overdose is of course a frequent complication of opiate dependence; overdoses are usually accidental, occuring in an attempt to achieve heightened effect, but may also occur because of loss of tolerance after a period of abstinence from drug-taking. Sometimes an overdose is taken deliberately in a suicidal attempt.

Mortality

The high mortality rate associated with opiate use has been known for many years and has been estimated at 20 to 28 times the rate expected for a non-dependent British population of similar demographic characteristics (James, 1967; Bewley, Ben Arie & James, 1968). Four studies that took place after the opening of the drug-dependence treatment clinics in 1968 demonstrated a mean mortality rate (of 642 opiate addicts) of 2 per cent after a follow-up of 12 months

(Boyd, Layland & Crickmay, 1971; Bewley *et al.* 1972; d'Orban, 1973; Stimson, 1973). With longer periods of follow-up this percentage rises progressively. Grimes (1977) studied all opiate addicts notified by hospitals from the time of the introduction of Notification of Addicts Regulations until the end of 1973. During the six years of the study 7 per cent of the notified drug-takers died and as the majority were young it is reasonable to conclude that nearly all did so prematurely: 9 per cent of all drug-takers notified in 1968 and 1969 had died by the end of 1973, compared with only 2 per cent of those notified in 1972 and 1973. A progressively increasing mortality rate was also shown in a follow-up study of 108 opiate addicts first seen between 1963 and 1965 and subsequently each year until 1971 (Chapple, Somekh & Taylor, 1972 a,b): 8 per cent were dead after one year, 12 per cent after two years, 16 per cent after three, four and five years, and 18 per cent after six years. Follow-up of 128 patients who formed a representative sample of addicts attending London drug-dependence treatment clinics in 1969 showed that 12 per cent had died during the 7–8 year follow-up period (Stimson, Oppenheimer & Thorley, 1978). The mean age at death was 28.9 and deaths were evenly distributed over the follow-up period yielding a death rate of 16.7/1000 heroin addicts yearly. This is appreciably lower than the rate quoted by James (1967) for male British addicts in the 1960s. The cause of death is usually drug overdose although this is not always an overdose of opiates alone. One or more other drugs may be taken simultaneously and, indeed, injected barbiturates are now a frequent cause of death of notified drug-takers (Ghodse *et al.*, 1978).

Abstinence syndrome

The symptoms of opiate withdrawal were accurately described a hundred years ago by Levinstein who was aware of the stereotyped nature of the abstinence syndrome. After opiate withdrawal the following symptoms and signs appear: craving for drugs, anxiety, yawning, lacrimation, rhinorrhoea, perspiration, muscle twitching, pilo-erection, anorexia, restlessness, irritability, diarrhoea, increased respiratory rate, mydriasis, and drug-seeking behaviour. In addition, there may be a raised blood pressure and pulse rate, vomiting, spontaneous ejaculation in males, and orgasm in females. Sapira and Cherubin (1975) emphasized that changes in pupil diameter and in the resting respiratory rate may be slight and difficult to observe but are of the greatest clinical significance in diagnosing the opiate abstinence syndrome. The timing of the opiate abstinence syndrome, its onset, peak, and duration vary with different opiate analgesics, with the dose on which the patient was dependent, and with the duration of dependence. For example, an abstinent heroin addict may be suffering from yawning, perspiration, and lacrimation only 8 hours after the last dose of heroin, whereas these features will not be apparent in an abstinent methadone addict until 34–48 hours after a dose. Generally, some symptoms and signs of withdrawal will be apparent within 24 hours of the last dose of opiate if the patient is truly dependent and is not receiving illicit supplies during intended drug withdrawal. The duration of the abstinence syndrome also varies enormously. That due to morphine or heroin withdrawal will peak on the second or third day and will then gradually subside, whereas that due to methadone withdrawal may not reach maximum intensity for several days or so. It is now recognized that the abstinence syndrome has two phases which merge into each other. There is an early, acute or primary phase in which the phenomena already described occur, and which lasts for four to ten weeks; in addition there is a protracted abstinence syndrome lasting for up to 26 weeks, during which certain physiological parameters, such as blood pressure, pulse rate, sensitivity of the respiratory centre to carbon dioxide, pupillary diameter, and so forth, all remain abnormal (Jaffe, 1975). The parallel between the protracted abstinence syndrome and the duration of tolerance for several months is obvious, and both of these observations may help to explain why relapse to opiate use occurs even after several months of abstinence.

The abstinence syndrome can also be induced in an opiate-dependent individual by the administration of an opiate antagonist such as naloxone.

Opiate antagonists

During the search for new opiate analgesics without the disadvantages of respiratory depression, tolerance, and dependence, many new compounds were synthesized, some of which, such as naloxone, naltrexone, cyclazocine and pentazocine have some antagonistic properties (Pradhan & Dutta, 1977). Of these, naloxone and naltrexone are pure antagonists. When administered to man in the absence of opiates, they have no important effects, even in high dosage. The main difference between these two drugs is that naltrexone has a somewhat longer duration of action.

If a small dose of naloxone (0.4–0.8 mg) is given either intramuscularly or intravenously to a non-dependent person, the effects of opiates can be prevented or abolished more or less immediately. For example, opiate-induced respiratory depression will be reversed within one or two minutes. This effect will last for several hours, depending on the dose of naloxone. If naloxone is given to opiate-dependent individuals, the abstinence syndrome is precipitated within minutes.

Cyclazocine, like nalorphine, is an agonist–antagonist and tolerance develops to the agonist but not the antagonist effects of these two drugs. In fact, after prolonged high dosage, withdrawal of nalorphine or cyclazocine produces a true abstinence syndrome characterized by light-headedness or fainting, lacrimation, rhinorrhoea, yawning, and diarrhoea; however, there is no craving or drug-seeking behaviour.

Uses of opiate antagonists
(1) Treatment of opiate overdose: see Treatment.
(2) Treatment of neonatal respiratory depression: if opiate analgesics are given to a woman during labour their depressant effect on the baby can be reversed by giving naloxone 0.4–0.8 mg to the mother, shortly before delivery. Alternatively, naloxone can be given to the baby although a therapeutic dose has not been established; 5 μg/kg has been suggested (Jaffe & Martin, 1975).
(3) Diagnosis of physical dependence on opiates: the use of opiate antagonists for this purpose is less important now that sensitive biochemical tests are available for drug-screening. However, the procedure is of theoretical interest.
The diameter of the pupils of the patient and the resting respiratory rate are measured in a dimly lit room; 3 mg of nalorphine are injected subcutaneously, and the measurements are repeated 30 minutes later. In an opiate-dependent patient, the antagonist effect of nalorphine will cause pupil dilatation of 0.5 mm or more, together with other withdrawal signs, such as increased respiration. In an opiate-naive individual the agonist effect of nalorphine may be manifest by pupillary constriction or there will be no change, in which case a further 5 mg of nalorphine are given, and if there is still no response, a third dose of 7 mg can be administered. If naloxone is used, the initial

dose is 0.16 mg i.m., and 0.24 mg can be given subsequently if necessary; in a dependent individual pupil dilatation will occur but no change occurs in a non-dependent individual (Sapira & Cherubin, 1975).

(4) Treatment of opiate dependence: see treatment.

Treatment

The treatment of dependence on opiates has two components. Firstly, there are the specific measures described below which are used to treat dependence on this particular group of drugs and its complications. Secondly, there are more general measures such as psychotherapy, therapeutic communities, and rehabilitation which are discussed in volume 4, chapter 10. The successful management of opiate dependence integrates both types of treatment as appropriate for the individual patient.

(1) *Opiate maintenance.* Three important practical questions have to be answered by any doctor treating opiate-dependent patients with opiates – for whom to prescribe, what to prescribe, and what dose to prescribe. In other branches of medical practice, the same therapeutic decisions are taken according to the needs of the individual patient's medical condition. In the field of drug dependence, the doctor's role in controlling the drug problem as a whole assumes importance and therapeutic decisions are made with an awareness of the existence of a black market from which the patient may obtain more or other drugs and in which he may sell the drugs prescribed for him. In no other field does a situation arise in which a patient, although voluntarily seeking treatment, may have very different treatment aims from those of his doctor, whose decisions are rarely accepted without argument. Indeed, bargaining about the drug and dose to be prescribed occurs uniquely in the drug dependence treatment clinics.

The decision about for whom to prescribe can be difficult because in these days of multiple drug abuse, the patient may be abusing a wide variety of drugs including opiates without being physically dependent on any. A regular supply of prescribed opiate might then be an important factor in causing dependence. Detailed enquiries should be made about the history of drug-taking, attention being given to whether the financial means of the patient could adequately account for the drug use claimed, and to the patient's familiarity with the drug scene.

A careful physical examination, particularly for signs of opiate withdrawal and of self-injection, together with repeated urine testing for the presence of drugs are also very important. In drug dependence treatment clinics the decision about prescription is taken only after a period of assessment of a few weeks, during which time the patient is interviewed on different occasions by different members of the therapeutic team. Obviously the value of assessment is vitiated if the patient is in receipt of prescribed methadone from a sympathetic practitioner, who accepts the patient's claim of dependence without question and before referral to the clinic. One factor among many affecting the decision about prescription is the knowledge that a refusal to prescribe opiates is followed by difficulty in holding the patient in treatment (Blumberg *et al.*, 1974).

Because of cross-tolerance, it is theoretically unimportant which opiate is prescribed to an opiate-dependent patient. In practice, in the UK the choice is between heroin and methadone. In the eleven years since the opening of the clinics, there has been a trend away from prescribing injectable drugs, and oral methadone mixture is now generally considered to be the drug of choice because its longer duration of action permits once-daily administration, because the complications of self-injection are avoided and because it has less black market potential.

Mitcheson and Hartnoll (1978) investigated the consequences of prescribing injectable heroin or oral methadone to opiate-dependent patients. Overall, those patients who received heroin continued to inject regularly and there appeared to be no improvement in either their social function or their use of illicit drugs, as is sometimes claimed. The prescription of oral methadone resulted in a higher abstinence rate after twelve months. However, it was also associated with a much lower re-attendance rate, the clinic failing to maintain contact with a group of patients who were highly involved in criminal activities to maintain their illicit drug use.

The dose of opiate to be prescribed has to be assessed on an individual basis. The aim should be to prescribe the minimum so that the patient has to take it all, personally, to prevent the abstinence syndrome and has no excess to produce euphoria or sedation, or to sell. This decision requires skill and experience to evaluate the claims made by the patient. In practice, nowadays, the dose of methadone prescribed to a new patient is usually between 40 and 60 mg daily. This represents an enormous reduction since the time when the clinics opened when daily doses of heroin of 200–300 mg were not uncommon.

Originally, it was understood that for most patients, opiate maintenance should be for a limited, although unspecified period, during which time it was hoped that a therapeutic relationship would develop between the patient and the staff of the clinic, and that this relationship would be used to encourage the gradual withdrawal of drugs. In practice, maintenance has become a long-term condition for many patients, and although this was envisaged by the Rolleston Committee in 1926 (Departmental Committee, Ministry of Health, 1926), they probably had no idea that it would be the therapeutic endpoint for so many young patients. What appears to be a useful approach for new patients is a 'treatment contract package' which is agreed between staff and patient before opiates are first prescribed. After a period of stabilization on oral methadone, the dose is gradually reduced over a realistic time scale until abstinence is achieved, when further follow-up and support is carried out at a 'non-prescribing' session of the clinic. The goal of drug withdrawal is coupled with others, such as getting a job, achieving a more stable life-style, and giving up the abuse of illicit drugs. This approach encourages the patient and the therapeutic team to be active in the same direction rather than allowing the clinic to become just a prescribing centre where the perpetual conflict between staff and patients produces frustration and attitudes of indifference. It also emphasizes the importance of other goals apart from drug abstinence and offers to all patients the opportunity to come off drugs, even if only for a short time. Obviously, the risk of relapse is accepted and there should always be the option of re-assessment.

(2) *High dose methadone maintenance*. An alternative form of methadone maintenance was pioneered in the USA by Dole and Nyswander (1965) in which the patient is prescribed a high dose of methadone (for example 80–120 mg), achieved gradually if necessary, by stepwise increments of dose, so that the craving for other opiates is lost. If the patient does experiment with them again, the euphoric effect is blocked, and drug-seeking behaviour should stop as a result of extinction of a previously conditioned response. Success has been reported with this type of treatment in terms of life-style, employment, and misuse of illicit drugs and Newman & Whitehill (1979) in Hong Kong reporting a double-blind comparison of meth-adone and placebo maintenance, have demonstrated the superiority of methadone. In the UK, although some patients are on high doses of methadone, they are those patients who were formerly injecting large doses of heroin and who require this level of methadone maintenance to prevent withdrawal symptoms; some still, however, abuse other opiates. High dose methadone maintenance specifically for its blockade effect has never really been assessed in this country and the differing drug scenes of the UK and the USA mean that the experience of one cannot necessarily be applied to the other. This treatment clearly carries the risk of diversion of prescribed drugs to the black market, unless daily visits are made to the clinic for drug consumption.

(3) *Opiate detoxification*. Although abstinence from opiate use is a fundamental and important goal in the treatment of a dependent individual, it can be attempted as a short-term project only with a patient whose motivation and co-operation is assured. It should be preceded by careful psychiatric assessment and physical examination. Occasionally, with a highly motivated, stable patient, it is carried out on an out-patient basis, but usually the patient is admitted to hospital.

The abrupt withdrawal of opiates results in the unpleasant, although rarely dangerous, abstinence syndrome – the 'cold turkey', so feared by the opiate-dependent patient. Usually opiates are withdrawn gradually, the first step being to establish the stabilization dose if the patient has not previously been receiving prescribed opiates. Methadone is the drug of choice and as an approximation, 1 mg methadone is equivalent to 1 mg heroin, 3 mg morphine, or 20 mg pethidine. A practical way to arrive at the stabilization dose is to observe the patient for signs of opiate withdrawal and then to administer methadone 15–20 mg; further methadone is given if the signs are not suppressed, or when they occur. After 24–36 hours, the daily stabilization dose can be calculated. Thereafter it can be reduced by 3–5 mg daily, although initial reduction can be higher if the patient is on a large dose to start with. Other drugs can be used to reduce the anxiety which is invariably experienced at this stage. Minor tranquillizers can be given, but phenothiazines are preferable because of the lack of evidence of any dependence liability.

(4) *Opiate antagonists*. The theoretical basis for the treatment of opiate dependence with antagonists,

rests on the observation that they abolish, or greatly reduce, the pleasurable effects of opiates which may be reinforcing drug-taking behaviour. Thus, if an abstinent opiate user maintained on an opiate antagonist experiences craving for opiates and obtains them, they are robbed of their reinforcing effect and drug-seeking behaviour will stop as a result of extinction of previously conditioned responses. Cyclazocine and naltrexone have been used for treating opiate dependent patients. Because of the dysphoria caused by cyclazocine, it is not wholly suitable, although this side effect can be minimized by gradual increments of dosage up to a total of 4–6 mg daily. Naltrexone, like naloxone, is a pure antagonist, but with a longer duration of action, blocking the effects of opiates for up to 72 hours. It can thus be administered on a thrice-weekly basis, providing a practical advantage over cyclazocine, and it also lacks the dysphoric side effects of the latter. Currently, an even longer-acting antagonist is being sought, and depot preparations of naltrexone are being tried in animal experiments to extend opiate blocking action for up to 60 days. The practical advantages of this scheme are obvious, as once the injection is given patient non-compliance cannot occur.

Although the use of narcotic antagonists in treating opiate dependence is theoretically simple and logical, the result of treatment is not predictable because of the widely different personalities and situations of the patients. Successful treatment depends on a high degree of patient motivation and there is a clear relationship between time on naltrexone and opiate-free status (Resnick, Resnick & Washton, 1979).

(5) *Acupuncture*. Although acupuncture has been practised in China for thousands of years, its use in the treatment of opiate dependence dates from 1972 when it was observed that during a course of acupuncture-induced analgesia, symptoms of opiate withdrawal were simultaneously relieved (Wen & Cheung, 1973). It was subsequently found that heroin addicts, treated with acupuncture specifically for the relief of withdrawal symptoms sustained a rise in CSF met-enkephalin levels although CSF endorphin remained constant. In contrast, in ten patients receiving low frequency electro-acupuncture for recurrent pain, CSF beta-endorphin levels rose, but not the enkephalin levels, while in a control group without pain, beta-endorphin levels did not rise.

Although the source of the increased endorphin in the CSF has not been established it has been suggested that it originates in the pituitary gland. However, as beta-endorphin can still be identified in the CSF of hypopituitary patients it is possible that the brain might (also) be a source.

The mechanism of acupuncture in the treatment of opiate dependence, or indeed of any condition is not yet understood but it has been suggested that the enkephalinergic system may be involved in addicts, the serotoninergic system in high frequency electro-acupuncture, and the endorphinergic system in low frequency electro-acupuncture.

(6) *Treatment of the opiate abstinence syndrome*. The features of the opiate abstinence syndrome have already been described. Although it is unpleasant, it is rarely dangerous and the diagnosis should only be made after the observation of specific signs of withdrawal and never on the basis of the history or symptoms alone. Although any opiate can be used in the treatment of the abstinence syndrome, oral methadone is the drug of choice: 10 mg should be given initially, followed by 20 mg one hour later if there is no improvement; a further 20 mg can be repeated two hours later if necessary, a total of 40–50 mg in divided doses being sufficient to relieve the symptoms of most opiate-dependent patients, while other arrangements for treatment are being made.

(7) *Treatment of opiate overdose*. The treatment of an overdose of an opiate drug is according to accepted medical principles. In the presence of severe respiratory depression, the use of an opiate antagonist may be considered. In an opiate-dependent patient, however, the abstinence syndrome will be precipitated, and cannot then be suppressed by the administration of opiates during the period of action of the antagonist. However, a small dose of naloxone (0.4–0.8 mg i.v.) should reverse respiratory depression without producing severe withdrawal symptoms; as the duration of action of naloxone is short, its administration may need to be repeated if respiratory depression and excessive sedation recur.

Prognosis

The proportion of opiate-dependent individuals who subsequently abstain from opiate use is not known. A recent report by Stimson, Oppenheimer and Thorley (1978) describes the status of 128 patients first interviewed in 1969 when they were receiving daily prescriptions of heroin. Seven years later, approximately one-third were abstinent and nearly half were still taking opiates, almost all of the latter still obtaining them on prescription. Wille (1980) interviewed the abstinent group a year later and concluded that changes in the socio-cultural environment play an important role in the process of recovery. Chapple, Somekh and Taylor (1972) also studied a large group of opiate addicts. After five years, the short-term addicts (those notified to the Home Office less than 18 months before first clinic attendance) were more likely to be opiate free than were "chronic' addicts and Chapple and colleagues believed that prognosis is more hopeful if drug withdrawal is effected within a year of treatment, preferably with minimal or no prescribing. Whether 'modern' opiate-dependent patients, with much lower levels of opiate use in a somewhat different drug scene will have a similar pattern of outcome is of course conjectural and many important questions remain to be answered. It is not clear, for example, what the effect of regular prescription of opiate is. It is possible, as Chapple and colleagues (1972a) suggest, that such a supply confirms a patient in his dependence or at any rate delays abstention. Similarly, little is known about opiate-dependent patients who have not (yet) attended a clinic although their numbers may be considerable, or about those who do not receive a regular prescription for opiates from the clinic and subsequently fail to re-attend. It is also not known how many people use opiates occasionally over a long period or whether this type of use ever succeeds dependence upon opiates. Certainly many factors apart from clinic-based treatment affect the outcome of opiate dependence which should not be assesssed only in terms of opiate use but in terms of life-style, physical health, criminal record, employment, misuse of illicit drugs, and so forth.

Barbiturates

All barbiturate drugs are chemical derivatives of barbituric acid. Traditionally, they are classified according to the duration of their hypnotic action in animals into long-acting, intermediate, and short-acting drugs, these differences being related to the rates of metabolism and excretion, and to the constitution of the molecular side-chains. The relevance of these observations to the action of barbiturates in man is not clear and a more useful and practical classification would be into sedative–hypnotic and anaesthetic barbiturates.

Effects

The central nervous system is very sensitive to the effects of barbiturates, which appear to have negligible effects on other organs. In the central nervous system there is a depressant effect at all levels, particularly on the cerebral cortex and the reticular activating system, varying from sedation to hypnosis, to general anaesthesia, and to death according to the particular barbiturate chosen, the dose, the individual's barbiturate tolerance, the route of administration, and the state of excitation of the nervous system.

Barbiturate-induced sleep differs from natural sleep in its reduced proportion of rapid eye movement (REM) sleep, an effect which is not always wholly desirable. Moreover, although subjective feelings of drowsiness may or may not be reported, some slowing of performance is detectable for at least 12 hours after a single dose of barbiturates (Malpas, Rowan, Joyce & Scott, 1970). It seems likely therefore that there may be many people driving or performing other skilled or potentially dangerous tasks while suffering from a mild hangover of which they may be unaware. At hypnotic and sedative doses, barbiturates have no obvious effects on the autonomic nervous system, but with increasing doses there is depression of the respiratory and vasomotor centres, producing respiratory depression and hypotension. At these doses there is also reduced urine volume because of increased secretion of antidiuretic hormone from the posterior pituitary.

The mortality rate of barbiturate overdose varies from centre to centre and, depending on the proportion of cases with severe poisoning, is reported to be between 0.8 per cent and 5 per cent, or even higher (Linton & Ledingham, 1966; *Lancet*, 1967). It has been estimated that about 2000 deaths occur each year in the United Kingdom from this cause, reflecting the frequency with which barbiturates are used in incidents of drug overdose (*British Medical Journal*, 1976).

Tolerance

Tolerance to some of the effects of barbiturates develops rapidly. For example, even with the therapeutic doses of barbiturates prescribed for the insomniac patient, there is increasing delay in the onset of sleep, reduction in the total sleep time, and within as short a period as five days, a return of the proportion of REM sleep to normal values (Evans, Lewis, Gibb & Cheetham, 1968). The habitual barbiturate user may show little sign of sedation and may only be sleeping for an hour or two more than usual while consuming daily doses of barbiturate that would be highly sedating for the barbiturate-naive individual.

Although it is difficult to compare tolerance toward different classes of drugs, it is fair to describe the tolerance that develops towards barbiturates as limited in extent when compared with tolerance to opiates. For the latter drugs, there is seemingly no upper limit to the dose that an opiate-tolerant individual may take because tolerance develops to the fatal, respiratory depressant effect, so that an opiate-dependent individual may be taking a dose of heroin, for example, 100 (or more) times greater than the usual, single, therapeutic dose. In contrast, the chronic barbiturate user may possibly be taking 2 g pentobarbitone daily, in divided doses, but more probably 1–1.2 g, which is only a few times greater than the normal therapeutic dose of pentobarbitone (0.1–0.2 g). At a dose level of 1.0 g per day, which would be profoundly sedating for a non-tolerant person, the dependent individual may show few, if any, signs of sedation or intoxication. However, once the point of maximum tolerance has been reached, even a small increase of dose beyond this point produces a state of intoxication, and a further increase is as likely to be fatal for the dependent individual as for the non-dependent. It will be appreciated that this represents one of the main hazards of barbiturate dependence – that the coexistent state of tolerance narrows the gap between the dose that can be taken without ill-effect and the lethal dose, so that a fatal overdose can easily occur.

Increased drug metabolism caused by the induction of hepatic microsomal enzymes by barbiturates themselves is one proposed mechanism of tolerance, thought to be of particular importance in tolerance to short-acting barbiturates such as hexobarbitone. This mechanism cannot wholly account for the development of tolerance as there is tolerance not only to the dose of barbiturate, but also to a given serum concentration; altered sensitivity of the central nervous system has therefore been suggested as an additional mechanism, although the exact nature of this change is not known. This second mechanism must assume greater importance in the development of tolerance to long-acting barbiturates such as barbitone, which is not metabolized significantly (Hug, 1972).

A considerable degree of cross-tolerance develops between different central nervous system depressants, even when they are from chemically different classes, such as the alcohols, barbiturates and benzodiazepines. The mechanisms underlying this cross-tolerance are not fully understood; it seems likely that enzyme induction is important in cross-tolerance among non-alcoholic CNS depressants, but that altered nervous system sensitivity is the basis of cross-tolerance between alcohol and other nervous system depressants. Cross-tolerance does not develop between barbiturates and opiates (Hug, 1972).

Dependence

Dependence on barbiturates has both physical and psychological components. Physical dependence is characterized by an abstinence syndrome that occurs on drug withdrawal and by the state of chronic intoxication that usually develops in the dependent individual. Animal experiments have demonstrated the reinforcing properties of barbiturates and other sedative-hypnotics, although most experiments involve intravenous rather than oral administration. These drugs appear to be less powerful reinforcers of behaviour than are stimulants and opiates, although the behavioural depressant properties of barbiturates may interfere with the self-administration of drugs (Kumar & Stolerman, 1977). It is difficult to define the threshold of dose and the duration of use that is necessary to produce physical dependence on barbiturates because it depends on the particular criteria of dependence that are adopted. When the symptoms and signs of the abstinence syndrome as described below are taken as the criteria for physical dependence, a dose of pentobarbitone of 0.6–0.8 g per day taken for two months is required, and it is only when 1 g or more is being taken daily that a majority suffer withdrawal convulsions and delirium (Sapira & Cherubin, 1975; Sutherland, 1977).

Abstinence syndrome

The symptoms and signs of the barbiturate abstinence syndrome develop progressively; they include weakness, anxiety, insomnia, anorexia, nausea and vomiting, sweating, tachycardia (pulse rate over 100 per minute) with an increase in pulse rate of more than 15 per minute on standing, orthostatic hypotension, increased muscle tone with muscle twitching and tremors, mydriasis, and increased reflexes. These so-called minor phenomena may be followed by the major phenomena of convulsions of a grand mal type, which may progress to status epilepticus, and by a psychotic condition that closely resembles alcoholic delirium tremens with disorientation, sensory clouding, and visual (and auditory) hallucinations.

The onset and duration of the abstinence syndrome are variable, depending on the duration of action of the barbiturate being taken, the dose, and the length of time for which it has been taken. The early symptoms of the abstinence syndrome may appear between 8 and 36 hours after the last dose of pentobarbitone, reach their peak on the second day, and decline in intensity over the next week or two. Convulsions may develop as early as 12 to 16 hours after withdrawal, or as late as the twelfth day.

Chronic intoxication

Because there is an upper limit to the dose of barbiturates to which tolerance develops, intoxication is a common feature of dependence on these drugs. Symptoms of intoxication include drowsiness, difficulty in thinking, emotional instability, and agitation and, according to the severity, progressive signs of intoxication may be observed: there is a fine, lateral gaze nystagmus, a decrease in alertness with coarse nystagmus, reduced reflexes, ataxia, slurred speech, positive Rombergism, thick speech, and nystagmus on forward gaze. With even greater levels of intoxication, marked ataxia occurs with falling, confusion, sleep with difficulty in arousing, miosis, respiratory depression, shock, mydriasis, and death.

Epidemiology

Barbiturates were first introduced into clinical practice in 1903 when barbitone became commercially available. Subsequently, as other barbiturates were synthesized, this group of drugs was prescribed with increasing frequency. One reason for their popularity was that they were apparently safe and effective hypnotics, shortening the delay until sleep occurred and increasing the total sleep time. At first the only common adverse effects that they appeared to produce were skin rashes and, occasionally, the precipitation of acute porphyria.

Despite early reports describing the similarity of symptoms following barbiturate withdrawal and those of alcoholic delirium tremens, nearly 50 years elapsed after the introduction of barbiturates before dependence upon them was described. In time, and with their increasing use in suicides and suicidal attempts, the other main drawback of barbiturates – their serious effects when taken in overdose – also became apparent. For example, in 1962, barbiturates

were used in 55 per cent of 522 episodes of deliberate self poisoning in Edinburgh (Kessel, 1965).

During the early 1960s, the number of prescriptions issued annually for barbiturate hypnotics remained fairly steady at just over 15 million per year, but from 1965 to 1970 this decreased by 24 per cent to 12.2 million (Williams, 1980) and since then the decrease has continued and accelerated so that only 4.8 million prescriptions were dispensed in 1976. Although any reduction in the available pool of barbiturates is encouraging, the possibility of a residual, 'hard-core' of barbiturate-dependent individuals, still able to maintain their supply from this reduced pool, should not be overlooked. In the early 1960s, it appeared that the 'typical' barbiturate-dependent individual was a middle-aged woman obtaining her drugs on prescription from her general practitioner, probably with neither of them acknowledging her dependence status. The size of this problem and the extent to which it still persists is not known, but by the late 1960s there was evidence of widespread barbiturate abuse by young people.

The problems of barbiturate abuse by young people

It has been suggested that the reduced availability of heroin in the late 1960s encouraged opiate addicts to resort to other drugs such as barbiturates, although at one clinic a more liberal prescription of opiates did not reduce barbiturate abuse by its patients (Aylett, 1978). It is more likely that barbiturate abuse by this group was (and is) one facet, albeit an extremely dangerous one, of the increasing interest shown by young people in drugs in general and of the trend towards multiple drug use. However, the regular use of barbiturates induces dependence on them and patients may become dependent on both opiates and barbiturates.

In this situation, it is common for barbiturates (and other drugs), although manufactured for oral use, to be injected. This practice is associated with a number of local complications principally due to the irritant action of barbiturate and often aggravated by infection.

One of the most frequent problems presented by these patients is that of drug overdose. During a month-long survey in accident and emergency departments in London, 395 drug-dependent individuals were identified and they accounted for 412 separate incidents of drug overdose. Barbiturates were used in more than half of these incidents, often in connection with other drugs. In 60 per cent of cases, the barbiturate had not been prescribed for the patient but had been obtained illicitly and nearly a quarter of these patients had injected the drugs. Many of these patients had previously been notified to the Home Office for dependence on opiates but attended hospital because of the complications of abuse of non-notifiable drugs, such as barbiturates (Ghodse, 1977).

Obviously, a serious drug overdose with loss of consciousness requires hospital admission and treatment is in accordance with accepted medical principles. Nowadays, doctors should be aware that anyone, and in particular a young patient who takes a barbiturate overdose, may be physically dependent on barbiturates and that recovery from the acute effects of the overdose may be followed by the manifestations of the withdrawal syndrome, which should be treated appropriately.

A more difficult situation to deal with is the state of chronic intoxication with barbiturates, in which the patient is often abusive and aggressive. Care should be taken not to provoke hostility, but physical restraint may be necessary if the patient is violent or injures himself. A sedative drug, such as chlorpromazine 50–100 mg, intramuscularly, may be required although it potentiates the effects of other central nervous system depressants.

Another difficult situation is that of the young drug-dependent individual in a general practitioner's surgery or hospital out-patient department who is demanding drugs, whether opiate or non-opiate (usually barbiturates) and who, if his demands are not met, becomes abusive and aggressive. Although it may seem easier to comply with his demands, this policy is unwise: the doctor will soon be visited by other drug abusers as word gets round that he will prescribe for them and the general pool of drugs available to addicts is continuously replenished by such lax prescribing. In this situation, even if a patient appears to be suffering from barbiturate withdrawal, the prescription of barbiturates is not recommended. The barbiturate withdrawal syndrome is a serious condition which should be managed in hospital; the prescription of barbiturates, on demand, on an out-patient basis merely perpetuates the problem for the dependent individual, the doctor, and the community.

The abuse of barbiturates by young, drug-dependent individuals is associated with a high mortality rate: soon after they began to be widely used in this way, they were found in significant quantities in autopsies and in London, in the early 1970s, more than half of the deaths of drug-dependent individuals were primarily attributable to barbiturates (Ghodse *et al.*, 1978).

Management of barbiturate withdrawal

Because the barbiturate abstinence syndrome may include the serious and potentially life-threatening condition of grand mal convulsions as well as psychosis, withdrawal of these drugs from an individual who is physically dependent upon them must be managed in a planned and careful way, in hospital and preferably in a closed ward.

Pentobarbitone is probably the most suitable drug, as its short duration of action permits a flexible regime of drug administration. Phenothiazines are contra-indicated; they are an illogical choice and may precipitate or potentiate convulsions. The first step is to decide the dose of pentobarbitone on which neither signs of withdrawal nor of intoxication are apparent. In practice, for most male patients and for female patients known to have had convulsions on drug withdrawal previously, a daily dose of 1000 mg pentobarbitone is required; this is given as an elixir in four doses, at 8 a.m, 12 noon, 5 p.m and 10 p.m. Most female patients, male patients who have been out of hospital for less than two weeks, and male patients previously intoxicated on 1000 mg per day should be started on 800 mg pentobarbitone daily. Higher doses may be needed if there is a definite history of larger daily doses. The starting dose is administered for three days. If signs of withdrawal occur, this stage should be prolonged and/or the dose increased. Thereafter, the dose should be reduced by 100 mg daily. Throughout this period, and for 48 hours after drug withdrawal, careful observation of the patient and in particular of pulse and blood pressure, both lying and standing, is required. Although this scheme may appear unnecessarily lengthy, it is a safe procedure and one which, because it is usually acceptable to the patient, is more likely to obtain his or her co-operation.

Non-barbiturate, sedative–hypnotic drugs

The description of many sedative–hypnotic drugs as 'non-barbiturate' implies that it is their differences from barbiturates that are important, rather than any intrinsic superiority. Since the disadvantages of barbiturates have become apparent, there has been a continuous search for new and safer drugs lacking the dependency liability of barbiturates and their serious effects when taken in overdose. Many new drugs have been synthesized which can be classified into two broad groups of benzodiazepines (diazepam, chlordiazepoxide, and so forth) and non-benzodiazepines (for example methaqualone, meprobamate, glutethimide, chlormethiazole). Although some of these drugs, particularly the benzodiazepines, do appear to be 'safer' than barbiturates, any differences are those of degree rather than of radical changes in the properties of the drugs.

The effects of these drugs when taken in overdose assumes great importance because of the frequency with which they are used in episodes of deliberate self-poisoning. Whereas barbiturates were once the group of drugs used most frequently, non-barbiturate tranquillizers and hypnotics are now the principal drugs of overdose and although the margin of safety between the therapeutic dose and the dose required for serious overdose or death is considerable for benzodiazepines, non-benzodiazepines have a much narrower margin which is encroached upon by the development of tolerance to the therapeutic, but not to the lethal, effects. When taken in overdose, all of these drugs show features of poisoning similar to those of barbiturate overdose, although some (e.g. glutethimide) are particularly dangerous. Although benzodiazepine overdose is rarely life-threatening, their effects are potentiated and may be fatal if they are taken, as they often are, together with other central nervous system depressants, such as alcohol. Despite early hopes and claims to the contrary, tolerance develops to some of the effects of all of these drugs, although it is thought to develop at a slower rate for benzodiazepines than for other sedative-hypnotics. Cross-tolerance is said to exist between these different central nervous system depressants, despite their chemical differences, although the mechanisms of tolerance and cross tolerance are not understood (Hug 1972).

Dependence, both physical and psychological, can also develop on all of these drugs (Lader, 1978; 1981). The fact that most reports of dependence are of isolated cases only, suggests that the dependence liability is indeed less than that of barbiturates, but the abstinence syndromes and states of chronic intoxication are very similar in kind to what is caused by barbiturates.

During recent years, the number of prescriptions for barbiturates has been falling, partly because of an awareness of the dangers and partly because of the availability of apparently safer alternatives, which have correspondingly been prescribed with increasing frequency (Williams, 1980; 1981). Given that these drugs possess a dependence liability too, it is not known how many of the millions of prescriptions dispensed are for individuals dependent upon them – in the sense that they are tolerant to some of the effects of the drugs and may exhibit at least mild symptoms on drug withdrawal. Neither the individual concerned, nor the doctor may be aware of their (mild) state of dependence, just as in the 1950s and 1960s there were many middle-aged housewives unaware of their dependence on their regular dose of barbiturates.

Certainly, non-barbiturate sedative-hypnotics are already used extensively in one form of drug misuse – that of drug overdose (Ghodse, 1981; Volans, 1981; Kreitman, 1981). They are also being used increasingly by those young drug-dependent individuals who abuse a wide variety of drugs, and if the trend towards reduced availability of barbiturates continues, it seems likely that these newer drugs will take the place of barbiturates in the drug abuser's 'repertoire'.

It has been suggested that some drugs may be drugs of dependence, but not of abuse, either because of unpleasant, initial effects, or because they do not produce a quick escape from reality (Oswald, Lewis, Březinová & Dunleavy, 1972). As yet, there is little evidence for the widespread use of some of these drugs and this may be related to pharmacokinetic properties, such as the onset of action and dose-response curve. Individual case reports of dependence often stress that the patient had previously abused other drugs such as barbiturates, implying that in these cases, an underlying propensity for drug abuse was more important than the properties of the drugs. It follows that the full dependence liability of these drugs may well be exposed if they become the frequent drugs of abuse of young, drug-dependent individuals deliberately exploring their psychic effects. On no account should the lessons of the last century be forgotten – that heroin was introduced as the 'heroic' cure for morphine dependence, that cocaine was used to treat the same condition, and that it took 30 years and 50 years respectively for the dependence-producing potential of amphetamines and barbiturates to be appreciated. In this context, claims for the lack of dependence liability of any psycho-active substance must be viewed with extreme scepticism.

Amphetamines

Amphetamine was first synthesized in 1927 and was introduced for the treatment of asthma and as a nasal decongestant. In the 1940s the effect of amphetamine in reducing appetite was noted so that it was used in the management of obesity and it was also prescribed for the treatment of mild depression.

Effects

Amphetamine is a synthetic sympathomimetic amine closely related chemically to adrenaline. It has comparatively weak effects on the sympathetic nervous system, manifested by tachycardia, palpitations, hypertension, dry mouth, sweating and so forth, but it has powerful central stimulant effects, because of which it has become a drug of abuse. Dextroamphetamine, the dextrorotatory isomer, is approximately twice as powerful as amphetamine as a central stimulant and is a less potent peripheral sympathomimetic. Amphetamine acts by interaction with the catecholamines, noradrenaline, and probably dopamine too, increasing their release from nerve terminals.

When taken orally, the amphetamine user experiences euphoria, self-confidence, and mental alertness with greater capacity for concentration. Feelings of hunger and fatigue are reduced, and with a feeling of greater energy, the user feels able to tackle any job. There may be increased talkativeness, restlessness, and even agitation. As the effects of the drug wear off, fatigue, drowsiness, and sleep supervene.

Tolerance and dependence

Tolerance develops to some of the effects of amphetamine, but not to others. Marked tolerance develops to amphetamine-induced euphoria so that chronic users may take 250–1000 mg d-amphetamine daily (as compared with 10–20 mg daily as the usual therapeutic dose) and intravenous users may inject up to 1000 mg methylamphetamine every few hours. Tolerance also develops to the cardiovascular effects of amphetamine and to its appetite suppressant effect. However, there is little tolerance to the awakening effect of amphetamine, which is therefore an effective treatment for narcolepsy. Cross-tolerance develops between different amphetamines but not between amphetamine and cocaine despite their many similarities.

Although psychological dependence on amphetamine is not disputed and animal experiments have shown that these drugs are powerful primary reinforcers of drug-seeking behaviour, the question of whether physical dependence develops has been the subject of much discussion (Kumar & Stolerman, 1977). Amphetamine-withdrawal from chronic users results in feelings of fatigue, prolonged periods of sleep, hunger, and depression. It has been suggested that these are physiological reactions to the lack of sleep and food that occurs during amphetamine use but it is more probable that they represent a true withdrawal symptom (Ellinwood & Petrie, 1977). Depression may be sufficiently profound for suicidal attempts to be made.

Epidemiology

Although there were reports of amphetamine misuse as early as the 1930s they were generally thought to be safe drugs and were widely available. Although many who took amphetamines regularly were undoubtedly dependent upon them, misuse did not represent a serious social problem until the 1950s when the demand for amphetamines by the general public was growing rapidly and amphetamine pills and inhalers were widely abused. They were frequently taken in combination with other drugs, usually sedatives, and there was a substantial black market. In an effort to combat this, there was a voluntary ban on the prescription of amphetamines by doctors, but in 1968 there was what can only be described as an epidemic of methylamphetamine injecting in London with many cases of amphetamine psychosis (Hawks, Mitcheson, Ogborne & Edwards, 1969). Until this time, amphetamine had been taken more or less exclusively orally (only opiate-dependent individuals administered drugs by injection), but in 1968, with the introduction of new legislation restricting the right to prescribe heroin and cocaine, some doctors prescribed methylamphetamine as a substitute for cocaine. The epidemic was rapidly curtailed when the manufacturers, by arrangement with the Ministry of Health and the British Medical Association, withdrew methylamphetamine from retail pharmacies.

During the 1960s when amphetamine use was very frequent, three patterns of misuse were described: (a) older tablet-users who were mostly middle-aged housewives who first received prescriptions from medical practitioners for depression or slimming, (b) young tablet-users; the majority started illicit use at weekends and this gradually spread through the week to counteract the withdrawal depression and irritability induced by amphetamine, (c) intravenous users – mostly using methylamphetamine.

The concern felt by most doctors in the 1960s about the prescription of amphetamines now extends to other stimulants and appetite suppressants, some of which have also been drugs of abuse, and during the last ten years, though the number of prescriptions for psychotropic drugs in general has continued to rise, those for stimulants and appetite suppressants (including amphetamines) have been falling both in relative and absolute terms. Some amphetamines still find their way into the market from 'slimming clinics', from illicit factories, and from illegal imports. However, the number of individuals found guilty of offences involving amphetamines during recent years remains fairly steady at 1500–1800 per year, again suggesting that the problem is being contained at a lower level than previously.

Morbidity

Amphetamines are relatively safe drugs in the physical sense; indeed, if it were not so, the widescale misuse of the 1960s would not have occurred. Because of the development of tolerance, chronic users rarely develop the physical overdose syndrome which is characterized by signs of sympathetic hyperstimulation (tachycardia, hyperthermia, arrhythmias, hypertensive crisis). In fact, even when taking high doses of amphetamine, in the absence of a psychotic reaction, the chronic user may appear to be suffering from little more than an anxiety state. Obviously it is the cardiovascular effects of these drugs that are potentially the most serious, particularly because of interactions with other drugs if several are abused simultaneously. Drug interactions, the complications of intravenous injection, and suicide during drug withdrawal are the three main causes of morbidity and mortality due to amphetamine dependence.

Psychosis. The most serious consequence of amphetamine abuse is the development of a psychotic illness. This was very common in 1968 during the epidemic of methylamphetamine injection but can also happen after the oral use of amphetamines. In fact, psychosis has been reported after single doses of amphetamine and so it is not surprising that it can develop in some individuals with a daily dose of only 50 mg or less of amphetamine and after a period of abuse of less than six months (Kalant, 1966; Connell, 1972). Usually, however, psychosis occurs in a setting of chronic drug use.

The illness is characterized by ideas of reference and paranoid delusions, often about the police or foreign agents. Auditory and visual hallucinations develop in a setting of clear consciousness and although the illness may be indistinguishable from schizophrenia, the predominance of visual hallucinations to an extent that is unusual for schizophrenia and the absence of thought disorder may be of value in the differential diagnosis. These symptoms remit on drug withdrawal, usually within one week, but may require treatment with phenothiazines or haloperidol in the interim period.

Stereotyped behaviour. Another feature of amphetamine abuse is the development of stereotyped behaviour; this may occur as part of an amphetamine-induced psychotic state or separately. It is characterized by automatic, stereotyped, repetitive behaviour in which some action such as tidying a handbag, fiddling with a radio, taking apart and reassembling some appliance may continue for hours. Some subjects will search compulsively for insects or parasites under their skin.

Brain damage. It has been suggested that the chronic use of amphetamine can cause brain damage but this question at present remains unanswered.

Other synthetic stimulants

Since the introduction of amphetamines into medical practice, many other drugs have been synthesized for their anorectic or stimulant effects. Most are chemically similar to amphetamine, have sympathomimetic effects, and have been drugs of abuse. They include methylphenidate (Ritalin), phenmetrazine, phentermine, diethylpropion (Apisate, Tenuate). Misuse of methylphenidate, phenmetrazine and diethylpropion have been reported and psychotic illnesses can occur (Connell, 1972). Fenfluramine, although chemically related to amphetamine is not a central stimulant and is not thought to be a drug of misuse although depression of mood may occur on drug withdrawal (Oswald *et al.*, 1971). Other sympathomimetic drugs, for example, those used as nasal decongestants (phenylpropanolamine, propyhexedrine) and as bronchodilators (ephedrine) are also widely available and are sometimes drugs of abuse.

Cocaine

Cocaine is an alkaloid found in the leaves of the coca shrub, Erythroxylon coca, which grows in South America.

Effects

The general pharmacological characteristics of cocaine are very similar to those of amphetamine; cocaine is a powerful, central nervous system stimulant producing increased wakefulness and activity, increased confidence, energy, and euphoria. Like amphetamine, it causes appetite suppression and has peripheral sympathomimetic effects. Although its chemical structure is different from that of amphetamine and similar drugs, it is likely that cocaine has an effect on brain catecholamines similar to amphetamine, both drugs blocking the re-uptake inactivation of brain amines (Snyder, 1972).

Tolerance and dependence

Although regular users may consume massive doses of cocaine, many times that used by the novice, it is not clear whether this escalation is due to the development of tolerance to the euphoric effects or to a search for even greater euphoria. As with dependence on amphetamine, there is no clear-cut withdrawal syndrome, although depression and apathy may occur with drug abstinence after a severe bout of abuse. Psychological dependence on cocaine is profound and it is a potent primary reinforcer of drug-taking behaviour (Kumar & Stolerman, 1977).

Epidemiology

In the United Kingdom, as elsewhere, cocaine has been recognized as a drug of abuse of the affluent and for the first half of this century there was probably a fairly constant, although unknown, number of individuals dependent upon it. In the 1960s, with the burgeoning interest in drugs by young people, there was a dramatic increase in the number of addicts using cocaine who were known to the Home Office. For example, in 1955, only six such people were known but by 1965 there had been a fifty fold increase to 311, and by 1968 there were 564. When the right to prescribe cocaine was severely restricted by the introduction of new legislation, the number of cocaine addicts fell immediately to 81, as the new drug-dependence treatment clinics did not prescribe cocaine liberally. Since then, there has been a steady fall in the number of notified cocaine addicts, to 17 in 1976. Although these figures might suggest that there is no longer a significant cocaine problem in the UK, the number of convictions for offences involving cocaine shows no such dramatic fall, and there is an increasing number of cocaine seizures, both domestically, and of imports and exports. Almost certainly the number of detected offences involving cocaine is an even greater underestimate of the total problem than usual, because the section of the population involved in cocaine abuse, by virtue of its social class and affluence, is not one which particularly attracts the attention of the police.

Morbidity

The abuse of cocaine may produce a toxic psychosis, similar in most respects to that produced by amphetamine, with paranoid delusions, stereotyped behaviour, and hallucinations which may be auditory, visual, or tactile; the latter produce the characteristic sensation of formication – of 'cocaine bugs' crawling under the skin. Drug withdrawal leads to an amelioration of symptoms, although phenothiazines may be needed acutely.

Cocaine inhalation may produce ischaemic ulceration of the nasal mucosa and ultimately septal perforation, because of repeated vasoconstriction. Its administration by subcutaneous injection frequently leads to abscesses, partly because of the lack of sterile precautions and partly because of prolonged ischaemia.

The mortality of cocaine dependence is not known. Fatal overdoses usually cause delirium and convulsions before respiratory depression and cardiac failure occur (Ellinwood & Petrie, 1977; Grinspoon & Bakalar, 1979).

Cannabis

Cannabis is prepared from the hemp plant, *Cannabis sativa*, which is grown commercially in many parts of the world as a source of rope fibre. *Cannabis sativa* contains many psycho-active compounds known collectively as cannabinoids and it is a selection of these organic compounds, unique to the cannabis plant, that make up the drug known as cannabis. Different preparations of leaves, flowers, and stems are known by different names in different countries (marihuana, hashish, bhang, ganja) but the flowering tops of the plants, together with the adjacent leaves, are said to contain the highest concentration of cannabinoids and therefore to have the highest potency. Potency is also affected by environmental factors, including the climate of the place where the plant was grown.

Effects

Many cannabinoids have now been isolated and identified and two isomers of tetra-hydrocannabinol are thought to possess the psycho-active properties responsible for the sought-after actions of cannabis. The major one is delta-9-tetrahydrocannabinol (Δ-9-THC); although delta-8-tetrahydrocannabinol is also psycho-active, it is present in very small amounts.

It has been estimated that cigarettes containing cannabis usually contain 300–500 mg of solid material of which, on average, only 1 per cent is Δ-9-THC. Even when smoked by an experienced user, only 50 per cent is actually absorbed and so the estimated dose of THC from one cigarette is of the order of 2.5 mg (Jaffe, 1975).

When cannabis is smoked its effects are experienced within seconds or minutes as THC is absorbed rapidly from the lungs. Alternatively, in some countries it may be consumed as a drink and in this case effects develop within thirty minutes to two hours. Traces of metabolites of cannabis can be detected in the urine for days or even weeks and although there is no biochemical evidence of accumulation in the tissues, it has been suggested, because of the lipid solubility of cannabis, that this does occur (Paton, 1973).

Physical effects. The physical effects of smoking cannabis include nausea, vomiting, diarrhoea, yawning, coughing, depressed respiration, diuresis, and mydriasis. The most significant physical effects occur in the cardiovascular system: a dose-related tachycardia; vasodilatation in the conjunctivae leading to characteristically blood-shot eyes, and with high doses some postural hypotension may occur. It has also been reported that dilatation of the pulmonary airways occurs (*Lancet*, 1975).

There appears to be no clear idea of what constitutes a toxic dose of cannabis, not only because of the development of tolerance but also because of uncertainties about the quantities of the active principle in any particular sample. In addition cannabis is so insoluble in water that it is probably difficult to achieve a fatal dose in the circulation unless the drug is given intravenously.

Psychological effects. The psychological effects of cannabis are very variable; among the many factors affecting the response are the dose, whether or not the subject is naive, his expectations, and the situation in which the drug is taken. The sought-after psychological effect is euphoria and this is often accompanied by feelings of relaxation and sleepiness. Changes in mood are followed with increasing dosage, by changes in perception, memory, motor co-ordination, and cognitive ability. Perceptual changes start with heightened sensory awareness and characteristically an altered perception of time but, with increasing dosage, hallucinations and depersonalization may occur. Impairment of short-term memory occurs, together with lapses of attention and disorganized thought so that there is increased difficulty in carrying out complex tasks. These observations are important because of the possible effect that cannabis smoking has on any individual's ability to drive safely.

Tolerance and dependence

The evidence that tolerance to the effects of cannabis can develop in animals is now unequivocal, and almost certainly tolerance develops in man too. In Eastern countries chronic users consume very high daily doses by Western standards, and in laboratory studies daily users of cannabis showed less impairment of perceptual and motor functions and smaller increases in heart rate than did naive subjects. Moreover, during the course of a long-term experiment there was a tendency to increase the number of cigarettes smoked or the oral consumption of synthetic cannabinoid (Edwards, 1974).

However, in the past, the picture has been confused by the phenomenon of so-called 'reverse tolerance', so that an experienced user may record more subjective effects than a novice. The explanation is probably that the effects of cannabis are affected by the experience of the user, his mental set, and the setting in which the drug is taken, and this may be more favourable for the experienced than for the naive user.

As with other drugs the development of tolerance to cannabis requires administration of the drug in sufficient dosage. In the UK, even an 'experienced' user may smoke only one or two cigarettes two or three times a week and at this dosage level may well have no demonstrable tolerance and continue to experience euphoria even after one cigarette.

The question of the development of dependence on cannabis remains controversial, individual opinions often being affected by the argument over the legalization (or decriminalization) of cannabis. Certainly, dependence on cannabis, if it occurs, is not of the same degree as dependence on opiates, barbiturates, or alcohol, and there is only weak evidence that cannabis has primary reinforcing properties (Kumar & Stolerman, 1977). However a mild cannabis withdrawal syndrome can occur and not surprisingly most reports of a dependence syndrome come from countries where cannabis is widely available and where it is often taken in large doses. It is in this situation in which states of chronic cannabis intoxication can be maintained for at least part of each day that the mild dependence liability (if it exists) of cannabis is most likely to be manifest, and observations on Western cannabis users who smoke only occasionally are unlikely to shed much light on this difficult question (Jones, 1972; Edwards, 1974).

Epidemiology

Because of the illegal status of cannabis, users are reluctant to declare themselves and there is little objective data about the prevalence of cannabis use in the UK. One indicator is the number of convictions for cannabis use, although this is based on the assumption that convictions accurately reflect use. It has been suggested (Bewley, 1966) that for each of these convictions there are ten to twenty individuals who are not convicted, and a further ten to twenty who may occasionally try cannabis. Bearing these reservations in mind, there were 626 convictions in 1965, 4683 in 1969, and 12 611 in 1972. From then until 1975, when there were 8837 convictions, the number decreased but this trend probably reflected changes in the attitude and activity of the police rather than in the prevalence of cannabis use. The last two years for which figures are available again show an increasing number of convictions (10 440 in 1977). These figures pale however before the results of a study carried out for the BBC Midweek programme based on random sampling of electoral registers in representative parliamentary constituencies; according to this survey nearly 4 million people had used cannabis at some time (*Drug Link*, 1978).

Morbidity

Adverse psychological effects of cannabis vary from feelings of mild panic to an acute psychotic reaction with disorientation, confusion, paranoid delusions, and auditory and visual hallucinations, although hallucinations are said to be uncommon and less distinct than in schizophrenia. The production of psychosis is probably dose-related, suggesting that this is a primary psychopharmacological effect of cannabis (although modified by personality, experience, and setting) and not merely a non-specific precipitating factor operating in a predisposed individ-

ual. The incidence of such reactions in the UK is not known. Most are transient, lasting only a few hours, and are probably dealt with in the situation in which they arise; some may last considerably longer and require hospital admission.

'Flashbacks' are also said to occur after cannabis use; this is a recurrence of hallucinations and perceptual disturbances similar to those experienced at the time of drug use, but occurring in the abstinent state. They occur more frequently when drugs such as LSD have been used too and because of the difficulties of obtaining accurate drug histories it is not clear whether they ever occur after the use of cannabis alone.

Amotivational syndrome. The long-term effects of cannabis, and in particular the development of an amotivational syndrome and of brain damage, have been the subject of much interest and controversy. These effects must be considered in the light of recently acquired information on the high-lipid solubility of tetrahydrocannabinol and its slow excretion rate. Both factors imply the possibility that any toxicity may be cumulative.

An association between the prolonged use of cannabis in high dosage and slothfulness, apathy, and loss of ambition, the so-called amotivational syndrome, has often been described. Early reports are based on observations from Eastern countries but similar accounts have also been presented recently about chronic cannabis users in the UK and the USA, and in most cases the reported dose of cannabis implies a high degree of tolerance to its effects. Most studies, however, can be criticized as methodologically unsound; many do not mention the use of other drugs, for example, nor take into account the possibility that cannabis use might be a consequence of social deterioration rather than its cause. Despite these reservations the possibility remains, based on a large number of clinical observations, that an amotivational syndrome can develop.

Brain damage. Brain damage due to the prolonged use of cannabis in high dosage was described by Campbell, Evans, Thomson and Williams (1971), following the findings of enlarged cerebral ventricles in ten cannabis smokers. Investigation of cannabis smokers using computerized axial tomography has not confirmed Campbell's observations (Kuehnle, Mendelson, Davis & New, 1977; Co *et al.*, 1977).

Escalation. A 'complication' of cannabis use that assumes importance in the debate about its legalization is the possibility of 'escalation' from cannabis use to other potentially more harmful drugs such as LSD or opiates. The 'evidence' for the phenomenon rests on flimsy logic about the number of heroin users who have previously used cannabis. Undoubtedly, in the world as a whole, cannabis users do not subsequently use opiates, and indeed there is no physiological nor pharmacological basis for the expectation that they should. In Western societies sociological explanations are obvious.

Lysergic acid diethylamide (LSD)

Lysergic acid diethylamide (LSD) was first synthesized in 1938. After its discovery it was used therapeutically throughout the 1950s and the 1960s, primarily as an aid to psychotherapy. It was used in the treatment of alcoholism and opiate dependence and for terminally-ill patients to induce feelings of tranquillity. However, it proved to be of little long-term value and although a licensing system still exists in the UK to allow doctors to use LSD if they wish, there are no therapeutic uses for it at present.

The illicit use of LSD reached a peak in the 1960s when it was widely used, particularly in the USA by students interested in mysticism and exploration of the inner world. In the UK, although the majority who used it were under the age of 25 years, they came from all social backgrounds. Its use was certainly part of the 'hippy' culture of the 1960s and was much in evidence at pop music festivals.

Effects

LSD is an extremely potent drug, producing effects in man with doses as small as 25 μg although a dose of about 150 μg is usually used when its psychoactive effects are desired.

After oral administration absorption into the blood is very rapid, peak plasma concentrations being reached in less than half an hour. It is distributed rapidly and widely throughout the body and although it has such profound psychological effects it has been estimated that only 1 per cent of the ingested dose enters the brain. LSD is completely and rapidly metabolized in the liver, its half-life in humans being approximately 3 hours. Somatic symptoms of LSD use are first perceived within a few minutes of oral administration. Psychic effects are experienced soon afterwards but may not be intense until after about 1 hour; they may persist for 8–12 hours. The exact mechanism of action of LSD is not known although it appears to have mixed agonist and antagonist actions to serotonin.

Physical effects. In comparison with its psychological effects, the somatic effects of LSD are mild and are usually those due to stimulation of the sympathetic nervous system. They include mydriasis, piloerection, hyperthermia, and tachycardia. Parasympathomimetic effects may also occur, such as lacrimation and salivation and there is a variable, mild effect on the blood pressure. There may also be nausea, loss of appetite, dizziness, paraesthesiae, tremor, hyperreflexia, and a mild leucocytosis. Epileptic fits have also been reported but the role of LSD in their causation is not definitely established (Malleson, 1971).

LSD appears to be a very safe drug from the point of view of drug toxicity. Although people have died by committing suicide or by accident during LSD intoxication, none have done so as a direct physical effect of drug overdose. The size of the lethal dose of LSD for human beings is not known but has been estimated, by extrapolation from animal studies, to be 0.2 mg/kg, or 14 mg for the average adult male. Overdosage in animals results in death due to respiratory failure.

Related to the possible teratogenic effects of LSD (see later) are neoplastic effects, and the presence of a Philadelphia chromosome (an abnormality that may occur in chronic myeloid leukaemia), in two LSD users is therefore of interest. Acute leukaemia in an LSD user has also been reported (*Lancet*, 1967; *British Medical Journal*, 1969).

Psychological effects. The psychological effects of LSD although very variable are well-documented. They depend not only on the dose of the drug that is taken but also on the mental set of the user and the setting in which the drug is taken. Changes in perception affect all sensory modalities, particularly vision, and there may be intensification and distortion of stimuli. Colours may appear more intense, stationary objects may appear to move and surfaces to undulate; there may be micropsia, and previously ignored detail may become overwhelming. In addition, synaesthesia, the merging of sensory modalities, may occur with colours being heard and sounds seen. Auditory perception is often enhanced. In the presence of all these amazing changes the drug-user is usually aware that they are not real but are due to the effects of LSD, and true hallucinations are less common. Changes in the perception of time are also common, and there may be a subjective feeling of time slowing profoundly. Changes in awareness of the self may occur so that depersonalization and derealization phenomena arise and there may be fear of self-disintegration.

The mood of the LSD user is often very labile, varying from anxiety and fear to depression and to euphoria. Often the subject is quiet and withdrawn, preoccupied with visions and thoughts, and may be so difficult to arouse as to appear stuporose or even catatonic. Less frequently there may be disorganized hyperactivity. Thought processes may also be disorganized by LSD and concentration impaired, so that conversation is illogical and often dominated by pseudophilosophical or mystical content.

Tolerance and dependence

In man, tolerance to the effects of LSD develops unusually rapidly; it is, in fact, evident when the second dose is given only 24 hours after the first and is more or less complete after only 3 or 4 daily doses, so that subsequent administration has no effect. Loss of tolerance is equally rapid, being evident after abstention for only 3–5 days, when full sensitivity to the original dose is regained. Cross-tolerance develops between LSD and mescaline and LSD and psilocybin; it does not occur between LSD and cannabis products despite many apparent similarities in their effects. The mechanism of tolerance for LSD and other hallucinogens is not known and no hypothesis accounts for the rapid and dramatic degrees of tolerance that develop (Hug, 1972).

It is generally agreed that physical dependence on LSD does not develop and an abstinence syndrome has not been described. Psychological dependence is probably also uncommon as chronic, frequent use of LSD is very rare, and there is no convincing evidence that LSD has primary reinforcing properties.

Epidemiology

The prevalence of LSD use is not known and it is difficult even to estimate how many people use it regularly or occasionally. Questionnaire surveys have been carried out, but usually on such highly selected groups that the results cannot be applied to the general population. National surveys of drug use, however, have suggested that approximately 1 per cent of the total population may have used LSD at some time.

A study based on the random sampling of electoral registers in representative parliamentary constituencies estimated that 657 000 people have used LSD but this sheds no light on the pattern of use of the drug or on how many people continue to use it regularly (*Drug Link*, 1978). It appears that the common pattern of use is intermittent, LSD being used a few times and then spontaneously discontinued, or else used only occasionally thereafter. Criminal statistics on convictions for offences involving LSD cannot be related directly to LSD use but may shed some light on prevailing trends. In 1968 there were 72 such convictions and the number rose to a peak of 1537 in 1971. Since then the numbers have fallen each year to 277 in 1977. In that year, however, a massive seizure of LSD from one illegal factory was made, so these figures should not give rise to complacency. Because it is easy for the competent chemist to synthesize LSD, illicit production is difficult to eliminate.

Morbidity

Three types of adverse response to LSD use have been described although they are not mutually exclusive (Bewley, 1967; Dewhurst & Hatrick, 1972).

Acute panic (bad trip). This is the most commonly experienced adverse reaction. Instead of the desired euphoria, the effects of LSD are so frightening that the user suffers an acute panic reaction.

'Flashbacks'. Flashbacks are the spontaneous recurrence of LSD effects occurring during abstinence from drug use. They may occur after LSD has been used only once or many times; any type of LSD experience may occur although perceptual changes, especially visual perceptual changes, are the most frequent. Usually flashbacks last for only a few minutes although they are sometimes more prolonged.

Psychosis. A wide variety of psychiatric symptoms may occur, including thought disorder, auditory and visual hallucinations, disturbed behaviour, and paranoid delusions, so that the differential diagnosis of LSD psychosis or schizophrenia may sometimes be very difficult. However certain features such as regression to childhood, loss of time sense, grandiose delusions of a pseudophilosophical nature, and visual hallucinations or other extraordinary perceptual disturbances are more likely to occur in LSD psychosis. It is, of course, difficult to assess the exact cause of symptoms such as these as the prior mental state of the individual is usually not known. It is possible for example that it was because of an impaired mental state that the individual took LSD which then exacerbated and prolonged the original condition. Suicide has been reported following LSD ingestion and receives much attention from the media; subjects may experience sudden, compulsive suicidal impulses in a setting of rapid mood changes; potentially suicidal actions such as flying or walking on water may also occur because of grandiose delusions, depersonalization and feelings of unreality (Sandison, 1968).

Treatment

Most adverse reactions to LSD are probably dealt with satisfactorily by companions participating in the drug-taking experience, so that only the more serious reactions ever come to medical attention. Patients suffering from acute panic reactions should be 'talked down', if possible by someone sympathetic to and with understanding of the LSD experience. If such reassurance is insufficient and the patient is severely agitated sedation may be necessary; chlorpromazine is probably the drug of choice although diazepam has also been used. Chlorpromazine may also be used in the treatment of LSD psychosis and flashbacks; the patient suffering from flashbacks should be warned against the further use of cannabis, LSD, or other hallucinogens.

Other hallucinogenic drugs

LSD is only one of the wide range of drugs which may cause changes in sensory perception, thought, and mood in those who take them. They have been described as hallucinogenic, psychotomimetic, psychotogenic, psychedelic, and so forth. Many are drugs that have been developed from plants, their original sources having been used for many years in religious rituals. There are reports of the sporadic abuse of substances such as nutmeg, morning glory seeds, and particular species of mushrooms. Psychological dependence on them is common but physical dependence is rare (*British Medical Journal*, 1966; Beattie, 1968).

Sniffing syndrome

The inhalation or 'sniffing' of volatile solvents is more often the subject of reports in the popular press than of systematic research. As a result relatively little is known about this form of drug misuse.

The substances involved include a wide range of commercial and domestic products such as paint thinners, glue and lacquer, which contain a variety of volatile hydrocarbons such as toluene, benzene and acetone. The usual method of sniffing is to put some of the chosen substance on to a piece of material or into a paper or plastic bag which is then held over the mouth and nose. A few deep breaths produce the desired 'high' which may last for a few minutes or even up to half an hour or so. The solvents are absorbed through the respiratory tract and because most are fairly lipid-soluble they are distributed rapidly to the nervous system. Some are excreted unchanged through the lung, causing a characteristic odour on the breath, while others are excreted in urine.

Effects

The desired effect of solvent sniffing is euphoria, which may be achieved with just a few deep breaths. Other effects vary according to the solvent being inhaled and the duration of inhalation and include giddiness, slurred speech, ataxia, impaired judgement, hallucinations, and delusions. If inhalation continues the subject becomes drowsy and eventually loses consciousness. Associated with the initial euphoria there may be feelings of omnipotence and of recklessness so that dangerous behaviour of an impulsive or destructive nature may occur.

A glue-sniffer's rash has been described; it is believed to be due to the repeated application of a plastic or polythene bag containing the solvent to the nose. The rash is symmetrical in distribution and consists of comedones, papules, and pustules extending from each nostril up the nasal fold and across the bridge of the nose (Watson, 1978).

Another dangerous consequence of solvent inhalation is suffocation, which is particularly likely to occur if the solvent is put into a plastic bag which is then placed over the subject's head. Deaths have also been reported as a result of cardiac arrhythmias which seem to occur most frequently when sniffing aerosol propellant gases, trichloroethane and other fluorinated hydrocarbons (*Drug Link*, 1976).

The toxic effects of many solvents are well known from industrial medicine but the relevance of the chronic, low-dose exposure of factory workers to repeated, acute, high-dose exposure of the adolescent 'sniffer' is not known. The chronic effects reported include hepatic and renal damage, bone marrow depression, anaemia, encephalopathy, and neuropathy. The consequence depends on the particular solvent that is inhaled (Cohen, 1977, 1979).

Tolerance and dependence

It appears that tolerance to the effects of a particular solvent can develop, increasing amounts being required to achieve the desired effects; true physical dependence with a defined withdrawal syndrome probably does not occur although psychological dependence is certainly possible (Hofmann & Hofmann, 1975).

Epidemiology

The prevalence of solvent inhalation is not known and because it involves a wide variety of substances which are not classified as drugs, even indirect evidence is difficult to obtain. Predominantly it is a phenomenon of schoolchildren, usually younger teenagers, and boys outnumber girls. It often seems to occur as a 'craze' in a particular school or locality and may involve a large proportion of children before it is replaced by another craze. Older teenagers tend to give up 'sniffing' and if drug abuse continues it is more likely to involve alcohol or other illicit drugs (*Drug Link*, 1976).

Morbidity and mortality

Little is known about the morbidity and mortality of solvent inhalation. Although the toxic effects of many solvents are well-known the relevance of this for the occasional 'sniffer' is not known. However, deaths do occur and in this respect aerosol propellants seem to be particularly hazardous.

Minor analgesics

The excessive consumption of minor analgesics, such as aspirin and phenacetin, is frequently overlooked in studies of drug abuse. There are at least two reasons for this attitude. Firstly, it involves a group of drugs which are freely available and secondly, it is easy to dismiss it as uninformed self-medication by a population ignorant of the dangers of excessive use of these drugs. In many ways, however, those who abuse analgesics resemble individuals who abuse restricted drugs: they often deny their drug abuse and indeed may go to considerable lengths to conceal it; moreover, many abuse other drugs too and admit that they take analgesics for the feeling of well-being that they induce and sometimes specifically for the dangerous state of salicylism which they find pleasurable.

The prevalence of analgesic abuse is not known, partly because there is no precise definition of what constitutes abuse. A useful, working definition is analgesic consumption of 1 g daily for three years or a total analgesic consumption during this period of 1 kg (Murray, 1972). Information comes almost entirely from medical case reports about the complications of abuse, such as analgesic nephropathy, and by definition this is a selected sample representing only a fraction of the total who abuse these drugs. However, in a door-to-door survey carried out in Glasgow, Murray found that 1.1 per cent of his subjects abused analgesics and it has been suggested that there may be as many as 250 000 analgesic abusers in Britain (Murray, 1972). Most studies report that more women than men abuse analgesics.

Complications of analgesic abuse

Probably the most frequent consequence of analgesic abuse is nephropathy and it has been estimated that there are at least 500 new cases in England and Wales each year (Koutsaimanis & de Wardener, 1970). The clinical features include urinary tract infection, renal colic, haematuria, sterile pyuria, hypertension, and chronic renal failure. It is a serious condition with a high mortality rate of 35 per cent or more, deterioration of renal function and death being associated with analgesic consumption that persists despite medical advice (Murray, Lawson & Linton, 1971).

In addition, analgesic abuse may cause gastro-intestinal disturbance with peptic ulceration, bleeding, and anaemia. It has also been suggested that other consequences include infertility, congenital deformities, and brain damage (Murray, Greene & Adams, 1971). Analgesics are also used frequently in episodes of deliberate self-poisoning.

Other drugs

In addition to the drugs already discussed there are many drugs each of which are abused by just a few people. Some, for example, anti-Parkinsonian drugs may be taken for their psychic effects (Stephens, 1967). Others, such as purgatives or anticoagulants, may be taken to produce fictitious disease, those who abuse them seeking and apparently enjoying intensive, repeated medical investigation and care (Sladen, 1972; Forbes, Prentice & Sclare, 1974). Many of these patients have worked in hospitals in medical or para-medical capacities and resemblances to patients with Munchausen's syndrome are obvious. Finally, some prescribed drugs may be taken excessively, primarily to avoid unpleasant withdrawal symptoms; for example, increasing doses of ergotamine may be taken to avoid withdrawal headache and increasing doses of steroids to avoid unpleasant psychological effects (Gethin-Morgan, Boulnois & Burns-Cox, 1973; Lucas & Falkowski, 1973).

Neonatal problems associated with drug dependence

The increased frequency of drug abuse during recent years has resulted in many obstetric departments being faced with this problem in their pregnant patients and, because of the phenomenon of multiple drug abuse and the higher prevalence of psychotropic drug use by women, drug dependence in pregnancy may involve a variety of drugs. In addition, the personality and life-style of the pregnant drug-dependent woman may be important in causing some of the commonly encountered problems (Neuberg, 1970; Tylden, 1973).

The effects of maternal drug abuse on the foetus and new-born child can be considered in three groups: general effects, teratogenic effects, and withdrawal effects.

General effects

The diagnosis of pregnancy may be unduly delayed in an opiate-dependent individual because of confusion with drug-induced amenorrhoea (Gaulden, Littlefield, Putoff & Seivert, 1964), and the infectious consequences of self-injection may adversely affect the growth and development of the foetus as will an inadequate diet without the usual supplements of iron and vitamins. In addition poor antenatal attendance gives less opportunity for these and other problems to be prevented, diagnosed, or promptly treated. The effect of injecting drugs contaminated with adulterants is unknown.

Teratogenic effects

LSD. The drug of abuse that has received most attention because of the possibility that it is a teratogen is LSD. The evidence for this is that minute amounts of LSD can produce chromosomal damage in human leucocytes in culture and that abortion and congenital malformation follow the injection of LSD into rats, mice, and hamsters (but not rabbits) (*British Medical Journal*, 1968). However, there is no firm evidence that LSD is teratogenic in man, either by damaging the germ cells or by the presence of a persistent metabolite affecting organogenesis (Fernandez, Brennan, Masterson & Power, 1974; Malleson, 1971).

Cannabis. It has been suggested that cannabis is a teratogenic agent causing limb deformities in human beings (Tylden, 1973). However, this is a condition of high background incidence and anecdotal accounts of its occurrence, although interesting, provide inconclusive evidence on this point.

Withdrawal effects

Opiates. Because of the passage of opiates across the placenta, the foetus of the opiate dependent mother is constantly exposed to these drugs, which are then abruptly withdrawn at birth. It is therefore not surprising that a characteristic neonatal withdrawal syndrome can be recognized. The infants are described as hyperactive, irritable, and restless, with tremors or even convulsions; there may be gastro-intestinal disturbance with retching and vomiting; they may have a fever (Reddy, Harper & Stern, 1971; Fraser, 1976). The proportion of infants at risk who subsequently develop signs of withdrawal depends on the dose of opiate taken by the mother, the duration of her dependence, and the timing of the last dose in relation to the time of delivery. In a large series of 384 infants, reported from the USA, two-thirds manifested withdrawal (Zelson, Rubio & Wasserman, 1971). The onset of withdrawal signs in an infant born to a heroin-dependent mother usually occurs within the first 24 hours but may be delayed until the second or third day. Because of the longer duration of action of methadone, the neonatal withdrawal syndrome does not usually start until 48–72 hours after birth and may be delayed even later (National Institute on Drug Abuse, 1979). A number of treatments have been tried including the inhalation of opium smoke and a variety of sedatives including paregoric, barbiturates, and chlorpromazine. Sometimes treatment is started prophylactically but it appears unjustifiable to expose those infants who are not going to manifest the withdrawal syndrome or those who will do so only mildly, to yet more unnecessary drugs (Ghodse, Reed & Mack, 1977). Similarly the use of opiates is not advocated, as any metabolic changes induced by intra-uterine exposure to opiates are likely to be accentuated by their continued use (Zelson et al., 1971). Chlorpromazine is generally recommended as the drug of choice; it should be started only if there is evidence of progression in the number or severity of the signs of withdrawal. The dose should subsequently be reduced in a step-wise fashion every two to three days.

Other drugs. With the increasing use of psychotropic drugs, many of which have a dependence-producing capacity, other withdrawal syndromes have been described in neonates (National Institute on Drug Abuse, 1979). The signs of barbiturate withdrawal on the new born are similar to those of opiate withdrawal although their onset may be delayed, often for up to 4–7 days after birth and sometimes even later. This delay can in itself be hazardous as mother and baby may be discharged from hospital before the abstinence syndrome is manifest. More recently, cases of benzodiazepine withdrawal have been described in infants (National Institute on Drug Abuse, 1979).

The effects of maternal amphetamine abuse on the neonate are not clear. Although withdrawal signs have been described it is not clear whether these were due to amphetamines or to concomitant (although denied) use of opiates (Neuberg, 1970).

Polydrug abuse

Multiple drug abuse by drug-dependent individuals is not a new phenomenon. There are many reports, for example, from the early 1960s, of notified heroin addicts also abusing cocaine, methedrine, barbiturates, cannabis and LSD, but following the establishment of the drug dependence treatment clinics in 1968, multiple drug abuse became more widespread. The adoption by the clinics of a prescribing policy sufficiently frugal to prevent overspill to the black market undoubtedly left that market underfed in terms of heroin and cocaine, and their scarcity, coupled with the availability of other drugs which were therefore cheaper, contributed to the addicts' willingness to experiment. Multiple drug use became the established pattern of drug abuse, with a wide range of psychoactive drugs being taken, often simultaneously according to their availability, in a search for heightened effect.

The changing pattern of drug abuse by drug-dependent individuals during the 1960s and 1970s cannot wholly be explained, however, by new legislation and the prescribing practices of the clinics. During the same period, there have also been marked changes in drug-taking by the general population. The most important phenomenon has been described by Trethowan (1975) as the 'relentless march of the psychotropic juggernaut'. For example, between 1965 and 1970 there was a 19 per cent increase in the prescription of psycho-active drugs in England and Wales, and a further 8.3 per cent from 1970 to 1975 (Williams, 1980). This includes drugs such as barbiturates and non-barbiturates, hypnotics, tranquillizers, stimulants, and appetite suppressants: all of which, and in particular barbiturates, are now being abused by drug-dependent individuals on a large scale.

Whereas dependence on opiates involves drugs with which the general population is unfamiliar, the current drugs of abuse are those whose names are often household words and which may be shared or borrowed rather like cigarettes or aspirin. They may be taken, like alcohol, purely for their psychic effects, and yet they are still regarded as medical and not social agents; in fact, not only are they used like alcohol, but they are often taken with alcohol as a cheap method of intoxication.

Although a proportion of the prescriptions for psychotropic drugs is for defined psychiatric illness, many are prescribed for personal and interpersonal problems. Obviously, the difference between this type of use by the non-dependent population and misuse for personal pleasure is far less than in pre-psychotropic days when non-dependent individuals took drugs only for specific physical conditions. Multiple drug use is similarly a phenomenon that involves not only drug-dependent individuals but the general population too, as many prescriptions are for combinations of hypnotics, tranquillizers, and anti-depressants.

It is apparent, therefore, that the boundary between drug use and drug misuse is now less clearly defined than formerly, and this point is emphasized by consideration of another aspect of drug misuse.

Drug overdose is now a problem of epidemic proportions and there is no evidence that the peak of the epidemic has yet been reached. Indeed, such is its continuing prevalence that it is probably more accurate to describe it as an endemic form of drug misuse involving both the dependent and the non-dependent. For example, in July 1975, 1641 cases of drug overdose were treated in London accident and emergency departments. In 412 incidents the patient was dependent on drugs, in 877 cases the patient was not dependent, and in the remainder the dependence status was not known. Obviously, there were differences between the dependent and non-dependent populations: drug-dependent individuals were more likely to have taken repeated overdoses during the previous year, took opiates and barbiturates more frequently, and more often obtained the drugs illicitly; the male:female ratio among drug-dependent individuals was 1:1, compared to 1:2 in the non-dependent group; finally, drug-dependent individuals were more likely to have taken the drug overdose accidentally in a search for heightened effect, whereas the non-dependent individuals usually did so deliberately in a suicidal attempt or gesture.

Despite these differences, there are also marked similarities between the two groups: approximately half of all overdoses, whether taken by dependent or non-dependent individuals, involved more than one drug, and these drugs are almost exclusively psychoactive drugs, albeit of different classes. The incidence of both types of patients is greatest in the 20–30 age group, the peak being particularly marked in the drug-dependent group (Ghodse, 1979).

The findings of this study have been quoted in some detail because they emphasize an important feature of current patterns of drug dependence. Whereas once it could be regarded as an isolated phenomenon, now it seems to be much more closely related to drug-taking in the general population, with the multiple use of psychotropic drugs a feature of the behaviour of both groups. The common emphasis on substance dependence, a fault which has been perpetuated in this chapter for the sake of convenience, involves a concept which is now out-of-date. To describe the drug-dependent individual as a 'heroin addict' and to attribute his problems to dependence on the drug for which he has been notified to the Home Office, when he may be dependent on and/or abusing a wide variety of other drugs, is to over-simplify a complex subject. Moreover, such preoccupation with a particular drug diverts attention away from consideration of important issues, such as the relationship of drug dependence to other forms of drug-taking behaviour (deliberate self-poisoning, accidental overdose, alcoholism), and to other forms of dependency, such as gambling and over-eating. It is more likely that a fundamental understanding of the whole phenomenon of drug dependence will be reached in this way, rather than in terms of the biochemical effects of a particular group of drugs.

PART IV
Severe subnormality

16
Severe subnormality

DEREK RICKS

A severely subnormal person has been usefully defined as 'incapable of living an independent life or of guarding himself against serious exploitation or will be so incapable when of an age to do so' (Mental Health Act, 1959). Such a definition emphasizes the severity of a handicapping condition and hence the management problem it imposes. From a different viewpoint, the severely subnormal are described as those people whose IQ is lower than 50. Reliable measurement of IQ at low levels of attainment is notoriously difficult but such a definition has administrative significance, at least for the child, because it categorizes him as a pupil of an ESN(S) school. Since most modern intelligence tests have a standard deviation of 15 points of IQ, the epidemiological consequences implied by a cut-off at an IQ of 50 is that such a level is greater than three standard deviations below the mean. Since practically the total population (99.75 per cent) falls within three standard deviations from the mean an IQ below 50 is effectively beyond the limit of normal variations. For all practical purposes, severe subnormality is likely to be the result of a departure not a deviation from the norm. In short, it should theoretically have a cause associated with some or other pathology. These two features – the severity of the handicap with its attendant burden of care, and the likelihood of a causative pathology – dominate the doctor's efforts to help the severely subnormal patient and his family. Unless specializing in the field, he will not usu-

Table 16.1. *Prevalence of severe subnormality*

	0–14 yr	15+ yr	Total
1. Rate per 100 000 population	69.20	167.84	237.04
2. Incapacity associated with SSN			
(a) Non-ambulant	16.59	10.41	27.00
(b) Behaviour difficulties requiring constant supervision	9.69	18.75	28.44
(c) Severely incontinent	8.65	8.66	17.35
(d) Needing assistance to feed, wash or dress	19.53	25.87	45.40
(e) No physical handicap or severe behaviour difficulties	14.48	103.26	117.74
(f) Incapacity not assessed	0.83	1.88	2.71
3. Place of residence			
(a) Home	49.24	71.65	120.89
(b) Hospital or other residential care	19.96	96.19	116.15

Source: DHSS (1971) Better Services for the Mentally Handicapped, p. 6, Cmnd. 4683. London: HMSO
These figures, quoted as rates per 100 000 normal population are averages of the findings of surveys carried out in the Wessex and Newcastle hospital regions and in the former metropolitan borough of Camberwell.

ally be involved with discovering, or initially explaining, the cause of the handicap – if it is known; but inevitably he will need to help the family come to terms with the feelings generated in them by this knowledge or its lack. He will certainly be confronted by the family's need to be guided on their management of their severely subnormal member, in identifying his assets as well as assessing his disabilities, in advising how his assets can be developed as well as his disabilities reduced, in teaching social constraint while encouraging his limited social response. It is likely that any doctor whose clinical responsibility extends over a NHS district with a population of about 200 000 but not containing a severe subnormality hospital, would find in that population about 240 families with an SSN member with various disabilities outlined in table 16.1 (Better Services for the Mentally Handicapped). Details of prevalence rate per hundred thousand normal population are to be found in this table together with a breakdown into: (a) numbers associated with different forms of handicap and (b) numbers living at home and in hospital or

other residential centres. A general practitioner with a practice of about 4000 would expect to have between 5 and 8 such families under his care. The number is not large but each family may be very time-consuming because the severity of the handicap imposes not only frequent medical problems but practical and social consequences for the whole family. As happens with the afflicted family, most professionals who work with the severely handicapped can, on occasions, be overwhelmed with a sense of helplessness or have to struggle with themselves to see the point of continuing strenuous efforts for so little apparent return. Maintaining realistic perspectives with continuing encouragement in a chronically harrassed family is a role the doctor must undertake, and he must come to terms with the stress it imposes on himself. Other demands on the doctor distinctive to practice with the severely subnormal relate to the diversity of aetiological factors and disabilities which may be present and the characteristic array of management problems produced by quite normal interaction between family members and their

SSN child or adult. It is in these two ways that helping the mentally handicapped and their family diverges from other forms of psychiatric practice, so it is on these aspects of management that the following pages will concentrate. Initially they will be broadly discussed to arrive at a few general guidelines of practice which will then be applied at different stages of the severely subnormal person's life, from babyhood onwards.

Confronted by a family with a severely mentally handicapped child the psychiatrist will need to help with three broad issues each of which in this type of practice will have a distinctive emphasis – on organic aetiology and disabilities, on practical everyday management of those disabilities, and on emotional problems which arise from essentially normal interaction between parents and child. The three broad issues confronting the doctor can be represented as questions typically asked by the family.

(1) *Problems of aetiology*: 'Why is my child handicapped?'
(2) *Problems of function*: 'How is my child handicapped; what sort of disabilities afflict him and how do they prevent him developing and affect his future?'
(3) *Problems of management*: 'What can I do about this and in particular what can I do to help reduce his disability?'

These questions tend to be presented to the clinician in this sequence. Initially the overwhelming concern of parents is to discover why their child is severely handicapped and the doctor will here at least be on familiar professional ground which enables him to give information, explain and interpret it, or have access to specialist colleagues who can do so in more detail. In addition to technical explanations which should never be undervalued, there is the need to treat the feelings generated by this tragedy. Later, sometimes as quickly as a few days, parents begin to enquire what these effects explained to them mean for their child; 'In what way and to what extent will he be handicapped?' Usually they compare the handicapped child's development with what they would have wished; they ask whether normally anticipated emotionally significant milestones will be reached. 'Will he walk, will he talk, will he go to a normal school, earn his own living, get married, have children', and so on. Some of these questions are clearly over-optimistic, some are unanswerable, so it is helpful at this stage to encourage the parents to concentrate their efforts on achieving simple, early skills,

to take each step at a time, hoping to establish a sequence of aims each within a practical, and tolerable time scale with, if possible, reasonably defined goals. In this way a family can move on to the third issue – 'What can be done, and in particular what can *we* do?' This is a vital shift in emphasis from questioning to action. In some cases this reduces the sense of helplessness which so demoralizes the parents and prevents their recovery from the combined feelings of loss, guilt, and anger at the realization of the severe handicap of their child. Some parents resist this transition and insist on protracted investigations or discussions, which is understandable and must be respected. But when this is combined with a reluctance or even refusal to take up advice on handling or stimulation, it is an indication that earlier more fundamental problems have not been adequately resolved. Perhaps they never will be. The extent of tragic impact on a parent, particularly a mother, of bearing a severely subnormal child is such that all professionals working with the family need to appreciate that in some cases the situation for her is unbearable and sympathetic steps must be taken which respect this. We cannot expect invariably the mother to accept such a child. We are obliged, however, to do our utmost to find solutions tolerable to her and this will be discussed later.

Problems of aetiology: 'Why is my child handicapped?'

At whatever stage the doctor makes his own first contact with the severely retarded patient he may expect that the family will need to establish with him an understanding why their child is so handicapped. This may, as is often the case, have been earlier discussed at length with paediatricians, geneticists, or any other doctor involved when the handicapping condition was discovered. The whole episode may have been such a painful experience that it has aroused feelings which may be unexpressed even within the family. On the other hand these may have been apparently resolved, or the parents may assert they have 'come to terms' with the tragedy. But usually, 'coming to terms' relates to the life-style imposed on them rather than its origins. The doctor can expect that these underlying feelings will re-emerge. He must be sensitive to their expression and encourage their discussion in the family's own choice of time and setting. As they are discussed he can gauge the depth of feeling, the conflict it may have generated, the avenues into which this conflict has been chan nelled, which may in its turn have provoked unproductive pressures on the child in, for example, incontinence training, response to noise, their anxiety about hyperactivity and the child's safety. All SSN children, with their many handicaps, impose a burden of care upon their family but it is interesting how a particular constellation of problems may develop in a given child because his distinctive disabilities have been modified or exaggerated by the attitudes they generate in individual family members caring for him. In this context careful and sympathetic questioning, and in particular, allowing the parents themselves to talk about the causes of his handicap as they themselves understand them can reveal how they regard his handicap not only as a consequence of factors described but as a divergence from what they would personally value in the child they would have had and which has been denied them.

An early dilemma of the doctor involved with the family at this stage is that his attempts to explain and clarify the subnormal patient's aetiology may well take him into specialized areas of expertise. An investigation of the diverse causes might have been carried out if the child's handicap has been evident at birth or shortly after, or it might have been undertaken at the request of the paediatricians or Local Authority Medical Officer, when the child's failure to develop normally became apparent. However, this may not have occurred or the child's gross disability may be confined to his social response and language development so that with only moderately retarded motor development he may not have aroused much suspicion earlier.

There are diverse causes of mental handicap (table 16.2) but for all it is important to emphasize that the identification of a handicapping condition is technically complicated except in obvious cases from appearance such as Down's syndrome, or from history such as perinatal episode of profound cerebral insult. The family's need for as much certainty and detail as possible must be respected but it may well be beyond the psychiatrist's experience to meet. Referral to a paediatric department or clinical geneticist is obviously indicated but in quite a few cases indications in the history or the child's appearance may be minimal. Useful reference can be made to authoritative texts (Kirman & Bicknell, 1975; Penrose, 1954).

For the psychiatrist confronted with this situation, there are a number of simple guidelines he can follow. As a first working approximation there are

Table 16.2. *Aetiology of severe subnormality*

	%
1. Pre-natal aetiology	73
(a) Chromosomal	36
(b) Mutant genes	7
(c) Acquired	10
(d) Unknown	20
2. Perinatal aetiology	10
3. Post-natal aetiology	3
4. Psychotic group	3
5. Untraceable	11

two broad groups of aetiological factors producing severe handicapping conditions – cerebral insult or developmental anomaly which may be associated with an identifiable syndrome.

The first group is various forms of cerebral insult disabling what is assumed would have been a normal child; these are often loosely referred to as 'brain damage'. Usually this results from a serious reduction in the nutrition of the brain by impaired blood supply and oxygenation with associated chemical and eventually structural changes. Periods in the developing baby's life when this is more likely to occur, are pre-natally in the final trimester of pregnancy, as with pre-eclamptic toxaemia producing usually diffuse damage of the cortex; with complications of birth, or perinatally, usually producing more acute localized damage; in early babyhood, particularly with premature babies, in which a less dramatic though more sustained hypoxaemia may damage vulnerable parts of the brain, such as the cerebellum or striatum. Later cerebral insult usually accompanied by fits may result from encephalopathies from a variety of causes, including childhood fevers, septicaemia, intracranial complications, protracted coma, or more rarely after trauma or accidental poisoning with, for example, coal gas or car fumes. The dehydrating effect and associated thrombosis and electrolyte disturbance of severe or prolonged infantile gastro-enteritis may produce mental retardation. Various toxic agents have been implicated (in particular, lead), which, as with nutritional deficiency, are thought to be most dangerous during the post-natal phase of rapid neuro-development from birth to two or three years. In the case of lead poisoning there is considerable controversy whether, for example, pica leading to continued high ingestion of lead results from poisoning or from another, perhaps undetectable, independent cause on which the effects of plumbism are superimposed. Similar doubts may occur in the case of birth injury which may result from the vulnerability of a pre-natally abnormal brain. Establishing the cause with any accuracy or certainty may be impossible but the parents of such a child will regard his condition as having an identifiable cause.

This is much less likely to be the case for the second broad group of the severely subnormal where the brain is thought to have grown or functioned abnormally from a very early stage in its development. In some examples such early maldevelopment may be the result of damage, such as produced in some embryonic viral encephalopathies like toxoplasmosis, cytomegalovirus, or rubella infection of the mother. These conditions could be regarded as an overlap of the first group since the damaging agent can be regarded as external and not the result of some in-born process. There is a rapidly growing array of documented pathological conditions or syndromes producing severe mental retardation associated with chromosome abnormalities, enzyme deficiencies, and other biochemical defects. Many affected cases have not only a specified defect but more or less recognizable features and a known mode of transmission. Details, including copious illustrations can be found in various texts of which the most informative is by Holmes and colleagues (Holmes *et al.*, 1972).

If suspicions are alerted to some inherited defect the problem then is to select from a vast array of possibilities one or two whose characteristics at least approximate to those found in the patient. It would be unreasonable to expect the psychiatrist, unless he has specialized experience, and often not even then, to recognize any combination of features as signifying one group of possible syndromes. He may be able to link particular signs with possible disorders, for example, proptosis with Greuzot or Apert's, polydactyly with Patau's, synophrys with de Lange's and so on, which would guide his examination of the copious literature, otherwise he has to read through a vast array of data to test his suspicions. Some paediatric texts render the task much easier for those with no access to specialist colleagues, particularly McKay (McKay, 1976), in which a range of diagnosis is tabulated according to particular signs, for example, various facial features, abnormalities of hair, feet, hands, or skin, and so on. The clinician, alerted by some particular features can refer to it in the text as a useful starting point. It must be always remembered that such searches should be discreet (much anxiety can be unnecessarily aroused by an unguarded comment) and above all that the vast majority of suspect signs can occur within the normal population. Caution and tact must override diagnostic zeal.

There are some simple points which should alert the doctor to the possibility of inherited disease, since obviously he will want to seek help to exclude this, as indeed will the affected child's parents, for whom this may well be a recurrent and severe anxiety. It should always be remembered that, although an episode of cerebral insult, certainly if profound, is likely to account for the handicap, it does not exclude the possibility of underlying inherited disease. The absence of such an episode should always alert the doctor of such a possibility. In addition to the lack of any apparent precipitating event, other factors in the history include consanguinity in the parents, or any known example of abnormal development in relatives. Poor obstetric histories should be enquired about, since a succession of miscarriages or indeed a single one may indicate abnormal foetal development. The recall of vague but identifiable illness or of taking tablets in early pregnancy should be noted. In the child's history, feeding difficulties, failure to thrive, apparent apathy, slow motor milestones (though these may not be marked), and apparent uncaused fits especially in the first year, are all suggestive. Examining the child should never be neglected, although, as with the history, examination in a suspect case often raises expectations marginally if at all. In other cases, later recognized as severely retarded, early development may seem quite normal, since many responses in the newborn may not of necessity require cortical control. It should be remembered that in many seriously retarded children the cause of handicap is usually not discovered in even the most erudite hospital department. However, an odd appearance is worth noting and exploring further for such features as simple primitive ears, particularly if low set; very widely set eyes, particularly if associated with strabismus or proptosis; a small or large head, particularly if asymmetrical or with a flattened occiput; epicanthic folds, high arched palate, grossly maloccluded teeth, a narrow philtrum, umbilical hernia, or small appendages on the hands which may be residual extra digits. The skin should be examined and, although some blemishes are likely and will be of no significance, certain features should not in a retarded child be disregarded, including a malar flush, unusual distribution of hair, especially over the sacral spine, which may indicate neural tube defect, birth marks which are haemangiomatous or pigmented, and, in particular, clearly demarcated patches of white skin, especially if present from birth and situated around the trunk below the rib cage, which may be possible achromic spots, or pink nodular spots over the cheeks, both of which may raise the suspicion of epiloia. It should always be remembered that a grossly retarded child with epiloia can be born to a parent carrying the gene who may him- or herself be of normal intelligence with perhaps a single achromic skin patch as the only indication of the condition, so variable is its penetrance. Such a situation is rare but because of its genetic implications for any mildly affected sibling it should never be missed.

Satisfying as best he can the needs of parents with a severely handicapped child to question why this tragedy has fallen on them and to facilitate expression of their anger and grief in as constructive a manner for them as possible, is a task for the physician to undertake with the utmost seriousness and with ample time. The shock and sense of personal affront or inadequacy suffered by parents has been well documented (Tizard & Grad, 1961; Gath, 1978; Cunningham & Sloper, 1977; Davis, 1979). The resentment which is quite understandably generated in them by an emerging grasp of the damage that the episode of cerebral insult has inflicted on their child and a sense of loss they feel for the child who might have been – these are feelings which a doctor must always be aware of and take into account. To some degree they are always present. The obligation of the doctor is to appreciate that this is an injured and angry family, deserving not only professional support but a personal sympathy which recognizes and accepts the bitterness or dismay which may underlie occasional sporadic, apparently irrational, anxieties or prejudices in even most coping families.

Problems of function: 'How is my child handicapped?'

One of the most basic assumptions underlying medical and psychiatric practice is that the diagnosis of a disease and associated pathology endows the doctor with reliable insight into resulting malfunction. Unfortunately, in mental handicap this is often a very tenuous connection. Not only is the pathology often unknown, but even when it is defined as in phenylketonuria, the disabilities and behaviour that

result are not distinctive; they vary in severity and resemble other forms of mental handicap. Specific symptoms may be connected with an aetiological factor, as self-mutilation with uricaemia, but these are rare, not only because the numbers involved are too small to establish a reliable constellation of symptoms, but more fundamentally because there is as yet no link between facets of behaviour and the biochemical or genetic level at which aetiological factors are defined. Even a reasonably clear understanding of the distribution of brain damage does not necessarily indicate a predictably related pattern of handicap except within broad limits. In the severely retarded a multiplicity of handicaps is common; their interaction and the efforts made by the child himself, related in turn to the effectiveness of those who help him can produce a sufficiently wide spectrum of eventual achievement to deter the experienced doctor from too confident a prediction of how seriously a child will be disabled.

It is for this reason important to try to reconcile an honest and realistic prognosis with encouragement as to what can reasonably be attempted stage by stage. The family is often caught in a vicious circle since their initial shock may be reinforced by a hopeless forecast which prevents their attempting any therapeutic programme, thereby ensuring that the child's lack of development confirms their fears. With support, most parents eventually want to make every effort on their child's behalf. They want to set about this with an understanding of how their child's handicapping conditions have disabled him – and they often want to know this in detail. Unfortunately, this is often extremely difficult. Here again a few guidelines may be helpful.

In an earlier section a broad contrast in aetiological factors was drawn between handicap resulting from some form of cerebral insult and handicap with no such apparent cause. These two groups do tend to produce somewhat contrasting symptom constellations. They can be said to produce an equally contrasting outlook within the family, that is, a syndrome child, whether active or crippled, without a clear episode of cerebral insult, will tend to generate family problems and to be disabled in a way rather different from the brain-damaged child. Of course, such an interpretation, outlined below, is very generalized indeed, since handicapped children and their families are as individual and contrasting as any other group, but however rough and ready, it is intended as a guide to the reader who, unless he is experienced in the field, will be perplexed at the multiplicity and severity of the problems which confront him. Faced with the task of helping any family with a severely retarded member to understand how he is handicapped, and thereby how to treat him, the doctor will soon appreciate that most advice is sought for one or two main reasons. For some SSN patients the main problem is their dependence, the burden of daily care they impose on their family. These patients usually have motor defects as well as being severely retarded. Other patients present a totally different problem which relates to their family's efforts to control or even contain them; although they may be clumsy these patients have no motor defect; on the contrary, the difficulties they present relate to their high level of activity. Which of these categories any given patient falls into when brought to the doctor is usually very clear. The greater difficulty is to judge whether such a patient belongs to the damaged or syndrome group.

The crippled, severely retarded patient may present with varying degrees of motor handicap from virtual immobility to some effort at activity hindered by distorted posture and gait or defective balance. Whether such disabilities are the result of brain damage involving the motor cortex, associated nuclei, and cortico-spinal pathways should be evident from the history, but a very similar level of motor defect can develop, particularly in long-untreated children without such a damaging episode. A number of contrasting features can help to distinguish the damaged from the syndrome child (syndrome is used here as a shorthand term, though often no syndrome is known). The damaged child's expression and facial response is usually more alert and socially appropriate, contrasting with the apathy, sluggish visual fixing, and infrequent blink of the syndrome child. The damaged child, if watched patiently in familiar surroundings, spontaneously moves or struggles to move more readily, though the syndrome child has a far wider range of available movement. Movement, when it does occur, tends to be asymmetrical in the damaged child, left more than right, or arms more than legs: it is also predictably distorted by reflex patterning depending on the position of the patient's head or trunk. With the syndrome child, movement has not only a wider range but is unaffected by head position and tends to be symmetrical; either arm or leg may be moved and in the young tends to be total, that is, both arms or legs rather like a baby. On handling, the patients feel different, for the resting tone of the damaged child may be abnormally high or low but increases rapidly with movement, with a tendency to spasm. This will be exaggerated if a child is excited or frightened or simply trying very hard to move. The resting tone of the syndrome child is normal or rather low but rises sluggishly when harnessed for movement: it is difficult to elicit brisk tone changes, no matter how the child is stimulated, in complete contrast to the hair-trigger tone response of a damaged child.

The broad relationship between origins of the handicap and the resulting disability is quite readily explained in such cases and the parents can be helped to appreciate the connection between cerebral palsy and brain damage in one case and severe retardation producing apathy and sluggish movement in the other. The very rough explanation that one group is 'motivated to move but prevented by their handicap, the more so the more they struggle', while the other is handicapped by lack of interest in moving, though equipped to do so, is valuable because it can counteract the unproductive parent–child interactions which build up.

Parents with a damaged child will have developed expectations of a normal baby during the pregnancy. They may compensate for the ensuing traumatic perinatal episode by retaining some conviction that he is to some extent normal, an attitude often reinforced by the child's apparent social responsiveness. In consequence, they are sometimes prone, after an initial phase of apprehensive hesitant handling, to pressurize the child in the belief that, given a great deal of incentive or encouragement, he can improve his performance. In fact, in such a child such an attitude may raise his tone and level of excitation, aggravate his spasms, and cause him distress, making him more than usually vulnerable in any stimulating or teaching situation. Other parents never emerge from their initial anxiety when their handling elicits spasm, so that they retreat into an indulgent round of activity in which the child is required to do very little for himself at all. A balance needs to be struck between these extremes. The doctor must help to establish it by enabling the parents to appreciate better the manner in which his motor handicap is vulnerable to both over- and understimulation. From this understanding more detailed practical suggestions on handling will follow, as described below.

In contrast, the parents with a syndrome child will learn gradually of their child's handicap. They are unlikely to know its cause, yet its severity daily becomes more apparent. Such parents become not only distressed but increasingly bewildered. They may take refuge from an emotionally intolerable reality by projecting skills into their child which are clearly not there. They may, for instance, vigorously encourage his pulling on a particular red jersey because he laughed, assuming he likes that colour or texture, or talk enthusiastically with him while watching a particular TV programme because through some slight gesture he has conveyed to them what they feel to be an interest. These enthusiasms eventually fade and the family may in the meantime have developed others so the child may lack from the parents the very management he most needs – a simple but above all consistent daily routine, which attempts by sheer repetition to establish some reliable response. The painfully slow feedback of such children quite reasonably promotes in parents a succession of defensive brief enthusiasms which they may well need in order to persevere at all. They will occasionally be punctuated by bouts of depressed realization of what they feel to be the utter futility of their efforts. For such families the doctor needs to set realistic goals and help towards an understanding of the time-span involved in any progress. He needs to ensure that the family knows how everyone appreciates the tedium imposed and to respect their need occasionally to pretend to achievements, though with steady support they can themselves cope with the realization that it is pretence.

With the active child, the relationship between aetiology and handicapping condition is less clear, indeed one of the least understood areas of the subject is the definition of distinctive behaviour patterns which contrast psychosis, autism, and retardation produced by defined cerebral insult or in some other way. Informative reviews are available (Wing & Gould, 1979) but there are no reliable contrasts between the behaviour of, for example, a phenylketonuric child and an equally retarded active child disabled by perinatal cerebral hypoxaemia. The activity level in both is high although in a damaged child its peaks may more predictably be related to being thwarted or to some stress such as confined space, whereas the syndrome child's outbursts may occur in protracted episodes apparently unrelated to change in circumstances or social pressure. Stereotypies and self-mutilating activities will occur in both groups; this is somewhat more likely to be due to boredom in the damaged child and thus to be relieved by distracting him, whereas such behaviour tends in some syndrome children to be maintained to shut out sensory input or social involvement and so becomes worse if attempts are made to distract them. Damaged active children tend to be clumsy, with poor fine motor control aggravated by brief attention span which hinders their effective monitoring of any motor act; syndrome children are often dextrous and may sustain quite skilful, though often socially inconvenient, activities, becoming preoccupied with them to an extent which would be rare in a damaged child. Both groups would be severely language-handicapped; though both may be echolalic, damaged children are more likely to have normally inflected vocal output and may more readily convey their wants or interests by using their voice in ways readily understood by those who care for them. Epileptic attacks are common in both groups, though there is a greater tendency for them to occur at physiologically vulnerable periods in the damaged child such as waking or falling asleep or suffering from systemic illness. The fits of syndrome children often occur in bouts with fit-free periods between; they seem unrelated to any physiological stress and are commonly more refractory to anticonvulsant treatment.

In general, the family with the exasperatingly active damaged child can be helped to see his behaviour as the product of poor inhibitory control. His clumsy movements, distractibility, and short attention span prevent him from focusing and sustaining his attention, all of which, if realized, suggest the type of management he will need. Parents of such a child are often partially compensated by his obvious, to them, naughtiness, which at least renders his behaviour comprehensible and enables them to take more or less the same precautions as they would with normal children only with more consistency and vigour. However, consistent management, so necessary for such a child, is quite often the one feature conspicuously lacking. Although at times accepting his mischief, both parents may frequently be exasperated yet will refrain from reprimand because they feel he cannot help it, regarding the term 'brain damage' as some licence to behave in that fashion, or quite often as implying some fragile intracranial state which must be safeguarded. As a result, they may tolerate a whole succession of misdeeds until their patience snaps and they may reprimand him severely. At this they may well feel remorse and consequently again indulge his behaviour, so from the child's point of view a *laissez-faire* attitude to some activities is suddenly and inexplicably punctuated by punishment. Such inconsistency is both common and understandable in such harassed families and the doctor could help greatly by drawing attention without criticism to its effects.

It is the lack of any apparent connection between the child's handicap and his behaviour which so depresses the parents of the active syndrome child. His odd skills are often as meaningless and unpredictable as his outbursts, so that the family may become resigned to developing day-to-day safeguards and precautions which form the framework of domestic management within which they can operate. These precautions may be quite illogical, such as never closing room doors or leaving shoes within reach. The doctor's support in this context must be confined to taking an interest in, and often admiring, tactics which the family develop, keeping them in perspective, and coping sympathetically with the array of anxieties which confront such a family in their efforts to understand their child's behaviour. They will often want to know what damage fits inflict on the brain and how best to reconcile adequate anticonvulsant cover with sedation. They will often question whether their child's pathology can cause this or that defect or deterioration, as when parents may be convinced that apparently failing visual interest in a child with epiloia is the result of a disease process. It is important to know the family well enough to judge whether reassurance or further investigation is indicated; for example, in epiloia retinal phakomata may be interfering with what limited macula vision the child has and consultation with an ophthalmological colleague is indicated. Respecting the efforts of such a family to make some sort of logic out of their child's gross disability is a crucial element in their doctor's support.

Problems of management: 'What am I to do to help?'

The basic aim of the psychiatrist's involvement so far described is to support the family through the crisis of discovering the nature and extent of their child's handicap and to explain to them fully its causes and nature and as far as possible the relationship between this and the child's emerging disabilities. The counselling, explanation, and examinations thus entailed are in turn aimed at equipping the family as far as possible with emotionally sound perspectives so they could and would wish to involve themselves realistically in their child's handling and stimulation.

We are trying to make the family ready to do things for their child. This raises a number of practical points: what to do and what aims are set; how much can the family do; who helps, complements and guides their efforts; and who evaluates progress towards defined aims with them? Eventually, the family will need now and again to take stock, to consider whether aims are realizable and, if not, whether alternative programmes are needed, or indeed alternative care and arrangements.

It is unlikely that many readers, unless specialized in the field, would be expected to formulate in any detail treatment programmes for a particularly severely handicapped child in their practice. They will, however, need to counsel the family, perhaps acting as arbiter on the effectiveness of the treatment as the family sees it. They may be asked, when treatment is questioned, to advise on investigations which test its appropriateness. Broad outlines of management will be dealt with below in sections relating to different age groups through the life of the severely retarded patient. Two aspects of organizing help can be generally discussed: investigations and the arrangements for counselling.

Diagnostic investigations are likely to have been carried out before the psychiatrist is involved in the case of children whose retardation was suspected in babyhood, either from behaviour or appearance or whenever an episode of cerebral insult had occurred. In some conditions, however, such as epiloia or neuro-lipidoses, the clinician may not suspect a specific disease until later, when the child and family are already in his care. Suspicions may be aroused for a variety of reasons: a suspect family history; stunted growth; failure to achieve even early motor milestones; an emerging odd appearance or epileptic attacks. Which, if any, of the ever widening array of syndromes is suspected will depend on the clinician's own earlier experience or a ready access to more detailed and well-illustrated texts. He may hesitate to refer the case immediately to colleagues in clinical genetics until more confident of some developmental anomaly, in which situation he will make some broad screening investigations, not unpleasant to the child nor alarming to the family. Urine amino-acid chromatography is useful though obtaining a urine specimen can be very difficult, so serum chromatography may be needed. X-rays of the skull for bony deformities or calcification, or of the wrists for bone age may be of value. In severe retardation an EEG is almost invariably abnormal, rarely in any way diagnostically specific. Indeed, as with skull X-rays, a succession of records is usually more valuable in showing, for example, progressive calcification in the X-ray or a changing pattern of localized EEG abnormality in epiloia.

In some situations the suspicions of the parents themselves may be aroused, whether through reading or concern at some stigmata, so the doctor can embark on investigations with their approval. In other cases the suspicions may be the doctor's alone, and obviously care must be taken not to alarm the parents, so the tests can be described as appropriate to help find out in more detail what may underlie their child's slow development. The doctor must use his own judgement to what extent and at which stage he confides specific suspicions to the parents; most would await the results of tests but, in the author's experience, the more frank the doctor is the better his developing relationship with the family. With the test results available he should explain them and their implications fully to the parents, or, if negative, not only that this is the case but what suspicions have been refuted.

In the continuing management of the severely retarded patient a certain minimum of investigations is necessary. Recurrent hip X-rays are imperative for the retarded child with motor defect, certainly with adductor spasm. Here the danger of subluxation can be easily averted if detected early, whereas, once the hips are dislocated, much more serious surgical procedures are required with their attendant psychological problems. Recurrent skull X-rays may be of value to check the progress of calcification or of intracranial pressure in cases with Spitz-Holter valves. Blood levels are advisable in the monitoring of anticonvulsant drugs. Although it must always be remembered that the effectiveness of treatment depends on controlling fit frequency, blood levels can reveal otherwise hidden problems such as the accumulation effect of phenobarbitone with associated drowsiness or confused behavioural disturbance, or a sudden escalation of the level of phenytoin perhaps with induced fits, as can happen when the dose exceeds about 6 mg/kg body weight. A series of EEGs are usually of far more value in guiding management than a single invariably abnormal record; their value has been discussed elsewhere. Periodic dental examinations are well worth the effort of finding a sympathetic colleague to provide them. The early detection of carious teeth is an obvious advantage, whilst preventative measures to offset severe malocclusion or overcrowding, can avoid serious problems later. The advisability of hearing and visual tests have been discussed elsewhere: here it is worth emphasizing the value of keeping a weather eye open with occasional simple clinical checks. It is quite surprising how much behaviour disturbance or failing language use can be precipitated by wax in the ears; its insidious development can virtually isolate the apathetic retarded child, particularly if he has poor vision. Yet it may well be overlooked. Occasionally testing pupil responses can alert to incipient visual changes, as with developing cataracts which may be dense or extensive enough to be quite visually disabling long before they are clearly apparent even to quite careful facial scrutiny. Formal psychological assessments tend to be unproductive in the severely retarded, not least because the results may be difficult to interpret or unreliable owing to the uncooperative or apathetic response of the patient. If successful, however, such tests, perhaps by suggesting a performance level or mental age, may be a concept the parents find helpful in giving some perspective to their child's retardation in comparing, for example, with a sibling. On occasions they may be of value as a base-line, particularly if performed in an equable, familiar setting, and may reveal unexpected assets in some performance subtests. Their value is greatly increased if teaching-orientated assessments are used to outline the profile of disabilities and also of achievements, however limited, for the purpose of establishing a teaching or training programme and as a basis of decisions and building confidence in the family.

The severely retarded present such a variety of problems in management, physiological, educational, therapeutic, and social, that it is inevitable that several professional workers will be involved in efforts to help them. Nowadays, in any residential setting a similarly diverse group will be either caring for them or advising those who do. An essential component of responsible clinical management of the patient and his family is to draw together these various agents so that a coherent, consistent body of information and advice is given. Parents of the handicapped are inevitably depressed, angry, and bewildered people who will seek and be gratuitously given, explanations and advice from an array of professionals, relatives, and acquaintances. If what they hear is emotionally unacceptable or inconsistent they will quite understandably ask elsewhere. They are immensely vulnerable to any recommendations, from old wives' tales from neighbours to expensive, time-consuming programmes from well-advertized commercial organizations. Their response may vary from total rejection to a dedication which prompts them to move house and totally disrupt their previous life, to pursue what they see to be beneficial to their handicapped child. Hence effective counselling is essential. To be consistent and supportive it must be a coherent group effort; everyone involved with the family must appreciate what the family members understand to be the handicap and what feelings this generates. This is unlikely to be achieved without an occasional group meeting which welds the group into a team. Arranging this may well fall on the doctor. If possible all who treat the patient or advise the family should attend: this will usually be quite a manageable number. Meetings may not need to be frequent but they should be regular, yet arranged with enough flexibility for urgent and *ad hoc* meetings to occur to meet crises. Usually a key figure will emerge from the group, often someone who is practically involved, such as a physiotherapist or nursery teacher, or any member who establishes a particular rapport. A valuable group member in this context, if judiciously selected, can be another parent with a similarly affected child, and some local parents' organizations have panels with parents who undertake this role.

Obviously, each member of the group or team will be pursuing his or her respective programme with the patient and family and this will dominate his or her own individual professional experience with them. However, occasional meetings as a team facilitate each professional's work in a number of ways. They can co-ordinate practical arrangements, for example, by enabling therapists to arrange their sessions conveniently or by minimizing awkward travelling. Progress or setbacks can be compared to suggest common problems or the success of a particular technique. Explanations and advice can be standardized or agreed between team members so that parents are not confused or tempted to play off one professional against another. The psychiatrist may have a crucial responsibility to the team: he may wish or be expected to counsel the family alone and must keep the team members informed whilst respecting the family's confidences. He may well need to discuss frankly with the family when, and how much, such confidences should be shared with team members. He will need periodically to take stock of progress, to re-assess with the team any change in the patient's disability, to suggest explanations for this, to secure (or avoid) further investigations which

would confirm such explanations. He must understand the results of such investigations and translate them into guide-lines for further action. At some team-meetings members may wish to discuss issues among themselves but it is imperative that the parents participate at least occasionally, particularly at reviews. At such reviews future aims should be set which may well mean choosing among alternatives or establishing priorities; obviously the parents must participate in these decisions. Often the doctor's role is to keep uppermost a recognition by all that the patient is regarded as a total person and not as a challenge to each team member's expertise (an attitude quite natural in any enthusiastic team), and above all that the patient is the parent's child.

Depending on where he practises, the psychiatrist may find such a team already functioning, indeed it is to be hoped that he will be part of it. In some situations, particularly with young children, day-to-day needs may be met by the primary care team and the psychiatrist will liaise with the family doctor, health visitor, or social worker. In paediatric practice, more specialized groups are being established as child handicap teams, usually convened by the specialist in community medicine for child health of the NHS district or area. Recommended by the Court Committee (Report of Committee on Child Health Services, 1976), they are closely linked to the paediatric department of the local district general hospital and/or with the network of the local authority child welfare services. In some cases, such teams work in conjunction with the staff of the appropriate subnormality hospital or of child psychiatric services. The National Development Team have recommended Community Handicap Teams (Development Team for the Mentally Handicapped, 1976–77): where these have been established, the psychiatrist's role is more clearly defined. They contrast with the above arrangement by offering a service to all age groups of the mentally hanidcapped. In whatever way the service is organized the teams are expected to comprise members of various professions, to have a flexible constitution as the handicapped patient's needs change, to establish links with parent organizations and other community services. The group should be consistent in respecting one another's idiosyncrasies and should develop experience of local facilities. The emergence of more formal arrangements should help ensure that families are not deprived of resources and that efforts on their behalf are administratively co-ordinated, but a crucial feature of a team, effective from the parents' viewpoint, is that its members should deal directly with their retarded child. There is perhaps the danger that more formalized groups have to concern themselves with arrangements rather than the details of the treatment itself. The doctor may be able to redress the balance but he will need to appreciate the treatment programme himself sufficiently if he is to do this.

With a severely subnormal patient the combination of disabilities, both physical and psychiatric, can be so varied that the reader is advised to consult appropriate practical texts (Finnie, 1971; Freeman, 1975; L. Wing, 1980; Simon, 1980). Here general guide-lines of management will be suggested for the severely subnormal child as he grows older.

Babyhood and the very young child

In almost all cases severe subnormality is detected early at birth or during babyhood. A few potentially subnormal children have neither evident stigmata nor seriously delayed motor milestones and so may present as a very unresponsive or bizarre toddler (see section on psychotic children). The psychiatrist therefore is rarely required to diagnose severe subnormality in a baby although he may be invited to confirm or refute clinical suspicions about, for example, a very backward 6-monther or the unresponsive, oddly behaved older child of about 2 years who has not yet developed speech. In this situation it is important to anticipate at the onset that this first meeting will be the culmination for the parents of months of growing anxiety, so the meeting must be conducted accordingly. It is often helpful not only to behave sympathetically but state openly one's recognition of how worrying their child's lack of progress must have been. Many parents, taking an odd suspect child to a variety of clinics, may become convinced that no one really believes their fears, so they interpret sensible professional caution as scepticism or disbelief. They will certainly wonder how much they have themselves contributed to their child's unresponsiveness, which may further undermine their confidence. The doctor may not initially be sure himself of the extent or even the existence of their child's retardation but it is vital to take their fears very seriously. It is also important to find out in what way *they* consider him backward. This may encourage them to be confiding and thus more realistic. Some parents are surprising because they may ignore much more seriously retarded behaviour yet concentrate on one aspect which seems significant to them, attributing everything else to it. If the family are to

be effectively involved, as they must be, in helping their child's progress, the treatment must respect and work from their own anxieties towards a more realistic balanced programme.

Taking a history can be an opportunity for observing the child in a leisurely way and his parents' reactions to him; whether they share holding or controlling him and so on. The obstetric history should be checked, including such points as vague illnesses 'like flu' in the first trimester, frequent vomiting, or in an experienced mother a sense that the baby was particularly still *in utero*. Details of various milestones are obviously important, as also are feeding difficulties including poor sucking, chewing, or swallowing, sudden changes in mood with screaming attacks or apparent fears, or sudden stilling may be significant as may be brief stomach cramps which may emerge retrospectively as infantile spasms.

The young child's facial appearance is a valuable clue to the extent of his retardation: a passive immobile face with little eye movement and a slow blink rate, or a face showing a studied preoccupied interest unrelated to his surroundings, are both sinister – hence the value of watching the child with his parents. Excessively brisk or sluggish responses which seem random or are shifting and unsustained are noteworthy, as is the amount of spontaneous motor activity, how well it is controlled and directed, whether it shows markedly asymmetrical limb use, or whether in, for example, a 6-monther it is total, involving always both arms or legs, or is broken up into discrete limb movements. In such a young child retained Moro or grasp reflexes should be tested and such reflexes as placing reactions and the Landau (response to ventral suspension) should be sought.

Should the young child be suspected as potentially SSN the parents must be told frankly but sympathetically as outlined in the previous sections of this chapter. It is valuable to describe this not only in terms meaningful to them but as confirming their own suspicions – hence the need initially to listen to these carefully. These fears are why they have come to their doctor. The various stages of discussion will then need to be taken up as described above, but from the beginning it is important to recognise something positive in the child, which the parents may themselves have alluded to in passing, and as quickly as possible to direct attention to a particular problem in which they can be involved, for example, working for visual interest or head control. Supportive management means not only a frank explanation of the handicap and of its possible effects at that moment, but the setting of aims, however rudimentary, which are feasible, which can be worked for with a realistic hope of achievement in an emotionally acceptable period such as six months, and above all which involve the parents themselves. How this involvement may be arranged as part of team effort has already been discussed.

With very young SSN children the aims of treatment will of necessity be very modest. If the child is so retarded as to show no visual interest, then, ocular defect having been carefully excluded, the establishment of visual interest should be the first target. Few mothers can relate to a child who does not look either at her or apparently anyone else. Simply visually stimulating such a child with bright noisy toys may well be fruitless for many months and thus totally demoralizing for a mother. Concentrating on establishing head control may be much more productive as well as more emotionally satisfying. The simple technique of this process has been described more fully elsewhere (Ricks, 1980), but, briefly, the mother holding the child facing her on her lap, supported in, for example, a large towel wrapped around him, the ends being gathered and held by the mother. The towel initially supports the child's back and head so that he can be moved readily: later the support is lowered so that the child practises balancing his head on his trunk as he is moved sideways or nearer or farther from his mother who with face-to-face contact can also protract his shoulders and encourage him to handle her face or hair while crooning or speaking to him. With this handling the child is more likely to begin looking, as will be noted by his mother when his eyes begin occasionally to converge or eye movements compensating his head movement gradually develop. Simple handling techniques like this are extremely important for the young potentially SSN child, because they aim at capturing and sustaining interest in, and attention to, a person, which becomes increasingly difficult to establish as the child gets older, and the absence of which is the most profound disability. With similar handling the parents can try to elicit some form of vocal exchange, however simple. Any forms of oral activity, producing noises which appear to interest the child, blowing raspberries, clucking, cooing, and so forth, can all be tried. Once his attention is gained the next stage is to suggest that the parents imitate any noise the child makes for the purpose of establishing some noise exchange between them, using vocal output which the child himself certainly can produce. These interaction games can be brief, indeed should be, lasting only a

few minutes to be gradually extended and so can be fitted casually into the day, making use of more responsive periods as they occur. They should be accompanied as far as practicable with plenty of handling, care being taken to alert the child beforehand and of course to respect that on some occasions he will enjoy contact, on others resist it. Talking to the child should similarly be encouraged; it should be heralded by reasonable close facial contact and be highly inflected. Of all the complex qualities of human vocal output, pitch changes are the most readily appreciated: they are the most reliable incentive to listening and comprehension at the simplest level as well as enabling the child to localize the source of sound. Giving as rich an experience as possible of change of posture and position through handling; encouraging thereby appropriate motor responses; establishing head control and some purposeful vision; encouraging rudimentary social and vocal exchange with appropriately modified use of voice by the parents – these are the bases of a programme for the very young, which aim above all at capturing and sustaining social response, however brief initially. The programme can be varied, and if the general guiding principles are understood the parents will often ingeniously develop their own handling strategies. This should be particularly encouraged. The episodes of treatment can be brief and performed with a frequency to suit the family's convenience, the best guide being the child's own response. He may reject virtually all their efforts and the psychiatrist's main concern will be in such cases to maintain some enthusiasm in the parents, allowing them with his reassurance to tail off when the child seems particularly restive. Bouts of crying, problems of constipation or vomiting, epileptic attacks, and fluctuating irritability will often intrude into the programme. These need not only appropriate medical management but to be put into perspective. Many of these problems seem intractable in early childhood of the SSN but in most cases they ease off by the age of three or four. One of the most supportive roles of the doctor in this context is to put this harrowing period into perspective. At the same time, he will obviously need to meet the family and support team much more frequently at times of stress.

The pre-school child

The pre-school period is probably the most crucial in determining the progress of any SSN child. By the age of 2 to 3 years the pattern of disabilities is becoming clear; at the same time nursery provisions are usually available and more professional staff such as physiotherapists and preschool advisory teachers will become involved. The child does not yet usually present serious management problems but the parents themselves are becoming more acutely aware of developmental delay. This is now much more evident in their SSN child as he is compared with contemporaries who are all mobile, acquiring self-help skills, playing, and talking. It is at this time that the full impact of retardation begins to be felt, so a growing sense of urgency or dismay will often intensify the parents' need for support from the team. The questions discussed at length earlier in the chapter will need to be frequently re-discussed and an effort made to reach workable solutions. This is the time when intensive training or therapy will be of greatest value, when the total push is most productive, so the child's progress must be regularly checked, programmes monitored, and the enthusiasm of team members maintained.

Reviewing progress in the pre-school SSN child should as far as possible occur within his home or at least in a familiar setting. At no other stage is it more important to discover what the child not only *can* do but how he himself is likely to set about it. This is the time to recognize and respect the child's own tactics of acquiring simple skills, modifying and building on them rather than superimposing standardized instructions to the family showing how it should be done. If the child is motor-handicapped it will be helpful to check how much he does move spontaneously; whether the patterns of movement are asymmetrical; how much effort he will make and what rewards motivate his efforts; how his tone reacts to effort and excitement and so on. If he is mobile, the child's activity will reveal how much he explores, how he uses and judges situational clues, how much he can stop or grade his activity. Obviously the extent of his awareness is important as shown by the extent he visually scans, seems to rely on touch to explore or identify, how much if at all he needs to fix visually to direct his movements, how distractible he is and whether to visual stimuli or sounds, particularly the human voice. His vocal output is extremely important; does he utter a sort of running chatter without any obvious communicating function; does he vocalize at all for any apparent purpose; if so is his vocal output inflected in a normal way or at least in a way recognizable as meaning something to his parents; is his vocalization dissonant and harsh, with marked pitch changes suggesting hearing defect, or musical

and repetitive suggesting a future echolalia? Above all should be noted the child's level of alertness and social awareness; do they fluctuate, if so with any recognizable pattern; are they replaced by periods of preoccupation with stereotypies, do these episodes relate to any detectable stress; does the child seem to enjoy certain situations; if so are these related to people and their behaviour towards him and are they to any reliable extent reproducible? At this stage it is vital to try and establish a clear picture of the child as a total person with likes and dislikes as well as disabilities and assets, for it seems that consistent handling, if sensitive to his needs, is most productive at this stage.

To these general points of assessment can be added others which relate to particular types of handicap and their particular needs in the pre-school phase. By this age three major groups of disabilities can be distinguished: a) retarded children with severe sensory defects, e.g., blind or blind/deaf children; b) motor-handicapped dependent children; c) active socially unresponsive children usually with profound language defect. They will be discussed in turn.

(a) *SSN children with severe sensory defects* need at this age as far as possible to be encouraged to bear their weight and to become mobile. This may well mean long hours spent getting them accustomed to an upright stance, developing their confidence in familiar and padded surroundings, helping them to mobilize themselves, which for a very long period they will do only with support. This in turn emphasizes the importance of encouraging hand use; simple tactile exploration is often vigorously resisted by these children, unlike the blind child of normal intelligence. It is valuable to help them move over set familiar pathways using fairly regular distances since they acquire confidence more readily by a sense of local distance and direction than by identifying objects by touch – which comes later. Simple self-help skills similarly need to be practised by touch and a regular pattern of movement, always remembering that smell is often also extremely important especially for types of food or clothing, for instance. Always be prepared for resistance and occasional panic responses in these children, who may be highly sensitive to environmental features which we largely ignore, such as smell of traffic or feel of wind on the face. If such a child lives or works in a setting of mixed blind and blind/deaf children then certain problems can be anticipated. Blind/deaf children, even if quite young, are often active once mobile and frequently vocalize in a rather repetitive monotonous way with occasional staccato bursts of sound. The retarded blind child who hears is usually more reluctant to explore or move around and is often upset by noise since much of his orientation depends on listening, so that the company of busy noisy peers confuses him. Most blind/deaf children have some visual and auditory awareness: if it is to be harnessed then the pre-school period is the time to try so that residual sensory input can be built into the child's perceptual apparatus when he is most likely to harness it, that is, when he begins to mobilize himself. Now is the time to press for a clear evaluation of hearing loss and visual acuity and to ensure that aids are appropriate, tolerated, and used.

(b) Programmes to help the *retarded motor-handicapped child* are described in detail elsewhere (Ricks, 1980). A distinction has been made earlier between the basically unresponsive child whose poverty of movement is the product of apathy (called the syndrome child), and the brain-damaged child who often wants to move but whose efforts are hindered and distorted by a spastic weakness and poor balance or co-ordination (called the damaged child). As stressed earlier this clinical distinction is important since appropriate management for one group is highly inappropriate for the other. Syndrome children need stimulation to excite their interest and raise their tone; they need handling which gives them as much practice as possible in head control and balance reactions which in them are sluggish; they need movement experience, however supplied, as long as they enjoy it, to help towards postural control and better trunk rotation; any spontaneous movement is to be encouraged and can be extended or modified later. A sequence of skills can be aimed at, from establishing head control and visual interest to stable sitting with gradually reduced support to secure trunk control, then to weight-bearing from stable sitting in order to prevent the child from being totally dependent and requiring lifting from bed to chair or lavatory. Any gross visual defect must be detected, including severe refractive error or hearing loss; if discovered the pattern of stimulation must be adapted accordingly. The eventual aim, which will not be reached in the pre-school period, is a stable sitting child with hands released for self-feeding, help in dressing, and some simple play or signing, able to bear weight so that he can be supported rather than lifted from place to place. The programme for the damaged child will depend on his type of cerebral

palsy but in general quite contrasting principles apply. For him sustained pressure of stimulation should be avoided; he needs handling that is predictable and carefully graduated, thus reducing his propensity to spasms; that aims at teaching him to grade his tone rather than to raise and sustain it. To stimulate, interest, or feed him this child should be approached from the front not from the side. In contrast, the syndrome child is helped by the stimulation from the side to encourage his trunk rotation. In general the syndrome child needs to be kept interested to make an effort, whereas the damaged child needs to be kept calm to help him keep trying. In coping with the first type of child, with his apathy and slow achievements, parents need support to maintain enthusiasm, to appreciate small gains however slow in appearing and to keep a realistic perspective. They need to be helped to see that the aims of treatment, though modest and perhaps distant, will rescue their child from being totally dependent. Parents of the damaged child, who is hair-trigger, not sluggish, in his responses and is irritable rather than apathetic, need help to act in a consistent calm and predictable way, and to curb their impatience in the belief that he could do it if he really tried. A more detailed account of such treatment programmes is described elsewhere.

(c) The major aim in the pre-school period should be to establish a sensible understanding of the child's handicap and capabilities, laying the foundations of effective therapeutic management which all involved in it appreciate. This is the time to get the basics right, to sort out functional disability and promote good habits of stimulation and day-to-day handling. In no group is this more important than in the *active SSN with problems of distractibility and effective communication.* These are the children who can become the most taxing burden of care to their family. Yet in no group is it more difficult to set the family early on the right road – for a number of reasons. In active SSN children, usually with no worrying motor delay, a full assessment of their disabilities is often delayed because there may be no real medical anxiety until they fail to speak, the timing of which is flexible in normal children. In addition, they are extremely difficult to investigate and assess in conventional clinical surroundings which can deter prompt action. Their parents are frequently alarmed by odd behaviour, which in the young child can be, and sometimes is, construed as a product of their anxiety, so that attention may be directed more to their reactions than to the possible disabilities in the child independent of the parents' concern. It is extremely important always to take very seriously the full functional assessment of such a child as a fundamental first step. Strained parent/child relationships there will be, and usually a good deal of domestic conflict, all of which will aggravate the child's handicap, but this should be regarded, as a first approximation, as the result, not the cause, of his disability. This may be revised later but it should not deflect attention from the child's handicapping condition.

The basic objective of management of this type of child is quite simple to state but extremely difficult to achieve: it is to equip him to focus and sustain his attention so that he is accessible to social constraints and can reliably respond to them. All these children are distractable with attention spans so brief that it hinders their attempt to listen selectively, or to abstract categories from their sensory input, so they do not recognize regularities in their experience, symbolize, embark on language, or develop representational play. As a result their daily activity remains exploratory and is not channelled into any protracted play other than repetitive mannerisms or stereotypies. A distinction has been suggested earlier between damaged and syndrome SSN children which is a good deal less marked in this group nor does it have quite the same indications for management. Those parents with a damaged child of this type tend to be able to regard their child's distractibility and outbursts as exaggerated versions of naughtiness, that is, that a more or less comprehensible and predictable reason can be recognized as a precipitating event, so that precautions can be taken. To the parents of the SSN syndrome or psychotic active child there is often no apparent logic whatever in their child's outburst or preferences, though they may be consistently triggered by some apparently quite unrelated event so that the parents can learn which situations to avoid and which are likely to be tolerated or enjoyed. Management of this type of child's behaviour has been discussed elsewhere. To combat their distractability and associated learning problems both groups require regular routine in their handling so that regularities emerge in their daily life by repetition; tasks in self-help or domestic skills should be demonstrated rather than instructed; speaking to them should be simplified, consistently worded, and with exaggerated inflection, and care is needed that all interaction is direct and not casual so

that the child has every chance to appreciate that contact is being made. Play and comforting experiences should be as quiet and private as possible but periods of exuberant play are needed, often frequently, but need organizing to occur in socially acceptable and largely accident-proof settings. In short the daily routine imposed on a family by such a child can be both tiring and regimented. They will find it hard to accept, as indeed will the SSN child's brothers and sisters. To sustain such a family will need not only counselling and support from all team members but an array of additional benefits and facilities. A few examples can be outlined.

Play groups and day nurseries can be of great value not only to give periods of relief but as an avenue of therapy or assessment outside the home. Some may employ part-time professional staff such as physio-, speech, or play therapists but, as with opportunity groups, some are run by non-professional staff sympathetic to and experienced with severe handicap. Some may be run in conjunction with parent groups or with libraries that lend toys. In some NHS districts paediatric or local authority child health and social work departments are establishing centres in which various therapists are periodically available, where parent groups are formed, and where the worried mother can gain much reassurance and practical tips from other mothers. The psychiatrist involved with the family should acquaint himself with local arrangements; there are also informative pamphlets available and organizations which can be contacted (Spain & Wigley, 1975; Russell, 1976). At this age even the seriously retarded child is generally acceptable in some local play group. In some cases the team may feel the child is over-excited by such an experience but this can usually be remedied by a graded involvement and local discussion. It is not uncommon for parents to raise a succession of apparently irrational objections to their SSN child's attendance at a play group, and much time may be taken on what appears to be fruitless negotiations with the staff to resolve these. Should this happen one should always be alert to the likelihood that it is the mother who finds the experience distressing probably because she is made uncomfortably aware in such a group of the severity of her child's handicap. This is understandably very painful and her reluctance to admit this to herself or to seem to decry the efforts made on her child's behalf may prompt her to excuse herself and her child from attending for what she feels will be acceptable reasons.

In some areas remedial or developmental programmes are taken into the child's home by peripatetic professionals such as pre-school advisory teachers, psychologists, or community nurses. These may formulate the therapeutic steps to be taken in conjunction with the parents and then visit regularly to check progress. This is another resource which needs to be known by the psychiatrist. Such a service has obvious advantages in that it is implemented in the best setting possible, involves the child's parents and so can be a regular daily experience, and endows the family with practical immediate aims and a real sense of involvement. Various such programmes are described (Portage Guide to Home Teaching; Cunningham & Sloper, 1978; Kiernan *et al.*, 1978). Although it is clear how supportive they are, the psychiatrist should be prepared to find in some cases that parents begin to resist them particularly if they are fairly rigidly prescribed or are conveyed to the family too dogmatically. Some parents, if given a clear understanding of their child's handicap and the way in which it interferes with his functioning, find that they become adept at trying out their own strategies, often elaborated on the spur of the moment from chance acts which they are able to extend to a profitable sequence, such as pulling himself up or loading a spoon. The success of such parents owes much to their spontaneous interaction with their child, which may be offset by a more self-conscious structured attack on the same problem. Tactful discussion within the team may be needed to resolve this, depending on how flexible the therapists involved are, but it is important to respect that the parents 'may well be right' if this method works and a basic component of the family's treatment is to maintain their confidence and enthusiasm. This may flag sadly even with a pre-school child, so the family's capacity to cope must always be sympathetically reviewed.

Even with such a young child, particularly a hyperactive one, the family may well need periods of relief from his care. These tend at this stage to be of maximum benefit if they are regular and predictable, since it is usually the dawning realization of how unremitting is the care and programme imposed on them which demoralizes the family. A break to look forward to would enable them to hang on and better sustain their enthusiasm. It does not need to be long – a weekend or a single night is often sufficient – indeed many parents at this stage will be very hesitant about taking or certainly asking for such relief. If it is to be offered it needs to be emotionally accept-able otherwise the break will be more anxiety-provoking than their continued efforts at home. A visit to the prospective unit is helpful and most parents will want to be reassured not only of its home-like domestic atmosphere but of the commitment of its staff and of their own acceptance as parents with the need to be involved. Voluntary societies and parent groups are developing such short-term care provisions in many parts of the country; a unit thus organized tends to be reassuring to anxious parents. Some NHS units provide short-term care, their acceptability depending to a large extent on the attitude of senior, particularly medical, staff who are likely to arrange admissions. Parents are often reassured by the confidence of nursing staff in such settings who are clearly familiar with the care of the seriously handicapped, though they may be disheartened or even alarmed at what may be their first contact with a large number of such children. Periodic residential care to relieve the family will be an important component of their management in the years ahead so it is imperative that great care is taken to help them cope with their early misgivings at first relinquishing their child temporarily.

A few parents will already have found it impossible to come to terms with caring for their SSN child. At this stage this is not usually the result of disappointment at his lack of progress or a sense of hopelessness at the task ahead. It is more likely to be the final resolution of conflicting feelings generated when their baby's handicap was first realized. With appropriate team support the psychiatrist should have been aware of this development although on some occasions its mention is strenuously avoided because of the shame the parents feel at being unable to cope, a shame ironically often intensified by the supportive efforts and expectations of the team. If the parents are continually sceptical about any improvement, or are increasingly hesitant in their handling, or recurrently forgetful about arrangements with team members then the doctor should suspect that such a conflict is occurring though there may be no overt expression of it from either parent. When this situation is developed the parents' attitude should be accepted and accepted promptly, clearly indicating sympathy for the conflict that they must have experienced. Little is to be gained on the child's behalf by attempting to persuade his parents differently, and they need a great deal of help to come to terms with the decision they have felt compelled to make. Decisions about future care will need to be discussed with them and their social worker: choice of placement will depend on the type and severity of handicap and associated need for medical care, on the provisions available and on the policy pursued by the relevant social service department on fostering or other child care arrangements. In any case it is helpful if some holding arrangement can be made which respects the parents' wishes and enables them, without any pressure being exerted, to take stock together in the absence of their child; this also provides an opportunity to involve them as much as they wish in planning future arrangements.

The school child

When their child is admitted to school the family will enter a new phase of their life. With the regular relief from his care for several hours each day mother finds herself enjoying an unaccustomed independence, able to shop or go out at short notice and to plan her day. Many schools become the main supporting agency for the child and his family, particularly those which encourage close parent liaison and even the participation in the home of school staff, for instance, allocated social workers or home support teachers or aides. How successful educational programmes are depends a great deal on how successfully handling methods, effective in school, can be transferred to the home after discussion, it is to be hoped, with the family. This is particularly true of procedures in self-help and communication, such as feeding and simple table manners, routines of dressing and undressing, for example during swimming or PE sessions, and the use of signs or a small vocabulary. It is well-known that some SSN children do not readily transfer either self-help skills or orderly social response from school to home or vice versa and a tendency to conduct different lives in each is common. This is to some extent due to the practical difficulty of ensuring consistency of management in both, largely because school staff are less emotionally and socially susceptible than parents. Where such obstacles to consistency can be overcome not only is the child able to progress but the parents feel supported and involved within the larger family of the school.

Certain common parental anxieties are to be expected during the period of the child's schooling. The psychiatrist must recognize them and be prepared, on the advice of the school staff, to help to resolve them. Many parents initially are apprehensive that school staff will not appreciate the idiosyncrasies of their child. In this they are, of course, like most other parents on first sending their child to school. In the case of the SSN child, however, this is likely to be not only a realistic concern but one with important therapeutic consequences. SSN children, often greatly dependent on familiar surroundings and routine, can be alarmed at any new situation, and the more effusive the welcome, the more distressed they may become. The motor-handicapped child needs to become accustomed to an array of different handling experiences; the active child to new routines, to new spatial opportunities and constraints. Another cause for anxiety is the discovery that many forms of misbehaviour, troublesome at home, do not appear at school or that the child tries harder or perseveres longer there than at home. Experienced teaching staff usually recognize and placate these anxieties by the sensible explanation that all children play up more at home, but it leads to the parents' first realization of how indulgent they are or to what extent their own child's hyperactivity, screaming bouts, or apparent inability to help himself may be to some extent contrived. This can arouse considerable resentment, sometimes directed not at the child but displaced to teaching staff. Other parents may become quite depressed with a sense of their own inadequacy, which may in turn regenerate the personal conflict which arose in the turbulent period when the family struggled to come to terms with their child's handicap. Occasionally parents invest school attendance with quite unrealistic expectations; they may hope that their child, however disabled, will be involved in 'real' school work and take exception to his training there in self-help skills or simple domestic tasks which they protest he could learn at home even though they know he does not do so. Everyday parental concern about being happy with his class peers or with his teacher is often exaggerated because the family invest so much in his schooling – that it will contribute to his level of content at home and hence his progress and ease their efforts to care or control him there. All these anxieties can usually be best resolved by informal discussion between parents and school staff, but at times the doctor may be able to help clear the air with a more formal, though sympathetic, group meeting. It should always be remembered that increased tension in the family, expressed as heightened concern over the handicapped school child, may be the result of some quite independent stress such as unemployment, marital difficulty, or dissatisfaction with housing, so that a home visit, arranged ostensibly to discuss their child, may be rewarding if it generates sufficient confidence for the parents to reveal their real difficulty. If they do this, it is rarely in response to questioning, however oblique, but often volunteered as one is leaving after a reassuring talk about their child.

With a growing school child the family will increasingly need practical help. Short-term respite care will be needed as will genuine holidays for their child. Few parents really accept the euphemism of their child going, say, into hospital 'for a holiday'; the sheer incongruity of this does not escape them though no other alternative may be available if they themselves are to have a holiday. Their enjoyment is more likely if their child can be provided with some episode at least resembling a holiday. Responsible organizations can be contacted which arrange this (Organizations: Break).

From the point of view of the child himself much of the therapeutic drive involving the doctor and the handicap team would at this phase be transferred to the school staff. The doctor can assist by recognizing or anticipating and helping to remedy parent anxieties as described above, but he can contribute in a number of other ways.

One major task during school years for the SSN child is to persevere with therapeutic programmes that, it is to be hoped, have been established in him as a pre-school child. The operative word here is persevere, because the change in, for instance, postural control or hand use in the cerebral palsied child, mobility in the seriously retarded, or the array of simple communicating signs in the active child is extremely slow. Fortunately staff in ESN(S) schools are well aware of this, but the doctor's interest and support through regular reviews, constructive suggestions or just simple thanks on behalf of the family are well worthwhile. Revising medication may also help: the introduction of an effective tranquillizer such as haloperidol or the benzodiazepines may not have only genuine pharmacological effects but may boost morale in a harassed special care unit staff: Lioresal may reduce spasms in a cerebral palsy child, thus not only improving the effects of physiotherapy but also making handling, changing, and toileting easier for staff and child alike. The review of anticonvulsants in the school child is needed, not only in response to his epilepsy but in the light of his weight change. Occasionally with increasing fits unwise polypharmacy may be embarked on simply because with increasing weight the decreasing effectiveness

of a given dose is not recognized. Other clinical changes related to increasing age may cause apparent deterioration, which is fairly easily remedied. Recurrent upper respiratory tract infections associated with catarrhal otitis, which may well not reveal itself with earache or discharge, can produce a steadily progressive conductive deafness the effects of which may be misconstrued, particularly in the Down's syndrome child, as behaviour disturbance, poor management at home, or just increased retardation. The child with perhaps a bilateral conductive deafness of about 30 to 40 dB can hear if shouted at and with some effort can still recognize vowels and the inflection of sentences spoken to him, though not key words in them. In consequence his limited comprehension diminishes though he can perhaps still understand more or less what is meant, for instance that what he hears is inflected as a command, reprimand, or question, and he may guess its content by situational clues. Thus disabled he easily gets the reputation that he can understand if he wants to, and this, together with a loss of the few words he may have, frustrates both him, parents, and staff, sometimes precipitating episodes of disturbed behaviour. Hearing loss should always be considered in catarrhal SSN children. Similar problems may arise in an epileptic SSN child, for example, with marked reduction in nocturnal major fits which may be associated partly with the effectiveness of the anticonvulsants used but partly with a change of fit pattern with age. This can result in more frequent minor attacks which are not clearly apparent particularly if the child has manneristic or stereotyped behaviour which may mask brief minor psychomotor fits. Inevitably the child's limited attention span will be further disrupted, so he too may present as a behaviour problem and the last clinical feature to arouse suspicion will be his fits, now apparently more effectively controlled. SSN children whose severe motor delay renders them immobile are prone during their school years to develop a spinal kyphosis and flexed posture. Those with cerebral palsy often suffer from worsening adductor spasm of their hips; the stiff flexed posture such children adopt eventually deteriorates into a windswept position. This is best prevented by the active programme described above but, in addition, by prone rather than supine lying. Unfortunately many of these children are left for long periods supine, lying on their backs on floor mats or sprawling in ill-supporting chairs which aggravates these postural defects. Advice and some tactful vigilance about positioning these children as well as encouraging their handling can effectively reduce the likelihood of further disability.

During his pre-school period and the earlier years of his school life, involved staff and parents will be aiming at progress towards a goal, often unspoken, which is as 'normal' a child as possible. In the course of time this goal may well need to be reconsidered. Although everyone's efforts towards improvement must be sustained, a time comes for considering whether pressure on the child or efforts on his behalf to establish more or less normal functioning should be diverted to helping him refine his own preferred ways of performing, however abnormal they may be. A point is sometimes reached when it is not only kinder but wiser to allow the child to be entrenched with the functions he makes use of rather than to continue to press him to modify these to achieve a normal pattern. Such a point will be earlier in some children than in others; it may, for example in the case of the enthusiastic cerebral palsy child, never be reached, or it may be reached at separate stages for different disabilities in the same child. Whenever and however it is tackled, the discussion may be crucial and is often painful to parents and staff alike. The doctor may well find himself as the arbiter, expected to decide what is 'right'. As with any other medical speciality, if he has extensive experience, particularly in following up cases, he should be able to advise sensibly, but with the SSN child it is unwise to be dogmatic. An SSN child's capacity to continue improving his performance tends to be irregular with encouraging steps forwards intermixed with plateaux. An aptly timed, frank discussion may release tensions which ironically can re-establish progress. There are many examples of such decisions facing staff and parents: whether to continue encouraging bimanual play and training in a hemiplegic child without dystereognosis or to promote his ingenuity in using virtually one hand; whether to insist on reasonably accurate signing in helping the communication of a child with hearing and visual defect or to respond more to his own particular gesture and odd vocal output; whether to aim at a sedated but virtually fit-free child or to permit fits in a more alert one and so on. It is quite reasonable that individual therapists, teachers, or doctors are keen to get their particular contribution right, but the child's programme can become a battleground and someone at some time has to take an honest look at priorities, respecting the child's right to his own

solutions. In some cases both parents and staff have been struggling to achieve a particular aim, for instance the use of a hemiparetic limb, in spite of convictions which remain unspoken because they are reluctant for the child or its parents' sake to admit giving up. However, when there is open discussion all may feel relief and the child may benefit far more from the changed attitude. It may fall to the doctor to make clear that all are aiming at a contented as well as an improving child.

The school-leaver: puberty, adolescence and the young adult

During the years of his school life the SSN child will have been cared for, treated, and educated by a group of people who will have seen their role primarily as helping him to progress and fulfil his potential towards as normal a life as possible. As time passed they would have accepted the slow and uneven course of his improvement and his need occasionally to find his own quite abnormal solutions to some disabilities. Up to now there has been an underlying assumption that it is the child's functioning that should be changed by improving his skills and self-control to fit within a normal environment. With adolescents an array of problems arise which may shift the emphasis from fitting the child to his environment to modifying the environment to meet his, by now, fairly entrenched needs. This is likely to be a contested decision, but a great deal of stress can be avoided if it is faced squarely. It is by no means necessarily the right decision for any individual adolescent, nor of course does it imply that further improvement should not be pursued, but the doctor should be prepared at this stage to view the patient's life-style in this new perspective and to equip his parents to do so too. By the time a family has cared for an active or dependent SSN member for sixteen years or more its own perspective will have inevitably changed. Enthusiasm for the total push of his childhood will be changing to a concern for settling him in a contented stable adult life. There is a realization, though often reluctant, that a number of uncomfortable issues are becoming crucial. These include: how much further progress can be expected; are there some ways in which he seems to be deteriorating; for how much longer can the family cope with his care; what arrangements can be made for his future if the family cannot cope particularly now that, as he is about to leave school different professionals will be involved? These issues can be taken in turn.

Ironically, continued progress for the SSN during adolescence is the less likely to be impressive the more effective earlier management has been. Patients, either dependent or very active, who improve in adolescence tend to do so as a result of a change of situation. The apathetic dependent patient who is moved from an indulgent or custodial situation where all is done for him including being lifted may respond well to a more energetic regime with movement experience and supported weight-bearing. The unsettled, obstreperous behaviour of the active SSN adolescent constrained within his own home may quickly subside in a more spacious and less anxious setting. These are quite common findings, but to the family, considering whether further progress will be sufficient to enable them to continue coping, they are no comfort because to them the appropriate remedies are not available. For them a novel, fresh management routine demanding more effort to mobilize their dependent adolescent or a more relaxed daily routine in open surroundings is not feasible. In addition to these situational obstacles the adolescent himself changes: his increase in size and weight add to the burden of his care and resistivity or his assertiveness. If motor-handicapped he needs to make more effort to overcome weight, leverage, and stiffening joints; his reluctance may develop into petulant stubbornness. If active he becomes increasingly able physically to assert himself so that confrontations provoke alarm in his parents, which in turn frighten him and add to his agitation. To what extent these difficulties result from physical changes or from an SSN equivalent of adolescent rebellious feelings is uncertain: pubertal hormonal changes may occur at the normal time, or later, or not at all in the SSN yet these saddening behaviour changes are found independently, for instance in SSN teenage girls without secondary sexual characteristics and not yet menstruating.

In addition to the physical and emotional development which may restrict the adolescent's progress, other changes associated with this age can cause deterioration. His increased weight and skeletal growth may result in spinal kyphosis or in a re-emerging postural asymmetry associated with lateralized brain damage so that a spinal scoliosis, pelvic tilt, and a more pronounced hemiparesis develop. In puberty his fits may increase in frequency or his visual acuity may alter markedly. With the onset of menstruation, hygiene problems will be aggravated and behaviour disturbance or fit frequency may increase pre-menstrually. The lack of social independence and consequent need for supervision and care should protect the SSN from sexual risk but a real social problem with emerging sexuality is masturbation which in some cases can be unremitting. Although distraction with other activities and trying to minimize social reaction may help if this, like some other mannerisms, is provocative or attention-seeking, in many cases particularly the profoundly retarded, social remedies are of little help. Anti-libidinal drugs can be prescribed including benperidol (which may sedate or provoke a dyskinesia, difficult to distinguish from an increase in the agitated over-activity already present), or, in the male, cyproterone both of which can be continued on a maintenance dose after an initial period of high-dose suppression of symptoms.

It is clear that adolescence is often a taxing period for the SSN patient's family. Of course some patients retain their self-help and social skills, diversifying and extending them at this age, but usually in the SSN a combination of increasing physical burden, emotional changes, and a growing tiredness in aging parents compels the family to question how much longer they can continue. The doctor must be sensitive to this potential crisis. He will need to explore the feelings of the whole family, since by this stage adolescent siblings may well be more assertive themselves and, although loyal and affectionate to the patient, more prepared to question the regime which the patient has imposed on the whole family. Their studying or social life may be seriously disrupted and their emerging hostility and embarrassment, however mollified, may confront the parents with a painful reality – that their retarded child becomes steadily less appealing and less tolerable as an adolescent. Family conflicts may escalate, with a brother or sister angrily leaving home or pressing for his removal. Meanwhile a number of tactical difficulties commonly arise in the home: strenuous attempts to correct or anticipate wilful behaviour are increasingly unsuccessful and therefore perhaps enjoyable to the adolescent who begins to take pleasure in confrontation; as increasingly physical restraint becomes alarming parents may argue or reason much more with their SSN adolescent which tends to make him worse; his need for company and above all activity is unlikely to be met, certainly whenever or for as long as he wants, so he becomes bored and more petulant. Some of these problems can be anticipated by school staff familiar with the patient at the school-leavers conference. This should be an opportunity to seek practical outlets and to establish social work contact if a social worker has not already been allocated.

It is when helping the family struggling with an SSN adolescent to decide if and in what way to continue his care and training that the doctor realizes in many cases how deficient community services still are. The alternatives available are few to the family who want to continue caring for their adolescent at home. Efforts can be made to support them by recognizing and as far as possible ameliorating the various problems clinical and social, that have been described earlier. A variety of aids and allowances are available to modify facilities in the home and to ease pressure on the family in caring or transporting their teenager; the local social services department will know of these but so should the doctor supporting the family. Regular attendance at a day centre is imperative if the family are to survive. Some social service departments organize special care groups in adult training or social education centres. Where this happens close liaison is essential with team members or school staff familiar with the adolescent so that workers in the centre can adjust their perspectives to his potential, be prepared for his idiosyncrasies, and respect his likes and dislikes. To achieve a reasonable transition from school to centre, a graded part-time attendance at both can be helpful since much of the apprehension or the agitation of the SSN adolescent relates to his entering the unfamiliar. Again close cooperation and discussion with parents is of great value to meet the same objectives.

In spite of aids, regular day-care programmes, and support from professionals the parents may be unable to continue caring for their teenager and seek residential placement. If local NHS or social service provision has already provided respite care, this decision will be eased if vacancies are available. In some cases the family must make this choice without previous experience. It is always a painful one and care should be taken at all ages to promote the feeling in the family that everyone appreciates to the full their previous efforts and that to continue struggling is unwise and unnecessary. Parents invariably blame themselves for giving up their child of whatever age to someone else's care: these feelings should be sympathetically but openly discussed if and when this seems acceptable to the parents. More than through discussion, their feelings of inadequacy at this stage can be helped by involvement as far as practicable in the new caring situation, so that as with the transfer from school to adult day centre the parents can comfort themselves that their teenager as a person is important in all his idiosyncrasies to the staff who now care for him.

Finding residential placement for the disturbed or very dependent SSN adolescent is particularly difficult. In recent years some voluntary parent societies have established residential training schemes for blind/deaf (Organizations: The Manor House), cerebral palsied (Organizations: Dene Park College), mentally handicapped (Organizations: Social Training Unit), and autistic teenagers (Organizations: Somerset Court) largely in response to their appreciation of the scarcity of facilities. The acceptability to parents of such placements is due partly to their sense of involvement since they are run by parent organizations, and partly to a positive sense of continuing their teenager's education rather than recognizing the, to them, negative fact that he needs someone somewhere to cope with him. This unpalatable fact is in some cases an obvious, inevitable need met in the vast majority by hospitals often struggling themselves with inadequate staff. Some hospital units however have established wards in which the community of patients living there can sympathetically absorb even the severely disturbed. They have in addition important environmental advantages, including plenty of space, distance from traffic hazards, a setting familiar with and therefore tolerant of noise and disruptive behaviour, an array of local social outlets appropriate to the SSN, and a population of patients from which to draw such a supportive resident group. Again close liaison with the patients' parents is essential; parents' groups are valuable and parents should always be invited to assessment meetings at which progress is reviewed and future objectives agreed. The aim of the family is a settled, as far as possible fulfilling, life for their now adult member; this is the topic for the next section.

The SSN adult: providing a settled life

The normal grown-up leaves home; his parents expect it. If it does not occur it presupposes the unhealthy extension of a mutually dependent relationship between parent and child. This can well happen with the SSN adult because his dependence, his limited understanding, and even his tantrums compel his parents to treat him as a child. They may also regard him as one. This is a trap which awaits them both. The SSN adult's everyday needs may command his parents' almost constant attention which exasperates and tires them yet caters for their unconscious need to make reparations to their affected child. Their indulgence comforts him yet makes him more dependent and demanding. This dilemma may be so anxiety-provoking that any discussion however gently introduced is resisted and the family are carried forward day by day through the momentum of a routine as oppressive as it is habitual. Its resolution through exhaustion or death of a spouse can be heartbreaking. To be able to help in the tragic and potentially disastrous situation the doctor needs to convey however gradually or patiently that the SSN member is an adult however limited his abilities and that his needs are an adult's and not the extension of the needs of a child. He may need to visit the family many times to gain their confidence, to recruit the help of other parents of handicapped adults and of a social worker. This is an extreme example and there are of course parents who cheerfully and realistically cope for years with the care of their SSN adult son or daughter. However, they contrast with the more psychiatrically vulnerable parents in their readiness to discuss and make eventual arrangements for the future and their wish to see their son or daughter settled in his own permanent home. They may also wish to ensure that their son or daughter is not abandoned but visited after their death and wish to absolve other siblings from this obligation: arrangements are available to ensure this (Organizations: NSMHC). Another contrast is their regarding daily attendance at a centre not only as an enjoyable interlude but as a further preparation for a life away from home.

Further education of the SSN in adult training or social education centres is presenting social service departments with considerable difficulties. Such centres usually cater for the full spectrum of the retarded which contains a very wide range indeed of competence and manageability. Staff training and expectations understandably are directed towards the more able majority so the staffing demands of the SSN may have been unrecognized. Some centres have developed special care units, others have attempted to integrate the SSN in small numbers into other groups. One important role of the doctor in this context is to support the centre staff in their efforts not only to educate but to contain its SSN members. Various practical points can be mentioned: staff in centres often do not appreciate the limited tolerance of noise or the poor spatial orientation of the SSN so the ready availability of a quiet room simply furnished can be helpful; there is a compassionate but unwise tendency to explain or instruct (whereas the SSN learn more easily by demonstration) and to reason rather than act in a challenging situation; often staff are not aware how helpful self-seclusion can be for the SSN if agitated, or how much they enjoy boisterous activity or simple, repetitive, apparently pointless tasks. They will often need to be reassured that a tantrum is usually simply a temper and not a 'fit' if the patient is epileptic, nor a psychotic episode if he is on tranquillizing drugs. Regular visits to the centre and its staff are essential, and in particular a reassurance that the parent will visit promptly if needed in a crisis. To provide a full daily programme for the SSN members of a busy centre is a taxing task and needs readily available medical support.

A few day centres have residential homes associated with them or there may be other hostels run by the local social services department. Some of these may admit SSN patients, particularly if they are aiming at a comprehensive residential service for their own locality, but as yet vacancies are few. Permanent settled care for the SSN is provided in the majority of cases either by hospital or in residential communities. These latter usually consist of a cluster of living units containing residents of varying ability but customarily needing to have reliable self-help with some simple domestic or horticultural skills. Maintaining the standard of care provided is the responsibility of the registering social service department, but the departments local to the SSN resident's original home have a similar responsibility on behalf of their client through the allocated social worker. Information and advice on such communities can be obtained from various reputable organizations, one of which, recently established, is attempting to formulate a code of practice and specific standards of care of member organizations (Organizations: Association of Residential Communities). For admission for hospital care the doctor will need to approach colleagues in the catchment area hospital servicing the locality in which the family live. The manner in which patients are grouped together in ward units either by disability, level of competence, or locality of their home, varies between hospitals as does provision of day programmes and leisure pursuits. Some hospitals have very active parent groups which organize social activities and transport to and from the hospital. These are a few of the details which parents may wish to know when contemplating permanent hospital care. Some hospitals provide brochures which give a great deal of practical information. The doctor can help parents by acquiring these and arranging visits to the hospital for discussion there with staff likely to be involved with their son or daughter.

Ageing, death and bereavement

Multiple handicaps, epilepsy, and anatomical malformation are common in the SSN so that ageing carries a higher than normal morbidity and mortality risk. Frailty increases the likelihood of early mortality of which most parents are aware, but their child's vulnerability to an array of accidents renders some of them liable to sudden, unpredictable death. Gastro-intestinal anomalies mean that, for example, volvulus seems common at a much younger age than in the normal population; foraging habits may result in intestinal obstruction; ingestion without chewing produces choking; severe epilepsy, present in many conditions, can result in a fatal status epilepticus; there are many examples of potentially lethal clinical conditions which are much more prevalent in the SSN than in the normal population.

When the family has a confident relationship with the team it is helpful to explore tactfully their own understanding of such risks and their attitude should a catastrophe occur. It is of course a subject that needs very sympathetic handling but for many parents it is a buried but constant dread, the more repressed because on occasions they regard such an event as a release from what they feel is an intolerable existence for their disabled child or an intolerable burden on themselves. They may dread even more the child or adult's surviving them leaving him with no one that they feel really cares for him, or to become an unwelcome burden on his siblings. Some parents wish to ensure regular visiting and continued personal interest in their child after their own deaths through trusteeship and insurance schemes; details of these are available. Opening up this topic can be of great value. By warning of such risks, parents can be spared the shock of sudden death, which is particularly traumatic if it follows closely on admission to a hospital or residential centre. This is not unlikely in situations where the parents cannot any longer cope with a patient's frailty or severe epileptic fits. A sudden death shortly after leaving home convinces them that they have, by abandoning his care, killed him. This is an acutely depressing conviction, which is extremely difficult to treat but which can be less-

ened by a sympathetic but realistic discussion at the time of admission. Frank discussion with parents at this level is likely to be a confidence enjoyed by the doctor or a key figure in the parents' eyes, perhaps a social worker, or ward sister, or another parent who may be acting as a supportive team member. When known, the parents feelings should, with their permission, be discussed with staff involved in the patient's care; it gives a humane perspective to the controversial question of how much effort is made to secure the survival of a profoundly disabled patient. All involved would agree to management which minimizes suffering and that the SSN have the same right to specialized medical resources as other patients, but this needs to be balanced against the benefit to the patient of survival perhaps with greatly increased disability. This often uncomfortable decision will be the responsibility of the doctor who will need to respect the feelings of other team members and in particular those of a patient's parents.

Although parental grief at the death of an SSN child may well be an ambiguous combination of sadness, guilt, and relief, it is accepted as a predictable, understandable reaction demanding the doctor's attention. The possibility of a grief reaction in the SSN at the death of their parent however is more likely to be overlooked. Indeed some parents, ageing and less able to visit a hospitalized son or daughter or dreading the prospect of his or her inevitable admission, comfort themselves with the conviction that their absence would not even be noticed. In the profoundly handicapped all evidence may suggest this belief since the patient's behaviour reveals an interest only in the pleasures accompanying a parental visit, for instance a bag of favourite food, a picnic, or a car ride, with an apparent unconcern about who actually comes providing. It is worthwhile remembering that the realistic acceptance that a helpless SSN son or daughter may really miss them can be so painful for parents that they may deny it to themselves and to each other: the converse belief that their child would really be indifferent to their death is equally distressing so that the doctor must keep an open mind about his SSN patient's reaction to the disappearance of their parents. Some patients accept a parent's death quite equably, particularly if the cause is explained to them sympathetically but simply: it seems that being bewildered is more distressing than being bereft. However a sense of loss may occur which may not present as grief but as some behaviour disturbance so that bereavement, however simple, can be disregarded and distress misinterpreted. When evaluating this situation it is worthwhile enquiring how the patient has reacted in the past to, for example, the departure of a long familiar nurse. To help the patient through this period trustee schemes can provide a continued personal support, if possible maintaining the same parental visiting pattern. Often nurses or care staff, if the patient's possible grieving is discussed with them, will themselves divert him on visiting days with treats that they know he enjoys, a gentle appreciative act which should always be duly recognized.

References

CHAPTER 1

Alexander, F., French, T. M. & Pollock, G. H. (1968) *Psychosomatic Specificity*, vol. 1, *Experimental Study and Results.* Chicago: University of Chicago Press

Andrews, G. & Tennant, C. (1978a) Becoming upset and becoming ill: an appraisal of the relationship between life events and physical illness. *Med. J. Aus.*, **1**, 324–7

— (1978b) Life event stress and psychiatric illness. *Psychol. Med.*, **8**, 545–9

Dohrenwend, B. S. & Dohrenwend, B. P. (1978) Some issues in research on stressful life events. *J. nerv. ment. Dis.*, **166**, 7–15

Evans, N. J. R., Baldwin, J. A. & Gath, D. (1974) The incidence of cancer among in-patients with affective disorders. *Brit. J. Psychiat.*, **124**, 518–25

Friedman, M., Rosenman, R. H., Straus, R., Wurm, M. & Kositchek, R. (1968) The relationship of behaviour pattern A to the state of the coronary vasculature. A study of fifty-one autopsy subjects. *Amer. J. Med.*, **44**, 525–37

Granville-Grossman, K. L. (1976) The relationship between physical and psychiatric disorder. In *Integrated Medicine: The Human Approach*, ed. Maxwell, H., chap, 6, pp. 78–88. Bristol: Wright

Greer, S. (1979) Psychological enquiry: a contribution to cancer research. *Psychol. Med.*, **9**, 81–9

Heine, B. (1970) Psychogenesis of hypertension. *Proc. R. Soc. Med.*, **63**, 1267–70

Hinkle, L. E. & Wolff, H. G. (1958) Ecological investigations of the relationship between illness, life experiences and the social environment. *Ann. int. Med.*, **49**, 1373–88

Hinton, J. M. (1963) The physical and mental distress of the dying. *Q. J. Med.*, **32**, 1–21

Holding, T. A. & Barraclough, B. M. (1977) Psychiatric morbidity in a sample of accidents. *Brit. J. Psychiat.*, **130**, 244–52

Holmes, T. H. & Rahe, R. H. (1967) The social readjustment rating scale. *J. psychosom. Res.*, **11**, 213–18

Kerr, T. A., Schapira, K. & Roth, M. (1969) The relationship between premature death and affective disorders. *Brit. J. Psychiat.*, **115**, 1277–82

Lewis, A. J. (1967) Aspects of psychosomatic medicine. In *Inquiries in Psychiatry*, pp. 193–212. London: Routledge & Kegan Paul

Lipowski, Z. J. (1976) Psychosomatic medicine: an overview. In *Modern Trends in Psychosomatic Medicine – 3*, ed Hill, O. W. London: Butterworths

Maguire, G. P. & Granville-Grossman, K. L. (1968) Physical illness in psychiatric patients. *Brit. J. Psychiat.*, **1**, 268–70

Maguire, G. P., Julier, D. L., Hawton, K. E. & Bancroft, J. H. J. (1974) Psychiatric morbidity and referral on two general medical wards. *Brit. med. J.*, **1**, 268–70.

Mann, A. H. (1977) Psychiatric morbidity and hostility in hypertension. *Psychol. Med.*, **7**, 653–9

Nemiah, J. C. & Sifneos, P. E. (1970) Affect and fantasy in patients with psychosomatic disorders In *Modern Trends in Psychosomatic Medicine – 2*, ed. Hill, O. W., London: Butterworths

Parkes, C. M. (1964) Recent bereavement as a cause of mental illness. *Brit. J. Psychiat.*, **110**, 198–204

Parkes, C. M., Benjamin, B. & Fitzgerald, R. G. (1969) Broken heart: a statistical study of increased mortality among widowers. *Brit. med. J.*, **1**, 740–3

Popper, K. R. & Eccles, J. C. (1977) *The Self and its Brain*. Berlin: Springer

Rosenman, R. H. & Friedman, M. (1971) The possible role of behaviour patterns in proneness and immunity to coronary heart disease. In *Coronary Heart Disease*, ed. Russek, H. I., & Zohman, B. L., pp. 77–84. Philadelphia: Lippincott

Ryle, G. (1949) *The Concept of Mind*. London: Hutchinson

Sifneos, P. E., Apfel-Savitz, R. & Frankel, F. H. (1977) The phenomenon of 'alexithymia'. *Psychother. Psychosom.*, **28**, 45–57

Sims, A. & Prior, P. (1978) The pattern of mortality in severe neuroses. *Brit. J. Psychiat.*, **133**, 299–305

Skinner, B. F. (1953) *Science and Human Behaviour*. New York: Macmillan

Whitlock, F. A. (1978) Suicide, cancer and depression. *Brit. J. Psychiat.*, **132**, 269–74

Wittkower, E. D. (1977) Historical perspective of contemporary psychosomatic medicine. In *Psychosomatic Medicine. Current Trends and Clinical Applications*, ed. Lipowski, Z. J., Lipsitt, D. R. & Whybrow, P. C., pp. 3–13. New York: Oxford University Press

World Health Organization (1964) Psychosomatic disorders: thirteenth report of the WHO expert committee on mental health. *WHO Technical Report Series*, No. 275. Geneva: WHO

CHAPTER 2

Ackerman, S. & Weiner, H. (1976) Peptic ulcer disease: Some considerations for psychosomatic research. In *Modern Trends in Psychosomatic Medicine – 3*, ed. Hill, O. W. London: Butterworth

Adsett, C. A. & Bruhn, J. C. (1968) Short term group psychotherapy for post-myocardial infarction patients and their wives. *Can. Med. Ass. J.*, **99**, 577–84.

Alexander, F. (1902) *Psychosomatic Medicine*. London: Allen & Unwin

Alexander H. de M. (1950) A few observations on the blood pressure in mental disease. *Lancet*, **ii**, 18–20

Alfrey, A. C. Le Gendre, G. R. & Kaehny, W. D. (1976) The dialysis encephalopathy syndrome. *New Eng. J. Med.*, **294**, 184–8

Altschule, M. D. (1953) *Bodily physiology in mental and emotional disorders*. New York: Grune & Stratton

Altshuler, K. Z. (1971) Studies of the deaf: relevance to psychiatric theory. *Amer. J. Psychiat.*, **127**, 1521–6

American Journal of Public Health (1969) Editorial, **59**, 1568

Ax, A. F. (1953) The physiological differentation between fear and anger in humans. *Psychosom. Med.*, **15**, 433–42

Bastiaans, J. & Groen, J. J. (1955) Psychogenics and psychotherapy of bronchial asthma. In *Modern Trends in Psychosomatic Medicine – 1*, ed. O'Neill, D. London: Butterworth

Benson, H., Shapiro, D., Tursky, B. & Schwartz, G. E. (1971) Decreased systolic blood pressure through operant conditioning techniques in patients with essential hypertension. *Science*, **173**, 740–1

Bickford, R. G. & Butt, H. R. (1955) Hepatic coma: the electroencephalographic pattern. *J. clin. Invest.*, **34**, 790–9

Bilodean, C. B. & Hackett, T. P. (1971) Issues raised in a group setting by patients recovering from myocardial infarction. *Amer. J. Psychiat.*, **128**, 73–8

Blachy, P. H. & Starr, A. (1964) Post cardiotomy delirium. *Amer. J. Psychiat.*, **121**, 371–5

Bloomer, H. A., Barton, L. J. & Maddock, R. K. (1967) Penicillin-induced encephalopathy in uraemia patients. *J. Amer. Med. Ass.*, **200**, 121–3

Bonfils, S., Mazet, P., de M'Uzan, M., Hachette, J. C. & Lewins, M. (1971) Étude corrélative de la sécrétion gastrique et des caractéristiques psychologiques des ulcéreux duodénaux. *Pathol. Biol. (Paris)*, **19**, 967–75

Boyle, E. J. (1970) Biological patterns in hypertension by race, sex, body weight and skin color. *J. Amer. Med. Ass.*, **213**, 1637–43

Brandt, D. J., Rosenman, R. H., Sholtz, R. I. & Friedman, M. (1976) Multivariant prediction of coronary heart disease in the Western Collaborative Group Study compared to the findings of the Frammingham Study. *Circulation*, **53**, 348–55

British medical journal (1969) Leading article, **i** 1–2

Brozek, J. (1966) Personality differences between potential coronary and non-coronary subjects. *Ann. N.Y. Acad. Sci.*, **134**, 1057–64

Bull, H. C. & Venables, P. H. (1974) Special perception in schizophrenia. *Brit. J. Psychiat.*, **125**, 350–4

Bulpitt, C. J., Hoffbrand, B. I. & Dollery, C. T. (1976) Psychological features of patients with hypertension attending hospital follow-up clinics. *J. psychosom. Res.*, **20**, 403–11

Carney, M. W. P. (1972) Hepatic porphyria with mental symptoms. *Lancet*, **ii**, 100–1

Cay, E. Philip, A. & Aitken, C. (1976) Psychological aspects of cardiac rehabilitation. In *Modern Trends in Psychosomatic Medicine – 3*, ed. Hill, O. W. London: Butterworths

Cay, E. L., Vetter, N., Philip, A. E. & Dugard, P. (1972a) Psychological status during recovery from an acute heart attack. *J. psychosom. Res.*, **16**, 425–35

— (1972b) Psychological reaction to a coronary care unit. *J. psychosom. Res.*, **16**, 437–47

— (1973) Return to work after a heart attack. *J. psychosom. Res.*, **17**, 231–42

Chazan, J. A. & Winkelstein, W., Jr. (1964) Household aggregation of hypertension. *J. chron. Dis.*, **17**, 9–19

Cochrane, R. (1973) Hostility and neuroticism among unselected essential hypertensives. *J. psychosom. Res.*, **17**, 215–18

Cooper, A. F. (1976) Deafness and psychiatric illness. *Brit. J. Psychiat.*, **129**, 216–26

Cooper, A. F. & Porter, R. (1976). Visual acuity and ocular pathology in the paranoid and affective psychoses of later life. *J. psychosom. Res.*, **20**, 107–14

Cramond, W. A. (1970) The psychological problems of renal dialysis and transplantation. In *Modern Trends in Psychosomatic Medicine – 2*, ed. Hill, O. W. London: Butterworths

Croog, S. H., Shapiro, D. & Levine, S. (1971) Denial among male heart patients: an empirical study. *Psychosom. Med.*, **33**, 385–97

Culpan, R. & Davies, B. (1959) Emotional stress and myocardial infarction. *N. Z. Med. J.*, **58**, 191–4

Davies, M. H. (1970) Blood pressure and personality. *J. psychosom. Res.*, **14**, 89–104

Dawber, T. R. & Kannel, W. B. (1962) Atherosclerosis and you: pathogenic implications from epidemiologic observations. *J. Amer. Geriat. Soc.*, **10**, 805–21

Denmark, J. C. (1966) Mental illness and early profound deafness. *Brit. J. med. Psychol.*, **39**, 117–24

Dominian, J. & Dobson, M. (1969) Study of patients' psychological attitudes to a coronary care unit. *Brit. med. J.*, **4**, 795–8

Doyle, A. E. & Fraser, J. R. E. (1961) Essential hypertension and the inheritance of vascular reactivity. *Lancet*, ii, 509–11

Dreyfuss, F., Shanan, J. & Sharon, M. (1966) Some personality characteristics of middle-aged men with coronary artery disease. *Psychother. Psychosoma.*, **14**, 1–16

Druss, R. G. & Kornfeld, D. S. (1967) The survivors of cardiac arrest. *J. Amer. Med. Ass.*, **201**, 291–6

Druss, R. G., O'Connor, J. F., Prudden, J. & Stern. L. O. (1968) Psychologic response to colectomy. *Arch. gen. Psychiat.*, **18**, 53–59

Druss, R. G., O'Connor, J. F. & Stern, L. O. (1969) Psychologic response to colectomy, 11. Adjustment to a permanent colostomy. *Arch. gen. Psychiat.*, **20**, 419–27

Dunbar, H. F. (1954) *Emotions and Bodily Change.* New York: Columbia University Press

— (1943) *Psychosomatic Medicine.* New York: Hoeber

Egerton, N. & Kay, J. H. (1964) Psychological disturbances associated with open heart surgery. *Brit. J. Psychiat.*, **110**, 433–9

Engel, G. L. (1971) Sudden and rapid death during psychological stress. *Ann. int. Med.*, **74**, 771–82

— (1974) Psychological aspects of gastrointestinal disorders. In *American Handbook of Psychiatry*, ed. Arieti, S. & Reiser, M. F. 2nd ed., vol. 4, pp. 653–92. New York: Basic Books

Engel, G. L., Reichsman, F. & Segal, H. (1956) A study of an infant with a gastric fistula. 1. Behaviour and the rate of total hydrochloric acid secretion. *Psychosom. Med.*, **18**, 374–98

Epstein, F. H. (1971) Epidemiologic aspects of atherosclerosis. *Atherosclerosis*, **14**, 1–11

Feldman, G. M. (1976) The effect of biofeedback training on respiratory resistance of asthmatic children. *Psychosom. Med.*, **38**, 27–34

Fessel, J. M. & Conn, H. O. (1973) Lactulose in the treatment of acute hepatic encephalopathy. *Amer. J. Med. Sci.*, **266**, 103–10

Fischer, J. E. & Baldessarini, R. J. (1971) False neurotransmitters and hepatic failure. *Lancet*, ii, 75–80

Fisher, S. H. (1963) Psychological factors and heart disease. *Circulation*, **27**, 113–17

French, Th. N. & Alexander, F. (1941) Psychogenic factors in bronchial asthma. *Psychosom. Med.*, monograph 4

Friedman, M., Byers, S. O., Rosenman, R. H. & Newman, R. (1971) Coronary prone individuals (type A behavioural pattern): growth hormone responses. *J. Amer. med. Ass.*, **217**, 929–32

Friedman, M. & Rosenman, R. H. (1959) Association of specific overt behaviour patterns with blood and cardiovascular findings. *J. Amer. Med. Ass.*, **169**, 1286–96

— (1971) Type A behaviour pattern: its association with coronary heart disease. *Ann. clin. Res.*, **3**, 300–12

Goldberg, D. (1970) A psychiatric study of patients with disorders of the small intestine. *Gut*, **11**, 459–65

Groen, J. J. (1976) Psychosomatic aspects of ischaemic (coronary) heart disease. In *Modern Trends in Psychosomatic Medicine – 3*, ed. Hill, O. W. London: Butterworth

— (1976) Present status of the psychosomatic approach to bronchial asthma. In *Modern Trends in Psychosomatic Medicine –3*, ed. Hill, O. W. London: Butterworths

Groen, J. J. & Pelser, H (1960) Experiences and results of group psychotherapy in patients with bronchial asthma. *J. psychosom. Res.*, **4**, 191–205

Groen, J. J., Van Der Vack, J. M. & Weiner, A. (1971) Psychological factors in the pathogenesis of essential hypertension. *Psychother. Psychosom.*, **19**, 1–26

Gundry, R. K., Donaldson, R. M., Punderhughes, C. A. & Barrabee, W. A. (1967) Patterns of gastric acid secretion in patients with duodenal ulcer: correlations with clinical and personality factors. *Gastroenterology*, **52**, 176–84

Hackett, T. P. & Cassem, N. H. (1969) Factors contributing to delay in responding to signs and symptoms of acute myocardial infarction. *Amer. J. Cardiol.* **24**, 651–8

Hall, R. C. W., Popkin, M. K., Devaul, R. A., Faillace, L. A. & Stickney, S. K. (1978) Physical illness presenting as psychiatric disease. *Arch. gen. Psychiat.*, **35**, 1315–21

Harburg, E., Schull, W. J. & Erfurt, J. C. (1970) A family set method of estimating heredity and stress. 1 A pilot study of blood pressure among negroes in high and low stress areas: Detroit 1966–1967. *J. chron. Dis.*, **23**, 69–81

Harris, R. E. & Forsyth, R. P. (1973) Personality and emotional stress in essential hypertension in man. In *Hypertension; Mechanisms and Management*, ed. Onesti, G. *et al.* New York: Grune & Stratton

Hay, D. R. & Turbott, S. (1970a) Rehabilitation after myocardial infarction and acute coronary insufficiencies. *N. Z. Med. J.*, **71**, 267

— (1970b) Changes in smoking habits in men under 65 years after myocardial infarction and coronary insufficiency. *Brit. Heart J.*, **32**, 738–40

Heine, B. E., Sainsbury, P. & Chynoweth, R. C. (1969) Hypertension and emotional disturbance. *J. psychiat. Res.*, **7**, 119–30

Hellerstein, H. K. & Friedman, E. H. (1970) Sexual activity and the post-coronary patient. *Arch. int. med.*, **125**, 987–99

Henry, J. P. & Cassel, J. C. (1969) Psychological factors in essential hypertension. Recent epidemiologic and animal experimental evidence. *Amer. J. Epidemiol.*, **90**, 171–200

Herbert, M. E. & Jacobson, S. (1967) Late paraphrenia. *Brit. J. Psychiat.*, **113**, 461–9

Herd, J. A., Morse, W. H., Kelleher, R. T. & Jones, L. G. (1969) Arterial hypertension in the squirrel monkey during behavioral experiments. *Amer. J. Physiol.*, **217**, 24–9

Herrmann, H. J. M., Rassek, M., Schäfer, N., Schmidt, Th. & von Uexküll, Th. (1976) Essential hypertension: problems, concepts and an attempted synthesis. In *Modern Trends in Psychosomatic Medicine – 3*, ed. Hill, O. W. London: Butterworth

Heyman, A., Patterson, J. L. & Jones, R. W. (1951) Cerebral circulation and metabolism in uraemia. *Circulation*, 3, 558–63

Innes, G., Miller, W. M. & Valentine, M. (1959) Emotions and blood pressure. *J. ment. Sci.*, 105, 804–51

Jenkins, C. D. (1971) Psychological and social precursors of coronary disease. *New Eng. J. Med.*, 284, 244–55, 307–17

Jenkins, C. D., Rosenman, R. H. and Zyganski, S. J. (1974) Predictors of clinical coronary heart disease by a test for the coronary prone behaviour pattern. *New Eng. J. Med.*, 290, 1271–5

Jenkins, C. D., Zyzanski, S. J., Rosenman, R. H. & Friedman, M. (1969) Recent developments in defining and measuring behavioural risk factors in coronary heart disease. *Psychosom. Med.*, 31, 446

Johnson, H. D. (1965) Gastric ulcer: classification, blood group characteristics, secretion patterns and pathogenesis. *Ann. Surg.*, 162, 996–1004

Jörgensen, G. (1969) Genetik des hohen Blutdrucks. In *Arterielle Hypertonie*, ed. Heintze, R. & Losse, H. Stuttgart: Thieme

Jost, H., Ruilmann, C. J. & Hill, T. S. (1952) Studies in hypertension. II: Central and autonomic nervous system reactions of hypertensive individuals to simple physical and psychological stress situations. *J. nerv. ment. Dis.*, 115, 152–62

Kasl, S. V. & Cobb, S. (1970) Blood pressure changes in men undergoing job loss: a preliminary report. *Psychosom. Med.*, 32, 19–38

Kay, D. W. K., Cooper, A. F., Garside, R. F. & Roth, M. (1976) The differentiation of paranoid and affective psychoses by patients' premorbid characteristics. *Brit. J. Psychiat.*, 129, 207–15

Kay, D. W. K. & Roth, M. (1961) Environmental and hereditary factors in the schizophrenias of old age ('late paraphrenia') and their bearings on the problems of causation in schizophrenia. *J. ment. Sci.*, 107, 649–86

Kessel, N. & Munro, A. (1964) Epidemiological studies in psychosomatic research. *J. psychosom. Res.*, 8, 67–81

Keys, A. (1957) Diet and the epidemiology of coronary heart disease. *J. Amer. Med. Ass.*, 164, 1912

Kimball, C. P. (1969) Psychological responses to the experience of open heart surgery. *Amer. J. Psychiat.*, 125, 348–59

— (1972) The experience of open heart surgery. III: towards a definition and understanding of post-cardotomy delirium. *Arch. gen. Psychiat.*, 27, 57–63

Kirk, R. V. (1968) Perceptual defect and role handicap: missing links in explaining the aetiology of schizophrenia. *Brit. J. Psychiat.*, 114, 1509–21

Klein, R. F., Dean, A., Wilson, M. & Bogdonoff, M. D. (1965) The physician and post-myocardial infarction invalidism. *J. Amer. Med. Ass.*, 194, 143–8

Klein, R. F., Kliner, V. A., Zipes, D. P., Troyer, W. G. & Wallace, A. G. (1968) Transfer from a coronary care unit. *Arch. int. Med.*, 122, 104–8

Kornfeld, D. S., Zimbers, S. & Malm, J. (1965) Psychiatric complications of open heart surgery. *New Eng. J. Med.*, 273, 287–292

Laidlaw, J. & Read, A. E. (1961) The electroencephalographic diagnosis of manifest and latent 'delirium' with particular reference to that complicating hepatic cirrhosis. *J. Neurol. Neurosurg. Psychiat.*, 24, 58–70

— (1963) The EEG in hepatic encephalopathy. *Clin Sci.*, 24, 109–20

Laidlaw, J., Read, A. E. & Sherlock, S. (1961) Morphine tolerance in hepatic disorder. *Gastroenterology*, 40, 389–96

Lamont, J. (1958) Psychosomatic study of asthma. *Amer. J. Psychiat.*, 114, 890

Layne, O. L. Jnr. & Yodofsky, S. C. (1971) Postoperative psychosis in cardiotomy patients. *New Eng. J. Med.*, 284, 518–20

Leigh, D. (1968) Recent advances in psychosomatic medicine. *Med. J. Austral.*, 1, 327–32

Leigh, H., Hofer, A., Cooper, J. & Reiser, M. F. (1972) A psychological comparison of patients in 'open' and 'closed' coronary care units. *J. psychosom. Res.*, 16, 449–55

Levi, L. (1961) Sympatho-adreno-medullary responses to emotional stimuli: methodologic, physiologic and pathologic considerations. In *An Introduction to Clinical Neuroendocrinology*, ed. Bajuaz, E. New York: Karger

Lewinsohn, P. M. (1956) Personality correlates of duodenal ulcer and other psychosomatic disorders. *J. clin. Psychol.*, 12, 296–298

Liebman, R., Minuchin, S. & Baker, L. (1974) The use of structural family therapy in the treatment of intractable asthma. *Amer. J. Psychiat.*, 131, 535–40

Lindemann, E. (1945) Psychiatric problems in conservative treatment of ulcerative colitis. *Arch. Neurol Psychiat.*, 53, 322–4

Lopez, R. I. & Collins, G. H. (1968) Wernicke's encephalopathy, a complication of chronic haemodialysis. *Arch. Neurol. (Chic.)*, 18, 248–259

Lowe, G. R. (1973) The phenomenology of hallucinations as an aid to differential diagnosis. *Brit. J. Psychiat.*, 123, 621–35

Lunzer, M. R., James, I. M., Weinman, J. & Sherlock, S. (1974) Treatment of chronic hepatic encephalopathy with levodopa. *Gut.*, 15, 555–61

MacDermott, J. R., Smith, A. I., Ward, M. K., Parkinson, I. S. & Kerr, D. N. S. (1978) Brain-aluminum concentration in dialysis encephalopathy. *Lancet*, i, 901–3

Mahapatra, S. B. (1974) Deafness and mental health: psychiatric and psychosomatic illness in the deaf. *Acta psychiat scand.*, 50, 596–611

Mahurkar, S. D., Dhar, S. K., Salta, R., Meyers, L., Smith, E. C. & Dunea, G. (1973) Dialysis dementia. *Lancet*, i, 1412–15

Mathé, A. A. & Knapp, P. H. (1971) Emotional and adrenal reactions to stress in bronchial asthma. *Psychosom. Med.*, 33, 323–40

Mawdsley, C. (1972) Neurological complications of haemodialysis. *Proc. R. Soc. Med.*, 65, 871–3

Mayou, R. (1973a) The patient with angina: symptoms and disability. *Postgrad. med. J.*, 49, 250–4

— (1973b) Chest pain, angina pectoris and disability. *J. psychosom. Res.*, 17, 287–91

Miller, W. P. & Rosenfeld, R. (1975) A psychological study of denial following acute myocardial infarction. *J. psychosom. Res.*, 19, 43–55

Minc, S. (1960) The civilised pattern of human activity and coronary heart disease. *Med. J. Austral.*, 2, 87

— (1965) Psychological factors in coronary heart disease. *Geriatrics*, 20, 747–55

Moldofsky, H. (1970) The significance of emotions in the course of rheumatoid arthritis. In *Modern Trends in Psychosomatic Medicine – 2.*, ed. Hill, O. W., pp. 217–225, London: Butterworths

Moore, N. J., (1965) Behaviour therapy of bronchial asthma: a controlled study. *J. psychosom. Res.*, 9, 257–76

Moos, R. H. & Solomon, G. F. (1964) Minnesota Multiphasic Personality Inventory response pattern in patients with rheumatoid arthritis. *J. psychosom. Res.*, **8**, 17–28

Morgan, D. H. (1971) Neuropsychiatric problems of cardiac surgery. *J. psychosom. Res.*, **15**, 41–7

Morgan, M. H. & Read, A. E. (1972) Antidepressants and liver disease. *Gut*, **13**, 697–701

Mutchnick, M. G., Lerner, E. & Conn, H. O. (1974) Portal-systemic encephalopathy and post aural anastomosis: A prospective, controlled investigation. *Gastroenterology*, **66**, 1005–19

Nagle, R., Gangola, R. & Picton-Robinson, I. (1971) Factors influencing return to work after myocardial infarction. *Lancet*, **ii**, 454–6

O'Connor, J. F. (1970) A comprehensive approach to the treatment of ulcerative colitis. In *Modern Trends in Psychosomatic Medicine – 2*, ed. Hill. O. W., pp. 172–188, London: Butterworths

O'Connor, J. F., Daniels, G., Flood, C. Karnsch, A., Moses, L. & Stern, L. O. (1964) An evaluation of the effectiveness of psychotherapy in the treatment of ulcerative colitis. *Ann. Int. Med.*, **60**, 587–602

Olin, H. G. & Hackett, T. P. (1964) The denial of chest pain in 32 patients with acute myocardial infarction. *J. Amer. med. Ass.*, **190**, 977–81

Ostfield, A. M. & Lebovitz, B. Z. (1960) Blood pressure liability: a correlative study. *J. chron. Dis.*, **12**, 428–39

Paffenbarger, R. S. Jnr., Notkin, J. & Krueger, D. E. (1966) Chronic disease in former college students. II: Methods of study and observations on mortality from coronary heart disease. *Amer. J. publ. Health.*, **56**, 962–71

Paffenbarger, R. S. Jnr., Wolf, P. A., Notkin, J. & Thorne, M. C. (1966) Chronic disease in former college students. I.: Early precursors of fatal coronary heart disease. *Amer. J. Epidem.*, **83**, 314–28

Parkes, J. D., Sharpstone, P. & Williams, R. (1970) Levodopa in hepatic coma. *Lancet*, ii, 1341–3

Pearson, H. E. S. & Joseph, J. (1963). Stress in occlusive coronary heart disease. *Lancet*, **i**, 415–18

Phear, E. A., Sherlock, G. & Summerskill, W. H. J. (1955) Blood ammonia levels in liver disease and hepatic coma. *Lancet*, **i**, 836–40

Pickering, G. W. (1955) *High blood pressure.* London: Churchill

Pierce, J. C., Madge, G. E., Lee, H. M. & Hume, D. M. (1972) Lymphoma, a complication of renal allotransplantation in man. *J. Amer. med. Ass.*, **219**, 1593–7

Platts, M. M. & Hislop, J. S. (1976) Aluminium and dialysis encephalopathy. *Lancet*, **11**, 98

Quinlan, D. M., Kimball, C. P. & Osborne, F. (1974) The experience of open heart surgery. IV: Assessment of disorientation and dysphoria following cardiac surgery. *Arch. gen. Psychiat.*, **31**, 241–4

Rahe, R. H. & Lind, E. (1971) Psychosocial factors and sudden cardiac death: A pilot study. *J. psychosom. Res.*, **15**, 19–24

Rahe, R. H. & Paasikivi, J. (1971) Psychosocial factors and myocardial infarction. II An outpatient study in Sweden. *J. psychosom. Res.*, **15**, 33–41

Rahe, R. H. & Theorell, T. (1971) Psychosocial factors and myocardial infarction. I: An inpatient study in Sweden. *J. psychosom. Res.*, **15**, 25–31

Read, A. E., Laidlaw, J. & McCarthy, D. F. (1969) Effects of chlorpromazine in patients with hepatic disease. *Brit. med. J.*, **3**, 497–9

Read, A. E., Sherlock, S., Laidlaw, J. & Walker, J. G. (1967) The neuropsychiatric syndromes associated with chronic liver disease and an extensive portal systemic collateral. *Q. J. Med.*, **36**, 135–50

Reiser, M. F., Rosenbaum, M. & Ferris, E. B. (1951) Psychologic mechanisms in malignant hypertension. *Psychosom. Med.*, **13**, 147–9

Reiser, M. F., Weiner, H. & Thaler, M. (1957) Patterns of object relationships and cardiovascular responsiveness in healthy young adults and patients with peptic ulcer and hypertension. *Psychosom. Med.*, **19**, 498

Richet, G. Lopez de Novales, E. & Verroust, P. (1970) Drug intoxication and neurological episodes in chronic failure. *Brit. Med. J.*, **1**, 394–5

Rimon, R. (1969) A psychosomatic approach to rheumatoid arthritis: a clinical study of 100 female patients. *Acta rheum. scand.* Supp. **13**

Robinson, J. O. (1964) A possible effect of selection on the test scores of a group of hypertensives. *J. psychosom. Res.*, **8**, 239–43

— (1969) Symptoms and the discovery of high blood pressure. *J. psychosom. Res.*, **13**, 157–61

Sainsbury, P. (1964) Neuroticism and hypertension in an outpatient population. *J. psychosom. Res.*, **8**, 235–8

Sandberg, B. & Bliding, A. (1976) Duodenal ulcer in army trainees during basic military training. *J. psychosom. Res.*, **20**, 61–74

Schachter, J. (1957) Pain, fear and anger in hypertensives and normotensives: A psychophysiological study. *Psychosom. Med.*, **19**, 17–29

Schiavi, R. C., Stein, M. & Sethi, B. B. (1961) Respiratory variables in response to a pain-fear stimulus and in experimental asthma. *Psychosom. Med.*, **23**, 485

Schucker, B. & Jacobs, D. R. (1977) Assessment of behavioural risk for coronary disease by voice characteristics. *Psychosom. Med.*, **39**, 219–28

Shapiro, A. P., Rosenbaum, M. & Ferris, E. B. (1951) Relationship therapy in essential hypertension. *Psychosom. Med.*, **13**, 140–6

Shekelle, R. B., Ostfeld, A. M. & Paul, O. (1969) Social status and incidence of coronary heart disease. *J. chron. Dis.*, **22**, 381–94

Sherlock, S. (1977) Hepatic encephalopathy. *Brit. J. hosp. Med.*, **17**, 144–59

Skelton, M. & Dominian, J. (1973) Psychological stress in wives of patients with myocardial infarction. *Brit. med. J.*, **2**, 101–3

Solomon, G. F. (1970) Psychophysiological aspects of rheumatoid arthritis and autoimmune disease. In *Modern Trends in Psychosomatic Medicine – 2*, ed. Hill, O. W. pp. 189–217 London: Butterworths

Steigman, F. S. & Clowdus, B. F. (1971) *Hepatic encephalopathy.* Springfield, Illinois: Thomas

Stenbäck, A. & Haapanen, L. (1967) Azotaemia and psychosis. *Acta psychiat. scand.* Supp. 197, 1–65

Summerskill, W. H. J., Davidson, E. A., Sherlock, S. & Steiner, R. E. (1956) The neuropsychiatric syndrome associated with hepatic cirrhosis and an extensive portal circulation. *Q. J. Med.*, **25**, 245–66

Tal, A. & Miklich, D. R. (1976) Emotionally induced diseases in pulmonary flow rates in asthmatic children. *Psychom. Med.*, **38**, 190–200

Thomas, C. B. (1951) Observations on some possible precursors of essential hypertension and coronary artery disease. *Bull. Johns Hopkins Hosp.*, **89**, 419–41

— (1968) On cigarette smoking, coronary heart disease and the genetic hypothesis. *Johns Hopkins med. J.*, **122**, 69–76

Thomas, C. B. & Greenstreet, R. L. (1973) Psychological characteristics in youth as predictors of five disease states: suicide, mental illness, hypertension, coronary heart disease and tumour. *Johns Hopkins med. J.*, **132**, 14–43

Tufo, H. M., Ostfeld, A. M. & Shekelle, R. (1970) Central nervous system dysfunction following open heart surgery. *J. Amer. Heart Ass.*, **211**, 1330–40

Tyler, H. R. (1976) Neurological disorders seen in renal failure. In *Handbook of Clinical Neurology.* ed. Vinken, P. J. & Bruyn, G. W., vol. 27, pp. 321–48. Amsterdam: North Holland

Valori, C., Thomas, M. & Shillingforth, J. (1967) Free noradrenaline and adrenaline excretions in relation to clinical syndromes following myocardial infarction. *Amer. J. Cardiol.*, **20**, 605–17

Verghese, A. (1967) Personality traits and coronary heart disease. *Austral., N. Z. J. Psych.*, **1**, 62

von Uexkull, Th., & Wick, E. (1962) Die Situationshypertonie. *Arch. Kreislaufforsch*, **39**, 236

Wallace, A. G. (1968) Catecholamine metabolism in patients with acute myocardial infarction. In *Acute Myocardial Infarction*, ed. Julian, D. G. & Oliver, M. F. Edinburgh: Livingstone

Weiner, H., Thaler, M., Reiser, M. F. & Mirsky, I. A. (1957) Aetiology of duodenal ulcer. I: Relators of specific psychological characteristics to rate of gastric secretion (serum pepsinogen). *Psychosom. Med.*, **19**, 1–10

WHO See World Health Organization

Whybrow, P. C. & Ferrell, R. B. (1973) Psychic factors in Crohn's disease. An overview. In *Emotional Factors in Gastrointestinal Disease*, ed. Lindner, A. E. New York: Elsevier, Excerpta Medica Amsterdam

Wishnie, M. A., Hackett, T. P. & Cassem, N. H. (1971) Psychological hazards of convalescence following myocardial infarction. *J. Amer. med. Ass.*, **215**, 1292–6

Wolf, S. (1953) Physiology of the mucous membranes and direct observations on gastric and colonic functions in man. In *Diseases of the Digestive System*, ed. Porkis, S. 3rd ed., pp. 183–208. Philadelphia: Lea & Feliger

Wolf, S., Pfeiffer, J. B. & Fipley, H. S. (1948) Hypertension as a reaction pattern to stress: summary of experimental data in variations in blood pressure and renal blood flow. *Ann. int. Med.*, **29**, 1056–76

Wolf, S. & Wolff, H. G. (1947) *Human Gastric Function*. London: Oxford University Press

— (1951) A summary of experimental evidence relating life stress to the pathogenesis of essential hypertension in man. In *Hypertension*, ed. Bell, E. T. Minneapolis: University of Minnesota Press

Wolff, H. G. (1953) *Stress and Disease*. Springfield, Illinois: Thomas

— (1955) Nocturnal gastric secretions of ulcer and non-ulcer patients under stress. *Psychosom. Med.*, **17**, 218–66

World Health Organization (1959) *Hypertension and coronary heart disease: Classification and criteria for epidemiological studies.* Tech. Rep. Ser. 168. Geneva: WHO

Wynn, A. (1967) Unwarranted emotional distress in men with ischaemic heart disease (IHD). *Med. J. Austral.*, **2**, 847–51

Wynn, D. (1969) Rehabilitation of men with ischaemic heart disease. *Israel J. med. Sci.*, **5**, 791

Zohman, L. R. & Tobis, J. (1970) *Cardiac rehabilitation*. New York: Grune & Stratton

CHAPTER 3

Asher, R. (1949) Myxoedematous madness. *Brit. med. J.*, **2**, 555–62

Ball, J. R. B. & Grounds, A. D. (1974) Head injury, hypopituitarism and paranoid psychosis. *Med. J. Austral.*, **2**, 403–5

Besser, M. (1978) The adrenal cortex. *Medicine (monthly add-on journal, 3rd series)*, **9**, 418–28

Bewsher, P. D., Gardiner, A. Q., Headley, A. J. & Maclean, H. C. S. (1971) Psychosis after acute alteration of thyroid status. *Psychol. Med.*, **1**, 260–2

Blau, J. N. & Hinton, J. M. (1960) Hypopituitary coma and psychosis. *Lancet*, i, 408–9

Bleuler, M. (1951) The psychopathology of acromegaly. *J. nerv. ment. Dis.*, **113**, 497–511

— (1954) *Endokrinologische Psychiatrie*. Stuttgart: Thieme

Brown, G. W., Sklair, F., Harris, T. O. & Birley, J. (1973) Life events and psychiatric disorders. Part I: some methodological issues. *Psychol. Med.*, **3**, 74–87

Carroll, B. J. (1969) Hypothalamic-pituitary function in depressive illness: insensitivity to hypoglycaemia. *Brit. med. J.*, **3**, 27–8

Clower, C. G., Young, A. J. & Kepas, D. (1969) Psychotic states resulting from disorders of thyroid function. *Johns Hopkins med. J.*, **124**, 305–10

Cohen, S. (1979) Personal communication

Cohen, S. I. & Marks, I. M. (1961) Prolonged organic psychosis with recovery in Addison's disease. *J. Neurol. Neurosurg. Psychiat.*, **24**, 366–8

Frerichs, H. & Creutzfeld, W. (1976) Hypoglycaemia I: Insulin secreting tumours. *Clin. Endocrin. Metab.*, **5**, 747–67

Furger, R. (1961) Psychiatrische Untersuchungen beim Cushing-Syndrom. *Schweiz. Arch. Neurol. Neurochir. Psychiat.*, **88**, 1–33

Granville-Grossman, K. (1971) *Recent Advances in Clinical Psychiatry*. London: Churchill

Greer, S. & Parsons, V. (1968) Schizophrenia-like psychosis in thyroid crisis. *Brit. J. Psychiat.*, **114**, 1357–62

Henschke, P. J. & Pain, R. W. (1977) Thyroid disease in a psychogeriatric population. *Age and Ageing*, **6**, 151–5

Hoffenberg, R. (1978) The thyroid. *Medicine (monthly add-on journal, 3rd series)*, **8**, 392–404

Ingbar, S. H. (1966) Thyrotoxic storm. *New Eng. J. Med.*, **274**, 1252–4

Jain, V. K. (1972) A psychiatric study of hypothyroidism. *Psychiat. clin.*, **5**, 121–30

Jeffcoate, W. J., Silverstone, J. T., Edwards, C. R. W. & Besser, G. M. (1979) Personal communication

Jellinek, E. H. (1962) Fits, faints, coma and dementia in myxoedema. *Lancet*, ii, 1010–12

Kind, H. (1958) Die Psychiatrie der Hypophyseninsuffizienz speziell der Simmondsschen Krankheit. *Fortschr. Neurol. Psychiat.*, **26**, 501–63

Kitis, G. (1976) Sheehan's syndrome with psychosis. *Proc. R. Soc. Med.*, **69**, 805–6

Knowlton, A. I. (1971) Addison's disease: a review of its clinical course and management. In *The Human Adrenal Cortex*, ed. Christy, N. P., pp. 329–58. New York: Harper and Row

McLarty, D. G., Ratcliffe, W. A., Ratcliffe, J. G., Schimmins, J. G. & Goldberg, A. (1978) A study of thyroid function in psychiatric in-patients. *Brit. J. Psychiat.*, **133**, 211–18

Marks, V. M. & Rose, F. C. (1965) *Hypoglycaemia*. Oxford: Blackwell

Marks, V. & Samols, E. (1974) Insulinoma: natural history and diagnosis. *Clini. Gastroenterol.*, **3**, 559–73

Marks, V. M. (1975) Hypoglycaemia II: Other causes. *Clin. Endocrin. Metab.*, **5**, 769–82

Michael, R. P. & Gibbons, J. L. (1963) Interrelationships between the endocrine system and neuropsychiatry. *Int. Rev. Neurobiol.*, **5**, 242–302

Olivarius, B. F., & Röder, E. (1970) Reversible psychosis and dementia in myxoedema. *Acta psychiat. scand.*, **46**, 1–13

Pitts, F. N. & Guze, S. B. (1961) Psychiatric disorders and myxoedema. *Amer. J. Psychiat.*, **118**, 142–7

Regestein, Q. R., Rose, L. I. & Williams, G. H. (1972) Psychopathology in Cushing's syndrome. *Arch. int. Med.*, **130**, 114–17

Reid, J. L. (1978) The adrenal medulla. *Medicine (monthly add-on journal: 3rd series)* **9**, 429–34

Ross, E. J. (1972) Phaeochromocytoma. *Proc. R. Soc. Med.*, **65**, 792–3

Ross, E. J., Marshall-Jones, P. & Friedman, M. (1966) Cushing's syndrome: diagnostic criteria. *Q. J. Med.*, **35**, 149–92

Sachar, E. J. (1974) Psychiatric disturbances in endocrine disease: some issues for research. *Res. Pub. Ass. Res. nerv. ment. Dis.*, **53**, 239–49

Schulte, D. B. (1976) Paranoid-halluzinatorische Psychosen bei Akromegalie. *Schweiz. Arch. Neurol. Neurochir. Psychiat.*, **118**, 357–77

Sheehan, H. L. & Summers, V. K. (1949) The syndrome of hypopituitarism. *Q. J. Med.*, **18**, 319–62

Smith, C. K., Barish, J., Correa, J. & Williams, R. H. (1972) Psychiatric disturbance in endocrinologic disease. *Psychosom. Med.*, **34**, 69–86

Sönksen, P. H. & Lowy, C. (1978) The hypothalamus and anterior pituitary. *Medicine (monthly add-on journal, 3rd series)*, **8**, 373–86

Stoll, W. A. (1953) *Die Psychiatrie des Morbus Addison*. Stuttgart: Thieme

Thomas, F. B., Massaferri, E. L. & Skillman, T. G. (1970) Apathetic thyrotoxicosis: a distinctive clinical and laboratory entity. *Ann. int. Med.*, **72**, 679–85

Trethowan, W. H. & Cobb, S. (1952) Neuropsychiatric aspects of Cushing's syndrome. *Arch. Neurol. Psychiat.*, **67**, 283–309

Wayne, E. J. (1960) Clinical and metabolic studies in thyroid disease. *Brit. med. J.*, **1**, 1–11 & 78–90

Whybrow, P. C., Prange, A. J. & Treadway, C. R. (1969) Mental changes accompanying thyroid gland dysfunction. *Arch. gen. Psychiat.*, **20**, 48–63

CHAPTER 4

Anderson, J. T., Lawler, A. & Keys, A. (1957) Weight gain from simple over-eating. *J. clin. Invest.*, **36**, 81–8

Březinová V. & Oswald, I. (1972) Sleep after a bedtime beverage. *Brit. med. J.*, **2**, 431–3

Carlander, O. (1959) Aetiology of pica. *Lancet*, ii, 569

Carney, M. W. P., Williams, D. G. & Sheffield, B. F. (1979) Thiamine and pyridoxine lack in newly-admitted psychiatric patients. *Brit. J. Psychiat.*, **135**, 249–54

Crammer, J. L. (1957) Rapid weight changes in mental patients. *Lancet*, ii, 259–62

— (1959) Water and sodium in two psychotics, *Lancet*, i, 1122–6

Crammer, J. L. & Elkes, A. (1969) Body weight in depression and the effect of desmethylimipramine. In *The Present Status of Psychotropic Drugs*, ed. Cerletti, A. & Bové, F. J., pp. 503–5. Excerpta Medica, ICS 180. Amsterdam: Elsevier

Crisp, A. H. & Stonehill, E. (1976) *Sleep, Nutrition and Mood*. Chichester: Wiley

Daniel, P. M., Pratt, O. E. & Wilson, P. A. (1977) The transport of l-leucine into the brain of the rat *in vivo*: saturable and non-saturable components of the influx. *Proc. R. Soc.*, B, **196**, 333–46; see also *Q. J. exper. Physiol.*, **62**, 163–73

Davidson, S., Passmore, R., Brock, J. F. & Truswell, A. S. (1975) *Human Nutrition and Dietetics*, 6th ed. London: Churchill Livingstone

Davies, I. J. T. (1972) *The Clinical Significance of the Essential Biological Metals*. London: Heinemann

Davison, A. N. (1973) Nutrition and amino acid imbalance as factors influencing brain development. In *Biochemistry and Mental Illness*, ed. Iversen, L. L. & Rose, S. P. R. London: Biochemical Society

Dickens, G. & Trethowan, W. H. (1971) Cravings and aversions during pregnancy. *J. psychosom. Res.*, **15**, 259–69

Dohan, F. C. (1966) Cereals and schizophrenia. Data and hypothesis. *Acta psychiat. scand.*, **42**, 125–52

Dohan, F. C., Grasberger, J. C., Lowell, F. M., Johnston, H. T. Jr. & Arbegast, A. W. (1969) Relapsed schizophrenics: more rapid improvement on a milk and cereal-free diet. *Brit. J. Psychiat.*, **115**, 595–6

Dohan, F. C. (1978) In *Antigen Absorption by the Gut*, ed. Hemmings, W. A., pp. 155–60. Lancaster: M.T.P. Press

Eilenberg, M. D. (1960) Psychiatric illness and pernicious anaemia: a critical re-evaluation. *J. ment. Sci.*, **106**, 1539–48

Fabrykant, M. (1960) Neuropsychiatric manifestations of somatic disease – a review. *Metabolism*, **9**, 413–26

Falkner, F. T. & Tanner, J. M. (1978) *Human Growth. 3: Neurobiology and Nutrition*. London: Baillière Tindall

Fink, R. & Rosalki, S. B. (1978) Clinical biochemistry of alcoholism. *Clinics in Endocrinol. Metabol.*, **7**, 297–319

Garb, J. L. & Stunkard, A. J. (1974) Taste aversion in Man. *Amer. J. Psychiat.*, **131**, 1204–7

Garrow, J. S. (1974) *Energy Balance and Obesity in Man*. Amsterdam: North-Holland

Goodhart, R. S. & Shils, M. E. (1973) *Modern Nutrition in Health and Disease*. 5th ed. Philadelphia: Lea & Febiger

Gopelan, C. & Rao, K. S. J. (1975) Pellagra and aminoacid imbalance. *Vitamins and Hormones*, **33**, 505–28

Gredden, J. F. (1974) Anxiety or caffeinism: a diagnostic dilemma. *Amer. J. Psychiat.*, **131**, 1089–92

Green, A. R. (1978) The effects of dietary tryptophan and its peripheral metabolism on brain serotonin synthesis and function. In *Essays in Neurochemistry and Neuropharmacology*, ed. Youdim, M. B. H., Lovenberg, W., Sharman, I F. & Lagnado, J. R., vol 3, 103–28, Wiley: Chichester

Handbook of Physiology (1967) Sec. 6, ed. Code, C. F., *Alimentary Canal*: vol. 1, *Control of Food and Water Intake*, pp. 387–98. Bethesda, Maryland: American Physiological Society

Hemmings, W. A. (1978) *Antigen Absorption by the Gut*. Lancaster: M.T.P. Press

Herzberg, B., Coppen, A. J. & Marks, V. (1968) Glucose tolerance in depression. *Brit. J. Psychiat.*, **114**, 627–30

Keys, A., Brozek, J., Herschel, A., Miekelson, D. & Taylor, H. (1950) *The Biology of Human Starvation*. Minneapolis: University of Minnesota Press

Klee, W. A., Zioudrou, C. & Streaty, R. A. (1979) Exorphins: peptides with opioid activity isolated from wheat gluten and their possible role in the aetiology of schizophrenia. In *Endorphins in Mental Health Research*, ed. Usdin, E., Bunney, W. E. & Kline, N. S. London: Macmillan

Lancet (1959) Aetiology of pica. *Lancet*, **ii**, 281

Lishman, W. A. (1978) *Organic Psychiatry*. Oxford: Blackwell

MacGregor, G. A., Maskandu, N. D., Roulston, J. E., Jones, J. C. & de Wardener, H. (1979) Is 'idiopathic' oedema idiopathic? *Lancet*, **i**, 397–400

Marks, J. (1975) *A Guide to the Vitamins*. Lancaster. M.T.P. Press

Marsh, M. N. (1981). The small intestine: mechanisms of local immunity and gluten sensitivity. *Clin. Sci.*, **61**, 497–503

Mudd, S. H. & Freeman, J. M. (1974) N-methylenetetrahydrofolate reductase deficiency and schizophrenia: a working hypothesis. *J. psychiat. Res.*, **11**, 259–62

Naylor, G. J., & Smith, A. H. W. (1981) Vanadium: a possible aetiological factor in manic-depressive illness. *Psychol. Med.*, **11**, 249–56

Park, L. C., Baldessarini, R. J. & Kety, S. S. (1965) Methionine effects in chronic schizophrenics. *Arch. gen. Psychiat.*, **12**, 346–51

Paul, A. A., & Southgate, D. A. T. (1978) *McCance & Widdowson's The Composition of Foods*. MRC special report No. 297, 4th ed. London: HMSO; Amsterdam: Elsevier North Holland

Pauling, L. (1974) On the orthomolecular environment of the mind. *Amer. J. Psychiat.*, **131**, 1251; with comments by Wyatt, R. J., p. 1258, Klein, D. F., p. 1263, and Lipton, M. A., p. 1266

Rennie, M. J., Edwards, R. H. T., Krywawych, S., Davies, C. T. M., Halliday, D., Waterlow, J. C. & Millward, D. J. (1981) Effect of exercise on protein turnover in man. *Clin. Sci.*, **61**, 627–39

Reynolds, E. H., Preece, J. M., Bailey, J. & Coppen, A. (1970) Folate deficiency in depressive illness. *Brit. J. Psychiat.*, **117**, 287–92

Robinson, R. G., Folstein, M. F. & McHugh, P. R. (1979) Reduced calorie intake following small bowel by-pass surgery: a systematic study of possible causes. *Psychol. Med.*, **9**, 37–54

Sargant, W., & Slater, E. (1963) *An Introduction to Physical Methods of Treatment in Psychiatry*, 4th ed., pp. 149–64. London: Livingstone

Seakins, J. W. T. (1974) Hartnup disease. In *Handbook of Clinical Neurology*, ed. Vinken, P. J. & Bruyn, G. W., vol. 29, part III, chap 9, pp. 149–70. Amsterdam: North Holland

Sprince, H. (1967) Metabolic inter-relationships of tryptophan and methionine in relation to mental illness. In *Amines and Schizophrenia*, ed. Himwich, H. E., Kety, J. S. & Smythies, J. R. pp. 97–114. Oxford: Pergamon Press

Thomson, A. D. (1978) Alcohol and nutrition. *Clinics in Endocrinol. Metabol.*, **7**, 405–28

Weil-Malherbe, H. & Szara, S. I. (1971) Carbohydrate metabolism in affective disorder. In *The Biochemistry of Functional and Experimental Psychoses*, chap. 6. Springfield, Ill.: Thomas

Winstead, D. K. (1976) Coffee consumption among psychiatric inpatients. *Am. J. Psychiat.*, **133**, 1447–50

Wurtman, R. J. & Wurtman, J. J. (1977) *Nutrition and the Brain*, vols. I & II. New York: Raven

CHAPTER 5

Adams, F. (1939) The Genuine Works of Hippocrates: Translated from the Greek. London: Baillière, Tindall & Cox

Arkle, J. (1957) Termination of pregnancy on psychiatric grounds. *Brit. med. J.*, **1**, 558–60

Baker, A. A. (1967) *Psychiatric Disorders in Obstetrics*. Oxford: Blackwell

Barglow, P. & Brown, E. (1972) Pseudocyesis. In *Modern Perspectives in Psycho-obstetrics*, ed. Howells, J. G., pp. 53–67. Edinburgh: Oliver & Boyd

Beard, R. W., Belsey, E. M., Lal, S., Lewis, S. C. & Greer, H. S. (1974) King's termination study II. Contraceptive practice before and after out-patient termination of pregnancy. *Brit. med. J.*, **1**, 418–21

Beecham, J. B., Braun, T. E., Clapp, J. F. & Lucey, J. F. (1973) Intrauterine diagnosis of fetal liver dysfunction. *Obstet. Gynecol.*, **41**, 556

Bivin, G. D. & Klinger, M. P. (1937) *Pseudocyesis*. Bloomington, Indiana: Principia Press

Bluglass, R. (1978) Infanticide. *Bull. R. Coll. Psychiatrists*, (Aug.) 139–41

Bratfos, O. & Haug, J. O. (1966) Puerperal mental disorders in manic-depressive females. *Acta psychiat. scand.*, **42**, 285–94

Brewer, C. (1977) Incidence of post abortion psychosis: a prospective study. *Brit. med. J.*, **1**, 476–7

British Medical Journal (1938) Charge of procuring abortion: Mr. Bourne acquitted. **2**, 199–205

Brockington, I. F., Schofield, E. M., Donnelly, P. & Hyde, C. (1978) A clinical study of post-partum psychosis. In *Mental Illness in Pregnancy and the Puerperium*, ed. Sandler, M., pp. 59–68. Oxford: Oxford University Press

Brown, G. & Harris, T. (1978) *Social origins of depression*, pp. 140–1. London: Tavistock

Bucove, A. D. (1968) A case of pre-partum psychosis and infanticide. *Psychiat. Q.*, **42**, 263–70

Carr, A. T. (1974) Compulsive neurosis: a review of the literature. *Psychol. Bull.*, **81**, 311–18

Clare, A. (1978) Observations on psychiatric morbidity and premenstrual distress in women. In *Current Themes in Psychiatry*, ed. Gaind, R. & Hudson, B. L., pp. 142–54. London: Macmillan

Cloninger, C. R., Christiansen, K. O., Reich, T. & Gottesman, I. I. (1978) Implications of sex differences in the prevalences of antisocial personality, alcoholism, and criminality for familial transmission. *Arch. gen. Psychiat.*, **35**, 941–51

Coles, R. (1975) A retrospective study of patients seeking pregnancy advice, January 1971 to June 1974. *J. biosoc. Sci.*, **7**, 357–66

Cook, R. J. & Dickens, B. M. (1978) A decade of international change in abortion law: 1967–1977. *Amer. J. pub. Health*, **68**, 637–44

Cooper, J. E., Kendell, R. E., Gurland, B. J., Sharpe, L., Copeland, J. R. M. & Simon, R. (1972) *Psychiatric Diagnosis in New York and London*. Maudsley Monograph, No. 20. London: Oxford University Press

Cooper, S. J. (1978) Poisoned people: psychotropic drugs in pregnancy: morphological and psychological adverse effects on offspring. *J. biosoc. Sci.*, **10**, 321–34

Coppen, A., Stein, G. & Wood, K. (1978) Postnatal depression and tryptophan metabolism. In *Mental Illness in Pregnancy and the Puerperium*, ed. Sandler, M., pp. 25–34. Oxford: Oxford University Press

Dalton, K. (1971) Prospective study into puerperal depression. *Brit. J. Psychiat.*, **118**, 689–92

Deutsch, H. (1945) *The psychology of women.* vol. II, *Motherhood.* New York: Grune & Stratton

DHSS (1977) Health and personal social services statistics for England 1976. London: HMSO

d'Orban, P. T. (1979) Women who kill their children. *Brit. J. Psychiat.*, **134**, 560–71

Dunnell, K. & Cartwright, A. (1972) *Medicine Takers, Prescribers and Hoarders.* London: Routledge & Kegan Paul

Eggermont, E., Raveschot, J., Deneve, V. & Casteels-Van Daele, M. (1972) The adverse influence of imipramine on the adaptation of the newborn infant to extrauterine life. *Acta paediat. belg.*, **26**, 197–204

Ekblad, M. (1955) Induced abortion on psychiatric grounds: a follow-up study of 479 women. *Acta psychiat. scand.* Supp., **99**, 1–238

Esquirol, E. (1838) *Des maladies mentales considérées sous les rapports médical, hygiénique et medico-légal.* Paris: Baillière

Essen-Möller, E. (1956) Individual traits and morbidity in a Swedish rural population. *Acta psychiat. scand.*, Supp. 100

Fairweather, D. V. (1968) Nausea and vomiting during pregnancy. *Obstet. Gynecol. Ann.*, **7**, 91–105

Forfar, J. O. & Nelson, M. M. (1973) Epidemiology of drugs taken by pregnant women: drugs that may affect the fetus adversely. *Clin. Pharmacol. Ther.*, **14**, 632–42

Forrest, J. M. (1976) Drugs in pregnancy and lactation. *Med. J. Austral.*, **2**, 138–41

Forssman, H. & Thuwe, I. (1966) One hundred and twenty children born after application for therapeutic abortion refused. Their mental health, social adjustment and education level up to the age of 21. *Acta psychiat. scand.*, **42**, 71–88

Fowkes, F. G. R., Catford, J. C. & Logan, R. F. (1979) Abortion and the NHS: the first decade. *Brit. med. J.*, **1**, 217–19

Fraser, A. C. (1976) Drug addiction in pregnancy. *Lancet*, **ii**, 896–9

Freeman, C. L. (1979) Electroconvulsive therapy: its current clinical use. *Brit. J. hosp. Med.*, **21**, 281–92

Fried, P. H., Rakoff, A. E., Schopbach, R. R. & Kaplan, A. J. (1951) Pseudocyesis: a psychosomatic study in gynecology. *J. Amer. med. Ass.*, **145**, 1329–34

Gelder, M. (1978) Hormones and post-partum depression. In *Mental Illness in Pregnancy and the Puerperium*, ed. Sandler, M. pp. 80–90. Oxford: Oxford University Press.

Ghodse, A. H., Reed, J. L. & Mack, J. W. (1977) The effect of maternal narcotic addiction on the newborn infant. *Psychol. Med.*, **7**, 667–75

Gooch, R. (1820). Observations on puerperal insanity. *Med. Trans.*, .**6**. London: Woodfall

Granville-Grossman, K. (1971) *Recent Advances in Clinical Psychiatry*, chap. 9. London: Churchill

Greer, H. S., Lal, S., Lewis, S. C., Belsey, E. M. & Beard, R. W. (1976) Psychosocial consequences of therapeutic abortion. King's termination Study III. *Brit. J. Psychiat.*, **128**, 74–9

Guze, S. B. & Perley, M. J. (1963) Observations on the natural history of hysteria. *Amer. J. Psychiat.*, **119**, 960–5

Hagnell, O. (1970) The incidence and duration of episodes of mental illness in a total population. In *Psychiatric Epidemiology*, ed. Hare, E. H. & Wing, J. K., pp. 213–24. London: Oxford University Press

Hamilton, J. A. (1962) *Post-partum psychiatric problems.* St Louis, USA: Mosby

Handley, S. L., Dunn, T. L., Baker, J. M., Cockshott, C. & Gould, S. (1977) Mood changes in puerperium, and plasma tryptophan and cortisol concentrations. *Brit. med. J.*, **2**, 18–20

Hill, R. M., Craig, J. P., Chaney, M. D., Tennyson, L. M. & McCulley, L. B. (1977) Utilisation of over-the-counter drugs during pregnancy. *Clin. Obstet. Gynecol.*, **20**, 381–94

Hill, R. M., Desmond, M. M. & Kay, J. L. (1966) Extrapyramidal dysfunction in an infant of a schizophrenic mother. *J. Pediat.*, **69**, 589–95

HMSO (1968) *A Glossary of Mental Disorders.* London: HMSO

Höök, K. (1963) Refused abortion: a follow-up study of 249 women whose applications were refused by the National Board of Health in Sweden. *Acta psychiat. neurol. scand.* Suppl., **168**

Horsley, S. (1972) Psychological management of the pre-natal period. In *Modern perspectives in Psycho-Obstetrics*, ed. Howells, J. G., pp. 291–313. Edinburgh: Oliver & Boyd

Illsley, R. & Hall, M. H. (1976) Psychosocial aspects of abortion. A review of issues and needed research. *Bull. WHO*, **53**, 83–106

Ingham, J. G., Rawnsley, K. & Hughes, D. (1972) Psychiatric disorder and its declaration in contrasting areas of South Wales. *Psychol. Med.*, **2**, 281–92

Johnson, D. A. W. (1973) An analysis of out-patient services. *Brit. J Psychiat.*, **122**, 301–6

Kendell, R. E., Wainwright, S., Hailey, A. & Shannon, B. (1976) The influence of childbirth on psychiatric morbidity. *Psychol. Med.*, **6**, 297–302

Kessel, N. (1977) The fetal alcohol syndrome from the public health standpoint. *Health Trends*, **9**, 86–9

Kessel, N. & Shepherd, M. (1962) Neurosis in hospital and general practice. *J. ment. Sci.*, **108**, 159–66

Kraepelin, E. (1906) *Lectures on Clinical Psychiatry.* 2nd ed. Rev. and ed. Johnstone, T. London: Baillière, Tindall & Cox

Kreitman, N. (1978) Social and clinical aspects of suicide and parasuicide (attempted suicide). In *Companion to Psychiatric Studies.* 2nd ed., ed. Forrest, A. D., Affleck, J. W. & Zealley, A. K., pp. 30–43. Edinburgh: Churchill Livingstone

Kumar, R. & Robson, K. (1978) Neurotic disturbance during pregnancy and the puerperium: preliminary report of a prospective survey of 119 primiparae. In *Mental Illness in Pregnancy and the Puerperium*, ed. Sandler, M., pp. 40–51. Oxford: Oxford University Press

— (1978) Previous induced abortion and ante-natal depression in primiparae: preliminary report of a survey of mental health in pregnancy. *Psychol. Med.*, **8**, 711–15

Lask, B. (1975) Short-term psychiatric sequelae to therapeutic termination of pregnancy. *Brit. J. Psychiat.*, **126**, 173–7

Levy, W. & Wisniewski, K. (1974) Chlorpromazine causing extrapyramidal dysfunction in newborn infant of psychotic mother. *New York State J. Med.*, **74**, 684

Lewis, E. (1976) The management of stillbirth: coping with an unreality. *Lancet*, **ii**, 619–20

Lewis, E. & Page, A. (1978) Failure to mourn a stillbirth: an overlooked catastrophe. *Brit. J. med. Psychol.*, **51**, 237–41

Lewis, P. (1978) The effect of psychotropic drugs on the foetus. In *Mental Illness in Pregnancy and the Puerperium*, ed. Sandler, M., pp. 99–111. Oxford: Oxford University Press

Marks, I. M. (1969) *Fears and Phobias.* London: Heinemann

Maudsley, H. (1899) *The Pathology of Mind.* New York: Appleton

McLaren, H. C. (1967) The Abortion Bill (letter). *Lancet*, **i**, 565–6

Meares, R., Grimwade, J. & Wood, C. (1976) A possible relationship between anxiety in pregnancy and puerperal depression. *J. psychosom. Res.*, **20**, 605–10

Moulton, R. (1942) Psychosomatic implication of pseudocyesis. *Psychosom. Med.*, **4**, 376–89

Nilsson, A. & Almgren, P. E. (1970) Paranatal emotional adjustment. A prospective investigation of 165 women. *Acta psychiat. scand.*, Supp. 220, 65–141

Nott, P. N., Franklin, M., Armitage, C. & Gelder, M. G. (1976) Hormonal changes and mood in the puerperium. *Brit. J. Psychiat.*, **128**. 379–83

Osofsky, J. D. & Osofsky, H. J. (1972) The psychological reaction of patients to legalised abortion. *Amer. J. Orthopsychiat.*, **42**, 48–60

Paffenbarger, R. S. (1964) Epidemiological aspects of parapartum mental illness. *Brit. J. prev. soc. Med.*, **18**, 189–95

Pare, C. M. B. & Raven, H. (1970) Follow-up of patients referred for termination. *Lancet*, **i**, 653–8

Patrick, M. J., Tilstone, W. J. & Reavy, P. (1972) Diazepam and breast feeding. *Lancet*, **i**, 542

Pitt, B. (1968) Atypical depression following childbirth. *Brit. J. Psychiat.*, **114**, 1325–35

— (1973) 'Maternity blues'. *Brit. J. Psychiat.*, **122**, 431–3

Priest, R. G. (1978) Introduction. In *Mental Illness in Pregnancy and the Puerperium*, ed. Sandler, M., pp. 7–8. Oxford: Oxford University Press

Protheroe, C. (1977) Mother–baby units in psychiatric hospitals. *Bull. R. Coll. Psychiatrists*, (August), 12–14

Pugh, T. F., Jerath, B. K., Schmidt, W. M. & Reed, R. B. (1963) Rates of mental disease related to childbearing. *New Eng. J. Med.*, **268**, 1224–8

Reed. J. L. (1971) Hysteria. *Brit. J. hosp. Med.*, **5**, 237–47

Reich, T. & Winokur, G. (1970) Post-partum psychoses in patients with manic depressive disease. *J. nerv. ment. Dis.*, **151**, 60–8

RMPA Memorandum on Therapeutic Abortion (1966) *Brit. J. Psychiat.*; **112**, 1071–3

Savage, G. H. (1875) Observations on the insanity of pregnancy and childbirth. *Guy's Hospital Rep.*, **20**, 83–117

Savage, R. L. (1976) Drugs and breast milk. *Adverse Drug Reaction Bull.*, **61**, 212–15

Schou, M. & Amdisen, A. (1973) Lithium and pregnancy III. Lithium ingestion by children breastfed by women on lithium treatment. *Brit. med. J.*, **2**, 138

Schou, M., Goldfield, M. D., Weinstein, M. R. & Villeneuve, A. (1973) Lithium and pregnancy I. Report from the register of lithium babies. *Brit. med. J.*, **2**, 135–6

Seiden, A. M. (1976) Overview: research on the psychology of women. I. Gender differences and sexual and reproductive life. *Amer. J. Psychiat.*, **133**, 995–1007

Seymour-Shove, R., Gee, D. J. & Cross, R. P. (1968) Schizophrenia during pregnancy associated with injury to the foetus. *Brit. med. J.*, **1**, 686

Shepherd, M., Cooper, B., Brown, A. C. & Kalton, G. W. (1966) *Psychiatric Illness in General Practice*. London: Oxford University Press

Sim, M. (1963) Abortion and the psychiatrist. *Brit. med. J.*, **2**, 145–8

Simon, N. M. & Senturia, A. G. (1966) Psychiatric sequelae of abortion: review of the literature 1935–1964. *Arch. gen. Psychiat.*, **15**, 378–89

Stafford-Clark, D. (1967) *Psychiatry for Students*. London: Allen & Unwin

Stein, G., Milton, F., Bebbington, P., Wood, K. & Coppen, A. (1976) Relationship between mood disturbance and free and total plasma tryptophan in post-partum women. *Brit. med. J.*, **2**, 457

Steinberg, A., Pastor, N., Winheld, E. B., Segal, H. I., Schechter,

F. R. & Cotton, N. H. (1946) Psychoendocrine relationships in pseudocyesis. *Psychosom. Med.*, **8**, 176–9.

Taylor, Lord & Chave, S. (1964) *Mental Health and Environment*. London: Longman

Tod, E. D. M. (1964) Puerperal depression, a prospective epidemiological study. *Lancet*, **ii**, 1264–6

Tonks, C. M. (1976) Differential aspects of psychiatry in the female. In *Recent Advances in Clinical Psychiatry*, ed. Granville-Grossman, K., vol. 2, pp. 147–68. Edinburgh: Churchill Livingstone

Trethowan, W. H. & Dickens, G. (1972) Cravings, aversions and pica of pregnancy. In *Modern Perspectives in Psycho-obstetrics*, ed. Howells, J. G., pp. 251–68. Edinburgh: Oliver & Boyd

Tunkel, V. (1979) Abortion: how early, how late, how legal? *Brit. med. J.*, **2**, 253–6

Tylden, E. (1966) Suicide risk in unwanted pregnancy. *Med. World*, January, 25–28

— (1968) Hyperemesis and physiological vomiting. *J. psychosom. Res.*, **12**, 86–93

— (1977) Psychiatric disorders including drug therapy and addiction. *Clin. Obstet. Gynecol.*, **4**, 435–49

Uddenberg, N., Nilsson, A. & Almgren, P. E. (1971) Nausea in pregnancy: psychological and psychosomatic aspects. *J. psychosom. Res.*, **15**, 269–76

Visram, S. A. (1972) A follow-up study of 95 women who were refused abortion on psychiatric grounds. In *Psychosomatic Medicine in Obstetrics & Gynaecology*, ed. Morris, N., pp. 561–3. Basel: Karger

Vorherr, H. (1974) Drug excretion in breast milk. *Postgrad. Med.*, **56**, 97–104

Weissmann, M. M. & Klerman, G. L. (1977) Sex differences and the epidemiology of depression. *Arch. gen. Psychiat.*, **34**, 98–111

Whitlock, F. A. & Edwards, J. E. (1968) Pregnancy and attempted suicide. *Compr. Psychiat.*, **9**, 1–12

WHO (1974) *Glossary of mental disorders and guide to their classification*. Geneva: WHO

Winokur, G., Rimmer, J. & Reich, T. (1971) Alcoholism IV: Is there more than one type of alcoholism. *Brit. J. Psychiat.*, **118**, 525–31

Wolkind, S. & Zajicek, E. (1978) Psycho-social correlates of nausea and vomiting in pregnancy. *J. psychosom. Res.*, **22**, 1–5

Yalom, I. D., Lunde, D. T., Moos, R. H. & Hamburg, D. A. (1968) Post-partum 'blues' syndrome. A description and related variables. *Arch. gen. Psychiat.*, **18**, 16–27

Ziv, G., Shani, J., Givant, Y., Buchman, O. & Sulman, F. G. (1974) Distribution of tritiated haloperidol in lactating and pregnant cows and ewes. *Arch. int. Pharmacodyn. Thér.*, **212**. 154–63

CHAPTER 6

Adam, K. (1977) Brain rhythm that correlates with obesity. *Brit. med. J.*, **2**, 234

Bakwin, H. (1970) Sleep-walking in twins. *Lancet*, **ii**, 446–7

Březinová, V. (1974) Effect of caffeine on sleep: EEG study in late middle age people. *Brit. J. clin. Pharmacol.*, **1**, 203–8

British Medical Journal (1975) Tranquillizers causing aggression. *Brit. med. J.*, **1**, 113–4

Broughton, R. & Ghanem, Q. (1976) In *Narcolepsy*, ed. Guilleminault, C., Dement, W. C. & Passouant, P., pp. 201–20. New York: Spectrum Publications

Castleden, C. M., George, C. F., Mercer, D. & Hallett, C. (1977) Increased sensitivity to nitrazepam in old age. *Brit. med. J.,* **1**, 10–12

Clift, A. D. (1972) Factors leading to dependence on hypnotic drugs. *Brit. med. J.* **3**, 614–17

Crisp, A. H., & McGuiness, B. (1976) Jolly fat: relation between obesity and psychoneurosis in general population. *Brit. med. J.,* **1**, 7–9

Crisp, A. H. & Stonehill, E. (1973) Aspects of the relationship between sleep and nutrition: a study of 374 psychiatric outpatients. *Brit. J. Psychiat.,* **122**, 379–94

Feinberg, I., Koresko, R. L. & Heller, N. (1967) EEG sleep patterns as a function of normal and pathological aging in man. *J. psychiat. Res.,* **5**, 107–44

Fisher, C., Kahn, E., Edwards, A., Davis, D. M. & Fine, J. (1974) A psychophysiological study of nightmares and night terrors. *J. nerv. ment. Dis.,* **158**, 174–87

Frankel, B. L., Coursey, R. D., Buchbinder, R., & Snyder, F. (1976) Recorded and reported sleep in chronic primary insomnia. *Arch. gen. Psychiat.,* **33**, 615–23.

Gaillard, J. M. (1978) Chronic primary insomnia: possible physiopathological involvement of slow wave sleep deficiency. *Sleep,* **1**, 133–47

Gentil, M. L. F. & Lader, M. (1978) Dream content and daytime attitudes in anxious and calm women. *Psychol. Med.,* **8**, 297–304

Guilleminault, C. & Dement, W. C. (1978) Sleep apnea syndromes and related sleep disorders. In *Sleep Disorders,* ed. Williams, R. L. & Karacan, I., pp. 9–28. New York: Wiley

Hällström, T. (1972) Night terror in adults through three generations. *Acta psychiatrica scandinavica,* **48**, 350–2

Kales, A., Jacobson, A., Paulson, M. J., Kales, J. D. & Walter, R. D. (1966) Somnambulism: psychophysiological correlates. *Arch. gen. Psychiat.,* **14**, 586–94

Karacan, I., Thornby, J. I., Anch, M., Holzer, C. E., Warheit, G. J., Schwab, J. J. & Williams, R. L. (1976) Prevalence of sleep disturbance in a primarily urban Florida county. *Soc. Sci. Med.,* **10**, 239–44

Kokkoris, C. P., Weitzman, E. D., Pollak, C. P., Spielman, A. J., Czeisler, C. A. & Bradlow, H. (1978) Long-term ambulatory temperature monitoring in a subject with a hypernychthemeral sleep-wake cycle disturbance. *Sleep,* **1**, 177–90

Kraepelin, E. (1906) Über Sprachstörungen im Traume. *Psychologische Arbeiten,* **5**, 1–104

Kripke, D. F., Simons, R. N., Garfinkel, L. & Hammond, C. E. (1979) Short and long sleep and sleeping pills. *Arch. gen. Psychiat.,* **36**, 103–16

Lacey, J. H., Crisp, A. H., Kalucy, R. S., Hartmann, M. K. & Chen, C. N. (1975) Weight gain and the sleeping electroencephalogram: study of 10 patients with anorexia nervosa. *Brit. med. J.,* **4**, 556–8

Legal Correspondent (1970) Sleepwalking and guilt. *Brit. med. J.,* **2**, 186

McGhie, A. (1966) The subjective assessment of sleep patterns in psychiatric illness. *Brit. J. med. Psychol.,* **39**, 221–30

McGhie, A. & Russell, S. M. (1962) The subjective assessment of normal sleep patterns. *J. ment. Sci.,* **108**, 646–54

Mendels, J. & Hawkins, D. R. (1971) Sleep and depression. IV. Longitudinal studies. *J. nerv. ment. Dis.,* **153**, 251–72

Miles, L. E. M., Raynal, D. M. & Wilson, M. A. (1977) Blind man living in normal society has circadian rhythms of 24.9 hours. *Science,* **198**, 421–23

Mitchell, S. W. (1890) Some disorders of sleep. *Int. J. med. Sci.,* **100**, 109–27

Oswald, I. (1964) Physiology of sleep accompanying dreaming. In *The Scientific Basis of Medicine Annual Reviews 1964,* ed. Paterson Ross, J., pp. 102–24. London: Athlone Press

Oswald, I., Adam, K., Borrow, S. & Idzikowski, C. (1979) The effect of two hypnotics on sleep, subjective feelings and skilled performance. In *Pharmacology of the States of Alertness,* ed. Passouant, P. & Oswald, I., pp. 51–63. Oxford: Pergamon Press

Oswald, I., Březinová, V. & Carruthers-Jones, I. (1975) Sleep disorders today. In *Eleventh Symposium on Advanced Medicine,* ed. Lant, A. F., pp. 109–18. Tunbridge Wells: Pitman Medical

Pai, M. N. (1946) Sleep-walking and sleep activities *J. ment. Sci.,* **92**, 757–65

Roth, B., Nevsimalova, S. & Rechtschaffen, A. (1972) Hypersomnia with 'sleep drunkenness'. *Arch. gen. Psychiat.,* **26**, 456–62

CHAPTER 7

The reader is referred to the following books and reviews for full information on aspects of headache and facial pain.

Headaches and Cranial Neuralgias. (1968) *Handbook of Clinical Neurology,* ed. Bruyn, G. W. & Vinken, P. J., vol. 5. Amsterdam: North Holland

Friedman, A. P., Von Storch, T. J. C. & Merritt, H. M. (1954) Migraine and tension headaches. A critical study of two thousand cases. *Neurology,* **4**, 773–88

Lance, J. W. (1976) *The Mechanisms and Management of Headache,* 2nd ed. London: Butterworths

Lishman, W. A. (1978) *Organic Psychiatry.* Oxford: Blackwell

Martin, M. J., Rome, H. P. & Swenson, W. M. (1967) Muscle contraction headache: a psychiatric review. *Res. clin. Stud. Headache,* **1**, 184–92

Pearce, J. (1969) *Migraine, Clinical Features, Mechanisms and Management.* Springfield, Ill: Thomas

Wolff, H. G. (1963) *Headache and other Head Pain.* London: Oxford University Press

CHAPTER 8

Arie, T. (1973) Psychiatric needs of the elderly. In *Needs of the Elderly for Health and Welfare Services,* pp. 37–44. Institute of Biometry and Community Medicine, University of Exeter. Publication No. 2.

Arie, T. & Isaacs, A. D. (1978) The development of psychiatric services for the elderly in Britain. In *Studies in Geriatric Psychiatry,* ed. Isaacs, A. D. & Post, F., pp. 241–61. Chichester: Wiley

Barraclough, B. M. (1971) Suicide in the elderly. In *Recent Advances in Psychogeriatrics,* ed. Kay, D. W. K. & Wall, N. London: Royal Medico-Psychological Association

Bergmann, K. (1978) Neurosis and Personality Disorder in Old Age. In *Studies in Geriatric Psychiatry,* ed. Isaacs, A. D. & Post, F., pp. 66–71. Chichester: Wiley

Botwinick, J. (1973) *Ageing and Behaviour.* New York: Springer

British Medical Journal (1979) Vasodilators in senile dementia, **2**, 511–2

Bromley, D. B. (1978) Approaches to the study of personality changes in adult life and old age. In *Studies in Geriatric Psychiatry,* ed. Isaacs, A. D. & Post, F., chap. 2, pp. 17–40. Chichester: Wiley

Brooke, E. M. (1965) The psychogeriatric patient: some statistical considerations. In *Psychiatric Disorders in the Aged*, pp. 214–224. WPA Symposium. Manchester: Geigy (UK) Ltd.

Brook, P., Degun, G. & Mather, M. (1975) Reality orientation – a therapy for psychogeriatric patients: A Controlled Study. *Brit J. Psychiat.*, **127**, 42–5

Carstairs, V. & Morrison, M. (1971) *The Elderly in Residential Care.* Scottish Health Services Studies. 19. Edinburgh: Scottish Home and Health Department

Castleden, C. M. & George, C. F. (1978) Increased sensitivity to benzodiazepines in the elderly. In *Drugs and the Elderly*, ed. Crook, J. & Silverson, I. H. London: Macmillan

Cattell, R. B. (1943) Measurement of adult intelligence. *Psychol. Bull.*, **3**, 153–93

Chown, S. M. (1962) Rigidity and age. In *Social and Psychological Aspects of Ageing*, ed. Tibbitts, C. & Donahue, W., pp. 832–5. New York: Columbia University Press

Cooper, A. F., Kay, D. W. K., Curry, A. R., Garside, R. F. & Roth, M. (1974) Hearing loss in paranoid and affective psychoses in the elderly. *Lancet*, **ii**, 851–61

Copeland, J. R. M. (1978) Evaluation of diagnostic methods: an international comparison. In *Studies in Geriatric Psychiatry*, ed. Isaacs, A. D. & Post, F. Chichester: Wiley

Crooks, J. & Stevenson, I. H. (1978) Eds. *Drugs and the Elderly.* London: Macmillan

Cumming, E. & Henry, W. E. (1961) *Growing Old.* New York: Basic Books

d'Alarcon, R. (1964) Hypochondriasis and depression in the aged. *Gerontol. clin.*, **6**, 266–77

DHSS (1974) *Hospital In-patient Enquiry, 1974.* London: HMSO
— (1975) *In-patient statistics from the Mental Health Enquiry for England.* London: HMSO
— (1976) *The Census of Residential Accommodation.* London: HMSO
— (1977) *Health and Personal Services. Statistics.* London: HMSO

Eysenck, H. J. (1957) *The Diagnosis of Anxiety and Hysteria.* London: Routledge & Kegan Paul

Folstein, M. F., Folstein, S. E. & McHugh, P. R. (1975) 'Mini-mental scale'. A practical method for grading the cognitive state of patients for the clinician. *J. psychiat. Res.*, **12**, 189–98

Glatt, M. M., Rosin, A. J. & Javhar, P. (1978) Alcoholic problems in the elderly. *Age and Ageing*, **7**, Supp., 64–6

Hare, M. (1978) Clinical checklist for the diagnosis of dementia. *Brit. Med. J.*, **2**, 266–7

Havighurst, R. J. (1968) Personality and patterns of ageing. *Gerontologist* **8**, 20–3

Hodkinson, H. M. (1973) Mental impairment in the elderly. *J. R. Coll. Physicians (London)* **7**, 305

Hunt, Audrey (1978) *The Elderly at Home.* London: HMSO

Isaacs, B. & Kennie, T. A. (1973) The Set Test as an aid to the detection of dementia in old people. *Brit. J. Psychiat.*, **123**, 467–70

Jolley, D. J. & Arie, T. (1978) Organisation of psychogeriatric services. *Brit. J. Psychiatr*, **132**, 1–11

Kay, D. W. K., Beamish, P. & Roth, M. (1964) Old age mental disorders in Newcastle upon Tyne. *Brit. J. Psychiat.*, **110**, 146–58

Kay, D. W. K. & Bergmann, K. (1966) Physical disability and mental health in old age. *J. psychosom. Res.*, **10**, 3–12

Leff, J. P. & Isaacs, A. D. (1978) *Psychiatric Examination and Clinical Practice.* 2nd ed. Oxford: Blackwell

Lehman, H. C. (1953) *Age and Achievement.* London: Oxford University Press

Lewis, A. J. (1946) Ageing and senility: a major problem of psychiatry. *J. ment. Sci.*, **92**, 150–70

Lishman, W. A. (1978) *Organic Psychiatry*, chap. 3, pp. 117–32. Oxford: Blackwell

Marsden, C. D. & Harrison, M. J. E. (1972) Outcome of investigation of patients with presenile dementia. *Brit. med. J.*, **1**, 164–6

Pasker, P., Thomas, J. P. R. & Ashley, J. S. A. (1976) The elderly mentally ill whose responsibility? *Brit. med. J.*, **2**, 164–6

Population Trends 11 (1978) Office of Population Censuses and Surveys. London: HMSO

Post, F. (1966) *Persistent Persecution States of the Elderly.* Oxford: Pergamon Press
— (1975) Dementia, depression and pseudodementia. In *Psychiatric Aspects of Neurological Disease*, ed. Benson, D. F. & Blumer, D. New York: Grune & Stratton

Post, F., Rees, W. L. & Schurr, P. (1968) An evaluation of bimedial leucotomy. *Brit. J. Psychiat.*, **114**, 1223–41

Quereshi, K. N. & Hodkinson, H. M. (1974) Evaluation of a 10 question test in institutionalised elderly. *Age and Ageing* **3**, 152–7

Rosin, A. J. & Glatt, M. M. (1977) Alcohol excess in the elderly. *Q. J. Stud. Alc.* **32**, 53–9

Roth, M. (1973) The principles of providing a Service for psychogeriatric patients. In *Roots of Evaluation*, ed. Edwin, J. K. & Haffner, H. London: Oxford University Press

Roth, M. & Morrissey, J. D. (1952) Problems in the diagnosis and classification of mental disorders in old age. *J. ment. Sci.* **96**, 66–80

Roth, M., Tomlinson, B. E. & Blessed, G. (1966) Correlation between scores for dements and of degenerative changes in the cerebral grey matter of elderly subjects. *Proc. R. Soc. Med.*, **60**, 254–60

Registrar General (1974) *Statistical Review for England and Wales 1972.* London: HMSO.

Savage, R. C. (1971) Recent developments in psychogeriatrics. *Royal Medico-Psychological Association, Brit. J. Psychiat.* Spec. Pub. no 6, 51–62

Wechsler, D. (1958) *The Measurement and Appraisal of Adult Intelligence.* Baltimore: Williams & Williams

Williamson, J., Stokoe, I. H., Gray, S., Fisher, M., Smith, A., McShee, A. & Stephenson, E. (1964) Old people at home: their unreported needs. *Lancet*, **i**, 1117–20

Woods, R. T. (1979) Reality orientation and staff attention: a controlled study. *Brit. J. Psychiat.*, **134**, 502–7

Woods, R. T. & Britton, P. G. (1977) Psychological approaches to treatment of the elderly. *Age and Ageing*, **6**, 104–11

CHAPTER 9

Avery, D. & Winokur, G. (1976) Mortality in depressed patients treated with electroconvulsive therapy and antidepressants. *Arch. gen. Psychiat.*, **33**, 1029–37

Barker, J. C. & Baker, A. A. (1959) Deaths associated with electroplexy. *J. ment. Sci.*, **105**, 339–48

Barraclough, B. M. & Mitchell-Heggs, N. (1978) Use of neurosurgery for psychological disorders in British Isles during 1974–76. *Brit. med. J.*, **2**, 1591–3

Bond, M. R. (1975) Assessment of the psychosocial outcome after severe head injury. In *Outcome of Severe Damage to the Cen-*

tral Nervous System. Ciba Foundation Symposium, No. 34 (new series), 141–57. Elsevier Excerpta Medica. Amsterdam, Oxford, New York: North Holland

Bond, M. R. & Brooks, D. N. (1976) Understanding the process of recovery as a basis for the investigation of rehabilitation for the brain injured. *Scand. J. rehab. Med.*, **8**, 127–33

Bridges, P. K. (1972) Psychosurgery today: psychiatric aspects. *Proc. R. Soc. Med.*, **65**, 40–4

Bridges, P. K. & Bartlett, J. R. (1977) Review article: Psychosurgery: Yesterday and Today. *Brit. J. Psychiat.*, **131**, 249–60

British Medical Journal (1980) see Leader (1980)

Carlsson, C. A., von Essen, C. & Löfgren, J. (1968) Factors affecting the clinical course of patients with severe head injuries. *J. Neurosurg.*, **29**, 242–51

Cartlidge, N. E. F. (1978) Post-concussional syndrome. *Scot. med. J.*, **23** (i), 103

Cronholm, B. & Molander, M. (1964) Memory disturbances after electroconvulsive therapy. *Acta psychiat. neurol. scand.*, **40**, 212–16

Dikmen, S. & Reitan, R. M. (1977) Emotional sequelae of head injury. *Ann. Neurol.*, **6**, 492–4

Donnelly, J. (1978) The incidence of psychosurgery in the United States, 1971–1973. *Amer. J. Psychiat.*, **135**, 1476–79

Eson, M. E., Yen, J. K. & Bourke, R. S. (1978) Assessment of recovery from serious head injury. *J. Neurol. Neurosurg. Psychiat.*, **41**, 1036–42

Fahy, T. J., Irving, M. H. & Millac, P. (1967), Severe head injuries. *Lancet*, **ii**, 475–9

Field, J. H. (1976) *A study of the epidemiology of head injury in England and Wales, with particular application to rehabilitation.* London: HMSO

Fortuny, L. A. I., Briggs, M., Newcombe, F., Ratcliff, G. & Thomas, C. (1980) Measuring the duration of post-traumatic amnesia. *J. Neurol. Neurosurg. Psychiat.*, **43**, 377–9

Freeman, C. P. L. (1979) Electroconvulsive therapy: its current clinical use. *Brit. J. hosp. Med.*, **21**, 281–92

Freeman, C. P. L. & Kendell, R. E. (1980) ECT: I: Patients' experiences and attitudes. *Brit. J. Psychiat.*, **137**, 8–16

Freeman, C. P. L., Weeks, D. & Kendell, R. E. (1980) ECT: II: Patients who complain. *Brit. J. Psychiat.*, **137**, 17–25

Freeman, W. & Watts, J. W. (1942) *Psychosurgery.* Springfield, Ill.: Thomas

Gill, D. & Lambourn, J. (1979) Indications for electric convulsion therapy and its use by senior psychiatrists. *Brit. med. J.*, **1**, 1169–71

Göktepe, E. O., Young, L. B. & Bridges, P. K. (1975) A further review of the results of stereotactic subcaudate tractotomy. *Brit. J. Psychiat.*, **126**, 270–80

Goldstein, K. (1942) *After Effects of Brain Injuries in War.* New York: Grune & Stratton

— (1952) The effect of brain-damage on personality. *Psychiat.*, **15**, 245–60

Gomez, J. (1975) Subjective side-effects of E.C.T. *Brit. J. Psychiat.*, **127**, 609–11

Grahame-Smith, D. G., Green, A. R., & Costain, D. W. (1978) Mechanism of the antidepressant action of electroconvulsive therapy. *Lancet* **i**, 254–6

Greenblatt, M., Grosser, G. H. & Wechsler, H. (1964) Differential response of hospitalised depressed patients to somatic therapy. *Amer. J. Psychiat.*, **120**, 935–43.

Harrison, M. S. (1956) Notes on the clinical features and pathology

of post-concussional vertigo with especial reference to positional nystagmus. *Brain*, **79**, 474–86

Heshe, J. & Roeder, E. (1976) Electroconvulsive therapy in Denmark. *Brit. J. Psychiat.*, **128**, 241–5

Jamieson, K. G. & Kelly, D. (1973) Crash helmets reduce head injuries. *Med. J. Austral.*, **2**, 806–9

Jane, J. & Rimel, R. (1979) An assessment of recovery following head trauma. (Personal communication)

Jennett, W. B. & Bond, M. R. (1975) Assessment of outcome after severe brain damage. *Lancet* **i**, 480–4

Jennett, W. B. & MacMillan, R. (1981) Epidemiology of head injury. *Brit. med. J.*, **282**, 101–4

Jennett, W. B. & Plum, F. (1972) Persistent vegetative state after brain damage. *Lancet* **i**, 734–7

Jennett, W. B. & Teasdale, G. (1981). Assessment of outcome. In *Management of Head Injuries*, chap. 13, 301–17, Philadelphia: Davis

Kelly, D. H. W. & Mitchell-Heggs, N. (1973) Stereotactic leucotomy – a follow-up study of thirty patients. *Postgrad. med. J.*, **49**, 865–82

Kelly, D. H. W., Richardson, A. & Mitchell-Heggs, N. (1973) Stereotactic limbic leucotomy, neurophysiological aspects and operative technique. *Brit. J. Psychiat.*, **123**, 133–40

Kendell, R. E. (1978) Electroconvulsive therapy. *Editorial. J. R. Soc. Med.*, **71**, 319–21

Kiloh, L. G., Child, J. P. & Latner, G. (1960) Endogenous depression treated with Iproniazid – a follow-up study. *J. ment. Sci.*, **106**, 1425–8

Knight, G. C. (1964) The orbital cortex as an objective in the surgical treatment of mental illness: the results of 450 cases of open operation and the development of the stereotactic approach. *Brit. J. Surg.*, **51**, 114–24

— (1973) Further observations from an experience of 660 cases of stereotactic tractotomy. *Postgrad. med. J.*, **49**, 485

Leader (1952) Frontal lobes of the human brain. *Lancet* **i**, 407

Leader (1980) Effects of electric convulsion therapy. *Brit. med. J.*, **281**, 1588

Le Beau, J. (1952) The cingular and precingular areas in psychosurgery (agitated behaviour, obsessive compulsive states, epilepsy.). *Acta psychiat. neurol. scand.*, **27**, 305–16

Levin, H. S., Grossman, R. G., Rose, J. E. & Teasdale, G. (1979) Long-term neuropsychological outcome of closed head injury. *J. Neurosurg.*, **50**, 412–22

Lishman, W. A. (1966) Psychiatric disability after head injury: the significance of brain damage. *Proc. R. Soc. Med.*, **59**, 261–6

Lishman, W. A. (1968) Brain damage in relation to psychiatric disability after head injury. *Brit. J. Psychiat.*, **114**, 373–410

— (1973) The psychiatric sequelae of head injury: a review. *Psychol. Med.*, **3**, 304–18

London, P. S. (1967) Some observations on the cause of events after severe injury of the head. *Ann. R. Coll. Surg. Eng.*, **41**, 460–79

McKinlay, W. W., Brooks, D. N., Bond, M. R., Martinage, D. & Marshall, M. M. (1981) Outcome of severe blunt head injury as reported by the relatives of the injured person. *J. Neurol. Neurosurg. Psychiat.*, **44**, 527–33

Mandelberg, I. A. & Brooks, D. N. (1975) Cognitive recovery after severe head injury. *J. Neurol. Neurosurg. Psychiat.*, **38**, 1121–6

Miller, H. (1961). Accident neurosis. *Brit. med. J.*, **1**, 919–25.

Mitchell-Heggs, N., Kelly, D. H. W. & Richardson, A. (1976) Stereotactic limbic leucotomy – a follow-up at 16 months. *Brit. J. Psychiat.*, **128**, 226–40

Moniz, E. (1936) Les premières tentatives opératoires dans le traitement de certaines psychoses. *L'Encéphale*, **31**, 1

Najenson, T., Mendelson, L., Schecter, I., David, C., Mintz, N. & Groswasser, Z. (1974). Rehabilitation after severe head injury. *Scand. J. Rehab.*, **6**, 5–14

Newcombe, F., Hiorns, R. W., Marshall, J. C. & Adams, C. B. T. (1975) Acquired dyslexia: patterns of deficit and recovery. In *Outcome of Severe Damage to the Central Nervous System. Ciba Foundation Symposium. No. 34 (new series)*, 227–44, Elsevier–Excerpta Medica. Amsterdam: North Holland

Oddy, M., Humphrey, M. & Uttley, D. (1978) Subjective impairment and social recovery after closed head injury. *J. Neurol. Neurosurg. Psychiat.*, **41**, 611–16

O'Dea, J. P. K., Gould, D., Halberg, M. & Wieland, R. G. (1978) Prolactin changes during electroconvulsive therapy. *Am. J. Psychiat.*, **135**, 609–11

Ota, Y. (1969) Psychiatric Studies on Civilian Head Injuries. In *The Late Effects of Head Injury*, ed. Walker, A. E., Caveness, W. F. & Critchley, M., chap. 9. Springfield, Ill.: Thomas

Ottossen, J. O. (1960) Experimental studies of the mode of action of electroconvulsive therapy. *Acta psychiat. neurol. scand.*, **35**, Supp. 145, 140

Panting, A. & Merry, P. H. (1970) Long term rehabilitation of severe head injuries – social and medical support for the patient's family. *Injury*, **2**, 33–6

Papez, J. W. (1937) A proposed mechanism of emotion. *Arch. Neurol. Psychiat., Chicago*, **38**, 725–43

Perrin, G. M. (1961) Cardiovascular aspects of E.C.T. *Acta psychiat. neurol. scand.*, **36**, Supp. 153

Post, F., Linford Rees, W. & Schurr, P. H. (1968) Evaluation of bimedial leucotomy. *Brit. J. Psychiat.*, **114**, 1223–46

Reitan, M. R. & Davison, L. A. (1974) *Clinical Neuropsychology: Current Status and Applications*. Washington, D.C.: Winston

Roberts, A. H. (1976) The long-term prognosis of severe accidental head injury. *Proc. R. Soc. Med.*, **69**, 137–41

Romano, M. D. (1974) Family response to traumatic head injury. *Scand. J. rehab.*, **6**, 1–4

Rosenbaum, M. & Najenson, T. (1976) Changes in life patterns and symptoms of low mood as reported by wives of severely brain-injured soldiers. *J. consult. clin. Psychol.*, **44**, 881–8

Royal College of Psychiatrists (1977) Memorandum on the use of electroconvulsive therapy. *Brit. J. Psychiat.*, **131**, 261–72

Russell, W. R. (1932) Cerebral involvement in head injury. *Brain*, **55**, 549–603

Russell, W. R. & Smith, A. (1961) Post-traumatic amnesia in closed head injury. *Arch. Neurol.*, **5**, 16–29

Scoville, W. B. (1949). Selective cortical undercutting as a means of modifying and studying frontal lobe function in man: a preliminary report of 43 operative cases. *J. Neurosurg.*, **6**, 65–73

Squire, L. R. & Chance, P. M. (1975) Memory functions six to nine months after electroconvulsive therapy. *Arch. gen. Psychiat.*, **32**, 1557–64

Ström-Olsen, R. & Carlisle, S. (1971) Bi-frontal stereotactic tractotomy: a follow-up study of its effects in 210 patients. *Brit. J. Psychiat.*, **118**, 141–54

Taylor, A. R. & Bell, T. K. (1966) Slowing of cerebral circulation after concussional head injury. *Lancet*, ii, 178–80

Teasdale, G. & Jennett, W. B. (1974) Assessment of coma and impaired consciousness: a practical scale. *Lancet*, ii, 81–3

Thomsen, I. (1974) The patient with severe head injury and his family. *Scand. J. rehab. Med.*, **6**, 180–3

Toglia, J. U. (1969) Dizziness after whiplash injury of the neck and closed head injury: electronystagmographic correlations. In *The Late Effects of Head Injury*, ed. Walker, A. E., Caveness, W. F. & Critchley, M., chap. 6. Springfield, Ill.: Thomas

Tow, P. M. (1952) Therapeutic trauma of the brain. *Lancet*, ii, 253–5

Valentine, M., Keddie, K. M. G. & Dunne, D. (1968) A comparison of techniques in electroconvulsive therapy. *Brit. J. Psychiat.*, **114**, 989–96

Weddell, R., Oddy, M. & Jenkins, D. L. (1979) Social adjustment after rehabilitation. A two year follow-up of patients with severe head injury. *Psychol. Med.*, **10**, 257–63

Weeks, D., Freeman, C. P. L. & Kendell, R. E. (1980) ECT: III: Enduring cognitive deficits? *Brit. J. Psychiat.*, **137**, 26–37

Whitty, C. W. M., Duffield, J. E., Tow, P. M. & Cairns, H. (1952) Anterior cingulectomy in the treatment of mental disease. *Lancet*, i, 475–81

Yen, J. K., Bourke, R. S., Nelson, L. R. & Popp, A. J. (1978). Numerical grading of clinical neurological status after serious head injury. *J. Neurol. Neurosurg. Psychiat.*, **41**, 1125–30

CHAPTER 10

Adams, R. D. & Victor, M. (1977) *Principles of Neurology*, p. 520. New York: McGraw Hill

Albert, M. L., Feldman, R. G. & Willis, A. L. (1974) The 'subcortical dementia' of progressive supranuclear palsy. *J. Neurol. Neurosurg. Psychiat.*, **37**, 121–30

Alzheimer, A. (1907) Über eine eigenartige Erkrankung der Hirnrinde. *Allg. Zeitschr. Psychiat.*, **64**, 146–8

Asnis, G. (1977) Parkinson's disease, a review and case study. *Amer. J. Psychiat.* **134**, 191–5

Bear, D. M. & Fedio, P. (1977) Quantitative analysis of interictal behavior in temporal lobe epilepsy. *Arch. Neurol.*, **34**, 454–67

Blessed, G., Tomlinson, B. E. & Roth, M. (1968) The association between quantitative measures of dementia and of senile change in the cerebral grey matter of elderly subjects. *Brit. J. Psychiat.*, **114**, 797–811

Bruyn, G. W. (1968) Huntington's chorea: Historical, clinical, and laboratory synopsis. In *Handbook of Clinical Neurology*, ed. Vinken, P. J. & Bruyn, G. W., vol. 6, pp. 298–378. Amsterdam: North Holland

Bruyn, G. W., Bots, G. Th. A. M. & Dom, R. (1979) Huntington's chorea: current neuropathological status. In *Advances in Neurology*, ed. Chase, T. N., Wexler, N. S. & Barbeau, A. vol. 23, *Huntington's Disease*, pp. 83–93 New York: Raven Press

Burch, P. R. J. (1979) Huntington's disease: types, frequency and progression. In *Advances in Neurology*, ed. Chase, T. N., Wexler, N. S. & Barbeau, A., vol. 23, *Huntington's Disease*, pp. 43–57. New York: Raven Press

Butters, N., Albert, M. S. & Sax, D. (1979) Investigations of memory disorders of patients with Huntington's disease. In *Advances in Neurology*, ed. Chase, T. N., Wexler, N. S. & Barbeau, A., vol. 23, *Huntington's Disease*, pp. 203–13. New York: Raven Press

Carlson, R. J. (1977) Frontal lobe lesions masquerading as psychiatric disturbances. *Can. Psychiat. Ass. J.*, **22**, 315–18

Constantinidis, J. (1978) Is Alzheimer's disease a major form of senile dementia? Clinical, anatomical and genetic data. In *Alzheimer's Disease: Senile Dementia and Related Disorders*, ed. Katzman, R., Terry, R. D. & Bick, K. L., pp. 15–27. New York: Raven Press

Dewhurst, K., Oliver, J., Trick, K. L. K. & McKnight, A. L. (1969) Neuro-psychiatric aspects of Huntington's disease. *Confin. neurol.*, **31**, 258–68

Flekkoy, K. (1976) Visual agnosia and cognitive defects in a case of Alzheimer's disease. *Biol. Psychiat.*, **11**, 333–44

Foix, C., & Nicolesco, J. (1925) *Les noyaux gris centraux et la région mésencéphalo-sous-optique.* Paris: Masson

Folstein, M. F., Maiberger, R. & McHugh, P. R. (1977) Mood disorder as a specific complication of stroke. *J. Neurol. Neurosurg. Psychiat.*, **40**, 1018–20

Folstein, S. E., Folstein, M. F. & McHugh, P. R. (1979) Psychiatric syndromes in Huntington's disease. In *Advances in Neurology*, ed. Chase, T. N., Wexler, N. S. & Barbeau, A. vol. 23, Huntington's Disease. pp. 281–9. New York: Raven Press

Froehlich, A. (1901) Ein Fall von Tumor der Hypophysis Cerebri ohne Akromegalie. *Klin. Rundschau (Wien)*, **15**, 833

Goldstein, K. (1975) Functional disturbances in brain damage. In *American Handbook of Psychiatry*, ed. Reiser, M. F., pp. 182–207. New York: Basic Books

Goodwin, F. K. (1971) Psychiatric side effects of levodopa in man. *J. Amer. Med. Ass.*, **218**, 1915–20

Gruenberg, E. (1978) Epidemiology. In Katzman, R., Terry, R. D. & Bick, K. L. (Eds.), *Alzheimer's Disease: Senile Dementia and Related Disorders*, ed. Katzman, R., Terry, R. D. & Bick, K. L., pp. 323–6. New York: Raven Press

Hachinski, V. C., Lassen, N. A. & Marshall, J. (1974) Multi-infarct dementia: a cause of mental deterioration in the elderly. *Lancet*, ii, 207–10

Hécaen, H. & Ajuriaguerra, J. De (1956) *Troubles mentaux au cours des tumeurs intracraniennes.* Paris: Masson

Hunter, R., Blackwood, W. & Bull, J. (1968) Three cases of frontal meningiomas presenting psychiatrically. *Brit. med. J.*, **3**, 9–16

Huntington, G. (1872) On chorea. *Med. Surg., Rep.*, **26**, 317–32

Jacob, H. (1970). Muscular twitchings in Alzheimer's disease. In *Alzheimer's Disease and Related Conditions*, ed. Wolstenholme, G. E. W. & O'Connor, M., pp. 75–93. London: Churchill

Larsson, T., Sjögren, T. & Jacobson, G. (1963) Senile dementia: a clinical sociomedical and genetic study. *Acta psychiatr. scand.*, Supp. **167**, 1–259

Lauter, H., & Meyer, J. E. (1968) Clinical and nosological concepts of senile dementia. In *Senile Dementia: Clinical and Therapeutic Aspects*, ed. Muller, C. H. & Ciompi, L., pp. 13–27. Berne: Huber

Levy, R. (1978) Neurophysiological disturbances associated with psychiatric disorders in old age. In *Studies in Geriatric Psychiatry*, ed. Isaacs, A. D. & Post, F., pp. 169–87. Chichester: Wiley

Lewin, K., Mattingly, D. & Millis, R. R. (1972) Anorexia nervosa associated with hypothalamic tumour. *Brit. med. J.*, **2**, 629–30

Lieberman, A., Dziatolowski, M., Neophytides, A., Kupersmith, M., Aleksic, S., Serby, M., Korein, J. & Goldstein, M. (1979) Dementias of Huntington's and Parkinson's disease. In *Advances in Neurology*, ed. Chase, T. N., Wexler, N. S. & Barbeau, A., vol. 23, *Huntington's Disease*, pp. 273–89. New York: Raven Press

Lhermitte, J. (1922) Syndrome de la calotte pédonculaire. *Rev. Neurol.*, **38**, 1359–65

Lishman, W. A. (1978) (Ed.), *Organic Psychiatry*, p. 753. Oxford: Blackwell

Loranger, A. W., Goodell, H., McDowell, F. H., Lee, J. E. & Sweet, R. D. (1972) Intellectual impairment in Parkinson's syndrome. *Brain*, **95**, 405–12

McHugh, P. R. (1964) Occult hydrocephalus. *Q. J. Med.*, **33**, 297–308

— (1966) Hydrocephalic dementia. *Bull. N.Y. Acad. Med.*, **42**, 907–17

McHugh, P. R. & Folstein, M. F. (1975) Psychiatric syndromes of Huntington's chorea: a clinical and phenomenologic study. In *Psychiatric Aspects of Neurologic Disease*, ed. Benson, D. F. & Blumer, D., pp. 267–85. New York: Grune & Stratton

— (1979) Psychopathology of dementia: implications for neuropathology. In *Congenital and Acquired Cognitive Disorders*, ed. Katzman, R., pp. 17–30. New York: Raven Press

McMenemey, W. H. (1966) The dementias and progressive diseases of the basal ganglia. In *Greenfield's Neuropathology*, ed. Blackwood, W., McMenemey, W. H., Meyer, A., Norman, R. M. & Russell, D. S., pp. 520–76. Baltimore: Williams & Wilkins

Malamud, N. (1967) Psychiatric disorder with intracranial tumor of the limbic system. *Arch. Neurol.*, **17**, 113–23

Marrtilla, R. J. & Rinne, U. K. (1976) Dementia in Parkinson's disease. *Acta neurol. scand.*, **54**, 431–41

Mindham, R. H. (1974) Psychiatric aspects of Parkinson's disease. *Brit. J. hosp. Med.*, **11**, 411–14

Mindham, R. H. S., Marsden, C. D. & Parkes, J. D. (1976). Psychiatric symptoms during L-dopa therapy for Parkinson's disease and their relationship to physical disability. *Psychol. Med.*, **6**, 23–33

Newton, R. D. (1948) The identity of Alzheimer's disease and senile dementia and their relationship to senility. *J. ment. Sci.*, **94**, 225–49

Parkinson, J. (1817) *An Essay on the Shaking Palsy*, pp. 1–66. London: Whittingham & Rowland

Reed, T. E. & Chandler, J. H. (1958) Huntington's chorea in Michigan. I. Demography and genetics. *Amer. J. hum. Genet.*, **10**, 201–25

Reeves, A. G. & Plum, F. (1969) Hyperphagia, rage, and dementia accompanying a ventromedial hypothalamic neoplasm. *Arch. Neurol.* **20**, 616–24

Robinson, R. G. & Szetela, B. (1981) Mood change following left hemispheric brain injury. *Ann. Neurol.*, (in press)

Sacks, O. W. (1976) *Awakenings.* Harmondsworth, Middlsex: Penguin Books

Shoulson, I. (1977) Clinical care of the patient and family with Huntington's disease. *Report, The Commission for the Control of Huntington's Disease and its Consequences.* Vol. II, Technical Report, pp. 421–42. US Dept. HEW

Sjögren, T., Sjögren, E. & Lindgren, A. G. H. (1952) Clinical analysis of morbus Alzheimer and morbus Pick. *Acta psychiat. neurol. scand.*, Supp. **82**, 69–118

Smith, R. A., Gelles, D. B. & Vanderhaeghen, J. J. (1971) Subcortical visual hallucinations. *Cortex*, **7**, 162–8

Streletzki, F. (1961) Psychosen in Verlauf der Huntingtonschen Chorea unter besonderer Berucksichtigung der Wahnbildungen. *Arch. Psychiat. Nerv.*, **202**, 202–14

Surridge, D. (1969) An investigation into some psychiatric aspects of multiple sclerosis. *Brit. J. Psychiat.*, **115**, 749–64

Sweet, R. D., McDowell, F. H., Feigenson, J. S., Lorranger, A. W. & Goodell, H. (1976) Mental symptoms in Parkinson's disease during chronic treatment with levodopa. *Neurology*, **26**, 305–10

Terry, R. D. (1979) Morphological changes in Alzheimer's disease – senile dementia: ultrastructural and quantitative studies. In *Congenital and Acquired Cognitive Disorders*, ed. Katzman R., pp. 99–105. New York: Raven Press

Weingartner, H., Caine, E. D. & Ebert, M. H. (1979) Encoding processes, learning and recall in Huntington's disease. In *Advances in Neurology*, ed. Chase, T. N., Wexler, N. S., & Barbeau, A., vol. 23, *Huntington's Disease*, pp. 215–26. New York: Raven Press

Wilson, R. S. & Garron, D. C. (1979) Cognitive and affective aspects of Huntington's disease. In *Advances in Neurology*, ed. Chase, T. N., Wexler, N. S. & Barbeau, A., vol. 23, *Huntington's Disease*, pp. 193–201. New York: Raven Press

CHAPTER 11

Ackner, B., Cooper, J. E., Gray, C. H. & Kelly M. (1962) Acute porphyria: a neuropsychiatric and biochemical study. *J. psychosom. Res.*, **6**, 1–24

Bademosi, O., Falase, A. O., Jaiyesimi, F. & Bademosi, A. (1976) Neuropsychiatric manifestations of infective endocarditis: a study of 95 patients at Ibadan, Nigeria. *J. Neurol. Neurosurg. Psychiat.*, **39**, 325–9

Bleuler, M. (1951) Psychiatry of cerebral disease. *Brit. med. J.*, **2**, 1233–8

Bonhoeffer, K. (1909) Zur Frage der exogenen Psychosen. Translated in *Themes and Variations in European Psychiatry*, ed. Hirsch, S. R. & Shepherd, M., pp. 47–52. Bristol: Wright

— (1917) Die exogenen Reaktionstypen. *Arch. Psychiat. Nervenkrankh.*, **58**, 58–70

Chedru, F. & Geschwind, N. (1972) Disorders of higher cortical functions in acute confusional states. *Cortex*, **8**, 395–411

Committee on Safety of Medicines (1974) *Register of Adverse Reactions*, vol. 3, p. 83. Medicine and Food Division of Department of Health and Social Security

Curran, F. J. & Schilder, P. (1935) Paraphasic signs in diffuse lesions of the brain. *J. nerv. ment. Dis.*, **82**, 613–36

Cutting, J. C. (1978) Study of anosognosia. *J. Neurol. Neurosurg. Psychiat.*, **41**, 548–55

— (1980) Physical illness and psychosis. *Brit. J. Psychiat.*, **136**, 109–19

Daroff, R. B., Deller, J. J., Kastl, A. J. & Blocker, W. W. (1967) Cerebral malaria. *J. Amer. med. Ass.*, **202**, 679–82

De Jong, R. N. (1977) CNS manifestations of diabetes mellitus. *Postgrad. Med.*, **61**, 101–7

de Wardener, H. E. (1946) Cholera epidemic among prisoners-of-war in Siam. *Lancet*, **i**, 637–40

Diefendorf, A. R. (1912) Mental symptoms of acute chorea. *J. nerv. ment. Dis.*, **39**, 161–72

Dixon, H. B. F. & Lipscombe, F. M. (1961) Cysticercosis: an analysis and follow-up of 450 cases. *Medical Research Council Special Report Series (London)* No. 299

Dongier, S. (1959) Statistical study of clinical and electroencephalographic manifestations of 536 psychotic episodes occurring in 516 epileptics between clinical seizures. *Epilepsia*, **1**, 117–42

Engel, G. L. & Romano, J. (1959) Delirium, a syndrome of cerebral insufficiency. *J. chron. Dis.*, **9**, 260–77

Gamper, E. (1929) Schlaf – Delirium Tremens – Korsakowsches Syndrom. *Zentralbl. Neurol. Psychiat.*, **51**, 236–9

Gross, M. M., Goodenough, D., Tobin, M., Halpert, E. Lepore, D., Perlstein, A., Sirota, M., Dibianco, J., Fuller, R. & Kischner,
I. (1966) Sleep disturbances and hallucinations in the acute alcoholic psychoses. *J. nerv. ment. Dis.*, **142**, 493–514

Guttmann, O. (1952) Psychic disturbances in typhus fever. *Psychiat. Q.*, **26**, 478–91

Halpern, H., Darley, F. L. & Brown, J. R. (1973) Differential language and neurological characteristics in cerebral involvement. *Speech Hear. Disord.*, **38**, 162–73

Hinton, J. & Withers, E. (1971) The usefulness of clinical tests of the sensorium. *Brit. J. Psychiat.*, **119**, 9–18

Ives, E. R. (1963) Mental aberrations in diabetic patients. *Bull. Los Angeles Neurol. Soc.*, **28**, 279–85

Jenkyn, L. R., Walsh, D. B., Culver, C. M. & Reeves, A. G. (1977) Clinical signs in diffuse cerebral dysfunction. *J. Neurol. Neurosurg. Psychiat.*, **40**, 956–66

Kanner, L. (1972) *Child Psychiatry*, 4th ed., pp. 329–33. Springfield, Ill.: Thomas

Kind, H. (1958) Die Psychiatrie der hypophyseninsuffizienz speziell der Simmondsschen Krankheit. *Fortschr. Neurol. Psychiat.*, **26**, 501–63

Kornfeld, D. S., Zimberg, S. & Malm, J. R. (1965) Psychiatric complications of open-heart surgery. *New Eng. J. Med.*, **273**, 287–92

Layne, O. L. & Yudofsky, S. C. (1971) Postoperative psychosis in cardiotomy patients. *New Eng. J. Med.*, **284**, 518–20

Lazarus, H. R. & Hagens, J. H. (1968) Prevention of psychosis following open-heart surgery. *Amer. J. Psychiat.*, **124**, 1190–5

Levin, M. (1956) Thinking disturbances in delirium. *Arch. Neurol. Psychiat.*, **75**, 62–6

Levine, P. M., Silberfarb, P. M. & Lipowski, Z. J. (1978) Mental disorders in cancer patients. *Cancer*, **42**, 1385–91

Lipowski, Z. J. (1967) Delirium, clouding of consciousness and confusion. *J. nerv. ment. Dis.*, **145**, 227–5

— (1978) Organic brain syndromes: a reformulation. *Compr. Psychiat.*, **19**, 309–22

Lishman, W. A. (1978) *Organic Psychiatry*. Oxford: Blackwell

McClelland, H. A. (1978) Drug-induced delirium. *Adverse Drug Reaction Bull.*, **72**, 256–9

Manson-Bahr, P. H. (1968) *Manson's Tropical Diseases*. London: Baillière, Tindall & Cassell

Mesulam, M. M., Waxman, S. G., Geschwind, N. & Sabin, T. D. (1976) Acute confusional states with right middle cerebral artery infarction. *J. Neurol. Neurosurg. Psychiat.*, **39**, 84–9

Morse, R. M. & Litin, E. M. (1969) Postoperative delirium: a study of etiologic factors. *Amer. J. Psychiat.*, **126**, 388–95

Obrecht, R., Okhomina, F. O. A. & Scott, D. F. (1979) Value of EEG in acute confusional states. *J. Neurol. Neurosurg. Psychiat.*, **42**, 75–7

Osuntokun, B. O., Bademosi, O., Ogunremi, K. & Wright, S. G. (1972) Neuropsychiatric manifestations of typhoid fever in 959 patients. *Arch. Neurol.*, **27**, 7–13

Pai, M. N. (1945) Changes in personality after cerebrospinal fever. *Brit. med. J.*, **i**, 289–93

Peters, U. H. & Gille, G. (1973) Über die körperlichen Gründe körperlich begründbarer Psychosen. *Deutsche med. Wochenschr.*, **98**, 967–70

Peterson, P. (1968) Psychiatric disorders in 1° hyperparathyroidism. *J. clin. Endocrinol.*, **28**, 1491–5

Roger, H. & Poursines, Y. (1951) Formes psychosiques des méningo-neuro-brucelloses. *Ann. méd.-psychol.*, **109**, 145–69

Service, F. J., Dale, A. J. D., Elveback, L. R. & Jiang, N-S. (1976) Insulinoma: clinical and diagnostic features of 60 consecutive cases. *Mayo Clinic Proc.*, **51**, 417–29

Shapiro, M. B., Post, F., Löfving, B. & Inglis, J. (1956) 'Memory function' in psychiatric patients over 60, some methodological and diagnostic implications. *J. ment. Sci.*, **102**, 233–46

Smith, J. S. & Brandon, S. (1970) Acute carbon monoxide poisoning – 3 years experience in a defined population. *Postgrad. med. J.*, **46**, 65–70

Stenbäck, A. & Haapanen, E. (1967) Azotaemia and psychosis. *Acta psychiat. scand., Supp.*, 197

Summerskill, W. H. J., Davidson, E. A., Sherlock, S. & Steiner, R. E. (1956) The neuropsychiatric syndrome associated with hepatic cirrhosis and an extensive portal collateral circulation. *Q. J. Med.*, **25**, 245–66

Titchener, J. L., Zwerling, I., Gottschalk, L., Levine, M., Culbertson, W., Cohen, S. & Silver, H. (1956) Psychosis in surgical patients. *Surg. Gynecol. Obstet.*, **102**, 59–65

Toro, G. & Roman, G. (1978) Cerebral malaria. *Arch. Neurol.*, **35**, 271–5

Wade, O. L. & Beeley, L. (1976) *Adverse Reactions to Drugs*. 2nd ed. London: Heinemann

Weinstein, E. A. & Kahn, R. L. (1952) Non-aphasic misnaming (paraphasia) in organic brain disease. *Arch. Neurol. Psychiat.*, **67**, 72–9

Williams, M. & Smith, H. V. (1954) Mental disturbances in tuberculous meningitis. *J. Neurol. Neurosurg. Psychiat.*, **17**, 173–82

Williams, R. (1973) Hepatic encephalopathy. *J. R. Coll. Physicians London*, **8**, 63–74

Wilson, L. M. (1972) Intensive care delirium. *Arch. int. Med.*, **130**, 225–6

Wolff, H. G. & Curran, D. (1935) Nature of delirium and allied states. *Arch. Neurol. Psychiat.*, **33**, 1175–215

CHAPTER 12

Abramowicz, M. (1976) Drugs for improvement of cerebral function in the elderly. *Med. Lett.*, **18**, 38–9

Adams, R. D. (1975) Recent observations on normal pressure hydrocephalus. *Schweiz. Arch. Neurol. Neurochim. Psychiat.*, **116**, 7–15

Adams, R., Fisher, C., Hakim, S., Ojemann, R. & Sweet, W. (1965) Symptomatic occult hydrocephalus with 'normal' cerebrospinal-fluid pressure. A treatable syndrome. *New Eng. J. Med.*, **273**, 117

Aderman, M., Giardina, W. J. & Koreniowski, S. (1972) Effect of cyclandelate on perception, memory, and cognition in a group of geriatric subjects. *J. Amer. Geriat. Soc.*, **6**, 268–71

Adolfson, R., Gottfries, C., Roos, B. & Winblad, B. (1979) Changes in the brain catecholamines in patients with dementia of Alzheimer type. *Brit. J. Psychiat.*, **135**, 216–23

Alzheimer, A. (1898) Neuere Arbeiten über die Dementia senilis und die auf atheromatoser Gefässerkrankung basierenden Gehirnkrankheiten. *Monatsschr. Psychiat. Neurol.*, **3**, 101–15
— (1911) Über eigenartige Krankheitsfälle des späteren Alters. *Zeitschr. ges. Neurol. Psychiat.*, **4**, 356–85

American Psychiatric Association (1952) *Diagnostic and Statistical Manual of Mental Disorder, 1st ed.* Washington, D.C.

American Psychiatric Association (1980) *Diagnostic and Statistical Manual of Mental Disorders, 3rd ed.* Washington, D.C.: APA

Asnis, A. (1977) Parkinson's disease, depression and ECT. *Amer. J. Psychiat.*, **134**, 191–5

Ball, M. (1977) Neuronal loss, neurofibrillary tangles and granulovacuolar degeneration in the hippocampus with ageing and dementia. *Acta neuropathol.*, **37**, 11–18

Baltes, M., & Zerbe, M. (1976) Independence training in nursing-home residents. *Gerontologist*, **16**, 428–32

Barnes, R., Raskind, M., Scott, M. & Murphy, C. (1981) Problems of families caring for Alzheimer patients: use of a support group. *J. Amer. Geriat. Soc.*, **29**, 80–5

Baron, S., Jacobs, L. & Kinkel, W. (1976) Changes in size of normal lateral ventricles during aging determined by computerized tomography, *Neurol.*, **26**, 1011–13

Bazo, A. J. (1973) An ergot alkaloid preparation (Hydergine) versus papaverine in treating common complaints of the elderly: double blind study. *J. Amer. Geriat. Soc.*, **21**, 63

Bergmann, K., & Eastham, E. (1974) Psychogeriatric ascertainment and assessment for treatment in an acute medical war setting. *Age and Ageing*, **3**, 174–88

Binder, R. L. & Dickman, W. A. (1980) Psychiatric manifestations of neurosyphilis in middle-aged patients. *Amer. J. Psychiat.*, **137**, 741–2

Binswanger, O. (1894) Die Abgrenzung der allgemeinen progressiven Paralyse. *Berliner klin. Wochenschr.*, **31**, 1137–9

Birkett, D. P. (1971) Vasodilators in geriatric psychiatry. *J. med. Soc. N.J.*, **68**, 619–23
— (1972) The psychiatric differentation of senility and arteriosclerosis. *Brit. J. Psychiat.*, **120**, 321–5

Birkett, D. P. & Boltuch, B. (1973a) Psychotropic drugs in old age. *J. Med. Soc. N.J.*, **70**, 647–8
— (1972) Chlorpromazine in geriatric psychiatry, *J. Amer. Geriat. Soc.*, **20**, 403–6
— (1973b) Remotivation therapy. *J. Amer. Geriat. Soc.*, **21**, 368–71

Birkett, D. P. & Raskin, A. Arteriosclerosis, dementia and infarcts. *J. Amer. Geriat. Soc.* (in press)

Birkett, D. P., Hirschfield, W. & Simpson, G. M. (1972) Thiothixene in the treatment of diseases of the senium. *Curr. ther. Res.*, **14**, 775–9

Blackman, D., Howe, M. & Pinkston, E. (1976) Increasing participation in social interaction in the institutionalized elderly. *Gerontologist*, **16**, 69

Blessed, G., Tomlinson, B. E. & Roth, M. (1968) The association between quantitative measures of dementia and of senile dementia in the cerebral grey matter of elderly subjects. *Brit. J. Psychiat.*, **114**, 797–811

Bowen, D. & Davison, A. (1980) Biochemical changes in the cholinergic system of the ageing brain and in senile dementia. *Psychol. Med.*, **10**, 315–19

Bowen, D., Smith, C., White, P. & Davison, A. (1976) Neurotransmitter-related enzymes and indices of hypoxia in senile dementia and other abiotrophies. *Brain*, **99**, 459–96

Bowen, D., White, P., Flack, R., Smith, C. & Davison, A. (1974) Brain-decarboxylase activities as indices of pathological change in senile dementia. *Lancet*, **i**, 1247–9

Bowen, D., White P., Spillane, J., Goodhardt, M., Curzon, G., Iwangoff, P., Meier-Ruge, W. & Davison, A. (1979) Accelerated ageing or selective neuronal loss as an important cause of dementia? *Lancet*, **i**, 11–14

Boyd, W. D., Graham-White, J., Blackwood, G., Glen, J. & McQueen, J. (1977) Clinical effects of choline in Alzheimer's disease. *Lancet*, **ii**, 711

Briggs, R., Castleden, C. & Alvarez, A. (1981) Normal pressure hydrocephalus in the elderly: a treatable cause of dementia? *Age and Ageing*, **10**, 254–8

Brody, H. (1955) Organization of the cerebral cortex, *J. comp. Neurol.*, **102**, 511–56

Brook, P., Degun, G. & Mather, M. (1975) Reality orientation, *Brit. J. Psychiat.*, **127**, 42–5

Buell, S. & Coleman, P. (1979) Dendritic growth in human brain and failure of growth in senile dementia. *Science*, **206**, 854–5

Burton, M. (1980) Evaluation and change in a psychogeriatric ward through direct observation and feedback. *Brit. J. Psychiat.*, **137**, 566–71

Caird, F. I. (1977) Computerized tomography (Emiscan). *Age and Ageing*, **6** (Supp.), 50–1

Carroll, K. & Gray, K. (1981) Memory development: an approach to the mentally impaired elderly in the long-term care setting. *Int. J. Aging hum. Devel.*, **13**, 15–35

Chierichetti, S., Ferrari, P., Sala, P., Vibelli, C. & Pietrzkowski, A. (1977) Effects of amantadine on mental status of elderly patients: a double blind comparison with placebo. *Curr. ther. Res.*, **22**, 158–65

Christie, J., Blackburn, I., Glen, A., Zeisel, S., Shering, A. & Yates, M. (1979) Effects of choline and lecithin on CSF choline levels and on cognitive function in patients with presenile dementia of the Alzheimer type. In *Nutrition and the Brain*, ed. Barbeau, A., Growdon, J. & Wurtman, R., vol. 5, pp. 377–87. New York: Raven Press

Christie, J. E., Shering, A., Ferguson, J. & Glen, A. I. M. (1981) Physostigmine and arecoline: effects of intravenous infusions in Alzheimer presenile dementia. *Brit. J. Psychiat.*, **138**, 46–50

Citrin, R. & Dixon, D. (1977) Reality orientation: a milieu therapy used in an institution for the aged. *Gerontologist*, **17**, 39–43

Cohen, D. & Eisdorfer, C. (1977) Behavioural immunologic relationships in older men and women. *Exp. Ageing Res.*, **3**, 225–9

Cohen, E. & Wurtman, R. (1975) Brain acetylcholine; increase after systematic choline administration. *Life Sci.*, **16**, 1095–102

Cohen, D., Zeller, E., Eisdorfer, C. & Walford, R. (1979) Alzheimer's disease and the main histocompatibility complex (HLA System). *Gerontologist*, **19**, 57

Commission on Professional and Hospital Activities. (1978) *International Classification of Diseases, 9th Edition; Clinical Modification*. Ann Arbor, Michigan: Commission on Professional and Hospital Activities

Corsellis, J. A. N. (1962) *Mental Illness and the Ageing Brain*. Maudsley Monograph No. 9 London: Oxford University Press

Crapper, D. R., Krishnan, S. S. & Dalton, A. J. (1973) Brain aluminum distribution in Alzheimer's disease and experimental neurofibrillary-degeneration. *Science*, **180**, 511–13

Crockard, H., Hanlon, K., Duda, E. & Mullan, J. (1977) Hydrocephalus as a cause of dementia: evaluation by computerized axial tomography and intracranial pressure monitoring, *J. Neurol. Neurosurg. Psychiat.*, **40**, 735

Crook, T. (1979) Central-nervous-system stimulants: appraisal of use in geropsychiatric patients. *J. Amer. Geriat. Soc.*, **27**, 476–8

Davies, P. & Maloney, L. (1976) Selective loss of central cholinergic neurones in Alzheimer's disease. *Lancet*, **ii**, 1403

Davies, P. & Verth, A. (1977/78) Regional distribution of muscarinic acetylcholine receptor in normal and Alzheimer's type dementia brains. *Brain Res.*, **138**, 385–92

Davis, K., Mohs, R., Tinklenberg, J., Pfefferbaum, A., Hollister, L. & Kopell, B. (1978) Physostigmine: improvement of long term memory processes in normal humans. *Science*, **201**, 272–4

Dennis, H. (1978) Remotivation therapy groups. In *Working With the Elderly: Group Process and Techniques*, ed. Burnside, I. M. North Scituate, Mass.: Duxbury Press

Ditch, M. & Resnick, O. (1971) An ergot preparation (Hydergine) in the treatment of cerebrovascular disorders in the geriatric patient, double blind study. *J. Amer. Geriat. Soc.*, **19**, 208–17

Drachman, D. A. (1978) Memory, dementia and the cholinergic system. In *Alzheimer's Disease: Senile Dementia and Related Disorders*, eds. Katzman, R., Terry, R. D. & Bick, K. L., pp. 141–8. New York: Raven Press

Drachman, D. & Sahakian, B. (1979) Effect of cholinergic agents on human learning and memory. In *Nutrition and the Brain*, ed. Barbeau, A., Growdon, J. & Wurtman, J., vol. 5, pp. 351–66 New York: Raven Press

Drachman, D. & Stahl, S. (1975) Extrapyramidal dementia and levodopa. *Lancet*, **ii**, 809

Drummond, L., Kirchoff, L. & Scarborough, D. (1978) A practical guide to reality orientation. *Gerontologist*, **18**, 563–73

Eisdorfer, C. & Cohen, D. (1980) Serum immunoglobulins and cognitive status in the elderly: 2. An immunological–behavioural relationship? *Brit. J. Psychiat.*, **136**, 40–5

Etienne, P., Gauthier, S., Johnson, G., Collier, B., Mendis, T., Dastoor, D., Cole, M. & Muller, H. (1978) Clinical effects of choline in Alzheimer's disease, *Lancet*, **i**, 508–9

Fine, G. W., Lewis, D., Villa-Lande, I. & Blakemore, C. G. (1970) The effect of cyclandelate on mental functions in patients with arteriosclerotic brain disease. *Brit. J. Psychiat.*, **117**, 157–61

Ford, C. & Winter, J. (1981) Computerized axial tomograms and dementia in elderly patients. *J. Geront.*, **36**, 164–9

Fox, J., Topel, J. & Huckman, S. (1975) Use of computerized tomography in senile dementia. *J. Neurol. Neurosurg. Psychiat.*, **38**, 948–53

Gadjusek, D. C. & Gibbs, C. J. (1975) Slow virus infections of the nervous system and the laboratories of slow, latent and temperate virus infections. In *The Clinical Neurosciences*, ed. Chase, T. N. & Tower, D. B., pp. 113–35. New York: Raven Press

Gadjusek, D. C., Gibbs, C. J., Asher, D. M., Brown, P., Divan, A., Hoffman, P., Memo, G., Rower, R. & White, L. (1977) Precautions in medical care of, and in handling materials from, patients with transmissible virus dementia (Creutzfelt–Jakob disease). *New Eng. J. Med.*, **297**, 1253–8

Geinisman, Y., Bondareff, W. & Telser, A. (1977) Transport of ^{3}H-glucose labelled glycoproteins in the septo-hippocampal pathway of young adult and senescent rats. *Brain Res.*, **125**, 182–6

Gerin, J. (1969) Symptomatic treatment of cerebrovascular insufficiency with hydergine. *Curr. ther. Res.*, **11**, 539–46

Goldfarb, A. I. (1956) The rationale for psychotherapy with older persons. *Amer. J. med. Sci.*, **232**, 181–5

Goldstein, S. E., Birnbom, F., Luncee, W. J. & Darke, A. C. (1978) Comparison of oxazepam, flurazepam, and chloral hydrate. *J. Amer. Geriat. Soc.*, **26**, 366–71

Gruenberg, E. (1978) Epidemiology. In *Alzheimer's Disease: Senile Dementia and Related Disorders*, ed. Katzman, R., Terry, R. D. & Bick, K. L., pp. 323–6. New York: Raven Press

Gunasekera, L. & Richardson, A. (1977) Computerized axial tomography in idiopathic hydrocephalus. *Brain*, **100**, 749

Gurland, B. (1980a) The borderlands of dementia: the influence of socio-cultural characteristics on rates of dementia occurring in the senium. In *Clinical Aspects of Alzheimer's Disease and Senile Dementia*, ed. Miller, Mancy & Cohen, Gene. New York: Raven Press

— (1980) Assessment of the mental health status of older adults. In *Handbook on Mental Health and Aging*, ed. Birren, J. E. & Sloane, R. Englewood, N.J.: Prentice-Hall

Gurland, B., Dean, L., Cross, P. & Golden, R. R. (1980) The epidemiology of depression and dementia in the elderly: the use of multiple indicators of these conditions. In *Psychopathology in the Aged*, ed. Cole, Jonathan O. & Barrett, James. New York: Raven Press

Gurland, B., Dean, L., Gurland, R. & Cook, D. (1978) Personal time dependency in the elderly of New York City: Findings from the US–UK Cross-National Geriatric Community Study. In *Dependency in the Elderly of New York City, Report of a Research Utilization Workshop*. New York: Community Council of Greater New York, March 23

Hachinski, V., Iliff, M., Zilkha, E., Du Boulay, G., McAllister, V., Marshall, J., Ross Russell, R. & Syman, L. (1975) Cerebral blood flow in dementia. *Arch. Neurol.*, **32**, 632–7

Hachinski, V. V., Lassen, N. A. & Marshall, J. (1974) Multi-infarct dementia: a cause of mental deterioration in the elderly. *Lancet*, **2**, 207–10

Hakim, S. & Adams, R. D. (1965) The special clinical problems of symptomatic hydrocephalus with normal cerebrospinal fluid pressure: observations on cerebrospinal fluid hydrodynamics. *J. neurol. Sci.*, **2**, 307–27

Hanley, I., McGuire, R. & Boyd, W. (1981) Reality orientation and dementia: trial of two approaches. *Brit. J. Psychiat.*, **138**, 10–14

Harris, C. & Ivory, P. (1976) An outcome evaluation of reality orientation therapy with geriatric patients in a state mental hospital. *Gerontologist*, **16**, 496–504

Harrison, M. & Marsden, C. (1977) Progressive intellectual deterioration. *Arch. Neurol.*, **34**, 199

Hellebrandt, F. (1978) Comment: The senile dement in our midst: a look at the other side of the coin. *Gerontologist*, **18**, 67–70

Henschke, P., Bell, D. & Cope, R. (1978) Alzheimer's disease and HLA. *Tissue Antigens*, **12**, 132–5

Hodkinson, H. (1973). Mental impairment in the elderly. *J. R. Coll. Physicians*, **7**, 305–17.

Hounsfield, G. (1973) Computerized transverse axial scanning (tomography): Part 1. Description of system. *Brit. J. Radiol.*, **46**, 1016–22

Hughes, C. P. (1978) Differential diagnosis of dementia in the senium. In *Senile Dementia: A Biomedical Approach*, ed. Nandy, Kalidas. New York: Elsevier

Ingram, C., Phegan, K. & Blumenthal, H. (1974) Significance of an ageing-linked neuron binding gammaglobulin fraction of human sera. *J. Geront.*, **29**, 20–27

Ingvar, D. H. & Gustafson, L. (1970) Regional cerebral blood flow in organic dementia with early onset. *Acta neurol. scand.*, **46**, 42–73, Supp. 43

Iqbal, K., Grundke-Iqbal, I., Wisniewski, H. M. & Terry, R. D. (1978) Neurofibers in Alzheimer dementia and other conditions. In *Alzheimer's Disease: Senile Dementia and Related Disorders. Aging*, ed. Katzman, R., Terry, R. D. & Bick, K. L., vol. 7. New York: Raven Press

Isaacs, B. (1977) Comprehensive care of the cognitively impaired elderly. In *Cognitive and Emotional Disturbance in the Elderly*, ed. Eisdorfer, Carl & Friedel, Robert. Chicago: Year Book Medical Publishers

Jacobs, E. A., Winter, P. M., Alvis, H. J. & Small, S. M. (1969) Hyperoxygenation effect on cognitive functioning in the aged. *New Eng. J. Med.*, **281**, 753–7

Jacoby, R. & Levy, R. (1980) Computed tomography in the elderly: 3. Affective disorder. *Brit. J. Psychiat.*, **136**, 270–5

Janota, I. (1981) Dementia deep white matter damage and hypertension: 'Binswanger's disease'. *Psychol. Med.*, **11**, 39–48

Jarvik, M. (1973) A survey of drug effects upon cognitive activities of the aged. In *Psychopharmacology and Aging*, ed. Eisdorfer, C. & Fann, W. E., New York: Plenum Press

Jellinek, E. (1980) Cerebral atrophy or hydrocephalus? *Brit. med. J.*, **280**, 1146

Jenkins, J., Felce, D., Lunt, B. & Powell, L. (1977) Increasing engagement in activity of residents in old people's homes by providing recreational materials. *Behav. Res. Ther.*, **15**, 429–34

Kahn, R., Goldfarb, A. I., Pollack, M. & Peck, A. (1960). Brief objective measures for the determination of mental status in the aged. *Amer. J. Psychiat.*, **117**, 326–8

Kannel, W. B. (1966) An epidemiological study of cerebrovascular disease. In *Cerebral Vascular Diseases: Transactions of the Fifth Conference held under the auspices of the American Neurological Association and the American Heart Association*, Princeton, New Jersey, ed. Siekert, R., Stralton, G. & Wisnant, J. P., pp. 53–66. New York

Kasziak, A., Fox, J., Gandell, D., Garron, D., Huckman, M. & Ramsey, R. (1978) Predictors of mortality in presenile and senile dementia. *Ann. Neurol.*, **3**, 246–352

Katz, S. & Akpom, C. (1976) A measure of primary socio-biological functions. *Int. J. health Serv.*, **6**, 493–508

Katzman, R. (1978) Normal pressure hydrocephalus. In *Alzheimer's Disease: Senile Dementia and Related Disorders*, ed. Katzman, R., Terry, R. D. & Bick, K. L., pp. 115–22. New York: Raven Press

Katzman, R. & Hussey, F. (1970) A simple constant-infusion test for measurement of CSF absorption: I. Rationale and method. *Neurology*, **20**, 534

Konigsmark, B. & Murphy, A. (1970) Neuronal populations in the human brain. *Nature*, **228**, 1335–6

Kraepelin, E. (1968) *Lectures on Clinical Psychiatry*. Trans. rev. and ed. Johnstone, Thomas (Facsimile of 1904 ed.: pub. Baillière, Tindall & Cox in London). New York, under auspices of Library of N.Y. Academy of Medicine: Haffner

Larsson, T., Sjögren, T. & Jacobson, G. (1963) Senile dementia: a clinical, sociomedical and genetic study. *Acta psychiat. scand.*, **39**, Supp. 167

Libow, L. S. (1977) Senile dementia and 'pseudosenility': clinical diagnosis. In *Cognitive and Emotional Disturbance in the Elderly*, ed. Eisdorfer, Carl & Friedel, Robert, pp. 75–88. Chicago: Year Book Medical Publishers

Lieberman, A., Dziatolowski, M., Kupersmith, M. *et al.* (1979) Dementia in Parkinson disease. *Ann. Neurol.*, **6**, 355–9

McAlpine, C., Rowan, J., Matheson, M. & Patterson, J. (1981) Cerebral blood flow and intelligence rating in persons over 90 years old. *Age and Ageing*, **10**, 247–53

McDermott, J. R., Smith, A., Iqbal, K. & Wisniewski, A. M. (1977) Aluminium and Alzheimer's disease. *Lancet*, **ii**, 710–11

MacDonald, M. L. & Butler, A. K. (1974) Reversal of helplessness: producing walking behavior in nursing home wheelchair residents using behavior modification procedures. *J. Geront.*, **29**, 97–101

MacDonald, M. L. & Settin, J. M. (1978) Reality orientation versus sheltered workshops as treatment for the institutionalized aging. *J. Geront.*, **33**, 416–21

Malamud, N. (1972) Neuropathology of organic brain syndromes associated with aging. In *Aging and the Brain*, ed. Gaitz, Charles M. New York: Plenum

Mann, D., Lincoln, J., Yates, P., Stamp, J. & Toper, S. (1980) Changes in the monoamine containing neurones of the human CNS in senile dementia. *Brit. J. Psychiat.*, **136**, 533–41

Marquadsen, J. (1969) The natural history of acute cerebrovascular disease. *Acta neurol. scand.*, **45**, Supp. 38

Mayer, P., Chugtai, M. & Cape, R. (1976) An immunological approach to dementia in the elderly. *Age and Ageing*, **5**, 164–70.

Miller, E. (1977) The management of dementia: a review of some possibilities. *Brit. J. soc. clin. Psychol.*, **16**, 77–83

Miller Fisher, C. (1978) Communicating hydrocephalus. *Lancet*, **i**, 37

Moody, L., Baron, V. & Monk, G. (1970) Moving the past into the present. *Amer. J. Nursing*, **70**, 2353–6

Morel, B. A. (1955) *Traité des Maladies Mentales*, Paris: Victor Masson, 1860 (cited in *Clinical Psychiatry* by Mayer-Gross, W., Slater, E. & Roth, M., p. 218 Baltimore: Williams & Wilkins)

Mueller, D. & Atlas, L. (1972) Resocialization of regressed elderly residents: a behavioral management approach. *J. Geront.*, **27**, 390–2

Muller, H. (1978) The electroencephalogram in senile dementia. In *Senile Dementia: A Biomedical Approach*, ed. Nandy, Kalidas. New York: Elsevier

Nandy, K. (1977) Immune reactions in the ageing brain and senile dementia. In *the Aging Brain and Senile Dementia*, ed. Nandy, K. & Sherwin, I. New York: Plenum

— (1978) Morphological changes in the aging brain. In *Senile Dementia: A Biomedical Approach*, ed. Nandy, Kalidas, New York: Elsevier

Nielsen, R., Petersen, O., Thygesen, P. & Willanger, R. (1966) Encephalographic ventricular atrophy: relationships between size of ventricular system and intellectual impairment. *Acta radiol. diag.*, **4**, 240–56

Oliver, J. E. & Restell, M. (1967) Serial testing in assessing the effect of meclofenoxate on patients with memory deficits. *Brit. J. Psychiat.*, **113**, 219–22

Ostfeld, A., Smith, D. M. & Stotsky, B. A. (1977) The systemic use of procaine in the treatment of the elderly: a review. *J. Amer. Geriat. Soc*, **25**, 1–19

Perry, E., Gibson, P., Blessed, G., Perry, R. & Tomlinson, B. (1977a) Neurotransmitter enzyme abnormalities in senile dementia. *J. neurol. Sci.*, **34**, 247–65

Perry, E., Perry, R., Blessed, G. & Tomlinson, B. (1977b) Necropsy evidence of central cholinergic deficits in senile dementia. *Lancet*, **i**, 189

Perry, E. K., Perry, R. H. & Tomlinson, B. (1977c) Dietary lecithin supplements in dementia of Alzheimer type. *Lancet*, **ii**, 242–3

Perry, E., Tomlinson, B., Blessed, G., Bergmann, K., Gibson, P. & Perry, R. (1978) Correlation of cholinergic abnormalities with senile plaques and mental test scores in senile dementia. *Brit. med. J.*, **2**, 1457–9

Petersen, R. (1977) Scopolamine induced learning failures in man. *Psychopharmacol.*, **52**, 283–9

Pollock, M. & Hornabrook, R. (1966) The prevalence, natural history and dementia of Parkinson's disease. *Brain*, **89**, 429–45

Powell, L., Felce, D., Jenkins, J. & Lunt, B. (1979) Increasing engagement in a home for the elderly by providing an indoor gardening facility. *Behav. Res. Ther.*, **17**, 127–35

Rao, D. B., Georgiev, E. L., Paul, P. D. & Guzman, A. B. (1978) Cyclandelate in the treatment of senile mental changes. A double-blind evaluation. *J. Amer. Geriat. Soc.*, **25** (12), 548–51

Raskin, A., Gershon, S., Crook, T. H., Sathananthan, G. & Ferris, S. (1978) The effects of hyperbaric and normobaric oxygen on cognitive impairment in the elderly. *Arch. gen. Psychiat.*, **35**, 50–6

Reichel, W. (1978) Organic brain syndrome In *The Geriatric Patient*, ed. Reichel, W. pp. 31–7. New York: H. P. Publishing

Reisine, T., Yamamura, H., Bird, E., Spokes, E. & Enna, S. (1978) Pre- and post-synaptic neurochemical alterations in Alzheimer's disease. *Brain Res.*, **159**, 477–81

Renvoize, E., Hambling, M., Pepper, N. & Rajah, S. (1979) Possible association of Alzheimer's disease with HLA-BW15 and cytomegalovirus infection. *Lancet*, **1**, 1238

Roseman, J. M. & Buckley, C. E. (1975) Inverse relationship between serum IgG concentrations and measures of intelligence in elderly persons. *Nature*, **254**, 55–6

Roth, M. (1971) Classification and aetiology in mental disorders of old age. In *Recent Developments in Psychogeriatrics. Brit. J. Psychiat.* Special Publication No. 6. Ashford, England: Headley

Roubicek, J., Geige, C. H. & Abt, K. (1972) An ergot alkaloid preparation (Hydergine) in geriatric therapy. *J. Amer. Geriat. Soc.*, **20**, 222–9

Sachs, D. (1975) Behavioral techniques in a residential nursing home facility. *J. Behav. Ther. exp. Psychol.*, **6**, 123

Sahs, A. L. Hartman, E. C. & Aronson, S. M. (1976) (Eds.) *Guidelines for Stroke Care*. Washington, D.C.: U.S. Department of Health, Education and Welfare

Scarborough, D. (1979) Reality orientation, a decade of progress. *The Rope.* Tuscaloosa, Alabama: Reality Orientation Training Programme Publication

Segal, J. L., Thompson, J. F. & Floyd, R. A. (1979) Drug utilization and prescribing patterns in a skilled nursing facility: the need for a rational approach to therapeutics. *J. Amer. Geriat. Soc.*, **27**, 117–22

Serby, M. (1980) Psychiatric issues in Parkinson's disease. *Compr. Psychiat.*, **21**, 315–22

Seymour, D., Henschke, P., Cape, R. & Campbell, A. (1980) Acute confusional states and dementia in the elderly: The role of dehydration/volume depletion, physical illness and age. *Age and Ageing*, **9**, 137–46

Shraberg, D. (1980) An overview of neuropsychiatric disturbances in the elderly. *J. Amer. Geriat. Soc.*, **28**, 422–5

Signoret, J., Whitely, A. & Lhermitte, F. (1978) Influence of choline on amnesia in early Alzheimer's disease. *Lancet*, **ii**, 837

Simchowicz, T. (1914) La maladie d'Alzheimer et son rapport avec la démence sénile. *Encéphale*, **9**, 218–31

Sitaram, N., Calne, E. & Gilling, J. (1978) Choline: selective enhancement of serial learning and encoding of low imagery words in man. *Life Sci.*, **22**, 1555

Smith, C. & Swash, M. (1978) Possible biochemical basis of memory disorder in Alzheimer's disease. *Ann. Neurol.*, **3**, 471–3

Snowden, P., Woodrow, J. & Copeland, J. (1981) HLA antigens in senile dementia and multiple infarct dementia. *Age and Ageing*, **10**, 259–63

Soukupová, B., Vojtěchovsky, M. & Šafratová, V. (1970) Drugs influencing the cholinergic system and the process of learning and memory in man. *Activ. nerv. sup.*, **12**, 91–3

Stam, F., Wigboldus, J. & Bots, G. (1980) Presenile dementia – a form of Lafora disease. *J. Amer. Geriat. Soc.*, **28**, 237–40

Steury, S. & Blank, M. L. (1977) (Eds.) *Readings in Psychotherapy with Older People*. Washington: US Dept. of Health Education and Welfare. Publication No. (ADM) 77–409

Suzuki, K., David, E. & Kutschmann, B. (1971) Presenile dementia with Lafora-like intraneuronal inclusions. *Arch. Neurol.*, **25**, 69

Symon, L. & Hinzpeter, T. (1977) The enigma of normal pressure hydrocephalus: tests to select patients for surgery and to predict shunt function. *Clin. Neurosurg.*, **24**, 285

Taulbee, L. R. (1976) *The A-B-C's of Reality Orientation: An Instruction Manual for Rehabilitation of Confused Elderly Persons*. New Port Richey, Florida

— (1978) Reality orientation: a therapeutic group activity for elderly persons. In *Working with the Elderly: Group Process and Techniques*, ed. Burnside, I. M. North Scituate, Mass.: Duxbury Press

Taulbee, L. & Folsom, J. C. (1966) Reality orientation for geriatric patients. *Hosp. commun. Psychiat.*, **17**, 133–5

Terry, R. D., Fitzgerald, C., Peck, A., Millner, J. & Farmer, P. (1977) Cortical cell counts in senile dementia. Abstract No. 118. 53rd Annual Meeting of the American Association of Neuropathologists. Chicago, Illinois

Tsuang, M. M., Lu, L. M., Stotsky, B. A. & Cole, J. O. (1971) Haloperidol versus thioridazine for hospitalized psychogeriatric patients: a double blind study. *J. Amer. Geriat. Soc.*, **19**, 593

U.S. Public Health Service (1968) *Syphilis, a Synopsis*. Washington: U.S. Department of Health, Education and Welfare, Public Health Service Publication, 1660

Valentine, A., Mosely, I. & Kendall, B. (1980) White matter abnormality in cerebral atrophy: clinicoradiological correlations. *J. Neurol. Neurosurg. Psychiat.*, **43**, 138–42

Voelkel, D. (1978) A study of reality orientation and resocialization groups with confused elderly. *J. geront. Nursing*, **4**, 13–18

Walford, R. & Hodge, S. (1980) HLA distribution in Alzheimer's disease. In *Histocompatibility Testing*, ed. Terasaki, P. I. Copenhagen: Munksgaard

Wang, H. S. (1977) Dementia of old age. In *Aging and Dementia*, ed. Lynn Smith, W. & Kinsbourne, M., pp. 1–24. New York: Spectrum

Wells, C. & Duncan, G. (1977) Dangers of over reliance on computerized axial tomography. *Amer. J. Psychiat.*, **134**, 811–13

Wyper, D., Lennox, G. & Rowan, J. (1976) Two minute slope inhalation technique for cerebral blood flow measurement in man: 1. Method. *J. Neurol. Neurosurg. Psychiat.*, **39**, 141–6

Yamaura, H., Ito, M., Kubota, K. & Matsuzawa, T. (1980) Brain atrophy during aging: A quantitative study with computed tomography. *J. Geront.*, **35**, 492–8

Yesavage, T. (1979) Dementia: Differential diagnosis and treatment. *Geriatrics*, **34**, 51–9

Zepelin, H., Wolfe, C. & Kleinplatz, F. (1981) Evaluation of a year-long reality orientation program. *J. Geront.*, **36**, 70–7

CHAPTER 13

Asuni, T. & Pillutla, V. S. (1967) Schizophrenia-like psychoses in Nigerian epileptics. *Brit. J. Psychiat.*, **113**, 1375–9

Bagley, C. (1972) Social prejudice and the adjustment of people with epilepsy. *Epilepsia*, **13**, 33–45

Bear, D. & Fedio, P. (1977) Quantitative analysis of interictal behaviour in temporal lobe epilepsy. *Arch. Neurol.*, **34**, 454–67

Betts, T. A. (1974) A follow-up study of a cohort of patients with epilepsy admitted to psychiatric care in an English city. In *Epilepsy, Proceedings of the Hans Berger Centenary Symposium*, ed. Harris, P. & Mawdsley, C., pp. 326–36. London: Churchill Livingstone

Betts, T. A., Merskey, H. & Pond, D. A. (1976) Psychiatry. In *A Textbook of Epilepsy*, ed. Laidlaw, J. & Richens, A. London: Churchill Livingstone

Birley, J. L. T. & Brown, G. W. (1970) Crisis and life changes preceding the onset of relapse of acute schizophrenia: clinical aspects. *Brit. J. Psychiat.*, **116**, 327–33

Bleuler, E. (1924) *Textbook of Psychiatry*. (Trans. Brill, A. A.) New York: Macmillan. Reissued by Dover Publications, 1951

Blumer, D. (1977) Treatment of patients with seizure disorder referred because of psychiatric complications. In *Psychiatric Complications in the Epilepsies: Current Research and Treatment*, ed. Blumer, D. & Levin, K. *McLean Hospital Journal*, special issue, pp. 53–73

Brain, W. R. (1962) *Recent Advances in Neurology and Neuropsychiatry*. London: Churchill

Brown, G. W., Harris, T. & Copeland, J. R. (1977) Depression and loss. *Brit. J. Psychiat.*, **130**, 1–18

Bruens, J. H. (1971) Psychoses in epilepsy. *Psychiat. Neurol. Neurochir.*, **74**, 174–92

Chadwick, D., Jenner, P. & Reynolds, E. H. (1975) Amines, anticonvulsants and epilepsy. *Lancet*, **ii**, 473–6

Clark, R. A. & Lesko, J. M. (1939–40) Psychoses associated with epilepsy. *Amer. J. Psychiat.*, **96**, 595–607

Clarke, L. Pierce (1931) The psychobiologic concept of epilepsy. In *Epilepsy and the Convulsive State*. Association for Research in Nervous and Mental Disease, vol. VII. Baltimore: Williams & Wilkins

Coatsworth, J. J. (1971) *Studies on the Clinical Efficacy of Marketed Antiepileptic Drugs*. NINDS Monograph No. 12. Washington: US Government Printing Office

Cooper, I. A. (1973) Effect of chronic stimulation of anterior cerebellum on neurological disease. *Lancet*, **i**, 206

— (1978) *Cerebellar stimulation in man*. New York: Raven Press

Currie, S., Heathfield, K. W. C., Henson, R. A. & Scott, D. F. (1971) Clinical course and prognosis of temporal lobe epilepsy. *Brain*, **94**, 173–90

Currier, R. D., Jackson, M., Little, S. C., Suess, J. F. & Andy, O. J. (1971) Sexual seizures. *Arch. Neurol.*, **25**, 260–4

Dalby, M. A. (1969) Epilepsy and 3 per sec. spike and wave rhythms. *Acta neurol. scand.*, **45**, supp. 40

Davison, K. & Bagley, C. R. (1969) Schizophrenia-like psychoses associated with organic disorders of the central nervous system: a review of the literature. In *Current Problems in Neuropsychiatry*, ed. Herrington, R. N. *British Journal of Psychiatry*, Special Publication No. 4, 113–94

Delasiauve, L. J. F. (1854) *Traité de l'épilepsie; histoire; traitement; médicine légale*. Paris: Masson

Dominian, J., Serafetinides, E. A. & Dewhurst, M. (1963) A follow-up study of late onset epilepsy. *Brit. med. J*, **1**, 431–5

Dongier, S. (1959) Statistical study of clinical and electroencephalographic manifestations of 536 psychotic episodes in 516 epileptics between clinical seizures. *Epilepsia*, **1**, 117–42

Driver, M. V. & MacGillivray, B. B. (1976) Electroencephalography in *A Textbook of Epilepsy*, ed. Laidlaw, J. & Richens, A. London: Churchill Livingstone

Falconer, M. A. (1973) Reversibility by temporal lobe resection of the behavioral abnormalities of temporal lobe epilepsy. *New Eng. J. Med.*, **289**, 451–5

Falconer, M. A., Serafetinides, E. A., & Corsellis, J. A. N. (1964) Etiology and pathogenesis of temporal lobe epilepsy. *Arch. Neurol., Chicago*, **10**, 233–48

Fenton, G. W. (1972) Epilepsy and automatism. *Brit. J. Hosp. Med.*, **7**, 57–64

— (1974) The straightforward E.E.G. in psychiatric practice. *Proc. R. Soc. Med.*, **67**, 911–19

— (1976) Rehabilitation problems in people with epilepsy. *Rehabilitation*, **96**, 15–21

— (1979) Electronic aids to the treatment of epilepsy. In *Scientific Aids in Treatment*, ed. Nicholson, J. P. Chertsey, Surrey: Reedbooks

— (1980) Epilepsy and automatism. Supplement to *Irish med. J.*, **73**, 11–20

Fenton, G. W. & King, D. J. (1979) Acute drug induced disorders of the nervous system. In *Drug Induced Emergencies*, ed. Darcy, P. F. & Griffen, J. P. Bristol: Wright

Fink, M. & Kahn, R. L. (1957) Relation of electroencephalographic delta activity to behavioral response in electroshock. *Arch. Neurol. Psychiat.*, **78**, 516–25

Flor-Henry, P. (1969) Psychosis and temporal lobe epilepsy. *Epilepsia*, **10**, 363–95

— (1972) Ictal and inter-ictal psychiatric manifestations in epilepsy: specific or non-specific. *Epilepsia*, **13**, 773–83

— (1974) Psychosis, neurosis and epilepsy: developmental and gender-related effects and their aetiological contributions. *Brit. J. Psychiat.*, **124**, 144–50

— (1976) Epilepsy and psychopathology. In *Recent Advances in Clinical Psychiatry*, ed. Granville-Grossman, K., pp. 262–96. London: Churchill Livingstone

Gastaut, H. (1954) Interprétation des symptômes de l'épilepsie 'psychomotrice' en fonction des données de la physiologie rhinencéphalique. *Presse méd.*, **62**, 1535–7

— (1969) Clinical and electroencephalographical classification of epileptic seizures. *Supp. to Epilepsia*, **10**, S2–21

— (1976) Conclusions: Computerized transverse axial tomography in epilepsy. *Epilepsia*, **17**, 337–8

Gastaut, H., Gastaut, J. L. (1976) Computerized transverse axial tomography in epilepsy. *Epilepsia*, **17**, 325–36

Geschwind, N. (1979) Behavioural changes in temporal lobe epilepsy. *Psychol. Med.*, **9**, 217–19

Gibbs, F. A. (1951) Ictal and non-ictal psychiatric disorders in temporal lobe epilepsy. *J. nerv. ment. Dis.*, **11**, 522–8

Glaser, G. H. (1964) The problem of psychosis in psychomotor temporal lobe epileptics. *Epilepsia*, **5**, 271–8

Gloor, P. (1978) Generalized epilepsy with bilateral synchronous spike and wave discharge. In *Contemporary Clinical Neurophysiology* (EEG Supp. No. 34), ed. Cobb, W. A. & Van Duijn, H. Amsterdam: Elsevier

Goldensohn, E. S. & Ward, A. A., Jr. (1975) Pathogenesis of epileptic seizures. In *The Nervous System. Vol. 2, The Clinical Neurosciences*, ed. Tower, D. B. New York: Raven Press

Goode, D. J., Penry, J. K. & Dreifuss, F. E. (1970) Effects of paroxysmal spike-wave on continuous visual-motor performance. *Epilepsia*, **11**, 241–54

Goodglass, H., Morgan, M., Folsom, A. T. & Quadfasel, F. A. (1963) Epileptic seizures, psychological factors and occupational adjustment. *Epilepsia*, **4**, 322–41

Gregoriades, A., Fragos, E., Kapslakis, Z., & Mandouvalos, B.

(1971) A correlation between mental disorders and EEG and AEG findings in temporal love epilepsy. *5th World Congress of Psychiatry*, Mexico, Prensa Medica Mexicana, 325

Gruhle, H. W. (1936) Uber den Wahn bei Epilepsie. *Zeitschr. ges. Neurol. Psychiat.*, **154**, 395–9

Grunberg, F. & Pond, D. A. (1957) Conduct disorders in epileptic children. *J. Neurol. Neurosurg. Psychiat.*, **20**, 65–8

Gudmundsson, D. (1966). Epilepsy in Iceland. *Acta neurol. scand.*, **43**, Supp. 25

Guerrant, J., Anderson, W. W., Fischer, A., Weinstein, M. R., Jaros, R. M. & Deskins, A. (1962) *Personality in Epilepsy*. Springfield, Ill.: Thomas

Gunn, J. (1979) Forensic psychiatry. In *Recent Advances in Clinical Psychiatry*, ed. Granville-Grossman, K. London: Churchill Livingstone

Gunn, J. & Fenton, G. W. (1969) Epilepsy in prisons: a diagnostic survey. *Brit. med. J.*, **4**, 326–8

— (1971) Epilepsy, automatism and crime. *Lancet*, **i**, 1173–6

Gustaffsson, G. & Prave, I. (1972) Active work for epileptics who would otherwise be institutionalised. *Epilepsia*, **13**, 75–7

Hauser, W. A. & Kurland, L. T. (1975) Epidemiology of epilepsy in Rochester, Minnesota. 1935 through 1967. *Epilepsia*, **16**, 1–66

Hill, D. (1953) Psychiatric disorders of epilepsy. *Med. Press*, **229**, 473–5

Hoenig, J. & Hamilton, C. M. (1960) Epilepsy and sexual orgasm. *Acta psychiat. scand.*, **35**, 448–56

Hooshmand, H. & Brawley, B. W. (1969) Temporal lobe seizures and exhibitionism. *Neurology*, **19**, 1119–24

Jasper, H. H. (1964) Some physiological mechanisms involved in epileptic automatisms. *Epilepsia*, **5**, 1–20

Jennett, W. B. (1965) Predicting epilepsy after blunt head injury. *Brit. med. J.*, **4**, 1215–18

Jensen, I. & Klinken, L. (1976) Temporal lobe epilepsy and neuropathology. *Acta neurol. scand.*, **54**, 391–414

Jensen, I. & Larsen, J. K. (1979) Psychoses in drug resistant temporal lobe epilepsy. *J. Neurol. Neurosurg. Psychiat.*, **42**, 948–54

Kiørboe, E. (1974) Medical prognosis of epilepsy. In *Handbook of Clinical Neurology*, ed. Vinken, P. J. & Bruyn, G. W., vol. 15. Amsterdam: North Holland Elsevier

Kligman, D. & Goldberg, D. A. (1975) Temporal lobe epilepsy and aggression. *J. nerv. ment. Dis.*, **160**, 324–41

Knox, S. J. (1968) Epileptic automatisms and violence. *Med. Sci. Law*, **8**, 96–104

Kraepelin, E. (1904) *Lectures on Clinical Psychiatry*. (Trans. Johnstone, T.) New York: Wood

Kristensen, O. & Sindrup, E. H. (1978) Psychomotor epilepsy and psychosis. I Physical aspects. *Acta neurol. scand.*, **57**, 361–9

— (1978) Psychomotor epilepsy and psychosis. II Electroencephalographic findings. *Acta neurol. scand.*, **57**, 370–9

Lamprecht, F. (1973) Biochemische Aspekte in der Psychosenforschung. In *Psychische Störungen bei Epilepsie*, pp. 85–105. Stuttgart, New York: Schattauer

Landolt, H. (1958) Serial EEG investigation during psychotic episodes in epileptic patients and during schizophrenia. In *Lectures on Epilepsy*, ed. de Hass, Lorentz, pp. 91–133. Amsterdam: Elsevier

Levi, R. N. & Waxman, S. (1975) Schizophrenia, epilepsy, cancer, methionine and folate metabolism. *Lancet*, **i**. 11–17

Levin, S. (1952) Epileptic clouded states. *J. nerv. ment. Dis.*, **116**, 215–25

Liddell, D. W. (1953) Observations on epileptic automatism in a mental hospital population. *J. ment. Sci.*, **99**, 732–48

Lishman, W. A. (1978) *Organic Psychiatry*. Oxford: Blackwell

Long, C. G. & Moore, J. R. (1979) Parental expectations for their epileptic children. *J. child Psychol. Psychiat.*, **20**, 299–312

MacIntyre, I. (1974) Employment of people with epilepsy. *The Candle*, Spring number, 2–6

Marks, I. M. (1969) *Fears and Phobias*. London: Heinemann

Mattson, R. H., Heninger, G. R., Gallagher, B. B. & Glaser, G. H. (1970) Psychophysiologic precipitants of seizures in epileptics. *Neurol.*, **20**, 407

Maudsley, H. (1874) *Responsibility in Mental Disease*. New York: Appleton

Mayeux, R., Brandt, J., Rosen, J. & Benson, D. F. (1980) Interictal memory and language impairment in temporal lobe epilepsy. *Neurol.*, **30**, 120–125

Meldrum, B. S. (1978) Photosensitive epilepsy in *Papio papio* as a model for drug studies. In *Contemporary Clinical Neurophysiology*, ed. Cobb, W. A. & van Duijn, H. Amsterdam: Elsevier

Merlis, J. K. (1972) Epilepsy in different age groups. In *The Epidemiology of Epilepsy: a Workshop*, ed. Alter, M., & Hauser, W. A. NINDS Monograph 14. Washington: US Government Printing Office

— (1974) Reflex epilepsy. In *Handbook of Clinical Neurology*, ed. Vinken, P. J. & Bruyn, G. W., vol. 15. Amsterdam: North Holland, Elsevier

Metrakos, K. & Metrakos, J. D. (1974) Genetics of epilepsy. In *Handbook of Clinical Neurology*, ed. Vinken, P. J. & Bruyn, G. W., vol. 15. Amsterdam: North Holland, Elsevier

Mirsky, A. F., Primac, D. W., Ajmone-Marsan, C., Rosvold, H. E. & Steven, J. R. (1960) A comparison of the psychological test performance of patients with focal and non-focal epilepsy. *Exp. Neurol.*, **2**, 75–89

Mulder, D. W. (1953) Paroxysmal psychiatric symptoms in epilepsy. *Proc. Mayo Clin.*, **28**, 31–5

Nawishy, S., Trimble, M. R. & Richens, A. (1980) Antidepressants and epilepsy. In *Nomifensine*, ed. Stonier, P. D. & Jenner, F. A. International Congress and Symposium Series No. 25, Royal Society of Medicine, New York: Academic Press and Grune & Stratton

Neugebauer, R. & Susser, M. (1979) Epilepsy: some epidemiological aspects. *Psychol. Med.*, **9**, 207–15

Nuffield, E. J. A. (1961) Neurophysiology and behaviour disorders in epileptic children. *J. ment. Sci.*, **107**, 438–58

Pahla, A., Fenton, G. W., Driver, M. V. & Fenwick, P. B. C. Epilepsy and psychiatric disorder. (In preparation.)

Penfield, W. & Jasper, H. (1954) *Epilepsy and the Functional Anatomy of the Human Brain*. Boston: Little, Brown

Penfield, W. & Kristiansen, K. (1951) *Epileptic Seizure Patterns*. Springfield, Ill.: Thomas

Pinel, J. P. J. & Van Oot, P. H. (1976) Generality of the kindling phenomenon: some clinical impressions. In *Kindling*, ed. Wada, J. A. New York: Raven Press

Pinto, R. (1972) A case of movement epilepsy treated successfully by flooding. *Brit. J. Psychiat.*, **121**, 287–8

Pond, D. A. (1957) Psychiatric aspects of epilepsy. *J. Ind. med. Profession*, **3**, 1441–51

Pond, D. A. & Bidwell, B. H. (1960) A survey of epilepsy in fourteen general practices. II Social and psychological aspects. *Epilepsia*, **1**, 285–99

Pond, D. A., Bidwell, B. H. & Stein, L. (1960) A survey of epilepsy

in 14 general practices. I. Demographic and medical data. *Psychiat. Neurol. Neurochir.*, **63**, 217–326

Porter, R. J., Penry, J. K. & Dreifuss, F. E. (1973) Responsiveness at the onset of spike-wave bursts. *Electroenceph. clin. Neurophysiol.* **34**, 239–245

Rasmussen, T. (1975) Surgical treatment of epilepsy. In *The Nervous System. Vol. 2. The Clinical Neurosciences*, ed. Tower, D. B. New York: Raven Press

Reitan, R. M. (1974) Psychological testing and epilepsy. In *Handbook of Clinical Neurology*, ed. Vinken, P. J. & Bruyn, G. W., Vol. 15, pp. 559–75. Amsterdam: North Holland

Reynolds, E. (1967) Schizophrenia-like psychoses of epilepsy and disturbances of folate and vitamin B12 metabolism induced by anticonvulsant drugs. *Brit. J. Psychiat.*, **113**, 911–19

— (1975) Chronic anti-epileptic toxicity: a review. *Epilepsia*, **16**, 319–52

Richens, A. (1976) *Drug Treatment of Epilepsy*. London: Kimpson

Rodin, E. A. (1968) *The prognosis of patients with epilepsy*. Springfield, Ill.: Thomas

— (1972) Medical and social prognosis in epilepsy. *Epilepsia*. **13**, 121–31

Roger, J., Lob, H. & Tassinari, C. A. (1974) Status epilepticus. In *Handbook of Clinical Neurology*, ed. Vinken, P. J. & Bruyn, G. W., vol. 15 pp. 145–88. Amsterdam: North Holland, Elsevier

Roy, A. (1977) Hysterical fits previously diagnosed as epilepsy. *Psychol. Med.*, **7**, 271–3

— (1979) Hysterical seizures. *Arch. Neurol.*, **36**, 447

Rutter, M., Graham, P. J. & Yule, W. (1970) A neuropsychiatric study in childhood. *Clin. dev. Med.* London: Heinemann

Sato, M., Hikasa, N. & Otsuki, S. (1979) Experimental epilepsy, psychosis and dopamine receptor sensitivity. *Biol. Psychiat.*, **14**, 537–40

Schwartz, M. S. & Scott, D. F. (1971) Isolated petit-mal status presenting *de novo* in middle age. *Lancet*, **ii**, 1399–401

Scott, D. F., (1978) Psychiatric aspects of epilepsy. *Brit. J. Psychiat.*, **132**, 417–30

— (1978) Psychiatric aspects of sexual medicine. In *Epilepsy '78*. Wokingham, England: British Epilepsy Association

Serafetinides, E. A. (1965) Aggressiveness in temporal lobe epileptics. *Epilepsia*, **6**, 33–42

Slater, E., Beard, A. W. & Glithero, E. (1963) The schizophrenia-like psychoses of epilepsy. *Brit. J. Psychiat.*, **109**, 95–150

Small, J. G., Milstein, V. & Stevens, N. R. (1962) Are psychomotor epileptics different? A controlled study. *Arch. Neurol.*, **7**, 187–94

Small, J. G. & Small, I. F. (1967) A controlled study of mental disorders associated with epilepsy. *Recent Adv. biol. Psychiat.*, **9**, 171–81

Small, J. G., Small, I. F. & Hayden, M. P. (1966) Further psychiatric investigations of patients with temporal and non-temporal lobe epilepsy. *Amer. J. Psychiat.*, **123**, 303–10

Standage, K. F. (1973) Schizophreniform psychosis among epileptics in a mental hospital. *Brit. J. Psychiat.*, **123**, 231–2

Standage, K. F. & Fenton, G. W. (1975) Psychiatric symptom profiles of patients with epilepsy. *Psychol. Med.*, **15**, 152–60

Stevens, J. F. (1966) Psychiatric implications of temporal lobe epilepsy. *Arch. gen. Psychiat.*, **14**, 461–71

Stevens, J. R. (1980) The biological background of psychoses in epilepsy. *Advances in Epileptology: The Xth Epilepsy International Symposium*, ed. Wada, J. A. & Penry, J. K. New York: Plenum Press

Stores, G. (1978) Schoolchildren with epilepsy at risk for learning and behaviour problems. *Dev. Med. child Neurol.*, **20**, 502–8

Stores, G. & Hart, J. (1976) Reading skills of children with generalized or focal epilepsy attending ordinary school. *Dev. Med. child Neurol.*, **18**, 705–16

Symonds, C. (1962) Contribution to discussion on The Schizophrenic-like Psychoses of Epilepsy, by Beard, A. W. & Slater, E. *Proc. R. Soc. Med.*, **55**, 311–16

Taylor, D. C. (1971) Ontogenesis of chronic epileptic psychosis: a re-analysis. *Psychol. Med.*, **1**, 247–53

— (1972) Psychiatry and sociology in the understanding of epilepsy. In *Psychiatric Aspects of Medical Practice*, ed. Mandelbrote, B. M. & Gelder, M. G. London: Staples Press

— (1972) Mental state and temporal lobe epilepsy. *Epilepsia*, **13**, 727–65

— (1975) Factors influencing the occurrence of schizophrenia-like psychoses in patients with temporal lobe epilepsy. *Psychol. Med.*, **5**, 249–54

— (1977) Epileptic experience, schizophrenia and the temporal lobe. In *Psychiatric Complications in the Epilepsies: Current Research and Treatment*, ed. Blumer, D. & Levin, K. *McLean Hospital Journal*, special issue, 22–39

Tizard, B. (1962) The personality of epileptics. *Psychol. Bull.*, **59**, 196–210

Toone, B. K. (1980) Personal Communication

Toone, B. K., Wheeler, M. & Fenwick, P. B. C. (1980) Sex hormone changes in male epileptics. *Endocrinol.*, **12**, 391–5

Tower, D. B. (1974) Neurochemistry of epilepsy. In *Handbook of Clinical Neurology*, ed. Vinken, P. J. & Bruyn, G. W., vol. 15. Amsterdam: North Holland, Elsevier

Trimble, M. (1977) Relationship between epilepsy and schizophrenia: a biochemical hypothesis. *Biol. Psychiat.*, **12**, 299–304

— (1979) The effect of anticonvulsant drugs on cognitive abilities. *Pharmac. Ther. vol. 4*. 677–85. Oxford: Pergamon Press

Trimble, M. R., Anlezark, G. & Meldrum, B. (1977) Seizure and activity in photosensitive baboons following antidepressant drugs, and the role of serotoninergic mechanisms. *Psychopharmacol.*, **51**, 159–61

Turner, W. A. (1907) *Epilepsy*. London: Macmillan

Wasterlain, C. G. & Plum, F. (1973) Vulnerability of developing rat brain to electroconvulsive seizures. *Arch. Neurol.*, **29**, 38–45

Weil, A. A. (1959) Ictal emotions occuring in temporal lobe dysfunction. *Arch. Neurol.*, **1**, 87–97

Williams, D. (1956) The structure of emotions reflected in epileptic experiences. *Brain*, **79**, 29–67

— (1968) Man's temporal lobe. *Proc. R. Soc. Med.*, **61**, 355–6

Wilson, P. J. E. (1970) Cerebral hemispherectomy for infantile hemiplegia. *Brain*, **93**, 147–80

CHAPTER 14

Adams, R. D. & Foley, J. M. (1953) The neurological disorder associated with liver disease. *Ass. Res. nerv. ment. Dis., Proc.*, **32**, 198–237

Albert, M. S., Butters, N. & Levin, J. (1979) Temporal gradients in the retrograde amnesia of patients with alcoholic Korsakoff's disease. *Arch. Neurol.*, **36**, 211–16

Alexander, L., Pijoan, M. & Myerson, A. (1938) Beriberi and scurvy. *Trans. Amer. Neurol. Ass.*, **64**, 135–9

Banay, R. S. (1944) Pathologic reaction to alcohol. I. Review of the literature and original case reports. *Q. J. Stud. Alcohol*, **4**, 580–605

Barbizet, J. (1963) Defect of memorizing of hippocampal–mammillary origin: a review. *J. Neurol. Neurosurg. Psychiat.*, **26**, 127–35

Benedetti, G. (1952) *Die Alkoholhalluzinosen (Alcoholic Hallucinoses).* Stuttgart: Thieme

Berman, L. H. (1956) The treatment of delirium tremens. *Q. J. Stud. Alcohol*, **17**, 28–34

Blass, J. P. & Gibson, G. E. (1977) Abnormality of a thiamine-requiring enzyme in patients with Wernicke–Korsakoff syndrome. *New Eng. J. Med.*, **297**, 1367–70

Bleuler, E. (1930) In *Textbook of Psychiatry*, authorized translation by Brill, A. A., p. 163; pp. 342–5. New York: Macmillan

— (1951) In *Textbook of Psychiatry*, authorized translation by Brill, A. A., p. 327. New York: Macmillan

Boedeker, J. (1892) Klinischer Beitrag zur Kenntniss der acuten alkoholischen Augenmuskellahmung. *Charité-Annalen*, **17**, 790–814

Bonhoeffer, K. (1901) Die akuten Geisteskrankheiten der Gewohnheitstrinker. *Eine klinische Studie VIII.* Jena: Fischer

— (1904) Der Korsakowsche Symptomenkomplex in seinen Beziehungen zu den verschiedenen Krankheitsformen. *Allg. Zeitschr. Psychiat.*, **61**, 744–52

Bostock, J. (1939) Alcoholism and its treatment. *Med. J. Austral.*, **1**, 136–8

Bowman, K. M., & Jellinek, E. M. (1941) Alcoholic mental disorders. *Q. J. Stud. Alcohol*, **2**, 312–90

Bowman, K. M., Wortis, H. & Keiser, S. (1939) The treatment of delirium tremens. *J. Amer. med. Ass.*, **112**, 1217–19

Bratz, D. (1899) Alkohol und Epilepsie. *Allg. Zeitschr. Psychiat.*, **56**, 334–86

Brewer, C. & Perrett, L. (1971) Brain damage due to alcohol consumption: an air-encephalographic, psychometric and electroencephalographic study. *Brit. J. Addiction*, **66**(3), 170–82

Bumke, O. & Kant, F. (1936) In *Handbuch der Neurologie*, ed. Bumke, O. & Foerster, O., vol. 13, pp. 828–915. Berlin: Springer

Butters, N. (1979) Amnesic disorders. In *Clinical Neuropsychology*, ed. Heilman, K. & Valenstein, E. S., pp. 439–74. New York: Oxford University Press

Butters, N. & Cermak, L. S. (1980) *Alcoholic Korsakoff's Syndrome: An Information Processing Approach to Amnesia.* New York: Academic Press

Cala, L. A., Jones, B., Mastaglia, F. L. & Wiley, B. (1978) Brain atrophy and intellectual impairment in heavy drinkers – a clinical, psychometric and computerized tomography study. *Austral. N. Z. J. Med.*, **8**, 147–53

Campbell, A. C. P. & Russell, W. R. (1941) Wernicke's encephalopathy: the clinical features and their probable relationship to vitamin B deficiency. *Q. J. Med.*, **10**, 41–64

Carlen, P. L., Wortzman, G., Holgate, R. C., Wilkinson, D. A. & Rankin, J. G. (1978) Reversible cerebral atrophy in recently abstinent chronic alcoholics measured by computed tomography scans. *Science*, **200**, 1076–8

Chafetz, M. E. (1975) Alcoholism and alcoholic psychoses. In *Comprehensive Textbook of Psychiatry*, ed. Kaplan, H. I. & Sadock, B. J., 2nd ed., p. 1343. Baltimore: Williams & Wilkins

Chernoff, G. F. (1975) A mouse model of the fetal alcohol syndrome. *Teratol.*, **11**, 14A

Cleckley, H. M., Sydenstricker, V. P. & Geeslin, L. E. (1939) Nicotinic acid in the treatment of atypical psychotic states associated with malnutrition. *J. Amer. med. Ass.*, **112**, 2107–10

Courville, C. B. (1955) *Effects of Alcohol on the Nervous System of Man.* Los Angeles: San Lucas Press

Cravioto, J., Delicardie, E. R. & Birch, H. C. (1966) Nutrition, growth and neurointegrative development: an experimental and ecologic study. *Pediat.*, **38** (supp. 2), 319–72

Czaja, C. & Kalant, H. (1961) The effect of acute alcoholic intoxication on adrenal ascorbic acid cholesterol in the rat. *Can. J. Biochem. Physiol.*, **39**, 327–34

Dreyfus, P. M. & Victor, M. (1961) Effects of thiamine deficiency on the central nervous system. *Amer. J. clin. Nutrition*, **9**, 414–25

Ecker, A. D. & Woltman, H. W. (1939) Is nutritional deficiency the basis of Wernicke's disease? Report of case. *J. Amer. med. Ass.*, **112**, 1794–6

Ellis, F. W. & Pick, J. R. (1970) Experimentally-induced ethanol dependence in rhesus monkeys. *J. Pharmacol. exp. Ther.*, **175**, 88–93

Elvehjem, C. A., Madden, R. J., Strong, F. M. & Wooley, D. W. (1937) Relation of nicotinic acid and nicotinic acid amide to canine black tongue. *J. Amer. chem. Soc.*, **59**, 1767

Elzholz, A. (1900) Ueber Beziehungen der Korsakoff'sschen Psychose zur Polioencephalitis acuta haemorrhagica superior. *Wien. klin. Wochenschr.*, **13**, 337–44

Epstein, P. S., Pisani, V. D. & Fawcett, J. A. (1977) Alcoholism and cerebral atrophy. *Alcoholism: clin. exp. Res.*, **1**, 61–5

Evans, C. A., Carlson, W. E. & Green, R. G. (1942) Pathology of Chastek paralysis in foxes: counterpart of Wernicke's hemorrhagic polioencephalitis of man. *Amer. J. Pathol.*, **18**, 79–91

Ewing, J. A. (1960) The first phase of alcohol rehabilitation. Report of a controlled study with benactyzin, paraldehyde, and pyridoxine. *Q. J. Stud. Alcohol*, **21**, 68–81

Fazekas, J. F., Shea, J. & Rea, E. (1955) Use of chlorpromazine in the management of acute and postalcoholic states. *Int. Rec. Med.*, **168**, 333–9

Féré, C. (1892) *L'Épilepsie*, p. 227. Paris: Gauthier-Villars

Field, J. B., Williams, H. E. & Mortimore, G. E. (1963) Studies on the mechanism of ethanol-induced hypoglycemia. *J. clin. Invest.*, **42**, 497–506

Fischer, J. E. & Baldessarini, R. J. (1976) Pathogenesis and therapy of hepatic coma. In *Progress in Liver Disease*, ed. Popper, H. & Schaffner, F., vol. 5, pp. 363–97. New York: Grune & Stratton

Flink, E. B., Stutzman, F. L., Anderson, A. R., Lontig, T. & Frasier, R. (1954) Magnesium deficiency after prolonged parenteral fluid administration and after chronic alcoholism complicated by delirium tremens. *J. lab. clin. Med.*, **43**, 169–83

Fox, J. H., Ramsey, R. G., Huckman, M. S. & Proske, A. E. (1976) Cerebral ventricular enlargement. Chronic alcoholics examined by computerized tomography. *J. Amer. med. Ass.*, **236**, 365–8

Freinkel, N., Singer, D. L., Arky, R. A., Bleicher, S. J., Anderson, J. B. & Silbert, C. K. (1963) Alcohol hypoglycemia. I. Carbohydrate metabolism of patients with clinical alcohol hypoglycemia and the experimental reproduction of the syndrome with pure ethanol. *J. clin. Invest.*, **42**, 1112–33

French, S. W. & Morris, J. R. (1972) Ethanol dependence in the rat induced by nonintoxicating levels of ethanol. *Res. Commun. chem. Pathol. Pharmacol.*, **4**, 221–33

Freund, G. (1969) Alcohol withdrawal syndrome in mice. *Arch. Neurol.*, **21**, 315–20

Friedhoff, A. J. & Zitrin, A. A. (1959) A comparison of the effects of paraldehyde and chlorpromazine in delirium tremens. *New York J. Med.*, **59**, 1060–3

Gamper, E. (1928) Zur Frage der Polioencephalitis haemorrhagica der chronischen Alkoholiker: anatomische Befund beim alkoholischen Korsakow und ihre Beziehungen zum klinischen Bild. *Deutsche Zeitschr. Nervenheilk.*, **102**, 122–9

Gessner, P. K. (1979) Drug therapy of the alcohol withdrawal syndrome. In *Biochemistry & Pharmacology of Ethanol*, vol. II, ed. Majchrowicz, E. & Noble, E. P. New York: Plenum Press

Ghez, C. (1969) Vestibular paresis: A clinical feature of Wernicke's disease. *J. Neurol. Neurosurg. Psychiat.*, **32**, 134–9

Giove, C. & Viani, F. (1965) Atrofie cerebrali negli etilisti cronici; considerazioni fisiopatogeniche e correlazioni dei dati clinici, elettroencefalografici, gammaencefalografici e pneumoencefalografici. *Neuropsichiat.*, **31**, 548–69

Girard, P. F., Devic, M. & Garde, A. (1956) L'encéphalopathie de Gâyet–Wernicke des alcooliques. *Rev. Neurol.*, Paris, **94**, 493–527

Godfrey, L., Kissen, M. D. & Downs, T. M. (1958) Treatment of the acute alcohol withdrawal syndrome. *Q. J. Stud. Alcohol*, **19**, 118–24

Golbert, T. M., Sanz, C. J., Rose, H. D. & Leitschuh, T. H. (1967) Comparative evaluation of treatments of alcoholic withdrawal syndromes. *J. Amer. med. Ass.*, **201**, 113–16

Goldsmith, G. A., Sarrett, H. P., Register, V. C. & Gibbens, J. (1952) Studies of niacin requirement in man: experimental pellagra in subjects on corn diets low in niacin and tryptophan. *J. clin. Invest.*, **31**, 533–42

Goldstein, D. B. (1972a) Relationship of alcohol dose to intensity of withdrawal signs in mice. *J. Pharmacol. exp. Ther.*, **180**, 203–15

— (1972) An animal model for testing effects of drugs on alcohol withdrawal reactions. *J. Pharmacol. exp. Ther.*, **183**, 14–22

Goldstein, D. B. & Pal, N. (1971) Alcohol dependence produced in mice by inhalation of ethanol: grading the withdrawal reaction. *Science*, **172**, 288–90

Goodwin, D. W., Crane, J. B., & Guze, S. B. (1969) Alcoholic 'blackouts': a review and clinical study of 100 alcoholics. *Amer. J. Psychiat.*, **126**, 191–8

— (1969) Phenomenological aspects of the alcoholic 'blackout'. *Brit. J. Psychiat.*, **115**, 1033–8

Goodwin, D. W., Othmer, E., Halikas, J. A. & Freemon, F. (1970) Loss of short-term memory as a predictor of the alcoholic 'blackout'. *Nature*, **227**, 201–2

Griffiths, P. J., Littleton, J. M. & Ortiz, A. (1973) A method for the induction of dependence to ethanol in mice. *Brit. J. Pharmacol.*, **47**, 669–70

Gruenwald, F., Hanlon, T. E., Wachsler, S. & Kurland, A. A. (1960) A comparative study of promazine and triflupromazine in the treatment of acute alcoholism. *Dis. nerv. Syst.*, **21**, 32–81

Haggard, H. W. & Jellinek, E. M. (1942) *Alcohol Explored.* Garden City, N.Y.: Doubleday, Doran

Hanson, J. W., Jones, K. L. & Smith, D. W. (1976) Fetal alcohol syndrome. Experience with 41 patients. *J. Amer. med. Ass.*, **235**, 1458–60

Hare, F. (1915) Alcohol and delirium tremens. *Brit. med. J.*, **1**, 446–7

Harper, C. (1979) Wernicke's encephalopathy: a more common disease than realised. *J. Neurol. Neurosurg. Psychiat.*, **42**, 226–31

Hart, W. T. (1961) A comparison of promazine and paraldehyde in 175 cases of alcohol withdrawal. *Amer. J. Psychiat.*, **118**, 323–7

Haug, J. O. (1968) Pneumoencephalographic evidence of brain damage in chronic alcoholics. A preliminary report. *Acta psychiat. scand.*, Supp., **203**, 135–43

Heaton, F. W., Pyrah, L. N., Beresford, C. C., Bryson, R. W. & Martin, D. F. (1962) Hypomagnesaemia in chronic alcoholism. *Lancet*, **ii**, 802–5

Henderson, P. K. (1914) Korsakoff's psychosis occurring during pregnancy. *Johns Hopkins Hosp. Bull.*, **25**, 261–70

Horel, J. A. (1978) The neuroanatomy of amnesia. A critique of the hippocampal memory hypothesis. *Brain*, **101**, 403–45

Horvath, T. B. (1975) Clinical spectrum and epidemiological features of alcoholic dementia. In *Alcohol, Drugs and Brain Damage*, ed. Rankin, J. G., pp. 1–16. Toronto: Alcoholism & Drug Research Foundation of Ontario

Hurd, A. W. (1905) Korsakoff psychosis – report of cases. *Amer. J. Insanity*, **62**, 63–76

Isbell, H., Fraser, H. F., Wikler, A., Belleville, R. E. & Eisenman, A. J. (1955) An experimental study of the etiology of 'rum fits' and delirium tremens. *Q. J. Stud. Alcohol*, **16**, 1–33

Jelliffe, E. S. (1908) The alcoholic psychoses. Chronic alcoholic delirium (Korsakoff's psychosis). *New York Med. J.*, **88**, 767–77

Jellinek, E. M. (1943) Classics of the alcohol literature: Magnus Huss' *Alcoholismus Chronicus*. *Q. J. Stud. Alcohol*, **4**, 85–92

— (1952) The phases of alcohol addiction. *Q. J. Stud. Alcohol*, **13**, 673–84

Johanson, E. (1964) Mild paranoia. *Acta psychiat. scand.*, **40**, Supp., **177**, 1–100

Jolliffe, N., Bowman, K. M., Rosenblum, L. A., & Fein, H. D. (1940) Nicotinic acid deficiency encephalopathy. *J. Amer. med. Ass.*, **114**, 307–12

Jolly, F. (1897) Ueber die psychischen Stoerungen bei Polyneuritis. *Charité-Annalen*, **22**, 579–612

Jones, K. L. & Smith, D. W. (1973). Recognition of the fetal alcohol syndrome in early infancy. *Lancet*, **ii**, 999–1001

Jones, K. L., Smith, D. W., Streissguth, A. P. & Myrianthopoulos, N. C. (1974) Outcome in offspring of chronic alcoholic women. *Lancet*, **i**, 1076–8

Jubb, K. V., Saunders, L. Z. & Coates, H. V. (1956) Thiamine deficiency encephalopathy in cats. *J. comp. Pathol.*, **66**, 217–27

Kaim, S. C., Klett, C. S. & Rothfeld, B. (1969) Treatment of the acute alcohol withdrawal state: a comparison of four drugs. *Amer. J. Psychiat.*, **125**, 1640–6

Kalant, H. (1975) Direct effects of ethanol on the nervous system. *Federation Proc.*, **34**, 1930–41

Kalinowsky, L. B. (1942) Convulsions in non-epileptic patients on withdrawal of barbiturates, alcohol, and other drugs. *Arch. Neurol. Psychiat.*, **48**, 946–56

Kalm, H., Luckner, H. & Magun, R. (1952) Klinik und Pathologie der neurologischen Stoerungen bei tierexperimenteller B₁ Avitaminose. *Deutsche Zeitschr. Nervenheilk*, **167**, 334–354

Kant, F. (1932) Die Pseudoencephalitis Wernicke der Alkoholiker (Polio-encephalitis haemorrhagica superior acuta). *Arch. Psychiat. Nervenkrankh.* (Berlin), **98**, 702–68

Keller, M. (1959) Other effects of alcohol. In *Drinking and Intoxication*. Part I: Physiological and psychological effects of alcohol, ed. McCarthy, R. G., pp. 13ff. Glencoe, Ill.: Free Press

Keller, M. & McCormick, M. (1968) *A Dictionary of Words About Alcohol*. New Brunswick, N.J.: Rutgers Center of Alcohol Studies

Keller, M. & Gurioli, C. (1976) *Statistics on consumption of alcohol and on alcoholism*. New Brunswick, N.J.: Journal on the Studies of Alcohol

Kessel, N. & Walton, H. (1965) *Alcoholism*, p. 39. Baltimore: Penguin Books

King, L. S. & Meehan, M. C. (1936) Primary degeneration of the corpus callosum (Marchiafava's disease). *Arch. Neurol. Psychiat.*, **36**, 547–68

Kolb, L. C. (1968) *Noyes Modern Clinical Psychiatry*, 7th ed., p. 206. Philadelphia: Saunders

Korsakoff, S. S. (1887) Disturbance of psychic function in alcoholic paralysis and its relation to the disturbance of the psychic sphere in multiple neuritis of nonalcoholic origin. *Vestnik Klin. Sudeb. Psikhiat. Nevropatol.*, vol. 4, fasc. 2

— (1889) A few cases of peculiar cerebropathology in the course of multiple neuritis. *Ejenedel. Klin. Gaz.*, Nos. 5, 6, 7

— (1889) Psychic disorder in conjunction with multiple neuritis (Psychosis Polyneuritica S Cerebropathia Psychica Toxaemica). *Med. Obozrenije*, **31**, No. 13

Kraepelin, E. (1946) In *Lectures on Clinical Psychiatry* (authorized translation from second German ed., rev.), ed. Johnstone, T., pp. 102–9, New York: Wood

Krusius, F. E., Vartia, K. O. & Forsander, O. (1958) Experimentelle Studien über die Biologische Wirkung von Alkohol: II. Alkohol und Nebennierenrinden-Funktion. *Ann. Med. exp. Biol. Fenn.*, **36**, 424–34

Lambert, A. (1934) In *Textbook of Medicine*, ed. Cecil, R., 3rd ed., pp. 568–78. Philadelphia: Saunders

Langfeldt, G. (1961) The erotic jealousy syndrome. A clinical study. *Acta psychiat. neurol. scand.*, **36**, Supp., **151**, 7–68

Laties, V. G., Lasagna, L., Gross, G. M., Hitchman, L. L., & Flores, J. (1958) A controlled trial of chlorpromazine and promazine in the management of delirium tremens. *Q. J. Stud. Alcohol*, **19**, 238–43

Lemoine, P., Harrousseau, H., Borteyru, J. P., & Menuet, J. C. (1968) Les enfants de parents alcooliques: anomalies observées: à propos de 127 cas. *Quest-Méd.*, **25**, 477

Leventhal, C. M., Baringer, J. R., Arnason, B. G. & Fisher, C. M. (1965) A case of Marchiafava-Bignami disease with clinical recovery. *Trans. Amer. Neurol. Ass.*, **90**, 87–91

Lewis, A. (1952) Alcoholic psychoses. *British Encyclopaedia of Medical Practice*, 2nd ed., vol. 10, 394–402

Lieber, C. S., & DeCarli, L. M. (1973) Ethanol dependence and tolerance: A nutritionally controlled experimental model in the rat. *Res. Commun. chem. Pathol. Pharmacol.*, **6**, 983–91

Lynch, M. J. G. (1960) Brain lesions in chronic alcoholism. *Amer. Med. Ass. Arch. Pathol.*, **69**, 342–53

McEntee, W. J. & Mair, R. G. (1978) Memory impairment in Korsakoff's psychosis: a correlation with brain noradrenergic activity. *Science*, **202**, 905–7

— (1980) Memory enhancement in Korsakoff's psychosis by clonidine: further evidence for a noradrenergic deficit. *Ann. Neurol.*, **7**, 466–70

Malamud, W. & Skillicorn, S. A. (1956) Relationship between Wernicke and Korsakoff syndrome. *Arch. Neurol. Psychiat.*, **76**, 585–96

Marchand, L. (1932) Les lésions du système nerveux, du foie, des reins et de la rate dans le 'delirium tremens' des alcooliques. *Ann. d'anat. pathol.*, **9**, 1026–30

Marchiafava, E. & Bignami, A. (1903) Sopra un' alterazione del corpo calloso osservata in soggetti alcoolisti. *Riv. Patol. nerv. ment.* (Firenze), **8**, 544–9

Mello, N. K. (1973) Short term memory function in alcohol addicts during intoxication. In *Alcohol Intoxication and Withdrawal: Experimental Studies.* Proc. 39th Int. Cong. Alcoholism Drug Dependence, ed. Gross, M. M. New York: Plenum

— (1976) Animal models for the study of alcohol addiction. *Psychoneuroendocrinol.*, **1**, 347–57

Mendelson, J. H. & LaDou, J. (1964) Experimentally induced chronic intoxication and withdrawal in alcoholics: II. Psychophysiological findings. *Q. J. Stud. Alcohol*, Supp., **2**, 14–39

Mendelson, J. H., Wexler, D., Kubzansky, P., Leiderman, H. & Solomon, P. (1959) Serum magnesium in delirium tremens and alcoholic hallucinosis. *J. nerv. ment. Dis.*, **128**, 352–7

Meyer, A. (1901) On parenchymatous systemic degenerations mainly in the central nervous system. *Brain*, **24**, 47–115

Mingazzini, G. (1922) In *Der Balken*. Berlin: Springer

Mooney, H. B. (1965) Pathologic jealousy and psychochemotherapy. *Brit. J. Psychiat.*, **111**, 1023–42

Muller, D. J. (1969) A comparison of three approaches to alcohol withdrawal states. *Southern med. J.*, **62**, 495–6

Mulvihill, J. J. & Yeager, A. M. (1976) Fetal alcohol syndrome. *Teratol.*, **13**(3), 345–8

Murawieff, W. (1897) Zwei Fälle von Polioencephalitis acuta haemorrhagica superieur (Wernicke). *Neurol. Zentralbl.*, **16**, 56–61; 106–15

Neuburger, K. (1936) Über die nichtalkoholische Wernickesche Krankheit, insbesondere über ihr Vorkommen beim Krebsleiden. *Virch. Arch. Abt. A: Pathol. Anat.* (Berlin), **298**, 68–86

— (1937) Wernickesche Krankheit bei chronischer Gastritis: Ein Beitrag zu den Beziehungen zwischen Magen und Gehirn. *Zeitschr. ges. Neurol. Psychiat.*, **160**, 208–25

Noyes, A. P. (1939) *Modern Clinical Psychiatry*, 2nd ed. Philadelphia: Saunders

Osler, W. (1928) *Principles and Practice of Medicine*, pp. 387–91. New York: Appleton-Century-Crofts

Owen, M. (1954) A study of the rationale of the treatment of delirium tremens with adrenocorticotrophic hormone: I. The eosinophil response of patients with delirium tremens, after a test with ACTH. II. Clinical correlations to responsiveness to ACTH in delirium tremens. *Q. J. Stud. Alcohol*, **15**, 384–6

Phillips, G. B., Victor, M., Adams, R. D. & Davidson, C. S. (1952) A study of the nutritional defect in Wernicke's syndrome: the effect of a purified diet, thiamine, and other vitamins on the clinical manifestations. *J. clin. Invest.*, **31**, 859–71

Piker, P. (1937) On the relationship of sudden withdrawal of alcohol to delirium tremens. *Amer. J. Psychiat.*, **93**, 1387–90

Prickett, C. O. (1934) The effect of a deficiency of vitamin B₁ upon the central and peripheral nervous systems of the rat. *Amer. J. Physiol.*, **107**, 459–70

Raimann, E. (1900) Polioencephalitis superior acuta und Delirium alkoholicum als Einleitung einer Korsakow'schen Psychose ohne Polyneuritis. *Wien. klin. Wochenschr.*, **13**, 31–7

Raimann, E. (1901) Beitrage zur Lehre von den alkilischen Augenmuskellaehmungen. *J. Psychol. Neurol.* (Leipsig), **20**, 36–76

Randall, C. L., Taylor, W. J., & Walker, D. W. (1977) Ethanol-induced malformations in mice. *Alcoholism*, **1**, 219–24

Randall, R. E., Rossmeisl, E. C. & Bleifer, K. H. (1959) Magnesium depletion in man. *Ann. int. Med.*, **50**, 257–8

Rinehart, J. F., Friedman, M. & Greenberg, L. D. (1949) Effect of experimental thiamine deficiency on the nervous system of the Rhesus monkey. *Arch. Pathol.*, **48**, 129–39

Ron, M. A. (1977) Brain damage in chronic alcoholism: a neuropathological radiological and psychological review. *Psychol. Med.*, **7**, 103–12

Rosenblum, W. I. & Feigin, I. (1965) The hemorrhagic component of Wernicke's encephalopathy. *Arch. Neurol.*, **13**, 627–32

Rosenfeld, J. E. & Bizzoco, D. H. (1961) A controlled study of alcohol withdrawal. *Q. J. Stud. Alc.*, Supp. **1**, 77–84

Rosett, H. L., Ouellette, E. M. & Weiner, L. (1976) A pilot prospective study of the fetal alcohol syndrome at the Boston City Hospital. Part 1. Maternal drinking. *Ann. N.Y. Acad. Sci.*, **273**, 118–22

Ryan, C., Butters, N., Montgomery, K., Adinolfi, A. & Didario, B. (1980) Memory deficits in chronic alcoholics: continuities between the 'intact' alcoholic and the alcoholic Korsakoff patient. In *Biological Effects of Alcohol*, ed. Begleiter, H., pp. 701–18 New York: Plenum

Sabot, L. M., Gross, M. M. & Halpert, E. (1968) A study of acute alcoholic psychoses in women. *Brit. J. Addiction*, **63**, 29–49

Sanders, H. I. & Warrington, E. K. (1971) Memory for remote events in amnesic patients. *Brain*, **94**, 661–8

Schuckit, M. A. & Winokur, G. (1971) Alcoholic hallucinosis and schizophrenia: a negative study. *Brit. J. Psychiat.*, **119**, 549–50

Schwob, R. A., Gruner, J., Foucquiner, E., Harl, J. M., Francon, J. & Guerre, J. (1953) Sur trois cas de syndrome confusionnel avec contracture chez des éthyliques: le problème des encéphalopathies carentielles. *Rev. Neurol.*, **88**, 174–90

Scott, D. F. (1967) Alcoholic hallucinosis – an aetiological study. *Brit. J. Addiction*, **62**, 113–25

Seltzer, B. & Sherwin, I. (1978) Organic brain syndromes: an empirical study and critical review. *Amer. J. Psychiat.*, **135**, 13–21

Sereny, G. & Kalant, H. (1965) Comparative clinical evaluation of chlordiazepoxide (Librium) and promazine in treatment of alcohol withdrawal syndrome. *Brit. med. J.*, **1**, 92–7

Sereny, G., Rapoport, A. & Husdon, H. (1966) The effect of alcoholic withdrawal on electrolyte and acid-base balance. *Metabolism*, **15**, 896–904

Shea, J. G., Schultz, J. D., Lewis, E., Jr. & Fazekas, J. F. (1958) Clinical and cerebral action of promethazine and methylphenidate hydrochloride. *Amer. J. med. Sci.*, **235**, 201–5

Shepherd, M. (1961) Morbid jealousy: some clinical and social aspects of a psychiatric symptom. *J. ment. Sci.*, **107**, 687–753

Sherlock, S., Summerskill, W. H. J., White, L. P. & Phear, E. A. (1954) Portal-systemic encephalopathy: neurological complications of liver disease. *Lancet*, **ii**, 453–7

Smith, C. (1947) Effects of maternal undernutrition upon the newborn infant in Holland (1944–1945). *J. Pediat.*, **30**, 229–43

Smith, J. J. (1950) The treatment of acute alcoholic states with ACTH and adrenocortical hormones. *Q. J. Stud. Alcohol*, **11**, 190–8

Sneed, R. C. (1977) The fetal alcohol syndrome. Is alcohol, lead, or something else the culprit? *J. Pediat.*, **90**(2), 324

Spillane, J. D. (1947) *Nutritional Disorders of the Nervous System*, p. 48. Baltimore: Williams & Wilkins

Stanley, C. E. (1909–10) A report of three cases of Korsakow's psychosis. *Amer. J. Insanity*, **66**, 613–22

Strecker, E. A., Ebaugh, F. G. & Ewalt, J. R. (1951) *Practical Clinical Psychiatry*, pp. 150–70. New York: Blakiston

Sullivan, W. C. (1899) A note on the influence of maternal inebriety on the offspring. *J. ment. Sci.*, **45**, 489–503

Summerskill, W. H. J., Davidson, E. A., Sherlock, S. & Steiner, R. E. (1956) The neuropsychiatric syndrome associated with hepatic cirrhosis and an extensive portal collateral circulation. *Q. J. Med.*, **25**, 245–66

Suter, C. & Klingman, W. (1955) Neurologic manifestations of magnesium depletion states. *Neurology*, **4**, 691–9

Talland, G. A. (1965) *Deranged Memory*. New York & London: Academic Press

Tamerin, J. S., Weiner, S., Poppen, R., Steinglass, P. & Mendelson, J. H. (1971) Alcohol and memory: amnesia and short-term memory function during experimentally-induced intoxication. *Amer. J. Psychiat.*, **127**, 1659–64

Tashiro, K. & Nelson, J. S. (1972) Hemorrhagic necrosis of superior cerebellar vermis associated with acute Wernicke's encephalopathy. *J. Neuropath. exp. Neurol.*, **31**, 185

Tavel, M. E., Davidson, W. & Batterton, T. D. (1961) A critical analysis of mortality associated with delirium tremens: review of 39 fatalities in a nine-year period. *Amer. J. med. Sci.*, **242**, 18–29

Thomas, D. W. & Freedman, D. X. (1964) Treatment of the alcohol withdrawal syndrome. *J. Amer. med. Ass.*, **188**, 244–6

Thompson, W. L., Johnson, A. D., Maddrey, M. D. & Osler Medical Housestaff. (1975) Diazepam and paraldehyde for treatment of severe delirium tremens. *Ann. int. Med.*, **82**, 175–80

Ulleland, C. (1972) The offspring of alcoholic mothers. *Annals of the N.Y. Acad. Sci.*, **197**, 167–9

Victor, M. (1966) Treatment of alcoholic intoxication and the withdrawal syndrome: a critical analysis of the use of drugs and other forms of therapy. *Psychosom. Med.*, **28**, 636–50

Victor, M. & Adams, R. D. (1953) The effect of alcohol upon the nervous system. *Res. Pub. Ass. Res. nerv. ment. Dis.*, **32**, 526–73

— (1956) Neuropathology of experimental vitamin B₆ deficiency in monkeys. *Amer. J. clin. Nutrition*, **4**, 346–53

— (1961) On the etiology of the alcoholic neurologic diseases: with special references to the role of nutrition. *Amer. J. clin. Nutrition*, **9**, 379–97

Victor, M., Adams, R. D. & Collins, G. H. (1971) *The Wernicke–Korsakoff Syndrome: A Clinical and Pathological Study of 245 Patients, 82 with Postmortem Examinations*. Philadelphia: Davis

Victor, M., Herman, K. & White, E. E. (1959) A psychological study of the Wernicke–Korsakoff syndrome: results of Wechsler–Bellevue Intelligence Scale and Wechsler Memory Scale testing at different stages in the disease. *Q. J. Stud. Alcohol*, **20**, 467–79

Victor, M. & Hope, J. M. (1958) The phenomenon of auditory hallucinations in chronic alcoholism. *J. nerv. ment. Dis.*, **126**, 451–81

Victor, M. & Laureno, R. (1978) The neurologic complications of alcohol abuse: epidemiologic aspects. In *Advances in Neurology: Neuroepidemiology*, ed. Schoenberg, B. S., vol. 19, pp. 603–17. New York: Raven Press

Victor, M., Talland, G. & Adams, R. D. (1959) Psychological studies of Korsakoff's psychosis: I. General intellectual functions. *J. nerv. ment. Dis.*, **128**, 528–37

Victor, M. & Wolfe, S. M. (1973) Causation and treatment of the alcohol withdrawal syndrome. In *Alcoholism, Progress in Research and Treatment*, ed. Bourne, P. G. & Fox, R., chap. 6, pp. 137–69. New York: Academic Press

Victor, M. & Yakovlev, P. I. (1955) S. S. Korsakoff's psychic disorder in conjunction with peripheral neuritis: a translation of Korsakoff's original article with brief comments on the author and his contribution to clinical medicine. *Neurology*, **5**, 395–406

Vilter, R. W., Mueller, J. F., Glazer, H. S., Jarrold, T., Abraham, J., Thompson, C. & Hawkins, V. R. (1953) The effect of vitamin B₆ deficiency induced by desoxypyridoxine in human beings. *J. lab. clin. Med.*, **42**, 335–57

Wacker, W. E. C. & Vallee, B. L. (1958) Magnesium metabolism. *New Eng. J. Med.*, **259**, 431–8

Wagener, H. P. & Weir, J. E. (1937) Ocular lesions associated with post-operative and gestational nutritional deficiency. *Amer. J. Ophthalmol.*, **20**, 253–9

Warner, R. H. & Rosett, H. L. (1975) The effects of drinking in offspring: An historical survey of the American and British literature. *J. Stud. Alcohol*, **36**(11), 1395–420

Wechsler, D. (1917) A study of retention in Korsakoff's psychosis. *Psychiat. Bull. New York State Hosp.*, **2**, 403–51

Wernicke, C. (1881) In *Lehrbuch der Gehirnkrankheiten fur Aerzte und Studirende*, vol. 2, pp. 229–42. Kassel: Fischer

— (1900) *Grundriss der Psychiatrie*. Leipzig: Thieme

Wexler, D., Leiderman, P. H., Mendelson, J., Kubzansky, P. & Solomon, P. (1958) The effect of cetadiol on delirium tremens, alcoholic hallucinosis and alcoholic withdrawal. *Amer. J. Psychiat.*, **114**, 935–6

Whitfield, C. L., Thompson, G., Lamb, A., Spencer, V., Pfiefer, M. & Browning, M. (1978) Detoxification of 1024 alcoholic patients without psychoactive drugs. *J. Amer. med. Ass.*, **239**, 1409–10

Wolfe, S. M., Mendelson, J. H., Ogata, M., Victor, M., Marshall, W. & Mello, N. (1969) Respiratory alkalosis and alcohol withdrawal. *Trans. Ass. Amer. Physicians*, **82**, 344–52

Wolfe, S. M., Victor, M. (1969) The relationship of hypomagnesemia and alkalosis to alcohol withdrawal symptoms. *Ann. N.Y. Acad. Sci.*, **162**, 973–84

Wortis, H. (1940) Delirium tremens. *Q. J. Stud. Alcohol*, **1**, 251–67

Wortis, H., Bueding, E., Stein, M. H. & Jolliffe, N. (1942) Pyruvic acid studies in the Wernicke syndrome. *Arch. Neurol. Psychiat.*, **47**, 215–22

CHAPTER 15

Aylett, P. (1978) Barbiturate misuse in hard drug addicts. *Brit. J. Addiction*, **73**, 385–90

Beattie, R. T. (1968) Nutmeg as a psychoactive agent. *Brit. J. Addiction*, **63**, 105–9

Bewley, T. H. (1966) Recent changes in the pattern of drug abuse in the United Kingdom. *Bull. Narcotics*, **XVIII 4**, 1–13

— (1967) Adverse reactions from the illicit use of lysergide. *Brit. med. J.*, **3**, 28–30

Bewley, T. H. & Ben-Arie, O. (1968) Morbidity and mortality from heroin dependence, 2: Study of 100 consecutive in-patients. *Brit. med. J.*, **1**, 727–30

Bewley, T. H., Ben-Arie, O. & James, I. P. (1968) Morbidity and mortality of heroin dependence, 1: survey of heroin addicts known to Home Office. *Brit. med. J.*, **1**, 725–32

Bewley, T. H., James, I. P., LeFevre, C., Maddocks, P. & Mahon, T. (1972) Maintenance treatment of narcotic addicts (not British nor a system but working now). *Int. J. Addictions*, **7**, 597–611

Bewley, T. H., James, I. P. & Mahon, T. (1972) Evaluation of effectiveness of prescribing clinics for narcotic addicts in the United Kingdom (1968–70). In *Drug Abuse: Proceedings of the International Conference*, ed. Zarajonetris, C. T. D., Philadelphia: Lea & Febiger

Blumberg, H. H., Cohen, S. D., Dronfield, B. E., Mordecai, E. A., Roberts, J. C. & Hawks, D., (1974) British opiate users: I. People approaching London Drug Treatment Centres. *Int. J. Addictions*, **9**, (1), 1–23

Boyd, P., Layland, W. R. & Crickmay, J. R. (1971) Treatment and follow-up of adolescents addicted to heroin. *Brit. med. J.*, **4**, 604–5

British Medical Journal, (1966) Hallucinogens in morning glory, **1**, 814–15

— (1968) LSD and chromosomes, **2**, 778–9

— (1969) Leukaemia and LSD, **2**, 775–6

— (1976) Glutethimide – an unsafe alternative to barbiturate hypnotics, **1**, 1424–5

Campbell, A. M. G., Evans, M., Thomson, J. L. G. & Williams, M. J. (1971) Cerebral atrophy in young cannabis smokers. *Lancet*, **ii**, 1219–25

Chapple, P. A. L., Somekh, D. E. & Taylor, M. E. (1972a) A five-year follow-up of 108 cases of opiate addiction: I: General findings and a suggested method of staging. *Brit. J. Addiction*, **67**, 33–8

— (1972b) Follow-up of cases of opiate addiction from the time of notification to the Home Office. *Brit. med. J.*, **2**, 680–3

Co, B. T., Goodwin, D. W., Gado, M., Mikhael, M. & Hill, S. Y. (1977) Absence of cerebral atrophy in chronic cannabis users. Evaluation by computerized axial tomography. *J. Amer. med. Ass.*, **237**, 1229–30

Cochin, J. & Kornetsky, C. (1964) Development & loss of tolerance to morphine in the prevention of morphine tolerance. *Brit. J. Pharmacol.*, **13**, 17–37

Cohen, S. (1977) Abuse of inhalants. In *Drug Abuse, Clinical and Basic aspects*, ed. Pradhan, S. H. & Dutta, S. N., pp. 290–302. St Louis: Mosby

— (1979) Inhalants. In *Handbook on Drug Abuse*, ed. Dupont, R. L., Goldstein, A. & O'Donnell, J:, pp. 213–20. National Institute on Drug Abuse

Connell, P. H. (1972) Central nervous system stimulants. In *Side Effects of Drugs. A Survey of Unwanted Effects of Drugs Reported in 1968–71*, ed. Meyler, L. & Herxheimer, A., 7, pp. 1–16. Amsterdam: Excerpta Medica

de Alarcon, R. & Rathod, N.H. (1968) Prevalence and early detection of heroin abuse. *Brit. med. J.*, **2**, 549–53

De Leon, G., Holland, S. & Rosenthal, M. S. (1972) Phoenix House: Criminal activity of dropouts. *J. Amer. med. Ass.*, **222**, 686–9

Departmental Committee, Ministry of Health (1926) *Report of the Department Committee on Morphine and Heroin Addiction.* London: HMSO

Dewhurst, K. & Hatrick, J. A. (1972) Differential diagnosis and treatment of lysergic acid diethylamide induced psychosis. *Practitioner*, **209**, 327–32

Dole, V. P. & Nyswander, M. E. (1965) A medical treatment for diacetyl morphine (heroin) addiction. *J. Amer. med. Ass.*, **193**, 646–50

Dole, V. P., Nyswander, M. E. & Warner, A. (1968) Successful treatment of 750 criminal addicts. *J. Amer. med. Ass.*, **206**, 2708

d'Orban, P. T. (1973) Female narcotic addicts: a follow-up study of criminal and addiction careers. *Brit. med. J.*, **4**, 345–7

— (1975) Criminality as a prognostic factor in opiate dependence. *Brit. J. Psychiat.*, **127**, 86–9

Drug Link (1976) 'Not to be sniffed at'. 2, issue 1–2. Institute for the Study of Drug Dependence

— (1978) *LSD – Recurrence of a Communal Nightmare.* Institute for the Study of Drug Dependence

Eddy, N. B., Halbach, H., Isbell, H. & Seevers, M. H. (1965) Drug dependence: its significance and characteristics. *Bull. WHO*, **32**, 721–33

Edwards, J. G. (1974) Cannabis and the criteria for legislation of a currently prohibited recreational drug: groundwork for a debate. *Acta psychiat. scand.*, Supp., 251

— (1978) Some years on. Evolutions in the 'British system'. In *Problems of Drug Abuse in Britain*, ed. West, D. J. pp. 1–45, II Institute of Criminology, Cambridge University

Ellinwood, E. H. & Petrie, W. M. (1977) Dependence on Amphetamine, Cocaine and other Stimulants. In *Drug Abuse, Clinical and Basic Aspects*, ed. Pradhan, S. N. & Dutton, S. N., pp. 248–62. St Louis: Mosby

Evans, J. I., Lewis, S. A., Gibb, I. A. M. & Cheetham, M. (1968) Sleep and barbiturates: some experiments and observations. *Brit. med. J.*, **4**, 291–3

Fernandez, J., Brennan, T., Masterson, J. & Power, M. (1974) Cytogenetic studies in the offspring of LSD users. *Brit. J. Psychiat.*, **124**, 296–8

Forbes, C. D., Prentice, C. R. M. & Sclare, A. B. (1974) Surreptitious ingestion of Warfarin. *Brit. J. Psychiat.*, **125**, 245–7

Fraser, A. C. (1976) Drug addiction in pregnancy. *Lancet*, **ii**, 896–9

Fraser, H. F. & Isbell, H. (1952) Comparative effects of 20 mg of morphine sulphate on non-addicts and former morphine addicts. *J. Pharmacol. exp. Ther.*, **105**, 498–502

Gaulden, E. C., Littlefield, D. C., Putoff, O. E. & Seivert, A. C. (1964) Menstrual abnormalities associated with heroin addiction. *Amer. J. Obstet. Gynaecol.*, **90**, 155–60

Gethin-Morgan, H., Boulnois, J. & Burns-Cox, C. (1973) Addiction to prednisone. *Brit. med. J.*, **2**, 93–4

Ghodse, A. H. (1977) Drug dependent individuals dealt with by London Casualty Departments. *Brit. J. Psychiat.*, **131**, 273–80

— (1977) Casualty departments and the monitoring of drug dependence. *Brit. med. J.*, **1**, 1381–2

— (1979) Drug overdoses: a comparison of drug dependent and nondependent individuals attending London Casualty Departments. *Int. J. Addictions*, **14**, No. 3, 365–76

— (1981) The London Casualty Survey. In *The Misuse of Psychotropic Drugs*, ed. Murray, R., Ghodse, A. H., Harris, C., Williams, D. & Williams, P., pp. 49–53. London: Gaskell

Ghodse, A. H., Reed, J. L. & Mack, J. W. (1977) The effect of maternal narcotic addiction on the newborn infant. *Psychol. Med.*, **7**, 667–75

Ghodse, A. H., Sheehan, M., Stevens, B., Taylor, C. & Edwards, G. (1978) Mortality among drug addicts in Greater London. *Brit. med. J.*, **2**, 1742–4

Goldstein, A. (1979) Recent advances in basic research relevant to drug abuse. In *Handbook on Drug Abuse*, ed. Dupont, R. I., Goldstein, A. & O'Donnell, J., pp. 439–46. Washington, D.C.: NIDA, US Department of Health Education and Welfare

Gordon, A. M. (1978) Drugs and delinquency: a four-year follow-up of drug clinic patients. *Brit. J. Psychiat.*, **132**, 21–6

Grimes, J. A. (1977) *Drug Dependence Study. A Survey of Drug Addicts attending for Treatment.* Statistics and Research Division, Department of Health and Social Security, London

Grinspoon, L. & Bakalar, J. B. (1979) Cocaine. In *Handbook on Drug Abuse*, ed. Dupont, R. L., Goldstein, A., & O'Donnell, J., pp. 241–7. National Institute on Drug Abuse

Hawks, D. (1974) The epidemiology of narcotic addiction in the United Kingdom. In *Drug Use: Epidemiological and Sociological Approaches*, ed. Josephson, E. & Carroll, E. E., pp. 45–63. New York: Wiley

Hawks, D., Mitcheson, M., Ogborne, A. & Edwards, G. (1969) Abuse of methyl-amphetamine. *Brit. med. J.*, **2**, 715–21

Hofmann, F. G. & Hofmann, A. D. (1975) Generalized depressants of the central nervous system. Volatile solvent and aerosol inhalation. In *Handbook on Drug and Alcohol Abuse*, pp. 129–48. New York: Oxford University Press

Hug, C. C. (1972) Characteristics and theories related to acute and chronic tolerance development. In *Chemical and Biological Aspects of Drug Dependence*, ed. Mulé, S. J. & Brill, H., pp. 307–58. Cleveland, Ohio: CRC Press

Hughes, J. (1975) Isolation of an endogenous compound from the brain with pharmacological properties similar to morphine. *Brain Res.*, *88*, 295–306

Hughes, J. & Kosterlitz, H. W. (1977) Opioid peptides. *Brit. med. Bull.*, **33**, (2), 157–62

Interdepartmental Committee (1961) *Report on Drug Addiction*. London: HMSO

— (1965) *The Second Report of the Interdepartmental Committee*. London: HMSO

Jaffe, J. H. (1975) Drug addiction and drug abuse. In *The Pharmacological Basis of Therapeutics*, ed. Goodman, L. S. & Gilman, A., 5th ed., pp. 284–324. New York: Macmillan

Jaffe, J. H. & Martin, W. R. (1975) Narcotic analgesics and antagonists. In *The Pharmacological Basis of Therapeutics*, ed. Goodman, L. S. and Gilman, A., 5th ed., pp. 245–83. New York: Macmillan

James, I. P. (1967) Suicide and mortality amongst heroin addicts in Britain. *Brit. J. Addiction*, **62**, 391–8

Jones, R. T. (1972) Cannabis. In *Chemical and Biological Aspects of Dependence*, ed. Mulé, S. J. & Brill, H., pp. 65–81. Cleveland, Ohio: CRC Press

Kalant, O. J. (1966) *The Amphetamines: Toxicity and Addiction*, pp. 37–76 Ontario: University of Toronto Press

Kessel, N. (1965) Self-poisoning – Part I. *Brit. med. J.*, **2**, 1265–70

Koutsaimanis, K. G. & de Wardener, H. E. (1970) Phenacetin nephropathy, with particular reference to the effect of surgery. *Brit. med. J.*, **4**, 131–4

Kreitman, N. (1981) Drugs used in parasuicide. In *The Misuse of Psychotropic Drugs*, ed. Murray, R., Ghodse, A. H., Harris, C., Williams, D. & Williams, P., pp. 29–33. London: Gaskell

Kuehnle, J., Mendelson, J. H., Davis, K. R.& New, P. F. J. (1977) Computed tomographic examination of heavy marijuana smokers. *J. Amer. med. Ass.*, **237**, 1231–2

Kumar, R. & Stolerman, I. P. (1977) Experimental and clinical aspects of drug dependence. In *Handbook of Psychopharmacology*, ed. Iverson, L. L., Iverson, S. D. & Snyder, S. H., vol. 7, pp. 321–67 New York: Plenum Press

Lader, M. (1978) Benzodiazepines – the opium of the masses? *Neuroscience*, **3**, 159–65

— (1981) Benzodiazepine dependence. In *The Misuse of Psychotropic Drugs*, ed. Murray, R., Ghodse, A. H., Harris, C., Williams, D. & Williams, P., pp. 13–16. London: Gaskell

Lancet (1967) Barbiturate poisoning. *Lancet*, **i**, 200–1

— (1967) Hallucinogen and teratogen. *Lancet*, **ii**, 504–5

— (1975) Therapeutic possibilities in cannabinoids. *Lancet*, **i**, 667–9

Linton, A. L. & Ledingham, I. McA. (1966) Severe hypothermia with barbiturate intoxication. *Lancet*, **i**, 24–6

Lucas, R. N. & Falkowski, W. (1973) Ergotamine and methysergide abuse in patients with migraine. *Brit. J. Psychiat.*, **122**, 199–203

Malleson, N. (1971) Acute adverse reactions to LSD in clinical and experimental use in the United Kingdom. *Brit. J. Psychiat.*, **118**, 229–30

Malpas, A., Rowan, A. J., Joyce, C. R. B., & Scott, D. F. (1970) Persistent behavioural and electroencephalographic changes after single doses of nitrazepam and amylobarbitone sodium. *Brit. med. J.*, **2**, 762–4

Martin, W. R. (1968) A homoeostatic and redundancy theory of tolerance to and dependence on narcotic analgesics. *Res. Pub. Ass. Res. nerv. ment. Dis.*, **46**, 206–25

Merton, R. K. (1957) *Social Theory and Social Structure*. Glencoe, Ill.: Free Press

Mitcheson, M., & Hartnoll, R. (1978) Conflicts in deciding treatment within drug dependency clinics. In *Problems of Drug Abuse in Britain*, ed. West, D. J., 74–8. University of Cambridge: Institute of Criminology

Murray, R. M. (1972) The use and abuse of analgesics. *Scot. med. J.*, **17**, 393–6

Murray, R. M., Greene, J. G. & Adams, J. H. (1971) Analgesic abuse and dementia. *Lancet*, **ii**, 242–5

Murray, R. M., Lawson, D. H., & Linton, A. L. (1971) Analgesic nephropathy: clinical syndrome and prognosis. *Brit. med. J.*, **1**, 479–82

National Institute on Drug Abuse (1979) *Drug dependence in pregnancy: Clinical Management of Mother and Child*. Services Research Monograph Series. Washington, D.C.: US Department of Health Education and Welfare

Neuberg, R. (1970) Drug dependence and pregnancy: a review of the problems and their management. *J. Obstet. Gynaecol. Brit. Commonwealth*, **77**, 1117–22

Newman, R. G. & Whitehill, W. B. (1979) Double-blind comparison of methadone and placebo maintenance treatments of narcotic addicts in Hong Kong. *Lancet*, **ii**, 485

Oppenheim, A. N. (1976) Towards a social psychology of dependence. In *Drugs and Drug Dependence*, ed. Edwards, J. G., Russell, M. A. H., Hawks, D. & MacCafferty, M., pp. 214–21. Farnborough: Saxon House

Oswald, I., Lewis, S. A., Březinová, V. & Dunleavy, D. L. F. (1972) Drugs of dependence though not of abuse. In *Drug Addiction, Clinical and Socio-legal Aspects*, ed. Singh, J. M., Miller, L. H. & Lal, H., vol. 2, pp. 75–82. New York: Futura

Oswald, I., Lewis, S. A., Dunleavy, D. L. F., Březinová, V. & Briggs, M. (1971) Drugs of dependence though not of abuse: Fenfluramine and Imipramine. *Brit. med. J.*, **3**, 70–3

Paton, W. D. M. (1969) A pharmacological approach to drug dependence and drug tolerance. In *Scientific Basis of Drug Dependence*, ed. Steinberg, H., pp. 31–47. London: Churchill Livingstone

— (1973) Cannabis and its problems. *Proc. R. Soc. Med.*, **66**, 718–21

Pradhan, S. N. & Dutta, S. N. (1977) Narcotic analgesics. In *Drug Abuse, Clinical and Basic Aspects*, ed. Pradhan, S. N. & Dutta, S. N., pp. 49–77 St. Louis: Mosby

Reddy, A. M., Harper, R. G. & Stern, G. (1971) Observations on heroin and methadone withdrawal in the newborn. *Paediatrics*, **41**, 353–8

Reed, J. L. & Ghodse, A. H. (1973) Oral glucose tolerance and hormonal response in heroin-dependent males. *Brit. med. J.*, **2**, 582–5

Resnick, R. B., Resnick, E. S., & Washton, A. M., (1979) Treatment of opioid dependence with narcotic antagonists: a review and commentary. In *Handbook on drug-abuse*, ed. Dupont, R. L., Goldstein, A. & O'Donnell, J., pp. 97–104. National Institute on Drug Abuse

Sandison, R. A. (1968) The hallucinogenic drugs. *Practitioner*, **200**, 244–50

Sapira, J. D., & Cherubin, C. E., (1975) *Drug Abuse. A Guide for the Clinician*. Amsterdam: Excerpta Medica

Sharpless, S. & Jaffe, J. (1969) Withdrawal phenomena as manifestations of disuse supersensitivity. In *Scientific Basis of Drug Dependence* ed. Steinberg, H., pp. 67–76. London: Churchill Livingstone

Sladen, G. E. (1972) Effects of chronic purgative abuse. *Proc. R. Soc. Med.*, **65**, 288–91

Snyder, S. H. (1972) CNS stimulants and hallucinogens. In *Chemical and Biological Aspects of Drug Dependence*, ed. Mulé, S. J. & Brill, H., pp. 55–9. Cleveland, Ohio: CRC Press

Snyder, S. H. (1977) Opiate receptors and internal opiates. *Sci. Amer.*, **236** (iii), 44–56

Stephens, D. A. (1967) Psychotoxic effects of Benzhexol Hydrochloride (Artane). *Brit. J. Psychiat.*, **113**, 213–18

Stimson, G. V. (1973) *Heroin & Behaviour*. Dublin: Irish University Press

Stimson, G. V., Oppenheimer, E. & Thorley, A. (1978) Seven year follow-up of heroin addicts: drug use and outcome. *Brit. med. J.*, **1**, 1190–2

Sutherland, E. W. (1977) Dependence on barbiturates and other CNS depressants, in *Drug Abuse, Clinical and Basic Aspects*, ed. Pradhan, S. N. & Dutta, S. N., pp. 235–47. St. Louis: Mosby

Trethowan, W. H. (1975) Pills for personal problems. *Brit. med. J.*, **3**, 749–51

Tylden, E. (1973). The effects of maternal drug abuse on the foetus and infant. *Adverse Drug Reaction Bull.*, **38**, 120–3

Volans, G. (1981) The poisons unit experience. In *The Misuse of Psychotropic Drugs*, ed. Murray, R., Ghodse, A. H., Harris, C., Williams, D. & Williams, P., pp. 35–40. London: Gaskell

Watson, J. M. (1978) Clinical and laboratory investigations in 132 cases of solvent abuse. *Med. Sci. Law*, **18**, No. 1, 40–3

Wen, H. L. & Cheung, S. Y. C. (1973) Treatment of drug addiction by acupuncture and electrical stimulation. *Asian J. Med.*, **9**, 138–41

Wiepert, G. D., d'Orban, P. T. & Bewley, T. H. (1979) Delinquency by opiate addicts at two London clinics. *Brit. J. Psychiat.*, **134**, 14–23

Wikler, A. (1972) Theories related to physical dependence. In *Chemical and Biological Aspects of Drug Dependence*, ed. Mulé, S. J. & Brill, H., pp. 359–77. Cleveland, Ohio: CRC Press

Wille, R. (1980) Processes of recovery among heroin users. In *Drug Problems in the Sociocultural Context*, ed. Edwards, G. & Arif, A. Geneva: WHO

Williams, P. (1980) Recent trends in the prescribing of psychotropic drugs. *Health Trends*, No. 1, **12**, 6–7

— (1981) Trends in the prescribing of psychotropic drugs. In *The Misuse of Psychotropic Drugs*, ed. Murray, R., Ghodse, A. H., Harris, C., Williams, D. & Williams, P., pp. 7–12. London: Gaskell

World Health Organization (1957) *Expert Committee on Addiction-Producing Drugs*. WHO Technical Report Series No. 116. Geneva: WHO

— (1964) *Expert Committee on Addiction-Producing Drugs*. WHO Technical Report Series, No. 273. Geneva: WHO

— (1974) *Expert Committee on Drug Dependence: Thirteenth Report*. WHO Technical Report Series No. 551. Geneva: WHO

Zelson, C., Rubio, E. & Wasserman, E. (1971) Neonatal narcotic addiction: 10 year observation. *Paediat.*, **48**, 178–89

CHAPTER 16

Better Services for the Mentally Handicapped (1971) Cmd. 4683 (Table I, p. 6). London: HMSO

Cunningham, C. C. & Sloper, P. C. (1977) Parents of Down's syndrome babies: their early needs. *Child Health, Care Devel.*, **5**, 325–47.

— (1978) *Helping your Handicapped Baby*. London: Souvenir Press

Davis, M. (1979) Helping parents of handicapped children. *Community Care*, Jan.

Development Team for the Mentally Handicapped. *First Report, 1976–1977*. Part III. London: HMSO

Finnie, N. (1971) *Handling the Young Cerebral Palsied Child at Home*. London: Heinemann

Freeman, P. (1975) *Understanding the Deaf/Blind Child*. London: Heinemann

Gath, A. (1978) *Down's Syndrome and the Family: the Early Years*. London: Academic Press

Holmes, L. B., Moser, H. W., Halldövssen, S., Mack, C., Pint, S. & Matzilevich, B. (1972). *Mental Retardation: An Atlas of Diseases with Associated Physical Abnormalities*. London: Collier Macmillan

Kiernan, C., Jordan, R. & Saunder, C. (1978) *Starting Off*. London: Human Horizon Series

Kirman, B. & Bicknell, J. (1975) *Mental Handicap*. London: Churchill Livingstone

McKay, R. I. (1976) *Mental Handicap in Child Health Practice*. London: Butterworths

Mental Health Act (1959) London: HMSO

Penrose, L. (1954) *The Biology of Mental Defect*. London: Sidgwick & Jackson

Portage Guide to Home Teaching. Portage Project Cooperation Educational Service Agency. Portage, Wisconsin, 53901, USA

Report of the Committee on Child Health Services (1976) *Fit for the Future*. London: HMSO

Ricks, D. M. (1980) Motor handicap. In *The Modern Management of Mental Handicap*, ed. Simon, G. B. Lancaster: MTP Press

Russell, P. (1976) *Help Starts Here: for Parents of Children with Special Needs*. Voluntary Council for Handicapped Children. London: National Children's Bureau

Simon, G. B. (1980) Ed. *The Modern Management of Mental Handicap*. Lancaster: MTP Press

Spain, B. & Wigley, G. (Eds.) (1975) *Right from the Start*. London: Mentally Handicapped Children

Tizard, J. & Grad, B. (1961) *The Mentally Handicapped and their Families*. London: Oxford University Press

Wing, L. (1980) *Autistic Children: A Guide for Parents*. London: Constable

Wing, L. C. & Gould, J. (1979) Severe impairments of social interaction and associated abnormalities in children. Epidemiology and classification. *J. Autism Dev. Disord.*, **9**, no. 1

ORGANIZATIONS

Association of Residential Communities. Enquire: Mencap (below)

Break. 100 First Avenue, Bush Hill Park, Enfield, Middx

Dean Park College, Tonbridge, Kent. Enquire: The Spastics Society, 12 Park Crescent, London W1N 4EQ

The Manor House, Market Deeping, Lincs. Enquire: The National Association for Deaf/Blind and Rubella Handicapped

NSMHC Trusteeship Scheme. Enquire: Mencap (below)

Social Training Unit, Dilston Hall Conbridge, Northumberland. Enquire: Mencap, 117–123 Golden Lane, London EC1 0RT

Somerset Court, Brent Knoll, Somerset. Enquire: National Society of Autistic Children, 1a Golders Green Road, London NW11 8EA

Cross-references to other volumes in the series

CROSS-REFERENCES

In addition to specific references given below, the reader is referred to volume 1 for a discussion of the concepts, descriptive and developmental phenomena, principles of classification, diagnosis, assessment, and treatment, and neuropsychological, socio-cultural, and forensic aspects of general psychopathology, to volume 3 for a study of psychoses of uncertain aetiology, with particular reference to schizophrenias, affective psychoses, paranoid states, and psychoses with origin specific to childhood, to volume 4 for a review of the neuroses and personality disorders, and to volume 5 for a discussion of the scientific foundations of psychiatry.

(See also the key to volumes and chapters.)

The lay-out of the cross-references to volume 2 of the *Handbook of Psychiatry* has been designed to take into account the fact that clinical readers who consult this volume will do so to obtain descriptive accounts of various syndromes and their distinguishing features and to ascertain how far psychiatric features are causal or secondary to physical disease. For this reason, cross-references to psychiatric symptoms or conditions are not narrowly related to particular somatic conditions.

Author Index

Subject index